Diagnostic Pathology and Molecular Genetics of the Thyroid

SECOND EDITION

Diagnostic Pathology and Molecular Genetics of the Thyroid

SECOND EDITION

EDITORS

Yuri E. Nikiforov, MD, PhD

Professor of Pathology
Director, Division of Molecular Anatomic Pathology
Department of Pathology
University of Pittsburgh Medical Center
Pittsburgh, Pennsylvania

Paul W. Biddinger, MD

Professor of Pathology
Chief of Anatomic Pathology
Department of Pathology
Georgia Health Sciences University
Augusta, Georgia

Lester D. R. Thompson, MD, FASCP, FCAP

Consultant Pathologist
Department of Pathology
Southern California Permanente Medical Group
Woodland Hills, California

Drawings by Marina N. Nikiforova, MD and Paul W. Biddinger, MD

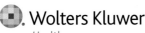 Wolters Kluwer | Lippincott Williams & Wilkins
Health

Philadelphia · Baltimore · New York · London
Buenos Aires · Hong Kong · Sydney · Tokyo

Senior Executive Editor: Jonathan W. Pine, Jr.
Product Manager: Marian Bellus
Vendor manager: Alicia Jackson
Senior Manufacturing Manager: Benjamin Rivera
Designer: Stephen Druding
Production Service: S4 Carlisle Publishing Services

Library of Congress Cataloging-in-Publication Data

Diagnostic pathology and molecular genetics of the thyroid / editor, Yuri E.
Nikiforov. — 2nd ed.
    p. ; cm.
  Includes bibliographical references and index.
  ISBN 978-1-4511-1455-3 (alk. paper)
  I. Nikiforov, Yuri.
  [DNLM: 1. Thyroid Neoplasms—diagnosis. 2. Molecular Diagnostic Techniques—methods.
  3. Pathology, Surgical—methods. 4. Thyroid Diseases—diagnosis. 5. Thyroid Diseases—
  genetics. 6. Thyroid Neoplasms—genetics. WK 270]
  616.99'444–dc23

                                                                    2011045972

Care has been taken to confirm the accuracy of the information presented and to
describe generally accepted practices. However, the authors, editors, and publisher are not
responsible for errors or omissions or for any consequences from application of the information in this book and make no warranty, expressed or implied, with respect to the currency,
completeness, or accuracy of the contents of the publication. Application of this information
in a particular situation remains the professional responsibility of the practitioner; the clinical treatments described and recommended may not be considered absolute and universal
recommendations.

The authors, editors, and publisher have exerted every effort to ensure that drug
selection and dosage set forth in this text are in accordance with the current recommendations and practice at the time of publication. However, in view of ongoing research, changes
in government regulations, and the constant flow of information relating to drug therapy and
drug reactions, the reader is urged to check the package insert for each drug for any change in
indications and dosage and for added warnings and precautions. This is particularly important
when the recommended agent is a new or infrequently employed drug.

Some drugs and medical devices presented in this publication have Food and Drug
Administration (FDA) clearance for limited use in restricted research settings. It is the responsibility of the health care provider to ascertain the FDA status of each drug or device planned
for use in his or her clinical practice.

Visit Lippincott Williams & Wilkins on the Internet at: LWW.COM. Lippincott Williams &
Wilkins customer service representatives are available from 8:30 am to 6 pm, EST.

9 8 7 6 5 4 3 2 1

DEDICATION

To Marina, Tanya, and Alexiy for all they mean to me.
To the memory of my father, Efim E. Nikiforov.

YURI E. NIKIFOROV

To the memory of my father, Robert W. Biddinger.

PAUL W. BIDDINGER

In a world with millions of competing priorities,
it is critical to focus on what is paramount:
The unwavering support and love of the most important
person in my life: my precious Sweet P.

LESTER D. R. THOMPSON

ACKNOWLEDGMENTS

This book contains illustrations provided by many individuals, and we thank all of them for their valuable contributions. Dr. Leon Barnes, Professor of Pathology at the University of Pittsburgh Medical Center, generously allowed us to use his outstanding collection of gross images and rare thyroid cases. Our special thanks to Dr. Mitchell E. Tublin, Associate Professor of Radiology at the University of Pittsburgh Medical Center, who contributed ultrasound images, and to Dr. James M. Mountz, Professor of Radiology at the University of Pittsburgh Medical Center, who provided thyroid scan images for the book. The following pathologists shared rare cases or microscopic and ultrastructural images used in the book:

Dr. J. Aidan Carney, Mayo Clinic, Rochester, Minnesota

Dr. Runjan Chetty, Oxford Radcliffe Hospitals NHS Trust and University of Oxford, Oxford, United Kingdom

Dr. Vincenzo Eusebi, University of Bologna, Bologna, Italy

Drs. Ronald Ghossein and JinRu Shia, Memorial Sloan-Kettering Cancer Center, New York, New York

Dr. A. Nihan Haberal, Baskent University School of Medicine, Ankara, Turkey

Dr. Clara S. Heffess, Endocrine Division, Armed Forces Institute of Pathology, Washington, District of Columbia

Dr. Ricardo V. Lloyd, University of Wisconsin, Madison, Wisconsin

Dr. Vânia Nosé, University of Miami, Miami, Florida

Dr. Robert L. Peel, University of Pittsburgh, Pittsburgh, Pennsylvania

Dr. Ales Ryška, Charles University Medical Faculty Hospital, Hradec Králové, Czech Republic

Dr. Manuel Sobrinho-Simões, IPATIMUP, Porto, Portugal

Dr. Giovanni Tallini, University of Bologna School of Medicine, Bologna, Italy

Drs. Marco Volante and Mauro Papotti, University of Turin, Italy.

The authors would like to thank staff members of the Molecular Anatomic Pathology Laboratory, Electron Microscopy Laboratory, Immunohistochemistry Laboratory, and In Situ Hybridization Laboratory at the Department of Pathology at the University of Pittsburgh Medical Center for help in preparing materials for many illustrations; Dr. Manoj Gandhi for fluorescence in situ hybridization images; and Mr. Frank Fusco for selected gross images.

We would like to recognize Ms. Angelique M. Hudec in Dr. Yuri Nikiforov's office for her help in coordinating the work on the book. We thank Ms. Tanya Nikiforova for her assistance with editing selected chapters of the book.

We would also like to acknowledge Dr. George K. Michalopoulos, Chair of the Department of Pathology at the University of Pittsburgh School of Medicine, and Dr. Samuel A. Yousem, Vice Chair for Anatomic Pathology at the University of Pittsburgh School of Medicine, as well as Dr. Amyn M. Rojiani, Chair of the Department of Pathology at Georgia Health Sciences University, and Dr. Jeffrey D. Shiffer, Chief of the Department of Pathology at the Woodland Hills Medical Center, for creating a supportive academic environment that enabled us to accomplish this challenging project.

Finally, we would like to express our appreciation to Mr. Jonathan W. Pine Jr., Senior Executive Editor at Lippincott Williams & Wilkins, for his guidance and invaluable help with the production of this book, and to Mr. Eric Johnson from Red Act Media Group, Mr. Kirubhagaran Palani and Mr. Joel Jones from S4 Carlisle Publishing Services, and Ms. Marian Bellus, from Lippincott Williams & Wilkins/Wolters Kluwer Health, for making the second edition possible.

CONTRIBUTORS

Paul W. Biddinger, MD

Professor of Pathology
Chief of Anatomic Pathology
Department of Pathology
Georgia Health Sciences University
Augusta, Georgia

Peter Kopp, MD

Associate Professor
Director ad interim Center for Genetic Medicine
Division of Endocrinology, Metabolism, and Molecular
    Medicine
Northwestern University
Chicago, Illinois

Yuri E. Nikiforov, MD, PhD

Professor of Pathology
Director, Division of Molecular Anatomic Pathology
Department of Pathology
University of Pittsburgh Medical Center
Pittsburgh, Pennsylvania

Marina N. Nikiforova, MD

Assistant Professor
Associate Director, Molecular Anatomic Pathology
Department of Pathology
University of Pittsburgh Medical Center
Pittsburgh, Pennsylvania

N. Paul Ohori, MD

Professor of Pathology
Medical Director of Cytopathology and Cytopathology
    Fellowship Program
Department of Pathology
University of Pittsburgh Medical Center
Pittsburgh, Pennsylvania

Christine Garcia Roth, MD

Assistant Professor
Department of Pathology
University of Pittsburgh Medical Center
Pittsburgh, Pennsylvania

Raja R. Seethala, MD, FASCP

Assistant Professor
Department of Pathology
University of Pittsburgh Medical Center
Pittsburgh, Pennsylvania

Lester D. R. Thompson, MD, FASCP, FCAP

Consultant Pathologist
Department of Pathology
Southern California Permanente Medical Group
Woodland Hills, California

PREFACE TO 1ST EDITION

Since the early 1990s, when several excellent textbooks devoted to thyroid pathology were published, the pathologic criteria for many thyroid lesions have been refined, new immunohistochemical markers have emerged, and a variety of novel genetic alterations responsible for the familial and sporadic forms of thyroid cancer have been discovered. Although some of these updates can be found in book chapters devoted to the pathology of thyroid tumors or nonneoplastic conditions, we felt a strong need for a book that is focused solely on the thyroid and provides the most current and complete information on nonneoplastic and neoplastic thyroid diseases. Most importantly, as molecular genetics has penetrated all fields of medicine and impacts more and more significantly on the practice of pathology, we believe that our times call for a book that provides a comprehensive description of classic morphology and molecular genetics side by side and in a single volume. In addition, as the incidence of thyroid cancer has increased dramatically in the United Sates and many other countries in the world over the last three decades, it would be beneficial to readers to find a description of the current knowledge of epidemiology, etiology, and molecular pathogenesis of each cancer type integrated with the discussion of the disease morphology.

To achieve these goals, most chapters in the book have a uniform structure and include sections dedicated to the incidence and epidemiology of a particular disease, etiology, pathogenesis and molecular genetics, and clinical presentation and imaging, followed by sections providing detailed discussions of gross and microscopic findings, as well as sections on immunohistochemistry, molecular diagnostics, electron microscopy, cytology, differential diagnosis, and treatment and prognosis. We expect that this organizational structure will allow readers to find all information pertinent to a particular disease in a single chapter and also easily search for a specific aspect of the disease, such as microscopic diagnostic features or immunohistochemistry, without reading the entire chapter.

Our intention was to provide a highly illustrated book, with ample illustrations of gross and microscopic features of every common thyroid disease, as well as drawings and diagrams summarizing diagnostic features and molecular characteristics. Two chapters are dedicated exclusively to the description of rare thyroid tumors. A separate chapter describes the principles of molecular diagnostics for those readers who wish to learn more about the general and technical aspects of molecular pathology.

We believe that the book will be useful to pathology trainees and practicing pathologists, endocrinologists, endocrine and head and neck surgeons, radiologists, internists, and scientists interested in thyroid diseases.

Yuri E. Nikiforov, MD, PhD
Paul W. Biddinger, MD
Lester D. R. Thompson, MD

The Second Edition of this book has been put together to capture recent advances in thyroid pathology, particularly the refinement of pathologic criteria for many thyroid lesions, description of new histopathologic variants of thyroid cancer, broader experience with use of immunohistochemical markers, and rapid progress in molecular genetics of the sporadic and familial forms of thyroid cancer.

The expanded Second Edition contains new information included to each chapter, as well as more than a hundred new illustrations, diagrams, and tables. To address a rapidly advancing diagnostic use of molecular markers, particularly in fine-needle aspiration material from thyroid nodules, a new chapter has been added to discuss in depth this important topic.

We intend for this book to be comprehensive, and it contains descriptions of non-neoplastic and neoplastic thyroid diseases, including thorough description of classic morphology and molecular genetics as well as a summary of the current knowledge of epidemiology, etiology, and molecular pathogenesis of each cancer type integrated with the discussion of the disease morphology. As in the First Edition, all main chapters in the book have a uniform structure and include sections discussing the incidence and epidemiology of a particular thyroid disease, etiology, pathogenesis and molecular genetics, clinical presentation and imaging, followed by

sections providing detailed discussions of gross and microscopic findings, as well as sections on immunohistochemistry, molecular diagnostics, electron microscopy, cytology, differential diagnosis, and treatment and prognosis. Many of the readers indicated that they find such a structure of the book very helpful, as it allows finding quickly the information pertinent to a particular aspect of a specific thyroid disease, and therefore the same structure of each chapter is preserved and even expanded in the Second Edition.

We hope that the readers will continue to find this text helpful in their everyday practice when dealing with challenging diagnostic cases, rare types of thyroid disease, or need to understand better the methodology and interpretation of various ancillary studies and novel molecular tests available for thyroid diseases. We hope that this book will be useful to practicing pathologists and pathology trainees, molecular pathologists, endocrinologists, endocrine and head and neck surgeons, radiologists, internists, and basic scientists interested in thyroid diseases.

Yuri E. Nikiforov, MD, PhD
Paul W. Biddinger, MD
Lester D. R. Thompson, MD

CONTENTS

CHAPTER 1

Paul W. Biddinger

Normal Anatomy and Histology

Descriptions of the thyroid and related diseases date back to antiquity. The thyroid was identified by European anatomists during the Renaissance including Vesalius who described the *glandulas ad laryngis radicem adnatas* in book six of his famous work *De Humani Corporis Fabrica* of 1543. Thomas Wharton is generally credited for first using the term *thyroid gland* in his 1656 treatise *Adenographia*. His use of this name seems to be because of the gland's proximity to the thyroid cartilage. The term *thyroid* has been applied to the major cartilage of the larynx dating back at least to the time of Galen. Thyroid derives from the Greek words *thyreos,* meaning shield, and *eidos,* meaning shape, form, or likeness. The *thyreos* is a narrow, oblong military shield, and its name derives from *thyra,* the Greek word for door. The thyroid cartilage indeed has a shield-like appearance.

Wharton considered the thyroid to be a pair of glands and described them as resembling an oblong fig or pear. He thought their principal function was uptake of superfluous fluids of the recurrent nerve. Other putative functions included warming the adjacent cartilages, lubricating the larynx, and contributing to the roundness and beautification of the neck.[1] Considerable advances in our understanding of the thyroid gland have occurred since the 17th century.

MACROANATOMY

Basic Anatomy

The thyroid gland is located in the lower anterior region of the neck at the level of C5–C7 vertebrae. It is a bilobed organ joined by an isthmus and encased in a thin fibrous capsule. The right and left lobes have a somewhat conical shape with convex anterior and lateral surfaces. The lobes tend to be about 4 to 5 cm in length, 2 to 3 cm in greatest transverse dimension, and 1.5 to 2 cm in greatest anterior–posterior dimension. The isthmus is about 1 cm in greatest transverse and vertical dimensions. The location of the isthmus is variable, but it usually joins the two lateral lobes at the level of the second and third tracheal rings.

Approximately half of all thyroid glands exhibit a pyramidal lobe, with most studies reporting an incidence in the 30% to 75% range (Fig. 1.1).[2] Some of the variation in incidence may relate to the variable size and prominence of the lobe, and hence threshold of recognition. The pyramidal lobe represents the remnant of the inferior portion of the thyroglossal duct. The lobe extends superiorly from the isthmus and may be attached to the hyoid bone by fibrous tissue. Pyramidal lobes are more frequently attached to the left side of the isthmus and in some cases attached to the left lobe itself.[2]

The tubercle of Zuckerkandl is a focal enlargement along the lateral border of the lateral lobes that is commonly observed during thyroid surgery.[3] It ranges from a slight thickening to a 1 cm or larger nodular structure. It can be found on either side or bilaterally. It has utility as a surgical landmark because the recurrent laryngeal nerve usually courses medially, sometimes in a cleft between the tubercle and the main substance of the lateral lobe. In addition, the superior parathyroid gland is commonly found just cephalad to the tubercle.

Normal Weight

Studies examining the weight of normal thyroid glands, either by direct measurement or by extrapolation from volume measurement, have yielded variable means and ranges, particularly the latter.[4–8] Distillation of these findings yields an average weight of about 18 g for adult men and 15 g for adult women. The reported distributions of thyroid weights tend to show a positive skew, with a broader range of weights above the mean than below. Most of the reported weights of normal adults lie within a range from 8 to 30 g. Glands with weights in excess of 50 g have also been reported, but these outliers raise questions regarding their normal status. The glands of adult women tend to be smaller than that of adult men, but the differences are modest and the ranges mostly overlap. Some studies have shown a positive correlation between thyroid weight and body weight, body mass index, or age.[4–9] Body weight or body mass index tends to show stronger correlation than age, but overall these correlations are weak. Thyroid weight tends to show a progressive increase in childhood and adolescence, stability in early to midadulthood, and gradual decline in older age.[7,8] An increase in thyroid size has been reported in pregnant women.[10,11] However, most cases of enlargement may reflect iodine deficiency as opposed to an invariable physiologic response to pregnancy.

Anatomic Relationships

The medial surfaces of the lobes abut the thyroid cartilage of the larynx and superior aspect of the trachea. The apices of the lobes are located near the oblique line of the thyroid cartilage and the bases at the level of the fourth, fifth, or sixth tracheal ring. The superomedial aspects of the lateral lobes are adjacent to the inferior pharyngeal constrictors and posterior portions of the cricothyroid muscles. The common carotid artery, internal jugular vein, and vagus nerve, encased within the carotid sheath, course along the posterolateral aspects of the lateral lobes (Fig. 1.2). The recurrent laryngeal nerves are located in the tracheoesophageal grooves in proximity to the posteromedial aspects of the lateral lobes. The superior branch of the external laryngeal nerve usually courses to the cricothyroid muscle immediately posterior to the superior poles of the lateral lobes.

The thyroid gland is encased by the pretracheal fascia, anchoring the gland to the trachea and correlating with the movement of the gland during swallowing. The sternothyroid muscle is located immediately anterior to the thyroid, spanning from the oblique line of the thyroid cartilage to the manubrium of the sternum. Muscles anterior to the sternothyroid are the sternohyoid, superior belly of the omohyoid, and the anterior border of the sternocleidomastoid. The thyrohyoid muscle is essentially a superior extension of the sternothyroid, extending from the oblique line of the thyroid cartilage to the hyoid bone.

Vascular Supply

The blood supply to the thyroid is through the right and left superior thyroid arteries and the right and left inferior thyroid

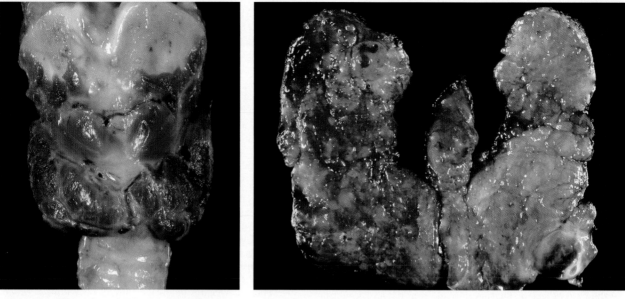

FIGURE 1.1. Gross photographs of thyroid glands. A: Bilobed thyroid and its relationship to the thyroid cartilage. **B:** Thyroid with prominent pyramidal lobe.

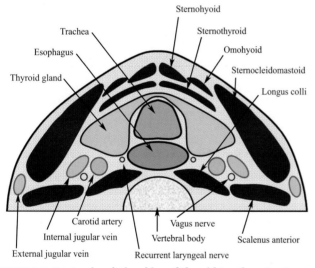

FIGURE 1.2. Anatomic relationships of thyroid to other structures of neck at the level of C6 vertebra.

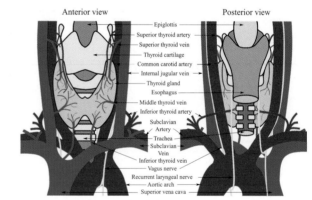

FIGURE 1.3. Vascular supply of thyroid.

arteries (Fig. 1.3). The superior thyroid arteries derive from the external carotid arteries, and the inferior thyroid arteries derive from the subclavian arteries through the thyrocervical trunks. An inconstant artery, the thyroidea ima, occasionally arises from the brachiocephalic trunk, aortic arch, or left common carotid and ascends along the anterior midline of the trachea to reach the thyroid in the region of the isthmus. Venous drainage is through a plexus that leads to the superior, middle, and inferior thyroid veins. The superior and middle veins drain into the internal jugular veins, and the inferior veins join the brachiocephalic veins. A dense capillary plexus encompassing the follicles lies between the arterial and venous vessels.

Lymphatic Drainage

The lymphatic drainage flows from vessels in the perifollicular connective tissue to a subcapsular network. Lymphatic vessels leave the gland in proximity to veins and extend to several regional lymph nodes (Fig. 1.4). The most proximate nodes are located in the anterior, or central, compartment of the neck and collectively compose the level VI nodes. These include those immediately adjacent to the thyroid gland (perithyroidal or pericapsular nodes), prelaryngeal, pretracheal, and paratracheal lymph nodes. A midline prelaryngeal node found anterior to the cricothyroid membrane and superior to the isthmus is known alternatively as the Delphian node. Lymphatic drainage involves other regional lymph nodes including the internal jugular (particularly levels III and IV), superior mediastinal, supraclavicular, spinal accessory, retropharyngeal, and, to a limited extent, the submandibular and submental (level I) lymph nodes.

Innervation

The thyroid is innervated by nerves originating from the superior and middle sympathetic cervical ganglia. These nerves release noradrenaline from interfollicular adrenergic nerve terminals.[12] Cholinergic nerve fibers also have been demonstrated in the thyroid, suggesting a role of the parasympathetic nervous system in the regulation of thyroid function.[13]

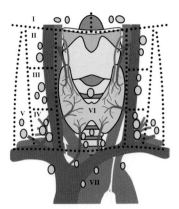

FIGURE 1.4. Regional lymph nodes draining thyroid with designation of levels I to VII. *Level I*, anterior triangle; *level II*, upper jugular; *level III*, middle jugular; *level IV*, lower jugular; *level V*, posterior triangle; *level VI*, central compartment; *level VII*, upper mediastinal.

 MICROANATOMY

The Follicle

The follicle is the distinctive basic unit of the thyroid gland (Fig. 1.5). It is a spherical structure that usually has a polyhedral appearance because of the abutment of adjacent follicles. Each follicle is lined by a single layer of follicular cells with apices in contact with a central extracellular collection of colloid. The bases of the follicular cells lie along a thin fibrovascular stroma rich in a capillary network that encompasses the follicle. Normal thyroid glands usually contain between 500,000 and 1.5 million follicles.[7] The size of most normal follicles lies in the range of 50 to 500 μm with an average size of about 200 μm. Thyroid lobules are formed by groups of 20 to 40 follicles. The lobules are invested by a thin layer of fibrous connective tissue, and each is supplied by small arterial branch. The fibrous tissue dividing the lobules is eventually contiguous with the capsule of the gland.

Colloid

The colloid within the central follicular space contains thyroglobulin, an iodinated glycoprotein that is the precursor of triiodothyronine (T_3) and thyroxine (T_4). Colloid has an amorphous eosinophilic appearance and is highlighted by periodic acid-Schiff and thyroglobulin stains. The intensity of staining with hematoxylin and eosin can vary. The colloid in follicles with low activity usually shows more intense eosinophilia compared with the colloid in follicles with a high level of hormone synthesis and release. Colloid in these latter follicles may also show scalloping or small vacuoles at the interface with follicular cells, a sign of endocytotic resorption. Larger, round to oval clear spaces are common within colloid, and some of these spaces may contain calcium oxalate crystals. Colloid generally has a homogeneous appearance. However, it can contain particulate-like clumps of material that are more intensely eosinophilic or slightly basophilic (Fig. 1.6). This histologic finding seems more common in active follicles, but it is unclear whether this is a manifestation of increased synthetic activity or a nonspecific artifact.[14]

Crystals

The presence of calcium oxalate crystals within colloid is a common finding.[15,16] Crystals appear as small clear refractile foci and are birefringent when viewed with polarizing filters (Fig. 1.7). These crystals begin to appear during childhood and adolescence and become more prevalent as adults age. Calcium oxalate crystals have potential utility in distinguishing thyroid from parathyroid tissue.[17]

Follicular Cells

Follicular cells have eosinophilic cytoplasm and round to slightly oval nuclei. The nuclei are located basally and have finely granular chromatin and inconspicuous nucleoli. Follicular cells vary in size and shape from low cuboidal to columnar, and this correlates with their level of thyroid hormone synthesis (Fig. 1.8). Cells with a low synthetic level have a low cuboidal appearance, and relatively abundant colloid occupies the lumen. This appearance of

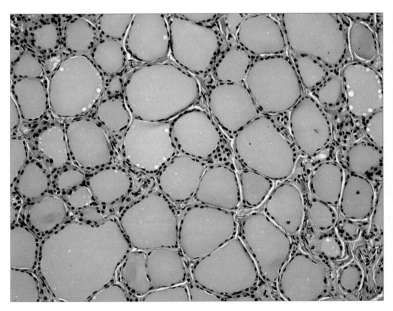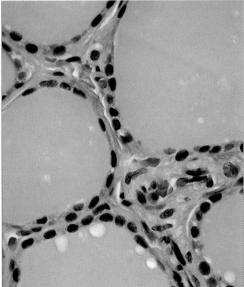

FIGURE 1.5. Low- and high-power photomicrographs of normal follicles.

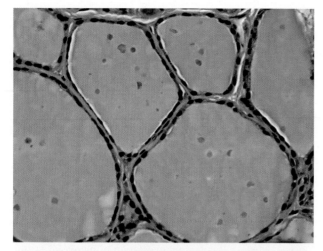

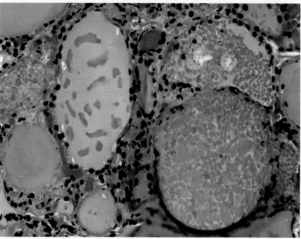

FIGURE 1.6. Photomicrographs showing particulate material within colloid. The top image shows a relatively subtle accumulation, whereas the bottom image is an extreme example of the phenomenon.

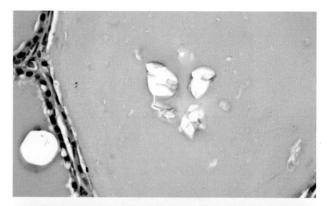

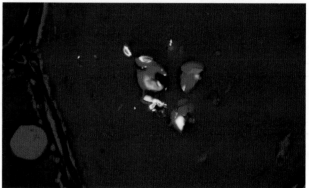

FIGURE 1.7. Calcium oxalate crystals within follicles. The crystals are birefringent when viewed through polarizing filters **(bottom)**.

Immunohistochemistry

Follicular cells exhibit cytoplasmic positivity in sections immunohistochemically stained for thyroglobulin and low molecular weight cytokeratins (Fig. 1.10).[18–21] Coexpression of vimentin has also been noted.[18–20] Normal follicular cells express transcription factors including thyroid transcription factor-1 (TTF1), TTF2, and paired box gene 8 (PAX8).[22,23] Thyroid stimulating hormone (TSH) receptor and thyroid peroxidase (TPO) can also be demonstrated immunohistochemically in normal follicular cells.[22,24,25] Growth factors and their receptors are also expressed, including epidermal growth factor (EGF), transforming growth factor (TGF(α)), and epidermal growth factor receptor (EGFR) (Table 1.1).[26,27]

C Cells

C cells, also known as parafollicular cells, are another component of the follicle. These cells, which produce calcitonin, are found singly or in small groups dispersed between or peripheral to the follicular cells. However, even those C cells that are peripheral to follicular cells and appear to be interfollicular are still encompassed by the basal lamina of the follicle.[28] C cells are separated from the colloid by the cytoplasm of overarching follicular cells.

C cells cannot be identified reliably in routine hematoxylin and eosin–stained sections. Histologic features suggestive of C cells include cytoplasm that is clear to faintly granular and nuclei that are larger and more finely granular than are adjacent follicular cells.[29] C cells vary in shape from polygonal to round to spindled. The C cells in glands of neonates and children tend to polygonal and relatively large compared with adults.[30,31]

Immunohistochemistry

Stains for argyrophilic granules highlight the cytoplasm of C cells, but the most specific and common method of identification is

follicles is sometimes designated the resting state. In contrast, follicular cells stimulated to produce more thyroid hormone exhibit columnar morphology. Histologic sections of normal adult thyroid glands usually show follicular cells with cuboidal to low cuboidal features.

Ultrastructure

Ultrastructural examination of follicular cells reveals junctional complexes of desmosomes and terminal bars linking cells along their lateral borders near the apices. The bases of the cells abut a basal lamina that separates them from the interstitial stroma and fenestrated capillary network (Fig. 1.9). The nuclei are basally located. Granular endoplasmic reticulum and mitochondria are readily identifiable components of the cytoplasm. The supranuclear region contains a Golgi complex that increases in prominence with increased activity. The apical region contains Golgi-derived dense secretory vacuoles, which transport glycoproteins to the plasmalemma for exocytosis into the follicular lumen. Lysosomes are prominent cytoplasmic components. This includes both primary and secondary lysosomes. The latter, also known as phagolysosomes, represents the fusion of primary lysosomes with colloid taken into the cytoplasm by endocytosis. Numerous apical microvilli are present, and their length increases when hormonal synthesis is stimulated.

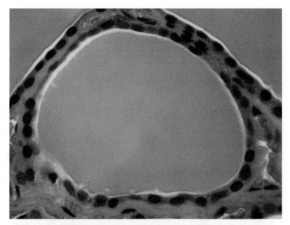

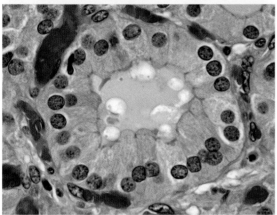

FIGURE 1.8. Photomicrographs of cuboidal (top) and columnar (bottom) follicular cells. The columnar cells are from a case of diffuse toxic hyperplasia (Graves disease).

an immunohistochemical stain for calcitonin (Fig. 1.11).[32,33] In addition to calcitonin, immunohistochemical studies of C cells have demonstrated positive staining for calcitonin gene-related peptide, low molecular weight cytokeratins, carcinoembryonic antigen (CEA), chromogranin, TTF1, cholecystokinin-2, helodermin, and several other neuroendocrine peptides.[33–38]

Distribution in Thyroid

C cells are relatively scant, comprising 0.1% or less of the total thyroid cell mass.[31,39] In addition, they are not evenly distributed throughout the thyroid. Most are found in the middle to upper-middle region of the lateral lobes, corresponding to the site of fusion of the ultimobranchial bodies with the medial thyroid anlage during embryogenesis (see Chapter 2).[29,31,40] Few, if any, C cells are present in the upper or lower poles or isthmus.

Ultrastructure

The most distinctive ultrastructural feature of C cells is membrane bound secretory granules within the cytoplasm. These electron-dense granules are the storage site of calcitonin. Type I granules measure 280 nm and the smaller, and denser type II granules are 130 nm in diameter.[41] The cytoplasm also contains rough endocytoplasmic reticulum, a distinct Golgi complex, numerous mitochondria, and free ribosomes. Nuclei are round to oval with finely granular chromatin. Proximity to capillary blood vessels, a characteristic of endocrine cells, is also evident at the ultrastructural level.

Solid Cell Nests

Solid cell nests (SCN) are interfollicular aggregates of cells resembling squamous or transitional epithelium. SCN are found in normal thyroid glands, and most investigators consider them to be remnants of the ultimobranchial bodies.[42–44] Evidence supporting this view includes histologic and ultrastructural

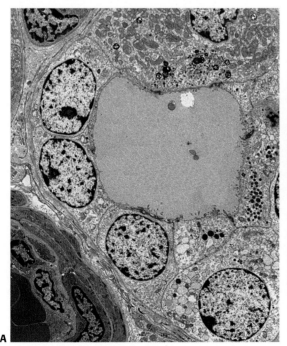

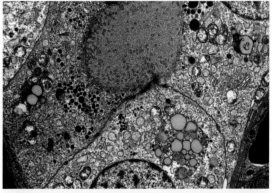

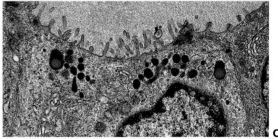

FIGURE 1.9. Electron photomicrographs of follicular cells. A: Low-power view showing follicular cells surrounding the central colloid-filled cavity. A blood vessel is evident in the lower left corner. **B:** Multiple follicular cells around central colloid **(upper center).** Numerous microvilli project into the colloid. Multiple lysosomes are evident in the apical cytoplasm of the centrally located follicular cell. **C:** High-power view showing luminal microvilli as well as dense secretory vacuoles and several phagolysosomes in the apical cytoplasm.

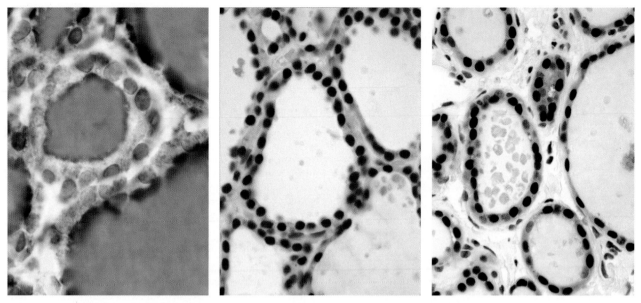

FIGURE 1.10. Follicular cells immunostained for thyroglobulin (left), TTF1 (center), and PAX8 (right).

Table 1.1	
Immunohistochemical Expression of Thyroid Cells	
Follicular Cells	**C Cells**
• Thyroglobulin	• Calcitonin
• Low molecular weight cytokeratins	• Low molecular weight cytokeratins
• TTF1	• Calcitonin gene-related peptide
• TTF2	• TTF1
• PAX8	• CEA
• Vimentin	• Chromogranin A
• TPO	• Synaptophysin
• TSH receptor	• Various neuroendocrine peptides
• EGF	
• EGFR	
• (TGF(α))	

similarities between SCN and ultimobranchial bodies, the presence of C cells within some SCN, and the relatively high density of C cells in the thyroid tissue surrounding SCN.[43,45] In addition, SCN are most frequently found in the middle third of the lateral lobes, a region corresponding to the usual site of fusion of the ultimobranchial bodies with the medial thyroid anlage during embryonic development.

Morphologic Features

SCN are microscopic findings and their incidence varies, in large part, depending on the extensiveness of sampling. They range from 50 to 1000 μm in greatest dimension.[46] SCN are interspersed between follicles and irregularly shaped although typically well demarcated (Fig. 1.12). Several investigators have reported a basal membrane around SCN, but this has not been a universal finding.[42–44,47] The cells range from polygonal to round to spindle shaped, and they have a compact arrangement. Distinct intercellular bridges are not typically seen; however,

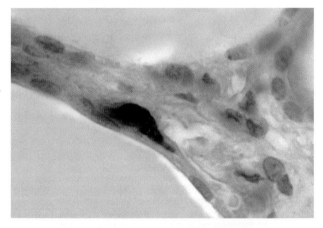

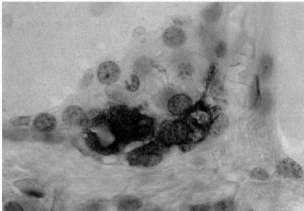

FIGURE 1.11. Photomicrographs of normal C cells (calcitonin immunostain).

desmosomes are evident ultrastructurally. The nuclei have finely granular chromatin, and nucleoli are absent or inconspicuous. Some nuclei exhibit longitudinal grooves. Most have relatively scant amphophilic cytoplasm, but cells with more abundant clear cytoplasm are also seen. Some SCN are associated with a cystic region (Fig. 1.12D) that may contain mucin. Follicular structures containing central colloid, an inner lining of follicular cells, and an outer rim of SCN type cells can be seen. Interpretations vary whether these represent mixed follicles derived entirely from SCN or SCN encircling follicles derived from the medial anlage.

Asioli et al.[48] have classified SCN into four types using morphologic features comparable with those used earlier by Vollenweider and Hedinger.[49] Type 1 is composed of "main" cells, characterized by round to oval or elongated cells with scant cytoplasm, centrally located oval to fusiform nuclei, and occasional nuclear grooves.

The cells form round to oval groups. Type 2 SCN are composed of larger, polygonal cells with an epidermoid appearance. Type 3 solid cell nests exhibit cystic architecture and cells that have a flattened or polygonal appearance. Type 4 solid cell nests, also known as mixed follicles, have a follicular appearance and contain both follicular epithelium and small "main" cells. This nomenclature, however, is relatively new and not widely used at this time. In addition, these different types of solid cell nests were identified in cases of Hashimoto thyroiditis and were present in high numbers (10 to 45 per slide),[48] raising the question whether they

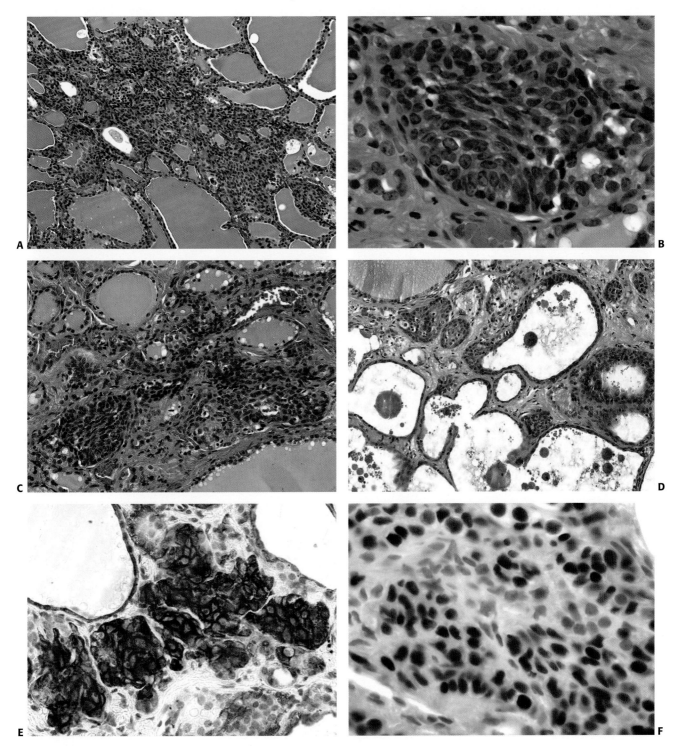

FIGURE 1.12. SCN. A: Low-power photomicrograph of relatively large SCN. **B:** High-power photomicrograph from the same SCN showing the squamoid appearance of the cells. **C:** Low-power photomicrograph of smaller SCN. **D:** SCN with cystic features. **E:** Section of SCN immunostained for low molecular weight cytokeratin (CAM 5.2 cytokeratin). **F:** Section of SCN immunostained for p63.

may represent foci of squamous metaplasia rather than being true remnants of the ultimobranchial bodies.

Immunohistochemistry

Immunohistochemical studies have shown consistently positive staining for low molecular weight cytokeratins (Fig. 1.12E) and variable staining for CEA. Variable results have also been reported for high molecular weight cytokeratins. The cells also express p63 (Fig. 1.12F).[45,50] Solid cell nests may contain a minority population of C cells that are highlighted by a calcitonin immunostain. The C cells correspond to cells with clear cytoplasm seen in hematoxylin and eosin–stained sections. The C cells also show nuclear staining for TTF1 in contrast to the main cells of the nests.[45,50] Most studies have not shown staining for thyroglobulin. Isolated cells positive for thyroglobulin have been reported and interpreted as suggesting that solid cell nests may be a source of follicular epithelium.[51] An alternative interpretation is thyroglobulin positive cells represent entrapped follicular epithelium.

Solid cell nests also exhibit staining for galectin-3.[45,52] Some may exhibit membranous staining for HBME1, particularly those composed of small cells characteristic of type 1 solid cell nests. The potential for galectin-3 and HBME1 to highlight solid cell nests should be borne in mind when using these stains to help evaluate lesions suspicious for malignancy.

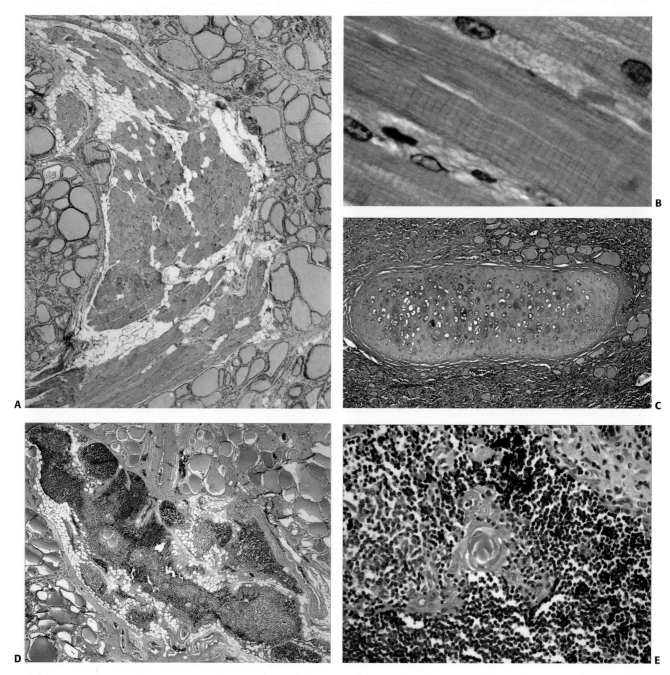

FIGURE 1.13. Heterologous tissues within thyroid. A: Focus of adipose tissue and skeletal muscle. **B:** High-power view of skeletal muscle. **C:** Focus of intrathyroidal cartilage. **D:** Intrathyroidal thymic tissue. **E:** High-power view shows Hassall corpuscle.

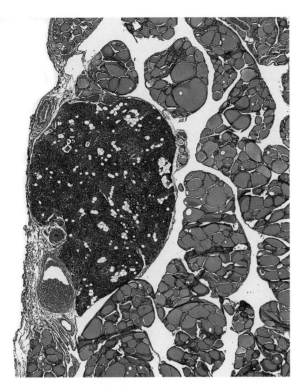

FIGURE 1.14. Parathyroid gland within thyroid. A parathyroid gland is enclosed by the thyroid capsule and largely surrounded by follicular tissue.

Differential Diagnosis

Solid cell nests are incidental findings. The differential diagnosis includes focal squamous metaplasia, intrathyroidal thymic remnant, primary or metastatic squamous cell carcinoma, thyroglossal duct cyst, C-cell hyperplasia, and papillary or medullary microcarcinomas. Squamous metaplasia is characteristically associated with chronic inflammation, and multiple scattered foci are common. The presence of Hassall corpuscles helps to identify thymic remnants. Solid cell nests do not exhibit the cytologic atypia characteristic of squamous cell carcinoma. Immunostaining for calcitonin can help distinguish solid cell nests from C-cell hyperplasia and medullary carcinoma because staining should be absent or only focal in solid cell nests. The absence of staining for p63 may also be useful to distinguish C-cell hyperplasia and medullary carcinomas, as well as papillary microcarcinomas, from solid cell nests.

Neoplastic Potential

Solid cell nests may play a role as the precursor for primary mucoepidermoid carcinomas of the thyroid (see Chapter 15).[53,54] Studies suggest the possibility that solid cell nests may be capable of hyperplasia and neoplastic transformation. If true, the risk of neoplastic transformation must be quite low given the relatively high frequency of solid cell nests and rarity of mucoepidermoid carcinomas of the thyroid.

Heterologous Tissues within Thyroid

Several tissues typically found external to the thyroid can be found within the substance of the gland. These include adipose, skeletal muscle, parathyroid, thymic, salivary, and cartilaginous tissues

(Figs. 1.13 and 1.14). These heterologous tissues are sometimes found in proximity to solid cell nests and may represent remnants of a pharyngeal pouch component.[14,55]

Intrathyroidal parathyroid glands account for small percentage of unintentional parathyroidectomies during thyroidectomies. Combining the findings of three studies with a total of 1,879 partial or total thyroidectomies, intrathyroidal parathyroid glands were found in 25 cases (1.3%).[56–58] An additional 24 parathyroid glands were reported within or just beneath the thyroid capsule. Parathyroid adenomas may develop within the thyroid gland and are a potential reason for failed surgical procedures. Combining the results of five studies of ectopic parathyroid adenomas associated with hyperparathyroidism, intrathyroidal parathyroid adenomas were found in 23 of 810 cases (2.8%).[59–63]

REFERENCES

1. Warton T. *Adenographia*. Freer S, translated from the Latin. Oxford: Clarendon Press; 1996.
2. Braun EM, Windisch G, Wolf G, et al. The pyramidal lobe: clinical anatomy and its importance in thyroid surgery. *Surg Radiol Anat*. 2007;29:21–27.
3. Gravante G, Delogu D, Rizzello A, et al. The Zuckerkandl tubercle. *Am J Surg*. 2007;193:484–485.
4. Hegedus L, Perrild H, Poulsen LR, et al. The determination of thyroid volume by ultrasound and its relationship to body weight, age, and sex in normal subjects. *J Clin Endocrinol Metab*. 1983;56:260–263.
5. Pankow BG, Michalak J, McGee MK. Adult human thyroid weight. *Health Phys*. 1985;49:1097–1103.
6. de la Grandmaison GL, Clairand I, Durigon M. Organ weight in 684 adult autopsies: new tables for a Caucasoid population. *Forensic Sci Int*. 2001;119:149–154.
7. Brown RA, Al-Moussa M, Beck J. Histometry of normal thyroid in man. *J Clin Pathol*. 1986;39:475–482.
8. Roberts PF. Variation in the morphometry of the normal human thyroid in growth and ageing. *J Pathol*. 1974;112:161–168.
9. Lee DH, Cho KJ, Sun DI, et al. Thyroid dimensions of Korean adults on routine neck computed tomography and its relationship to age, sex, and body size. *Surg Radiol Anat*. 2006;28:25–32.
10. Nelson M, Wickus GG, Caplan RH, et al. Thyroid gland size in pregnancy. An ultrasound and clinical study. *J Reprod Med*. 1987;32:888–890.
11. Berghout A, Wiersinga W. Thyroid size and thyroid function during pregnancy: an analysis. *Eur J Endocrinol*. 1998;138:536–542.
12. Melander A, Ljunggren JG, Norberg KA, et al. Sympathetic innervation and noradrenaline content of normal human thyroid tissue from fetal, young, and elderly subjects. *J Endocrinol Invest*. 1978;1:175–177.
13. Van Sande J, Dumont JE, Melander A, et al. Presence and influence of cholinergic nerves in the human thyroid. *J Clin Endocrinol Metab*. 1980;51:500–502.
14. Rosai J, Carcangiu ML, DeLellis RA. *Tumors of the Thyroid Gland. Atlas of Tumor Pathology, 3rd Series, Fascicle 5*. Washington, DC: Armed Forces Institute of Pathology; 1992.
15. Reid JD, Choi CH, Oldroyd NO. Calcium oxalate crystals in the thyroid. Their identification, prevalence, origin, and possible significance. *Am J Clin Pathol*. 1987;87:443–454.
16. Katoh R, Suzuki K, Hemmi A, et al. Nature and significance of calcium oxalate crystals in normal human thyroid gland. A clinicopathological and immunohistochemical study. *Virchows Arch A Pathol Anat Histopathol*. 1993;422:301–306.
17. Isotalo PA, Lloyd RV. Presence of birefringent crystals is useful in distinguishing thyroid from parathyroid gland tissues. *Am J Surg Pathol*. 2002;26:813–814.
18. Henzen-Logmans SC, Mullink H, Ramaekers FC, et al. Expression of cytokeratins and vimentin in epithelial cells of normal and pathologic thyroid tissue. *Virchows Arch A Pathol Anat Histopathol*. 1987;410:347–354.
19. Buley ID, Gatter KC, Heryet A, et al. Expression of intermediate filament proteins in normal and diseased thyroid glands. *J Clin Pathol*. 1987;40:136–142.
20. Viale G, Dell'Orto P, Coggi G, et al. Coexpression of cytokeratins and vimentin in normal and diseased thyroid glands. Lack of diagnostic utility of vimentin immunostaining. *Am J Surg Pathol*. 1989;13:1034–1040.
21. Lima MA, Gontijo VA, Schmitt FC. Thyroid peroxidase and thyroglobulin expression in normal human thyroid glands. *Endocr Pathol*. 1998;9:333–338.
22. Katoh R, Kawaoi A, Miyagi E, et al. Thyroid transcription factor-1 in normal, hyperplastic, and neoplastic follicular thyroid cells examined by immunohistochemistry and nonradioactive in situ hybridization. *Mod Pathol*. 2000;13:570–576.
23. Nonaka D, Tang Y, Chiriboga L, et al. Diagnostic utility of thyroid transcription factors Pax8 and TTF-2 (FoxE1) in thyroid epithelial neoplasms. *Mod Pathol*. 2008;21:192–200.
24. Mizukami Y, Hashimoto T, Nonomura A, et al. Immunohistochemical demonstration of thyrotropin (TSH)-receptor in normal and diseased human thyroid tissues using monoclonal antibody against recombinant human TSH-receptor protein. *J Clin Endocrinol Metab*. 1994;79:616–619.

25. Weber KB, Shroyer KR, Heinz DE, et al. The use of a combination of galectin-3 and thyroid peroxidase for the diagnosis and prognosis of thyroid cancer. *Am J Clin Pathol.* 2004;122:524–531.

26. van der Laan BF, Freeman JL, Asa SL. Expression of growth factors and growth factor receptors in normal and tumorous human thyroid tissues. *Thyroid.* 1995;5:67–73.

27. Westermark K, Lundqvist M, Wallin G, et al. EGF-receptors in human normal and pathological thyroid tissue. *Histopathology.* 1996;28:221–227.

28. DeLellis RA, Nunnemacher G, Wolfe HJ. C-cell hyperplasia. An ultrastructural analysis. *Lab Invest.* 1977;36:237–248.

29. Wolfe HJ, Voelkel EF, Tashjian AH Jr. Distribution of calcitonin-containing cells in the normal adult human thyroid gland: a correlation of morphology with peptide content. *J Clin Endocrinol Metab.* 1974;38:688–694.

30. Wolfe HJ, DeLellis RA, Voelkel EF, et al. Distribution of calcitonin-containing cells in the normal neonatal human thyroid gland: a correlation of morphology with peptide content. *J Clin Endocrinol Metab.* 1975;41:1076–1081.

31. Gibson WG, Peng TC, Croker BP. Age-associated C-cell hyperplasia in the human thyroid. *Am J Pathol.* 1982;106:388–393.

32. DeLellis RA, Wolfe HJ. The pathobiology of the human calcitonin (C)-cell: a review. *Pathol Annu.* 1981;16:25–52.

33. Schmid KW, Kirchmair R, Ladurner D, et al. Immunohistochemical comparison of chromogranins A and B and secretogranin II with calcitonin and calcitonin gene-related peptide expression in normal, hyperplastic and neoplastic C-cells of the human thyroid. *Histopathology.* 1992;21:225–232.

34. Kodama T, Fujino M, Endo Y, et al. Identification of carcinoembryonic antigen in the C-cell of the normal thyroid. *Cancer.* 1980;45:98–101.

35. Katoh R, Miyagi E, Nakamura N, et al. Expression of thyroid transcription factor-1 (TTF-1) in human C cells and medullary thyroid carcinomas. *Hum Pathol.* 2000;31:386–393.

36. Blaker M, de Weerth A, Tometten M, et al. Expression of the cholecystokinin 2-receptor in normal human thyroid gland and medullary thyroid carcinoma. *Eur J Endocrinol.* 2002;146:89–96.

37. Sundler F, Christophe J, Robberecht P, et al. Is helodermin produced by medullary thyroid carcinoma cells and normal C cells? Immunocytochemical evidence. *Regul Pept.* 1988;20:83–89.

38. Neuhold N, Wimmer M, Braun OM, et al. Reactivity of monoclonal islet cell antibodies on normal hyperplastic and neoplastic thyroid C-cells. *Cell Tissue Res.* 1989;257:437–443.

39. Tashjian AH Jr, Wolfe HJ, Voelkel EF. Human calcitonin. Immunologic assay, cytologic localization and studies on medullary thyroid carcinoma. *Am J Med.* 1974;56:840–849.

40. McMillan PJ, Hooker WM, Deptos LJ. Distribution of calcitonin-containing cells in the human thyroid. *Am J Anat.* 1974;140:73–79.

41. Nadig J, Weber E, Hedinger C. C-cell in vestiges of the ultimobranchial body in human thyroid glands. *Virchows Arch B Cell Pathol.* 1978;27:189–191.

42. Nadig J, Weber E, Hedinger C. C-cell in vestiges of the ultimobranchial body in human thyroid glands. *Virchows Arch B Cell Pathol.* 1978;27:189–191.

43. Janzer RC, Weber E, Hedinger C. The relation between solid cell nests and C cells of the thyroid gland: an immunohistochemical and morphometric investigation. *Cell Tissue Res.* 1979;197:295–312.

44. Harach HR. Solid cell nests of the thyroid. *J Pathol.* 1988;155:191–200.

45. Rios Moreno MJ, Galera-Ruiz H, De Miguel M, et al. Inmunohistochemical profile of solid cell nest of thyroid gland. *Endocr Pathol.* 2011;22:35–39.

46. Autelitano F, Santeusanio G, Di Tondo U, et al. Immunohistochemical study of solid cell nests of the thyroid gland found from an autopsy study. *Cancer.* 1987;59:477–483.

47. Yamaoka Y. Solid cell nest (SCN) of the human thyroid gland. *Acta Pathol Jpn.* 1973;23:493–506.

48. Asioli S, Erickson LA, Lloyd RV. Solid cell nests in Hashimoto's thyroiditis sharing features with papillary thyroid microcarcinoma. *Endocr Pathol.* 2009;20:197–203.

49. Vollenweider I, Hedinger C. Solid cell nests (SCN) in Hashimoto's thyroiditis. *Virchows Arch A Pathol Anat Histopathol.* 1988;412:357–363.

50. Reis-Filho JS, Preto A, Soares P, et al. p63 expression in solid cell nests of the thyroid: further evidence for a stem cell origin. *Mod Pathol.* 2003;16:43–48.

51. Harach HR. Solid cell nests of the thyroid. An anatomical survey and immunohistochemical study for the presence of thyroglobulin. *Acta Anat (Basel).* 1985;122:249–253.

52. Faggiano A, Talbot M, Baudin E, et al. Differential expression of galectin 3 in solid cell nests and C cells of human thyroid. *J Clin Pathol.* 2003;56:142–143.

53. Harach HR. A study on the relationship between solid cell nests and mucoepidermoid carcinoma of the thyroid. *Histopathology.* 1985;9:195–207.

54. Baloch ZW, Solomon AC, LiVolsi VA. Primary mucoepidermoid carcinoma and sclerosing mucoepidermoid carcinoma with eosinophilia of the thyroid gland: a report of nine cases. *Mod Pathol.* 2000;13:802–807.

55. Williams ED, Toyn CE, Harach HR. The ultimobranchial gland and congenital thyroid abnormalities in man. *J Pathol.* 1989;159:135–141.

56. Lee NJ, Blakey JD, Bhuta S, et al. Unintentional parathyroidectomy during thyroidectomy. *Laryngoscope.* 1999;109:1238–1240.

57. Sakorafas GH, Stafyla V, Bramis C, et al. Incidental parathyroidectomy during thyroid surgery: an underappreciated complication of thyroidectomy. *World J Surg.* 2005;29:1539–1543.

58. Abboud B, Sleilaty G, Braidy C, et al. Careful examination of thyroid specimen intraoperatively to reduce incidence of inadvertent parathyroidectomy during thyroid surgery. *Arch Otolaryngol Head Neck Surg.* 2007;133:1105–1110.

59. Feliciano DV. Parathyroid pathology in an intrathyroidal position. *Am J Surg.* 1992;164:496–500.

60. McIntyre RC Jr, Eisenach JH, Pearlman NW, et al. Intrathyroidal parathyroid glands can be a cause of failed cervical exploration for hyperparathyroidism. *Am J Surg.* 1997;174:750–753; discussion 3–4.

61. Phitayakorn R, McHenry CR. Incidence and location of ectopic abnormal parathyroid glands. *Am J Surg.* 2006;191:418–423.

62. Mendoza V, Ramirez C, Espinoza AE, et al. Characteristics of ectopic parathyroid glands in 145 cases of primary hyperparathyroidism. *Endocr Pract.* 2010;16:977–981.

63. Herden U, Seiler CA, Candinas D, et al. Intrathyroid adenomas in primary hyperparathyroidism: are they frequent enough to guide surgical strategy? *Surg Innov.* 2011.

Embryology and Developmental Lesions

 EMBRYOLOGY

Embryologic Origination

Knowledge of the embryologic development of the thyroid is key to understanding several abnormalities of the thyroid gland. The gland originates from the embryonic foregut, the same structure from which the pharynx, lungs, and upper digestive tract develop. The gland eventually contains two different types of hormonally active cells, follicular and C cells, and each type develops from a different embryologic structure. Follicular cells, which constitute the largest cell population, derive from the medial thyroid anlage. The C cells migrate to join the medial anlage through the lateral anlagen, also known as the ultimobranchial bodies (Fig. 2.1).

Medial Thyroid Primordium

The medial primordium, or anlage, is first visible near the end of the third week of embryonic life (Fig. 2.2). It appears as a thickening of endodermal epithelium of the cranial portion of the foregut, also known as the pharyngeal gut or pharynx.[1] The epithelial thickening develops in the ventral midline of the embryonic pharynx between the tuberculum impar and the copula (or hypobranchial eminence). This site, at the level of the second pharyngeal (or branchial) arch, eventually becomes the foramen cecum. The medial primordium soon invaginates to form a pit.

Migration

The invagination becomes more pronounced, yielding a flask-like diverticulum that begins to migrate caudally by the middle of the fourth week, concomitant with the descent of the heart. The migration of the thyroid anlage occurs through the loose mesenchyme ventral to the foregut. The cells continue to proliferate, and bilobation is evident early in the fifth week. The anlage, initially a hollow structure, solidifies with cells. It remains connected to the floor of the pharynx by the thyroglossal duct until the latter part of the fifth week when the duct begins to break down. The duct generally disappears between the sixth and eighth week, but portions may persist as fibrous cords or fine tubular structures with epithelial lining. Persistence of the latter into postnatal life can be the nidus of a thyroglossal duct cyst. As the medial anlage migrates, two lobes joined by an isthmus become visible during the sixth week. It reaches its final position anterior to the proximal region of the trachea during the seventh week of gestation.

Folliculogenesis

Formation of follicles begins in the 8th to 10th week as the thyroid transforms from solid cords of cells into rounded aggregates with small central lumina. Colloid is initially seen between the 10th and 12th week, and thyroid hormone is detectable in the fetal serum by the 11th to 12th week.[2–4] After the 13th week, the follicular cells appear morphologically well developed at the ultrastructural level,[4] and by the 14th week, distinct follicles are seen throughout the thyroid.

Growth and Maturation

The weight of the thyroid gland increases in a nearly linear manner from about 5 to 20 mg to 250 to 500 mg between the 10th and 20th week of gestation. The height of follicular cells stays between 12 to and 13 μm during the 10th to 20th week.[5] During this period of active folliculogenesis, the number of follicles per unit area initially increases and then declines, reflecting an increase in follicle size and colloid content. The follicular epithelium to colloid ratio declines until the 17th to 18th week. This ratio then remains fairly constant up to about the 29th week, suggesting the attainment of structural maturity early in the second trimester.[5,6] Proliferative activity in the thyroid as measured by Ki-67 (MIB-1) immunostaining of nuclei is relatively high between the 10th and 20th week, with averages ranging between 12% and 16% (Fig. 2.3).[7] The rate diminishes throughout the latter half of gestation, dropping to <0.5% at the time of birth. The average proliferative rate remains a fraction of a percentage throughout the pediatric and adult periods of life.

The thyroid increases in size throughout gestation, showing the highest relative rate of growth during the second trimester.[8] During the second trimester, the gland weight increases 7- to 8-fold, increasing from approximately 100 to 125 mg to 700 to 800 mg.[5,6,9] Follicular cell height increases to reach a maximum of 18 μm at about 30 weeks.[5] After the 29th week, fetal thyroids tend to show a gradual increase in the epithelial:colloid ratio as epithelial growth outpaces colloid accumulation. The size of follicles decreases and the number of follicles per unit area increases, reflective of the relatively small volume of colloid.

Thyroid glands of newborn full-term infants have a variable appearance in terms of colloid content. A significant number shows no appreciable colloid, and some consider this a physiologic response to labor.[10] Desquamation of follicular epithelium and aggregates of pyknotic nuclei can be seen, and some have attributed this to physiologic changes.[10] However, in most cases, these latter changes probably represent postmortem autolysis. At end of 40 weeks of gestation, the thyroid gland attains a weight in the range of 1 to 4 g.[5,9]

Lateral Thyroid Primordia

The ultimobranchial bodies constitute the lateral thyroid primordia that fuse with the medial anlage to form the complete thyroid gland (Fig. 2.1). The ultimobranchial bodies populate the thyroid gland with C cells.[11] The precursors of the C cells have been considered derivatives of the neural crest. The neural crest is a transient tissue initially found at the junction of the neural groove and ectoderm. After the neural groove fuses to form the neural tube, the neural crest forms an intermediate zone between the surface ectoderm and neural tube.

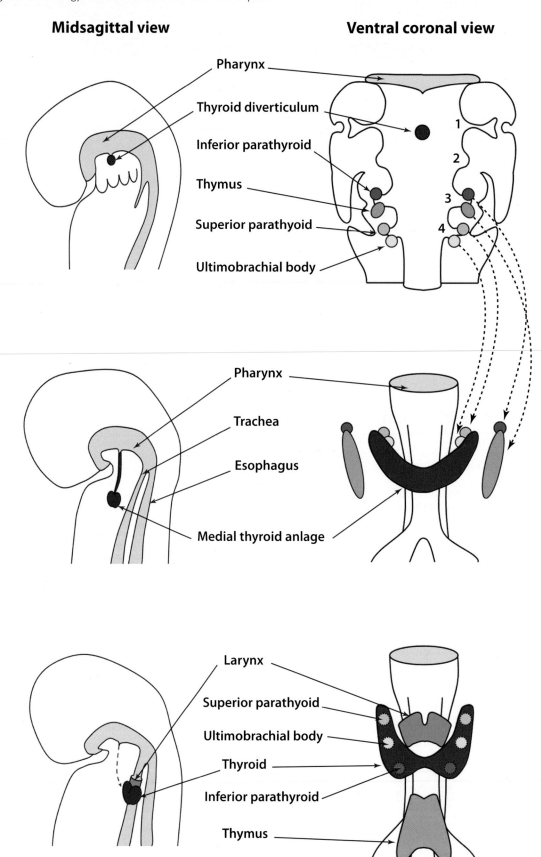

Midsagittal view

Ventral coronal view

Pharynx

Thyroid diverticulum

Inferior parathyroid

Thymus

Superior parathyroid

Ultimobrachial body

Pharynx

Trachea

Esophagus

Medial thyroid anlage

Larynx

Superior parathyroid

Ultimobrachial body

Thyroid

Inferior parathyroid

Thymus

FIGURE 2.1. Embryonic thyroid development from the fourth week through the seventh to eighth week. The midsagittal images on the left side show the origin of the medial anlage from the pharynx and the migration to final site adjacent to the larynx and trachea. The ventral coronal view images on the right side show the origin and migration of the inferior parathyroids and thymus (from the third pharyngeal pouches) and the superior parathyroids and ultimobranchial bodies (from the fourth pouches) to their final locations.

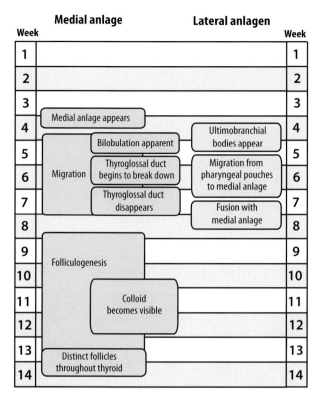

Medial anlage | **Lateral anlagen**

Week						Week
1						1
2						2
3						3
4	Medial anlage appears			Ultimobranchial bodies appear		4
5		Bilobulation apparent		Migration from pharyngeal pouches to medial anlage		5
6	Migration	Thyroglossal duct begins to break down				6
7		Thyroglossal duct disappears		Fusion with medial anlage		7
8						8
9	Folliculogenesis					9
10						10
11		Colloid becomes visible				11
12						12
13	Distinct follicles throughout thyroid					13
14						14

FIGURE 2.2. Timeline of thyroid developmental events during embryonic life.

The pleuripotent cells of the neural crest migrate extensively throughout the body and differentiate into a wide range of cells including sensory neurons, postganglionic autonomic neurons and Schwann cells of the peripheral nervous system, melanocytes, chondrocytes, and catecholamine-secreting cells of the adrenal medulla.[12]

Using chick–quail chimeras, Le Douarin and Le Lièvre demonstrated that avian C cells ultimately derive from the neural crest.[13] They engrafted sections of quail neural primordium into chick embryos and traced the migration of the quail cells, distinguishable by their large nucleoli. Quail cells subsequently proved to be the predominant component of the ultimobranchial bodies and formed the C cells.

The assumption that mammalian C cells derive from the neural crest has been challenged recently. The ultimobranchial bodies of birds and lower vertebrates do not fuse with the medial anlage. Avian ultimobranchial bodies are innervated structures containing C cells separate from the thyroid gland, in contrast to mammalian ultimobranchial bodies, which fuse with the medial thyroid and disperse C cells within the gland.[14] It is of note that a recent study of mice found that neural crest cells populate pharyngeal arches but not the pouches including the site of the ultimobranchial bodies.[15] These findings suggest the origin of murine C cells from the endodermal epithelium as opposed to the neural crest. However, at this time, the orthodox view remains that C cells ultimately derive from the neural crest.

The ultimobranchial bodies become apparent during the fourth to fifth week of gestation as stratified endodermal tissue in contact with the embryonic pharyngeal space.[16] The ultimobranchial bodies are located in the most caudal pharyngeal pouches. Because the fifth pouch is rudimentary in humans, controversy exists whether it should be considered a separate fifth pouch or a component of the fourth pharyngeal pouch. Thus, the region containing the ultimobranchial body is sometimes referred to as the fourth–fifth branchial pouch complex.[16] For practical purposes

in this chapter, ultimobranchial bodies will be considered part of the fourth pouch, acknowledging that they arguably constitute separate fifth pouches.

Migration and Fusion

The ultimobranchial bodies separate from the pharyngeal pouches and migrate centrally to fuse with the medial thyroid usually by the seventh to eighth week of gestation. Fusion typically occurs in the middle or midsuperior regions of the lateral lobes. After fusion with the larger medial anlage, the ultimobranchial bodies undergo dissolution with dispersal of C cells into the surrounding follicular tissue. Portions of the ultimobranchial bodies may persist in fetal or postnatal thyroid glands as small cystic structures or solid cell nests.[16–19]

 # GENES INVOLVED IN THYROID DEVELOPMENT

Early Development

Several genes that appear to play critical roles in thyroid development have been identified (Table 2.1).[20,21] The signal that initiates the development of the medial anlage is unknown. However, *TTF1 (NKX2-1), TTF2 (FOXE1), PAX8,* and *HHEX* are genes that are involved in the early embryologic stages of thyroid development by cell-autonomous mechanisms. *TBX1* has been identified as a gene that also plays an important role in early thyroid development, but, by a cell-nonautonomous mechanism involving the surrounding mesoderm. Much of our knowledge about their roles derives from studies of transgenic mice lacking these genes, the so-called knockout mice.

TTF1

TTF1, also known as *NKX2-1, TITF1,* or *T/EBP,* codes for a homeodomain-containing transcription factor, thyroid transcription factor 1 (TTF1), that is able to bind to the promoters of the thyroglobulin gene (*Tg*) and the thyroperoxidase gene (*TPO*). It maps to chromosome 14q13 and is a member of the NKX2 family of transcription factors.[22] Its expression is coincidental with the appearance of the initial endodermal thickening, and the medial anlage is the only location in the embryonic pharynx that shows TTF1 expression. It remains expressed in the thyroid throughout embryonic and fetal development and into adulthood. TTF1 is also expressed in C cells.[23] TTF1 seems to be necessary for the survival of the follicular precursors. Knockout mice lacking this gene show loss of the medial thyroid anlage through apoptosis along with the absence of C cells.[24,25] TTF1 does not appear to be necessary for formation and migration of ultimobranchial bodies but is essential for the survival of its cells during migration and for successful fusion with the medial anlage.[26]

NKX2-5 is another homeobox-containing gene that expresses its protein in the early medial thyroid anlage. NKX2-5 is a transcription factor that has a major role in cardiac development,[27] and recent data suggest that it may also play a role in cases of thyroid dysgenesis.[28]

PAX8

The *PAX8* gene codes for a member of a family of transcription factors with a 128 amino acid paired binding domain.[29,30] It is located on chromosome 2q12, and it derives its name from paired box gene 8. This transcription factor seems to have synergistic action with TTF1 and is critical for the development of the medial anlage past the early invagination stage.[31] Like TTF1, PAX8

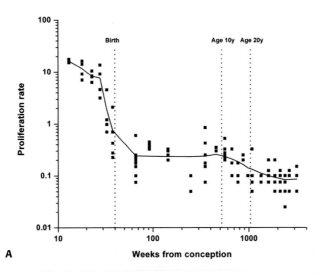

A

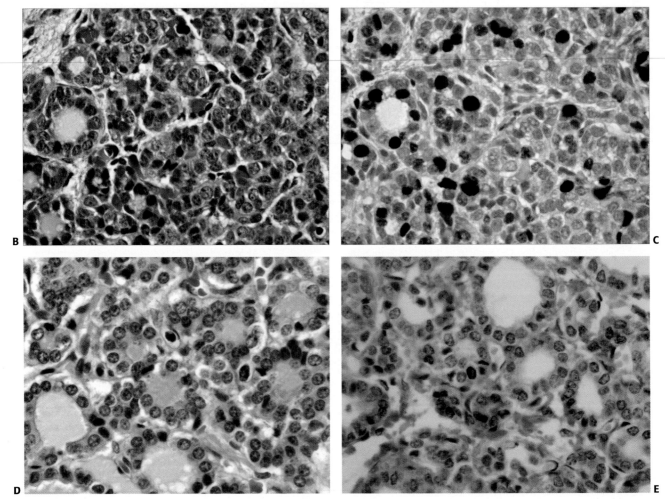

FIGURE 2.3. A: Change in the proliferative rate of human thyroid cells by weeks from conception based on immunostaining for Ki-67 (MIB-1), a marker of active cell proliferative cycle. (From Saad AG, Kumar S, Ron E, et al. Proliferative activity of human thyroid cells in various age groups and its correlation with the risk of thyroid cancer after radiation exposure. *J Clin Endocrinol Metab.* 2006;91:2672–2677, with permission. Copyright 2006, *The Endocrine Society.*) **B–E:** Comparison of thyroid of 13-week fetus **(B and C)** with that of a full-term infant **(D and E)**. **(B)** and **(D)** are photomicrographs of hematoxylin and eosin–stained sections, whereas **(C)** and **(E)** show immunostaining for Ki-67. The 13-week fetal thyroid shows staining of 16% of nuclei, whereas <1% of nuclei of full-term infant thyroid express Ki-67.

Table 2.1

Genes Involved in Thyroid Development

Gene	Chromosome Location	Functions
TTF1 (NKX2-1)	14q13	• Transcription factor able to bind to promoters of *Tg* and *TPO* • Necessary for survival of follicular precursors • Necessary for survival of C cells
PAX8	2q12	• Transcription factor having synergistic action with *TTF1* • Necessary for survival of medial anlage • Important for follicular development
TTF2 (FOXE1)	9q22	• Transcription factor able to bind to promoters of *Tg* and *TPO* • Essential role in medial anlage migration
HHEX	10q23	• Unclear; possible maintenance of expression of *TTF1*, *PAX8*, and *TTF2*
TBX1	22q11	• Transcription factor with nonautonomous mechanism involving the surrounding mesoderm • Appears to regulate the size of early medial anlage through control of *FGF8*
TSHR	14q31	• Codes for thyroid-stimulating hormone receptor
Tg	8q24	• Codes for thyroglobulin
TPO	2p25	• Codes for thyroperoxidase
NIS	19p13	• Codes for sodium-iodide symporter
HOXA3	7p15	• Transcription factor with essential role in the development of pharyngeal glandular tissues • Important for the development and/or interaction of medial anlage and ultimobranchial bodies
HASH1	12q22-23	• Transcription factor important in the development of C cells • Important role in the differentiation of neurons derived from neural crest

appears to be necessary for survival of the anlage but does not initiate its development. PAX8 also appears to play an important role in follicular differentiation. Disruption of both *PAX8* alleles in mice results in severe congenital hypothyroidism because of the absence of follicular cells.[32] Monoallelic mutations in *PAX8* have been documented in patients with sporadic and familial thyroid hypoplasia or ectopy.[33,34]

TTF2

The gene *TTF2*, also known as *FOXE1*, *TITF2*, or *FKHL15*, codes for a member of the forkhead/winged helix family of transcription factors and maps to chromosome 9q22.[35] This transcription factor is a nuclear protein that binds to *Tg* and *TPO* promoters. It is expressed when the medial thyroid anlage first appears. Like TTF1 and PAX8, expression continues throughout development and into adulthood. However, it has a wider area of foregut expression, being detected in the developing thyroid, tongue, epiglottis, palate, and esophagus. TTF2 seems to play an essential role in the migration of the medial anlage.

HHEX

The gene *HHEX* codes for a homeodomain-containing transcription factor that is expressed in the foregut before and after the appearance of the thyroid anlage. The gene is located on chromosome 10q23, and its name derives from hematopoietically expressed homeobox because it was first identified in hematopoietic tissue.[36,37] Expression of HHEX is seen in the primordial tissue of thyroid, liver, thymus, pancreas, and lungs. It shows the highest degree of expression in developing and adult thyroid. The role of *HHEX* is not defined at this time. In particular, it is unclear whether the factor is necessary for maintaining expression of TTF1, TTF2, PAX8, or vice versa.[20]

TBX1

The gene *TBX1*, also known as *T-box 1*, is a member of the family of T-box genes that code for transcription factors involved in the regulation of developmental processes. The gene is located on chromosome 22q11.[38] *TBX1* plays an important role in the development of pharyngeal structures and is a major gene associated with DiGeorge syndrome.[39,40] TBX1 is not expressed in the thyroid primordium but instead is expressed in the surrounding mesoderm, and it appears to regulate the size of the early thyroid primordium through the control of the fibroblast growth factor 8 gene (*FGF8*) expression.[40]

Later Development

Genes involved in the later stages of thyroid development include *TSHR, Tg, TPO, NIS, HOXA3, FGFR2*, and others from the *NKX2* family.[20] *TSHR* maps to chromosome 14q31 and is one of the superfamilies of G protein–coupled receptors.[41] TSHR, or thyroid-stimulating hormone receptor, is initially expressed in the medial thyroid anlage after the completion of migration but before follicular development. It seems to be important for follicular development because knockout mice with null or loss of function show severe hypothyroidism. These mice have hypoplastic thyroid glands as adults, even though the glands are of normal size at birth.

Tg, TPO, and NIS

Thyroglobulin (*Tg*), thyroperoxidase (*TPO*), and sodium-iodide symporter (*NIS*) are three critical genes involved in thyroid hormone production. Expression of these genes begins after the completion of thyroid anlage migration and continues through prenatal development and throughout postnatal life. Soon after initial expression in the embryonic thyroid, primitive follicles begin to appear. *Tg* maps to chromosome 8q24 and codes for thyroglobulin, the major product of follicular cells and precursor of thyroid hormone.[42] *TPO* is located on chromosome 2p25 and codes for thyroperoxidase (*TPO*).[43] This enzyme, located at apical microvilli, catalyzes the addition of iodide to tyrosine residues on thyroglobulin. *NIS* codes for the sodium-iodide symporter (NIS), which is located at the basilar aspect of the follicular cell and transports iodide from the bloodstream into the cell. *NIS* maps to chromosome 19p13.[44]

HOX

HOXA3 is a member of a family of 39 known genes that code for homeodomain-containing transcription factors that regulate regional development along the major axes of the embryo. The human *HOXA3* gene is located at chromosome 7p15.2.[45] Studies suggest that multiple *HOX* genes may function jointly to control development of a given tissue, but *HOXA3* appears to play the major role in the development of the pharyngeal glandular tissues.[46] HOXA3 is expressed in the neural crest, the mesenchyme of pharyngeal arches, and the pharyngeal endoderm, including the sites of the medial and lateral thyroid primordia. Mice lacking *HOXA3* are athymic and exhibit abnormalities of the thyroid gland including hypoplasia or absence of a lobe.[46] Persistent, ectopic ultimobranchial bodies containing C cells have been identified on the sides with the hypoplastic or absent lobes, raising the question whether interaction between the medial and lateral anlagen is important for the normal development of the thyroid gland.

HASH1

HASH1, also known as *hASH1, ASH1*, or *MASH1*, codes for a basic helix-loop-helix transcription factor and maps to chromosome 12q22-23.[47] This transcription factor plays an important role in the development of C cells and is a mammalian homolog of the protein coded by the Drosophila achaete-scute complex gene (*ASCL1*). It has a key role in the differentiation of neurons derived from the neural crest, and knockout mice show a marked reduction in C cells.[48–50]

The identification of genes and their products that play important roles in thyroid development is still in progress. There seems little doubt that thyroid development is affected by more genes than those discussed in this section. As time progresses, we should gain further insight into the full symphony of genes controlling thyroid development, their specific roles, and understanding what is a complex interplay of numerous genes and their products.

DEVELOPMENTAL LESIONS

Thyroid Dysgenesis

Thyroid dysgenesis encompasses a group of congenital thyroid abnormalities including absence of thyroid tissue (agenesis or athyreosis), hemiagenesis, ectopic thyroid tissue, and hypoplasia of an orthotopic gland (Table 2.2). Collectively, these abnormalities account for approximately 85% of cases of congenital hypothyroidism in iodine-sufficient regions.[20,51–53] The relative proportion of these abnormalities is variable and reflective of the detection methodology of a given study. Thyroid ectopia is usually the most frequent cause, particularly if assessment is by scintigraphy as opposed to sonography.[20] Most cases of ectopia are because of abnormal migration of the medial thyroid anlage, and ectopic tissue is almost always hypoplastic compared with an orthotopic gland. The reason why ectopic thyroid glands are hypoplastic is unclear, but one hypothesis relates to failure of the

Table 2.2

Forms of Thyroid Dysgenesis

Type of Dysgenesis	Definition	Usual Thyroid Function
Ectopia	Abnormal location of thyroid follicular tissue because of defective migration	Hypothyroid
Agenesis (athyreosis)	Absence of thyroid follicular tissue in orthotopic or ectopic location	Hypothyroid
Hemiagenesis	Absence of one of the lateral lobes	Euthyroid
Hypoplasia	Hypoplastic gland in orthotopic location	Hypothyroid

medial anlage to fuse with the lateral anlagen (ultimobranchial bodies).[20,46,54] Interaction between cells of the ultimobranchial bodies and medial anlage may be necessary for normal thyroid development. The ultimobranchial bodies have even been cited as a source of follicular cells, but this possibility is not widely accepted.[55]

Agenesis

Agenesis, or athyreosis, is the absence of thyroid follicular tissue in an orthotopic or ectopic location. Most studies report agenesis as the second most common abnormality comprising thyroid dysgenesis.[52] The absence of thyroid tissue may reflect failure to initiate formation of the medial anlage or failure to maintain it during its growth and migration. Defective expression of *TTF1, TTF2, PAX8*, and/or *HHEX* could explain agenesis. Bamforth–Lazarus syndrome, characterized by athyroidal hypothyroidism, spiky hair, choanal atresia, cleft palate, and bifid epiglottis, has been associated with loss of function of *TTF2*.[56]

Hypoplasia

Hypoplasia of an orthotopic thyroid is the least common phenotype of thyroid dysgenesis, comprising about 5% of cases.[20,51,52] Defects of any of the genes that control thyroid development and function can result in hypoplasia. Sometimes a gland may be so small and hypofunctional that it eludes detection by scintigraphy or sonography and appears to be a case of agenesis.[57]

Hemiagenesis

Thyroid hemiagenesis is a rare congenital abnormality in which one of the lateral lobes fails to develop. Its prevalence is in the range of 0.05% to 0.2% of births, with a slight female predominance.[58,59] By far most cases of hemiagenesis show absence of the left lobe. Hemiagenesis may be viewed as a form of dysgenesis, but unlike the other abnormalities described above in this section, individuals with hemiagenesis are typically euthyroid.[58] Some familial cases have also been reported, but no specific gene defect has clearly emerged as the cause of familial or sporadic cases.[60]

Thyroid Tissue in Abnormal Locations

Thyroid tissue can be found grossly or microscopically in various locations aside from its normal site. Many instances represent metastatic well-differentiated carcinoma, but some cases are bona fide ectopia of nonneoplastic thyroid tissue. Distinguishing between metastatic and truly ectopic thyroid tissue can be challenging, and this issue has been debated in medical literature for more than a century. Several terms and conflicting opinions have arisen. Unfortunately, the nomenclature has not always been well defined or applied uniformly, leaving us with overlapping terms. In addition, our knowledge and classification of thyroid neoplasia has evolved, particularly elimination of papillary adenoma as a diagnostic entity and recognition of the follicular variant of papillary carcinoma. Interpretation of some older literature is difficult because of this evolution in classification. The differential diagnosis of thyroid tissue in abnormal locations includes metastatic carcinoma, ectopic nonneoplastic thyroid tissue, thyroid neoplasia arising in ectopic tissue, and teratoma (Table 2.3).

Table 2.3

Differential Diagnosis of Thyroid Tissue with Abnormal Location in Neck

General Category	Specific Entity	Gross Features	Microscopic Features
Ectopic nonneoplastic thyroid	Ectopia because of abnormal descent of medial anlage	• Most commonly located at base of tongue (lingual thyroid) • Present somewhere along midline descent tract • Borders may be well or ill defined • Normal orthotopic thyroid usually absent if ectopic tissue grossly evident	• Follicles range in size; normofollicular and/or microfollicular patterns most common • Absence of nuclear features of papillary carcinoma • May be admixed with skeletal muscle or other soft tissues
	Thyroglossal duct cyst	• Cyst usually in 1–5 cm range • Smooth outer surface • Usually mucoid or gelatinous contents • Thyroid tissue usually not grossly identifiable	• Cyst lining variable: ciliated columnar, squamous, and/or cuboidal epithelium, or granulation tissue • About half contain foci of follicular tissue in wall • Variable acute and chronic inflammation
	Benign lymph node inclusions	• Inclusions not grossly evident • Lymph node medial to jugular vein	• Lack features of papillary carcinoma
	Parasitic nodule	• Separate nodule from thyroid gland; may be attached by thin fibrous strand • Thyroid gland usually has nodular hyperplasia	• Usually shows nodular hyperplasia or similar changes as seen in thyroid gland • Lacks features of malignant thyroid neoplasm • No evidence of lymph node
Thyroid neoplasia	Metastatic carcinoma	• Found within one or more lymph nodes; may be grossly apparent • Involved lymph nodes may show cystic change • Lateral or medial to jugular vein • Primary neoplasm in thyroid	• Follicular and/or papillary architecture • Psammoma bodies may be present • Cells show nuclear features of papillary carcinoma • Immunopositivity for galectin-3 and HBME-1
	Thyroid neoplasm arising in ectopic nonneoplastic tissue	• Usually associated with thyroglossal duct cyst; usually confined to cyst • Rare complication of lingual thyroid	• Papillary carcinoma most common • Squamous cell carcinoma may occur • Follicular and anaplastic carcinomas very rare; medullary carcinoma should not occur
	Teratoma	• Pediatric cervical teratomas may involve thyroid • Adult teratomas of thyroid extremely rare (see Chapter 16)	• Teratomas occurring in neck rarely have thyroid tissue as a component

Ectopic Thyroid Tissue

True Thyroid Ectopia

Truly ectopic tissue may be the sole thyroid tissue in an individual, or accessory tissue associated with an orthotopic thyroid. Ectopic tissue is usually found along the track of medial anlage descent somewhere between the base of tongue and the normal thyroid location (Fig. 2.4). Ectopic tissue has also been reported elsewhere in the neck and mediastinum including the submandibular region, trachea, esophagus or paraesophageal region, heart and great vessels, and superior mediastinum.[61–68] Thyroid tissue of most legitimate cases of ectopia is found within an inverted pyramidal region extending from the edges of the mandible inferiorly to the aortic arch. Several other unexpected sites have also been reported including lung, duodenum, gallbladder, porta hepatis, pancreas, small intestinal mesentery, adrenal gland, parotid gland, sella turcica, and skin.[69–78]

An embryologic basis for some of the ectopic sites listed above can be reasonably envisioned. Thyroid tissue may descend too far and develop in the lower neck or mediastinum. The heart, great vessels, and thymus originate very near to the primordial site of the thyroid, and attachment of thyroidal tissue may occur before their caudal migration. Developmental anomalies of the foregut may explain ectopia in the thorax and upper gastrointestinal tract. Although heteroplasia has been invoked to explain some cases of ectopia, application of this concept and proof of its validity is problematic. The possibility of metastasis should be considered and excluded before accepting aberrant thyroid tissue as ectopic.

Lingual Thyroid

The tongue is the most common site for total thyroid ectopia.[79] Most lingual thyroids are asymptomatic. Symptomatic lingual ectopia can present at any time in life but is most common during puberty, pregnancy, or menstruation. Patients may experience dysphagia, otalgia, dysphonia, dyspnea, and even overt upper airway obstruction. About 70% of individuals with *symptomatic* lingual thyroid lack other functional tissue, and about 70% have some degree of hypothyroidism.[80]

Lingual thyroids are usually located at or quite near the mucosal surface at the base of tongue, corresponding to the site of the foramen cecum. Less often they are found deeper within the musculature. The size of a lingual thyroid ranges from a few millimeters to several centimeters. The prevalence of grossly visible lingual thyroid is estimated to be 1 per 10,000 individuals, although the microscopic prevalence may be as high as 1 per 10.[80,81]

Clinically apparent lingual thyroids usually appear as a smooth, dome-shaped mucosal mass at the base of tongue. The lesion may appear well or ill defined on sectioning. Microscopically, the follicles can show a range of size and colloid content. The ectopic tissue typically has a normofollicular or microfollicular pattern, or a mixture of both (Fig. 2.5). Skeletal muscle is usually admixed with the thyroid tissue.

Follicular, oncocytic, and papillary thyroid carcinomas have been reported arising in lingual thyroids.[82–85] About 40 cases have been reported. Follicular carcinoma is the most frequent diagnosis, but this is difficult to confirm in some reports. The majority of more recently reported cases are papillary carcinomas, and this probably reflects greater recognition of the follicular variant of papillary carcinoma. Distinguishing follicular neoplasia in a lingual thyroid is challenging given the common intermingling of ectopic tissue with skeletal muscle. The diagnosis of follicular carcinoma in a lingual site requires vascular invasion, unequivocal infiltration with desmoplastic response, and/or metastasis in the absence of another primary site.[84] The incidence of malignancy in ectopic thyroid tissue does not appear to exceed that of orthotopic thyroid.[79,83]

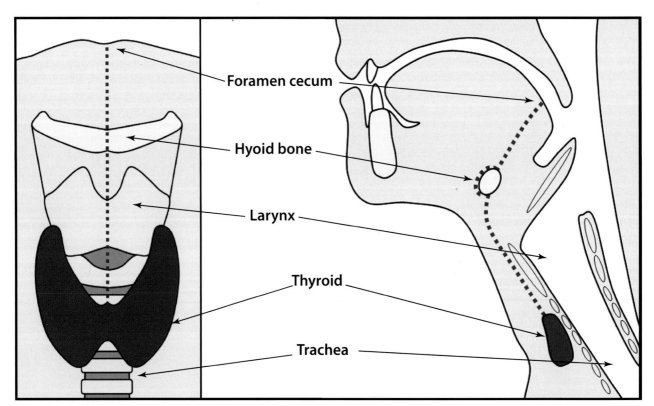

FIGURE 2.4. Diagram showing track of medial anlage descent from the foramen cecum to the normal location in the neck (*dotted line*)**.** Thyroid ectopia typically occurs along this midline track. Persistent portions of the thyroglossal duct and thyroglossal duct cysts are also found along this track.

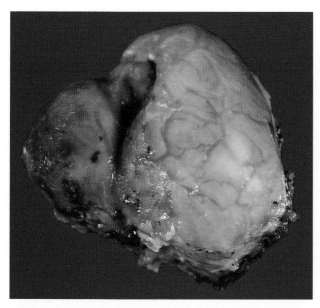

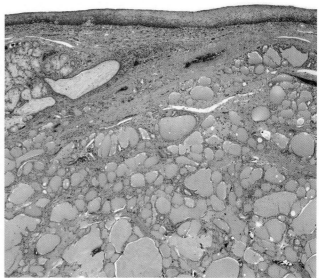

FIGURE 2.5. Gross photograph (left) and photomicrograph (right) of excised lingual thyroid. This lingual thyroid is well circumscribed and is located just below the squamous mucosa of the tongue. The intact mucosal surface is shown in the gross photograph and at the top of the photomicrograph. Minor salivary gland tissue is present in the upper left region of the photomicrograph.

Thyroglossal Duct Cyst

Remnants of the thyroglossal duct can develop into cysts. The cysts develop in the midline of the neck along medial anlage's

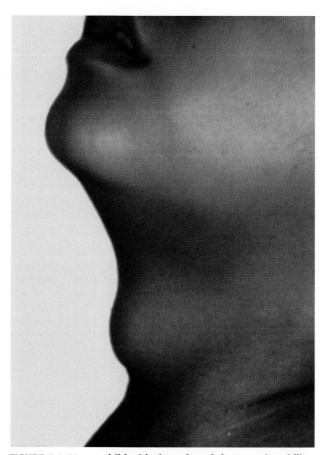

FIGURE 2.6. Young child with thyroglossal duct cyst in midline of neck.

track of descent between the foramen cecum and final location of the thyroid (Fig. 2.6). Cysts can be linked to the foramen cecum or skin by a sinus tract. During embryonic descent, the thyroglossal tract courses ventrally to the hyoid bone, a derivative of the second and third pharyngeal arches. As the hyoid bone moves to its final position, the tract is pulled with it posteriorly and cranially. The tract may run anterior, posterior, or within the hyoid bone.[86] Most cysts are located near the hyoid bone and connected to it by a solid fibrous or tubular remnant of the thyroglossal duct. Owing to this connection, the central portion of the hyoid bone is commonly removed during resection of a thyroglossal duct cyst in a procedure named after Sistrunk, who described surgical management of these cysts in 1920.[87]

Thyroglossal duct cysts can manifest during any time of life. Approximately half of thyroglossal duct cysts are detected during childhood and adolescence, commonly before the age of 5, and a significant number of cysts are evident at the time of birth. However, about one-third manifest after the age of 30.[88,89] The male:female ratio is about equal. Rare cases of hereditary thyroglossal duct cysts have been identified.[90] Most have an autosomal dominant pattern and, in contrast to sporadic cases, show female predominance. The explanation for the latter is unclear but may be because of genetic imprinting.

Morphologic Features

Thyroglossal duct cysts usually have a rounded, smooth external surface and measure from 1 to 5 cm in diameter with an average of about 2.5 cm (Fig. 2.7).[91,92] The interior usually contains mucoid or gelatinous material having a broad range of color (clear, yellow-tan, red-brown, and gray-white) and degree of opacity. Purulent exudate may fill the cavity if a cyst becomes infected. Thyroid tissue is usually not evident grossly but if present appears as a reddish-tan or reddish-brown focus.

Microscopically, cysts exhibit variable linings ranging from ciliated pseudostratified columnar epithelium to nondescript cuboidal or stratified squamous cells (Fig. 2.8). Sometimes the cyst is denuded of epithelium, at least focally, and this may reflect epithelial damage by inflammation. Granulation tissue can

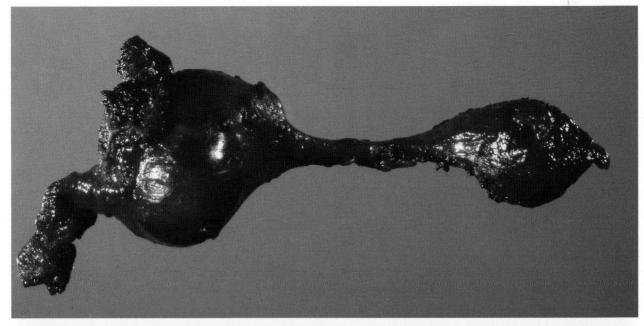

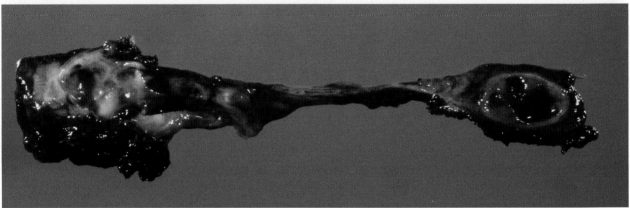

FIGURE 2.7. Thyroglossal duct cysts. The intact cysts are shown in the upper photograph and the bisected specimen in the lower. The cyst on the left side was located adjacent to the hyoid bone, and the cyst on the right was located just above the isthmus. The cysts are connected by the thyroglossal duct remnant.

be seen in these denuded regions. Squamous epithelium is more common in suprahyoid cysts, whereas columnar epithelium is seen more often in those below the hyoid.[79] Combinations of the above linings can be seen in a single cyst. The walls of cysts exhibit variable thickness and are composed of fibrous tissue that may contain thyroid follicles and/or mucous or seromucous glands. The frequency of salivary-type glands increases with proximity to the tongue.[79] Thyroid follicular tissue is seen in about 50% of cases, typically as irregular foci (Fig. 2.9). A significant number will not have identifiable follicular tissue, and its absence does not preclude the diagnosis of thyroglossal duct cyst. Variable degrees of acute and/or chronic inflammation may be seen in the wall.

Cytopathology
Fine needle aspiration of thyroglossal duct cysts typically yields sparsely cellular specimens with macrophages, either foamy or hemosiderin-laden, in a background of amorphous proteinaceous material resembling colloid (Fig. 2.10).[92,93] The colloid-like material ranges from thick and fragmented to thin and watery. Inflammatory cells, predominated by either lymphocytes or neutrophils, are common and usually outnumber epithelial cells. Ciliated

columnar or squamous cells may be seen along with anucleate squames. Thyroid follicles are seen in about 10% of fine needle aspirates. Aspirates often contain cholesterol crystals, which may be quite numerous.[94]

Differential Diagnosis
The differential diagnosis of thyroglossal duct cyst includes various cystic and solid lesions including dermoid cyst, epidermoid cyst, ranula, midline cervical cleft, cystic degeneration of a colloid nodule, lymph node metastasis with cystic degeneration, branchial cleft cyst, lymphangioma, lymph node with reactive hyperplasia, and teratoma. Branchial cleft cyst, discussed below in the section on lateral aberrant thyroid tissue, is generally distinguishable by its lateral location (Table 2.4).

Complications and Neoplasia
Complications of thyroglossal duct cysts include infection and malignant transformation. Residual thyroglossal duct connection to the foramen cecum may permit contamination with bacteria from the oral cavity. Carcinoma is a rare complication arising in 1% or less of thyroglossal duct cysts.[79,95] The vast majority are papillary thyroid carcinoma.[96] Papillary carcinoma occurring in

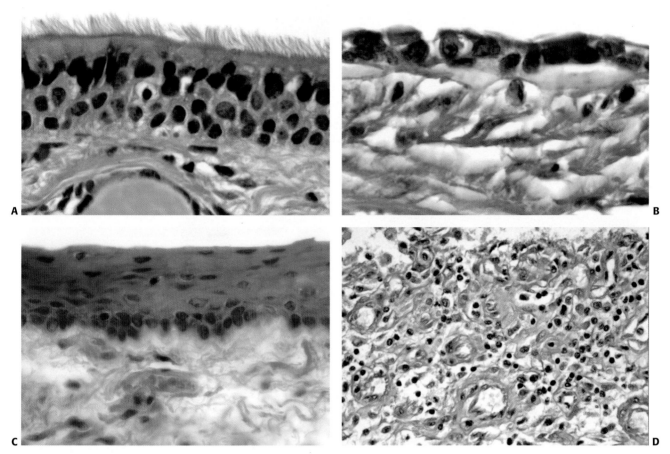

FIGURE 2.8. Photomicrographs showing different linings of thyroglossal duct cysts. A: Ciliated pseudostratified columnar epithelium. **B:** Nondescript cuboidal epithelium. **C:** Squamous epithelium. **D:** Inflamed granulation tissue.

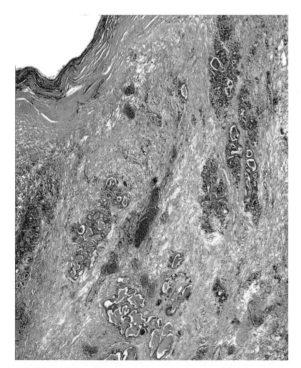

FIGURE 2.9. Low-power photomicrograph of thyroglossal duct cyst showing follicular tissue in wall. Cyst lumen is present in upper left region.

thyroglossal duct cysts has histologic features comparable with those occurring in the thyroid gland (Fig. 2.11). Both papillary and follicular architecture can be seen along with the diagnostic nuclear features. Squamous cell carcinoma (Fig. 2.12), although rare, is the second most common malignancy in thyroglossal duct cysts, whereas follicular and anaplastic thyroid carcinomas are even more rare.[97–100] Medullary carcinoma has not been reported, consistent with derivation of C cells from the ultimobranchial bodies. Most malignancies are identified after resection of a thyroglossal duct cyst, and resection is usually curative.

Lateral Aberrant Thyroid Tissue

The issue of lateral aberrant thyroid tissue has a long history of controversy. The crux of debate is whether all lateral thyroid tissue should be considered metastatic or whether some could be ectopic nonneoplastic tissue. A derivative of this issue is whether thyroid neoplasms can develop primarily in laterally located ectopic tissue.

The definition of lateral aberrant thyroid tissue is not explicitly stated in much of the literature but generally seems to refer to tissue found lateral to the thyroglossal tract. LiVolsi[101] has specifically defined lateral aberrant thyroid tissue as thyroid tissue lateral to the jugular vein. Of key consideration is whether the lateral thyroid tissue is associated with a lymph node. If so, the tissue probably represents metastatic papillary thyroid carcinoma, even if the tissue consists of normal-appearing follicles. There may be exceptions to this rule (see Thyroid Inclusions in Lymph Nodes section below). If the thyroid tissue is unassociated with a lymph node, true ectopia can be considered.

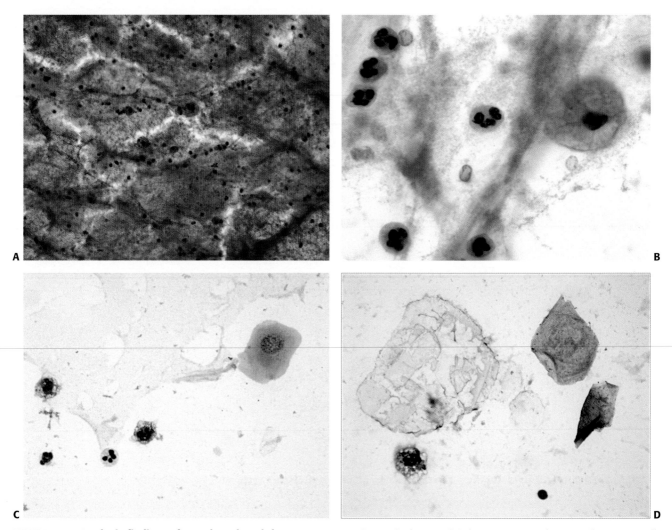

FIGURE 2.10. Cytologic findings of two thyroglossal duct cysts. Case 1 (Papanicolaou stain): low-power view showing inflammatory cells amidst mucoid material **(A)** and high-power view showing neutrophils and macrophage **(B)**. **Case 2 (Diff-Quik stain):** High-power views showing macrophages, neutrophils, mucoid material, nucleated squame **(C)**, and anucleate squames **(D)**.

A focus of the lateral aberrant thyroid debate concerns reports of thyroid carcinoma arising within branchial cleft cysts. Multiple instances of papillary carcinoma arising in branchial cleft cysts have been reported[102–106]; however, the proof of primary origin is tenuous in most cases.

During embryogenesis, the transient lateral cervical sinuses are formed as the second pharyngeal arches grow caudally to fuse with the cardiac eminences and cover the second, third, and fourth branchial (or pharyngeal) clefts. The cervical sinus may persist as a cyst in the lateral aspect of the neck. The cyst may be connected by a fistula externally to the skin and/or internally to the pharynx. Second branchial cleft and pouch abnormalities are the most common, whereas involvement of the third or fourth pouches is rare.[107] Thus, there is, at least theoretically, an embryologic explanation for tissue of the ultimobranchial body being part of a lateral neck cyst. This possibility, combined with reports of follicular tissue deriving from the ultimobranchial body, has been used to explain lateral ectopic thyroid tissue and associated follicular-derived neoplasms.[108,109] However, the question whether follicular tissue can derive from ultimobranchial bodies seems unsettled at this time.

Evaluation of neoplasia in putative branchial cleft cysts is problematic because of the presence of lymphoid tissue in their walls. Determining whether a lesion represents a branchial cleft

cyst or a lymph node metastasis with cystic change can be challenging, although the odds heavily favor the latter interpretation (Fig. 2.13). Thyroid carcinoma arising in a lateral aberrant thyroid seems to be more of theoretical possibility than a practical consideration. The presence of thyroid follicular tissue in a lateral cyst containing lymphoid tissue is best considered metastatic papillary carcinoma that warrants a careful search of the thyroid gland for a primary site.

Thyroid Inclusions in Lymph Nodes

The presence of thyroid tissue within distinct lymph nodes of the neck can pose a diagnostic challenge, particularly when the nodes have been removed during surgery unrelated to the thyroid. When inclusions exhibit definite features of papillary thyroid carcinoma, the diagnosis of metastatic carcinoma is made readily. However, when the thyroid tissue appears benign, a diagnostic challenge now confronts the pathologist.

Some have interpreted all thyroid tissue within lymph nodes as metastatic foci of papillary thyroid carcinoma.[110–112] Others have accepted the possibility of benign inclusions.[113,114] It seems reasonable at least to consider the possibility given that benign tissue such as nevus cells and salivary glands are seen within lymph nodes.

Table 2.4

Thyroglossal Duct Cyst versus Branchial Cleft Cyst

	Thyroglossal Duct Cyst	Branchial Cleft Cyst
Origin	• Thyroglossal duct	• Usually second branchial cleft or pouch
Location	• Midline • Usually near hyoid bone with connection through fibrous remnant of thyroglossal duct	• Lateral • Usually along anterior border of sternocleidomastoid muscle near angle of mandible • May be associated with cutaneous or mucosal sinus or fistula
Cyst contents	• Mucoid or gelatinous material • Purulent exudate if infected	• Serous, mucoid, or pasty • Purulent exudate if infected

Microscopic features	• Variable lining
	  ○ Ciliated respiratory epithelium
	  ○ Stratified squamous epithelium
	  ○ Cuboidal epithelium
	  ○ Granulation tissue secondary to inflammation
	• Variable acute or chronic inflammation in wall
	• About half contain thyroid follicles in wall
		• Usually stratified squamous epithelium
		  ○ Ciliated respiratory epithelium may be seen
		  ○ Granulation tissue secondary to inflammation
		• Lymphoid tissue in wall
		• Variable acute or chronic inflammation in wall

Age	• Usually children to young adults	• Usually children to young adults
Gender ratio	• Even	• Even
Neoplasia	• Occurs in 1% or less • Usually papillary carcinoma	• Extremely rare • Putative cases usually metastatic squamous cell carcinoma from primary in head or neck

Recognizing that most thyroid tissue within lymph nodes represents metastatic tumor, a set of criteria has evolved that should be met before diagnosing intranodal tissue as a benign inclusion (Table 2.5).[115,116] A benign inclusion should consist of a small, microscopic focus within a single lymph node and be located in or immediately subjacent to the capsule. The follicles should resemble those found in normal thyroid glands and not appear crowded. The nuclei should be normal size and lack cytologic features of papillary carcinoma. Papillary architecture, psammoma bodies, and/or reactive stromal proliferation are disqualifying features. Some advocate the additional restriction that lymph node location must be medial to the jugular veins.[101]

Are there additional studies that may augment the basic examination of hematoxylin and eosin–stained sections? Clonal analysis using the X chromosome–linked human androgen (HUMARA) technique was performed in a case with thyroid tissue in both the tongue and multiple cervical lymph nodes.[117] Investigators found polyclonality of all tissues, concluding they were consistent with ectopic tissue rather than malignant neoplasia. However, the involvement of 9 out of 54 lymph nodes is problematic.

Incidental thyroid tissue within cervical lymph nodes has been studied using immunohistochemical analysis for galectin-3 and HBME-1 expression and molecular analysis for *BRAF* and *RAS* mutations.[118,119] A high level of concordance has been observed between positive results for galectin-3 and HBME-1 expression and the presence of two or more nuclear features of papillary carcinoma (enlargement, crowding/overlapping, irregularity of contours, chromatin clearing, pseudoinclusions, and grooves) (Fig. 2.14). The absence of staining for both galectin-3 and HBME-1 was limited to tissue exhibiting none or only one of the nuclear features of papillary carcinoma (Fig. 2.15). These foci ranged from 0.8 to 2.1 mm in greatest dimension, were located in

or immediately subjacent to the capsule, and were only found in one lymph node. In addition, no mutations of *BRAF* or *RAS* were found, whereas either a *BRAF* or a *RAS* mutation was found in 85% of control cases of metastatic papillary carcinoma. Although not irrefutable evidence for benign thyroid inclusions, the findings did not eliminate the possibility and suggest that ancillary studies may be helpful in the evaluation of these challenging lesions.

Parasitic Nodule

A parasitic nodule is a nodule of nonneoplastic thyroid tissue separate from the main thyroid gland and is usually seen in the setting of nodular hyperplasia (multinodular goiter).[116] Parasitic nodules are also known as sequestered nodules. These nodules develop either by enlargement of nonneoplastic thyroid tissue located outside of the main gland or by separation of a portion of the thyroid from the main gland.

Separation of a portion of the thyroid by the mechanical action of neck muscles has been postulated to occur during the development of a nodular goiter.[120,121] Perhaps lending support to this concept is the report of separate nodules of thyroid tissue following surgical or blunt trauma.[122] Some examples of parasitic nodule show connection to the main thyroid gland by a fibrous strand, but most published cases report no connection. Although some parasitic nodules may occur because of mechanical separation from the main gland, others probably represent concurrent hyperplastic changes in accessory thyroid tissue.[120,123,124] Multiple studies have reported the presence of small nodules of normal-appearing thyroid tissue in proximity to thyroid glands that lack significant pathologic changes.[125] If these small nodules enlarge as part of the process of nodular hyperplasia, they could present as clinically apparent nodules or at least be found during thyroid surgery.

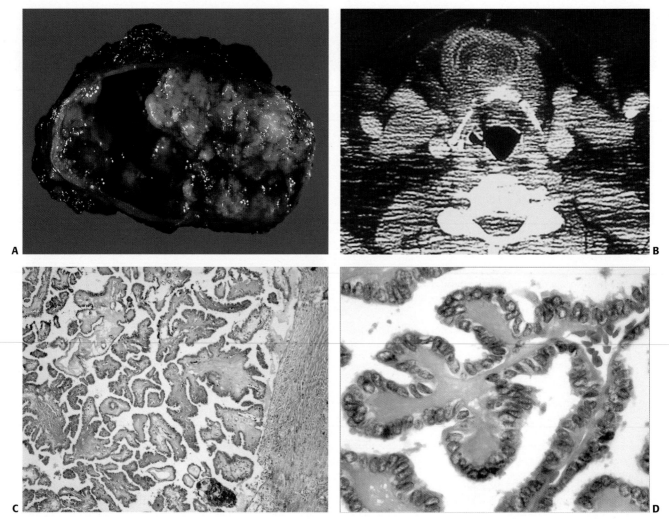

FIGURE 2.11. Papillary carcinoma arising in a thyroglossal duct cyst. A: Gross photograph of specimen sectioned to reveal intracystic mass. **B:** CT scan of cyst before resection. Note that cyst is contiguous with the hyoid bone. **C:** Low-power view showing papillary architecture and a portion of cyst wall along the right side. **D:** High-power view showing characteristic nuclear features of papillary carcinoma.

As with other abnormally located thyroid tissue, the main differential diagnosis of parasitic nodule is metastatic thyroid carcinoma. Criteria for the diagnosis of parasitic nodule include (1) absence of cytologic or architectural features of papillary carcinoma, (2) no evidence of a lymph node, (3) no primary carcinoma in the thyroid gland, and (4) the nodule and thyroid gland show similar nonneoplastic pathologic features, in particular nodular hyperplasia (multinodular goiter), Graves disease, or chronic lymphocytic (Hashimoto) thyroiditis (Fig. 2.16).[116] Cases of chronic lymphocytic thyroiditis can be very challenging, with the lymphoid component simulating a lymph nodes and cytologic features simulating papillary carcinoma. The absence of galectin-3 and HBME-1 immunoreactivity supports the diagnosis of parasitic nodule, whereas positive staining is generally consistent with carcinoma. The notable exception is chronic lymphocytic (Hashimoto) thyroiditis, in which follicular cells may show staining, particularly for galectin-3.

Teratoma and Struma Ovarii

Thyroid tissue can be a component of teratoma, but this is more of a consideration when abnormally located thyroid tissue is found outside the neck. Thyroid tissue as a component of teratoma is unusual with the exception of ovarian teratomas. Primary teratoma of the thyroid is discussed in Chapter 16.

Struma ovarii is a mature teratoma of the ovary composed exclusively or predominately of thyroid tissue. It accounts for approximately 3% of ovarian teratomas and is the most common type of monodermal ovarian teratoma.[126] Thyroid tissue can also be present as a minor component of mature cystic teratomas (Fig. 2.17). Macroscopically, struma ovarii usually exhibits solid, gelatinous sectioned surfaces ranging from reddish brown to greenish brown (Fig. 2.18). Thyroid tissue in struma ovarii can exhibit the same range of histologic features as seen in the thyroid gland. Usually, the tissue exhibits variably sized follicles lined by normal-appearing epithelium. Sometimes the follicular epithelium exhibits a microfollicular or solid growth pattern that may be difficult to recognize as thyroidal, but immunostains for thyroglobulin or TTF1 can help to confirm the diagnosis.

About 5% to 10% of struma ovarii exhibit features of malignant thyroid neoplasms.[127] Both typical and follicular variants of papillary carcinoma, conventional and oncocytic variants of follicular carcinoma, and poorly differentiated carcinoma occur. However, neither anaplastic nor medullary carcinomas have been reported in struma ovarii. As with primary thyroid neoplasms, papillary carcinoma is the most common type.[128–130]

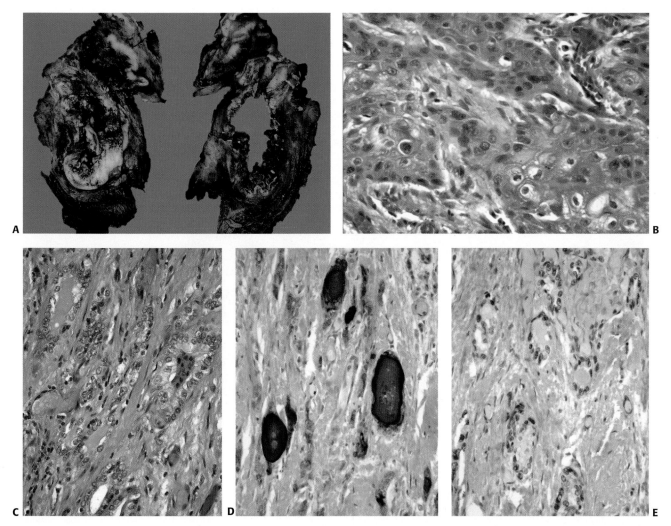

FIGURE 2.12. Squamous cell carcinoma arising in a thyroglossal duct cyst. A: Gross photograph of sectioned specimen showing cystic structure partially filled with tumor. **B:** High-power view of mass showing squamous cell carcinoma. **C–E:** High-power views of a focus of thyroid follicular tissue in the cyst wall. **(C)** is a hematoxylin and eosin–stained section, **(D)** is a thyroglobulin-immunostained section, and **(E)** is a TTF1-immunostained section.

Thyroid tissue can also be part of composite ovarian neoplasms including carcinoid (strumal carcinoid), Brenner tumor, and mucinous cystadenoma. To distinguish malignant struma ovarii from other related neoplasms such as strumal carcinoid, the term *thyroid-type carcinoma arising in struma ovarii* has been advocated.[128,129]

The criteria used to determine histologic malignancy are comparable with those used for primary thyroid malignancies.[127,130,131] The diagnosis of follicular carcinoma can be problematic given the lack of a tumor capsule. In addition to intraovarian vascular invasion or extraovarian spread, growth onto the ovarian serosa may be considered indicative of malignancy.[130] Not all histologically malignant struma ovarii exhibit malignant biologic behavior. Contrastingly, some cases of struma ovarii may appear innocuous when first encountered, and their malignant behavior not appreciated until a later recurrence.[131–133] Some investigators advocate the term *highly differentiated follicular carcinoma of ovarian origin* for this form of struma ovarii that histologically resembles nonneoplastic thyroid tissue yet spreads to the peritoneum or more distant sites.[132] Prediction of behavior is difficult, and a long period of follow-up may be necessary to make this determination. Fortunately, most thyroid malignancies arising in the ovary do not spread to extraovarian sites.[129]

Molecular analysis has been performed on several follicular variants of papillary thyroid carcinoma arising in the ovary. The analyses have revealed *RAS* mutations in two cases and a rare type of *BRAF* mutation (K601E) in another.[134–136] These mutations are comparable with those known to occur in primary thyroid carcinomas.

Pyriform Sinus Fistula/Sinus Tract

Pyriform sinus fistula or sinus tracts typically extend in an antero-inferior direction from the pyriform sinus through the cricothyroid muscle, ending blindly in the thyroid or perithyroidal tissue, where it may exhibit cyst-like dilation. Most of these lesions are sinuses instead of fistulae, in which case the term *pyriform sinus* sinus seems more appropriate, albeit somewhat awkward. Alternate terms include third or fourth branchial sinus/fistula/anomaly.

Classically, these tracts have been considered developmental remnants of the third or fourth pharyngeal (branchial) pouches. The theoretical courses of these tracts based on embryologic development of the third and fourth branchial arches do not match the clinical findings in most cases, and investigators have suggested that these tracts derive from the thymopharyngeal duct.[137,138] The thymopharyngeal duct is a structure that forms as the thymus descends from the third pharyngeal pouch during fetal

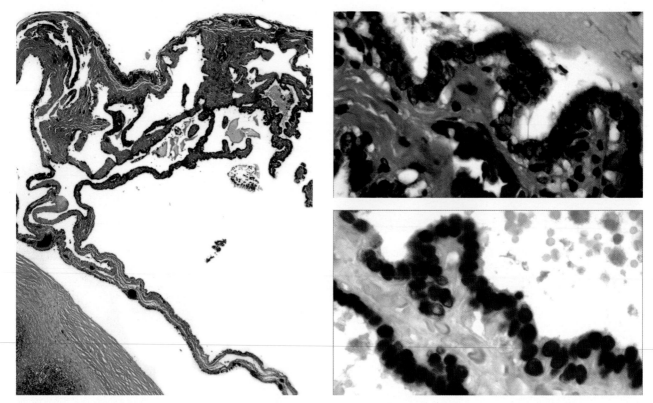

FIGURE 2.13. Lymph node of neck with metastatic papillary thyroid carcinoma associated with marked cystic change. The low power view on the left shows the cystic spaces. The right upper high-power view shows that the cells lining the cystic spaces have nuclear features of papillary carcinoma. The right lower high-power view shows nuclear staining for TTF1. The thyroid gland contained multifocal papillary carcinoma with extensive lymphatic invasion.

Table 2.5
Features of Benign Thyroid Inclusions in Lymph Node of Neck

- Microscopic focus
- Limited to one lymph node
- Lymph node located medial to jugular vein
- Intracapsular or immediately subcapsular
- Uncrowded, normal-appearing follicles
- Nuclei normal size
- Nuclei lack features of papillary carcinoma
- Absence of psammoma bodies
- Absence of stromal reaction
- Absence of staining for galectin-3 or HBME-1
- Absence of *BRAF, RET/PTC, RAS* mutations

development. Thymic tissue can be found in or adjacent to the thyroid, and if the thymopharyngeal duct failed to close, a sinus tract extending from the pyriform sinus to the thyroid could persist.

Most cases occur on the left side.[137,139–141] Left-sided predominance is thought to be related in some way to the asymmetric development of the fourth pharyngeal arches because the left becomes part of the aortic arch and the right forms the right subclavian artery. However, the mechanism for left-sided predominance is unclear.

The most significant clinical aspect of pyriform sinus fistulae/sinuses is their association with inflammatory lesions and abscesses in the neck. Acute thyroiditis, particularly in children, is frequently associated with a pyriform sinus tract lesion (see Chapter 4).

Cystic Remnant of Ultimobranchial Body

Remnants of the ultimobranchial body associated with the thyroid gland usually take the form of solid cell nests. Although typically solid, these remnant foci can exhibit cystic architecture and are usually microscopic findings or barely visible grossly.[142] Larger cysts in the range of 2 to 5 cm have been reported.[143,144] The cysts are usually lined by a thin layer of stratified squamous cells that is highlighted by immunostains for keratin (Fig. 2.19). Ciliated columnar cells may also be present.[142–144] Solid cell nests are common in the surrounding tissue and serve as a diagnostic clue.

A recent study reported the observation of cystic changes in the ultimobranchial bodies of mice with *NKX2-1/TTF1* (–/–) null genotype.[145] The relevance of this molecular aberration to cystic remnants in humans is unclear at this time.

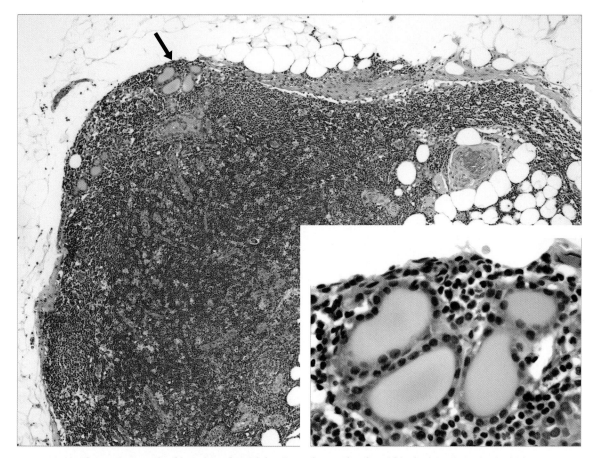

FIGURE 2.14. Photomicrograph of lymph node with benign subcapsular thyroid inclusions *(arrow)*. The high-power inset shows that the follicles are lined by normal-appearing follicular cells. The cells did not stain for galectin-3 or HBME-1. The lymph node was removed because of squamous cell carcinoma of the larynx. No carcinoma was found within the thyroid gland.

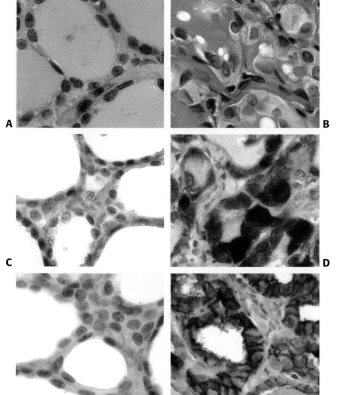

FIGURE 2.15. Photomicrographs comparing benign thyroid inclusion in lymph node (left side) with metastatic papillary carcinoma in lymph node (right side). A: Benign inclusion. **B:** Metastatic papillary carcinoma. **C:** Benign inclusion immunostained for galectin-3. **D:** Metastatic papillary carcinoma immunostained for galectin-3. **E:** Benign inclusion immunostained for HBME-1. **F:** Metastatic papillary carcinoma immunostained for HBME-1 showing membranous staining.

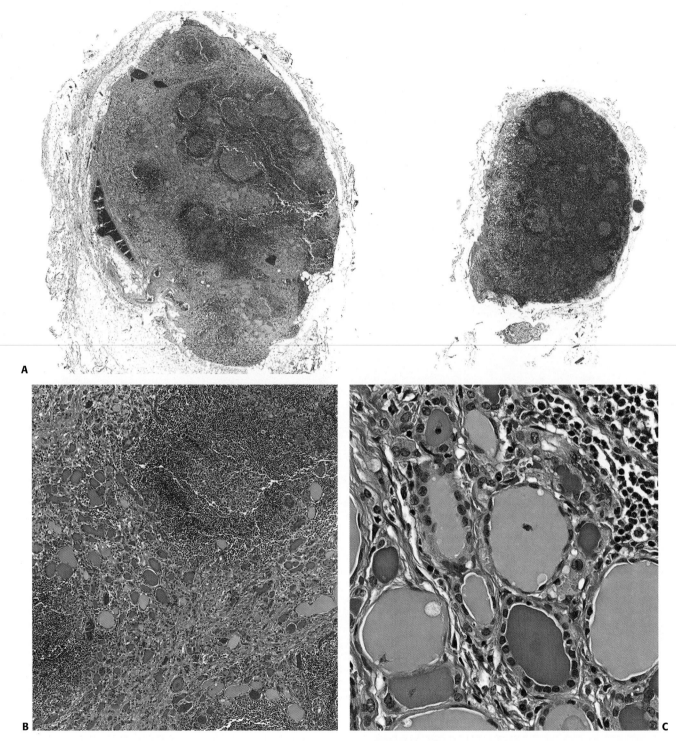

FIGURE 2.16. Photomicrographs of parasitic nodule. A: Low-power photomicrograph of parasitic nodule **(left)** and lymph node **(right)** removed from central neck compartment during thyroidectomy. Medium-power **(B)** and high-power **(C)** photomicrographs of parasitic nodule showing features of chronic lymphocytic (Hashimoto) thyroiditis. Similar features were found in the thyroidectomy specimen.

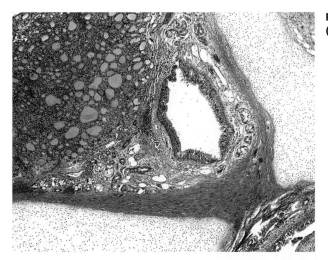

FIGURE 2.17. Thyroid tissue in ovary. Low-power view of thyroid follicular tissue **(upper left)** as a minor component of a mature ovarian teratoma.

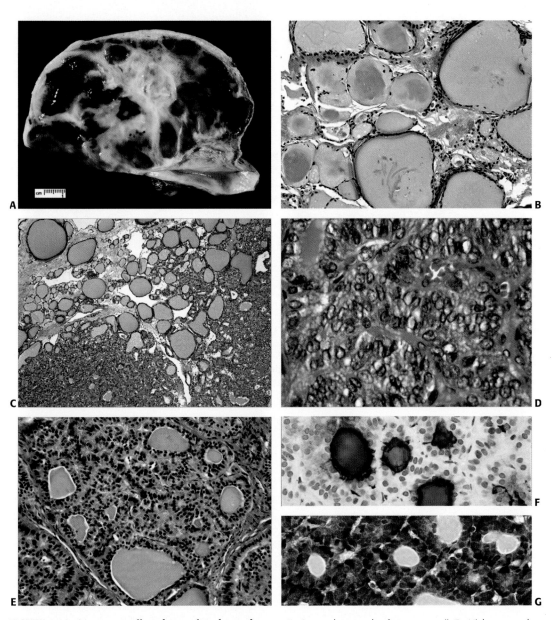

FIGURE 2.18. Struma ovarii and associated neoplasms. A: Gross photograph of struma ovarii. **B:** High-power photomicrograph of struma ovarii. **C and D:** Low- and high-power views of papillary thyroid carcinoma arising in struma ovarii. **E–G:** Photomicrographs of ovarian strumal carcinoid (**F**, thyroglobulin immunostain; **G**, chromogranin A immunostain).

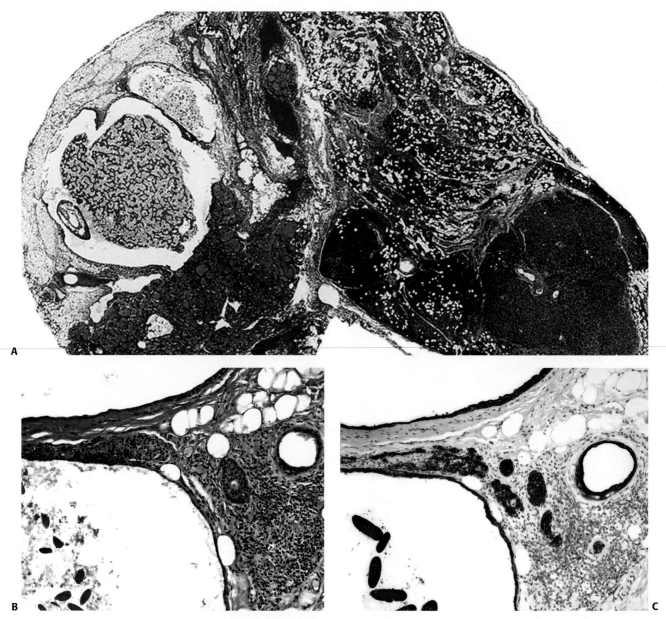

FIGURE 2.19. Cystic remnant of an ultimobranchial body. A: Low-power photomicrograph showing multiloculated cystic remnant **(upper left)** adjacent to thyroid tissue **(lower left)** and parathyroid adenoma **(lower right)**. **B and C:** Medium-power views of the cyst wall (**B**, hematoxylin and eosin stain; **C**, pankeratin immunostain). The cells lining the cyst are highlighted by the cytokeratin immunostain, as are cell nests in the adjacent tissue.

REFERENCES

1. O'Rahilly R. The timing and sequence of events in the development of the human endocrine system during the embryonic period proper. *Anat Embryol (Berl)*. 1983;166:439–451.
2. Shepard TH. Onset of function in the human fetal thyroid: biochemical and radioautographic studies from organ culture. *J Clin Endocrinol Metab*. 1967;27:945–958.
3. Greenberg AH, Czernichow P, Reba RC, et al. Observations on the maturation of thyroid function in early fetal life. *J Clin Invest*. 1970;49:1790–1803.
4. Chan AS. Ultrastructural observations on the formation of follicles in the human fetal thyroid. *Cell Tissue Res*. 1983;233:693–698.
5. Bocian-Sobkowska J, Wozniak W, Malendowicz LK. Morphometric studies on the development of the human thyroid gland. II. The late fetal life. *Histol Histopathol*. 1997;12:79–84.
6. Bocian-Sobkowska J, Malendowicz LK, Wozniak W. Morphometric studies on the development of human thyroid gland in early fetal life. *Histol Histopathol*. 1992;7:415–420.
7. Saad AG, Kumar S, Ron E, et al. Proliferative activity of human thyroid cells in various age groups and its correlation with the risk of thyroid cancer after radiation exposure. *J Clin Endocrinol Metab*. 2006;91:2672–2677.

8. Radaelli T, Cetin I, Zamperini P, et al. Intrauterine growth of normal thyroid. *Gynecol Endocrinol*. 2002;16:427–430.
9. Guihard-Costa AM, Menez F, Delezoide AL. Organ weights in human fetuses after formalin fixation: standards by gestational age and body weight. *Pediatr Dev Pathol*. 2002;5:559–578.
10. Sagreiya K, Emery JL. Perinatal thyroid discharge. A histological study of 1225 infant thyroids. *Arch Dis Child*. 1970;45:746–754.
11. Pearse AG, Carvalheira AF. Cytochemical evidence for an ultimobranchial origin of rodent thyroid C cells. *Nature*. 1967;214:929–930.
12. Le Douarin N. *The Neural Crest*. Cambridge, England: Cambridge University Press; 1982.
13. Le Douarin N, Le Lièvre C. [Demonstration of neural origin of calcitonin cells of ultimobranchial body of chick embryo]. *C R Acad Sci Hebd Seances Acad Sci D*. 1970;270:2857–2860.
14. Kameda Y, Okamoto K, Ito M, et al. Innervation of the C cells of chicken ultimobranchial glands studied by immunohistochemistry, fluorescence microscopy, and electron microscopy. *Am J Anat*. 1988;182:353–368.
15. Kameda Y, Nishimaki T, Chisaka O, et al. Expression of the epithelial marker E-cadherin by thyroid C cells and their precursors during murine development. *J Histochem Cytochem*. 2007;55:1075–1088.
16. Sugiyama S. The embryology of the human thyroid gland including ultimobranchial body and others related. *Ergeb Anat Entwicklungsgesch*. 1971;44:3–111.

17. Nadig J, Weber E, Hedinger C. C-cell in vestiges of the ultimobranchial body in human thyroid glands. *Virchows Arch B Cell Pathol.* 1978;27:189–191.
18. Harach HR. Histological markers of solid cell nests of the thyroid. With some emphasis on their expression in thyroid ultimobranchial-related tumors. *Acta Anat (Basel).* 1985;124:111–116.
19. Fraser BA, Duckworth JW. Ultimobranchial body cysts in the human foetal thyroid: pathological implications. *J Pathol.* 1979;127:89–92.
20. De Felice M, Di Lauro R. Thyroid development and its disorders: genetics and molecular mechanisms. *Endocr Rev.* 2004;25:722–746.
21. Fagman H, Nilsson M. Morphogenetics of early thyroid development. *J Mol Endocrinol.* 2011;46:R33–R42.
22. Guazzi S, Price M, De Felice M, et al. Thyroid nuclear factor 1 (TTF-1) contains a homeodomain and displays a novel DNA binding specificity. *Embo J.* 1990;9:3631–3639.
23. Katoh R, Miyagi E, Nakamura N, et al. Expression of thyroid transcription factor-1 (TTF-1) in human C cells and medullary thyroid carcinomas. *Hum Pathol.* 2000;31:386–393.
24. Kimura S, Hara Y, Pineau T, et al. The T/ebp null mouse: thyroid-specific enhancer-binding protein is essential for the organogenesis of the thyroid, lung, ventral forebrain, and pituitary. *Genes Dev.* 1996;10:60–69.
25. Kimura S, Ward JM, Minoo P. Thyroid-specific enhancer-binding protein/thyroid transcription factor 1 is not required for the initial specification of the thyroid and lung primordia. *Biochimie.* 1999;81:321–327.
26. Kusakabe T, Hoshi N, Kimura S. Origin of the ultimobranchial body cyst: T/ebp/Nkx2.1 expression is required for development and fusion of the ultimobranchial body to the thyroid. *Dev Dyn.* 2006;235:1300–1309.
27. Benson DW, Silberbach GM, Kavanaugh-McHugh A, et al. Mutations in the cardiac transcription factor NKX2.5 affect diverse cardiac developmental pathways. *J Clin Invest.* 1999;104:1567–1573.
28. Dentice M, Cordeddu V, Rosica A, et al. Missense mutation in the transcription factor NKX2-5: a novel molecular event in the pathogenesis of thyroid dysgenesis. *J Clin Endocrinol Metab.* 2006;91:1428–1433.
29. Plachov D, Chowdhury K, Walther C, et al. *Pax8*, a murine paired box gene expressed in the developing excretory system and thyroid gland. *Development.* 1990;110:643–651.
30. Poleev A, Fickenscher H, Mundlos S, et al. PAX8, a human paired box gene: isolation and expression in developing thyroid, kidney and Wilms' tumors. *Development.* 1992;116:611–623.
31. Miccadei S, De Leo R, Zammarchi E, et al. The synergistic activity of thyroid transcription factor 1 and Pax 8 relies on the promoter/enhancer interplay. *Mol Endocrinol.* 2002;16:837–846.
32. Mansouri A, Chowdhury K, Gruss P. Follicular cells of the thyroid gland require *Pax8* gene function. *Nat Genet.* 1998;19:87–90.
33. Macchia PE, Lapi P, Krude H, et al. *PAX8* mutations associated with congenital hypothyroidism caused by thyroid dysgenesis. *Nat Genet.* 1998;19:83–86.
34. Congdon T, Nguyen LQ, Nogueira CR, et al. A novel mutation (Q40P) in *PAX8* associated with congenital hypothyroidism and thyroid hypoplasia: evidence for phenotypic variability in mother and child. *J Clin Endocrinol Metab.* 2001;86:3962–3967.
35. Chadwick BP, Obermayr F, Frischauf AM. *FKHL15*, a new human member of the forkhead gene family located on chromosome 9q22. *Genomics.* 1997;41:390–396.
36. Hromas R, Radich J, Collins S. PCR cloning of an orphan homeobox gene (*PRH*) preferentially expressed in myeloid and liver cells. *Biochem Biophys Res Commun.* 1993;195:976–983.
37. Crompton MR, Bartlett TJ, MacGregor AD, et al. Identification of a novel vertebrate homeobox gene expressed in haematopoietic cells. *Nucleic Acids Res.* 1992;20:5661–5667.
38. Chieffo C, Garvey N, Gong W, et al. Isolation and characterization of a gene from the DiGeorge chromosomal region homologous to the mouse *Tbx1* gene. *Genomics.* 1997;43:267–277.
39. Stoller JZ, Epstein JA. Identification of a novel nuclear localization signal in *Tbx1* that is deleted in DiGeorge syndrome patients harboring the 1223delC mutation. *Hum Mol Genet.* 2005;14:885–892.
40. Lania G, Zhang Z, Huynh T, et al. Early thyroid development requires a Tbx1-Fgf8 pathway. *Dev Biol.* 2009;328:109–117.
41. Libert F, Passage E, Lefort A, et al. Localization of human thyrotropin receptor gene to chromosome region 14q3 by in situ hybridization. *Cytogenet Cell Genet.* 1990;54:82–83.
42. Berge-Lefranc JL, Cartouzou G, Mattei MG, et al. Localization of the thyroglobulin gene by in situ hybridization to human chromosomes. *Hum Genet.* 1985;69:28–31.
43. Endo Y, Onogi S, Umeki K, et al. Regional localization of the gene for thyroid peroxidase to human chromosome 2p25 and mouse chromosome 12C. *Genomics.* 1995;25:760–761.
44. Smanik PA, Ryu KY, Theil KS, et al. Expression, exon-intron organization, and chromosome mapping of the human sodium iodide symporter. *Endocrinology.* 1997;138:3555–3558.
45. Hillier LW, Fulton RS, Fulton LA, et al. The DNA sequence of human chromosome 7. *Nature.* 2003;424:157–164.
46. Manley NR, Capecchi MR. Hox group 3 paralogs regulate the development and migration of the thymus, thyroid, and parathyroid glands. *Dev Biol.* 1998;195:1–15.
47. Renault B, Lieman J, Ward D, et al. Localization of the human achaete-scute homolog gene (*ASCL1*) distal to phenylalanine hydroxylase (PAH) and proximal to tumor rejection antigen (TRA1) on chromosome 12q22-q23. *Genomics.* 1995;30:81–83.
48. Sommer L, Shah N, Rao M, et al. The cellular function of *MASH1* in autonomic neurogenesis. *Neuron.* 1995;15:1245–1258.
49. Lanigan TM, DeRaad SK, Russo AF. Requirement of the MASH-1 transcription factor for neuroendocrine differentiation of thyroid C cells. *J Neurobiol.* 1998;34:126–134.

50. Kameda Y, Nishimaki T, Miura M, et al. *Mash1* regulates the development of C cells in mouse thyroid glands. *Dev Dyn.* 2007;236:262–270.
51. Gillam MP, Kopp P. Genetic regulation of thyroid development. *Curr Opin Pediatr.* 2001;13:358–363.
52. Polak M, Sura-Trueba S, Chauty A, et al. Molecular mechanisms of thyroid dysgenesis. *Horm Res.* 2004;62(suppl 3):14–21.
53. Trueba SS, Auge J, Mattei G, et al. PAX8, TITF1, and FOXE1 gene expression patterns during human development: new insights into human thyroid development and thyroid dysgenesis-associated malformations. *J Clin Endocrinol Metab.* 2005;90:455–462.
54. Xu PX, Zheng W, Laclef C, et al. *Eya1* is required for the morphogenesis of mammalian thymus, parathyroid and thyroid. *Development.* 2002;129:3033–3044.
55. Kameda Y, Shigemoto H, Ikeda A. Development and cytodifferentiation of C cell complexes in dog fetal thyroids. An immunohistochemical study using anti-calcitonin, anti-C-thyroglobulin and anti-19S thyroglobulin antisera. *Cell Tissue Res.* 1980;206:403–415.
56. Castanet M, Park SM, Smith A, et al. A novel loss-of-function mutation in TTF-2 is associated with congenital hypothyroidism, thyroid agenesis and cleft palate. *Hum Mol Genet.* 2002;11:2051–2059.
57. Park SM, Clifton-Bligh RJ, Betts P, et al. Congenital hypothyroidism and apparent athyreosis with compound heterozygosity or compensated hypothyroidism with probable hemizygosity for inactivating mutations of the TSH receptor. *Clin Endocrinol (Oxf).* 2004;60:220–227.
58. Maiorana R, Carta A, Floriddia G, et al. Thyroid hemiagenesis: prevalence in normal children and effect on thyroid function. *J Clin Endocrinol Metab.* 2003;88:1534–1536.
59. Shabana W, Delange F, Freson M, et al. Prevalence of thyroid hemiagenesis: ultrasound screening in normal children. *Eur J Pediatr.* 2000;159:456–458.
60. Castanet M, Leenhardt L, Leger J, et al. Thyroid hemiagenesis is a rare variant of thyroid dysgenesis with a familial component but without *Pax8* mutations in a cohort of 22 cases. *Pediatr Res.* 2005;57:908–913.
61. Zieren J, Paul M, Scharfenberg M, et al. Submandibular ectopic thyroid gland. *J Craniofac Surg.* 2006;17:1194–1198.
62. Byrd MC, Thompson LD, Wieneke JA. Intratracheal ectopic thyroid tissue: a case report and literature review. *Ear Nose Throat J.* 2003;82:514–518.
63. Bowen-Wright HE, Jonklaas J. Ectopic intratracheal thyroid: an illustrative case report and literature review. *Thyroid.* 2005;15:478–484.
64. Salam MA. Ectopic thyroid mass adherent to the oesophagus. *J Laryngol Otol.* 1992;106:746–747.
65. Porto G. Esophageal nodule of thyroid tissue. *Laryngoscope.* 1960;70:1336–1338.
66. Porqueddu M, Antona C, Polvani G, et al. Ectopic thyroid tissue in the ventricular outflow tract: embryologic implications. *Cardiology.* 1995;86:524–526.
67. Williams RJ, Lindop G, Butler J. Ectopic thyroid tissue on the ascending aorta: an operative finding. *Ann Thorac Surg.* 2002;73:1642–1643.
68. Kantelip B, Lusson JR, De Riberolles C, et al. Intracardiac ectopic thyroid. *Hum Pathol.* 1986;17:1293–1296.
69. Bando T, Genka K, Ishikawa K, et al. Ectopic intrapulmonary thyroid. *Chest.* 1993;103:1278–1279.
70. Takahashi T, Ishikura H, Kato H, et al. Ectopic thyroid follicles in the submucosa of the duodenum. *Virchows Arch A Pathol Anat Histopathol.* 1991;418:547–550.
71. Harach HR. Ectopic thyroid tissue adjacent to the gallbladder. *Histopathology.* 1998;32:90–91.
72. Ghanem N, Bley T, Altehoefer C, et al. Ectopic thyroid gland in the porta hepatis and lingua. *Thyroid.* 2003;13:503–507.
73. Eyuboglu E, Kapan M, Ipek T, et al. Ectopic thyroid in the abdomen: report of a case. *Surg Today.* 1999;29:472–474.
74. Gungor B, Kebat T, Ozaslan C, et al. Intra-abdominal ectopic thyroid presenting with hyperthyroidism: report of a case. *Surg Today.* 2002;32:148–150.
75. Shiraishi T, Imai H, Fukutome K, et al. Ectopic thyroid in the adrenal gland. *Hum Pathol.* 1999;30:105–108.
76. Mysorekar VV, Dandekar CP, Sreevathsa MR. Ectopic thyroid tissue in the parotid salivary gland. *Singapore Med J.* 2004;45:437–438.
77. Ruchti C, Balli-Antunes M, Gerber HA. Follicular tumor in the sellar region without primary cancer of the thyroid. Heterotopic carcinoma? *Am J Clin Pathol.* 1987;87:776–780.
78. Maino K, Skelton H, Yeager J, et al. Benign ectopic thyroid tissue in a cutaneous location: a case report and review. *J Cutan Pathol.* 2004;31:195–198.
79. Batsakis JG, El-Naggar AK, Luna MA. Thyroid gland ectopias. *Ann Otol Rhinol Laryngol.* 1996;105:996–1000.
80. Baughman RA. Lingual thyroid and lingual thyroglossal tract remnants. A clinical and histopathologic study with review of the literature. *Oral Surg Oral Med Oral Pathol.* 1972;34:781–799.
81. Sauk JJ Jr. Ectopic lingual thyroid. *J Pathol.* 1970;102:239–243.
82. Singh HB, Joshi HC, Chakravarty M. Carcinoma of the lingual thyroid. Review and case report. *J Laryngol Otol.* 1979;93:839–844.
83. Massine RE, Durning SJ, Koroscil TM. Lingual thyroid carcinoma: a case report and review of the literature. *Thyroid.* 2001;11:1191–1196.
84. Seoane JM, Cameselle-Teijeiro J, Romero MA. Poorly differentiated oxyphilic (Hürthle cell) carcinoma arising in lingual thyroid: a case report and review of the literature. *Endocr Pathol.* 2002;13:353–360.
85. Kennedy TL, Riefkohl WL. Lingual thyroid carcinoma with nodal metastasis. *Laryngoscope.* 2007;117:1969–1973.
86. Podoshin L, Fradis M, Goldstein J, et al. Intrahyoid thyroglossal cyst. *J Laryngol Otol.* 1989;103:539–542.
87. Sistrunk WE. The surgical treatment of cysts of the thyroglossal tract. *Ann Surg.* 1920;71:121–122.2.
88. Hurley DL, Katz HH, Tiegs RD, et al. Cosecretion of calcitonin gene products: studies with a C18 cartridge extraction method for human plasma PDN-21 (katacalcin). *J Clin Endocrinol Metab.* 1988;66:640–644.

89. Josephson GD, Spencer WR, Josephson JS. Thyroglossal duct cyst: the New York Eye and Ear Infirmary experience and a literature review. *Ear Nose Throat J.* 1998;77:642–644, 646–647, 651.

90. Greinwald JH Jr, Leichtman LG, Simko EJ. Hereditary thyroglossal duct cysts. *Arch Otolaryngol Head Neck Surg.* 1996;122:1094–1096.

91. Dedivitis RA, Camargo DL, Peixoto GL, et al. Thyroglossal duct: a review of 55 cases. *J Am Coll Surg.* 2002;194:274–277.

92. Shahin A, Burroughs FH, Kirby JP, et al. Thyroglossal duct cyst: a cytopathologic study of 26 cases. *Diagn Cytopathol.* 2005;33:365–369.

93. Shaffer MM, Oertel YC, Oertel JE. Thyroglossal duct cysts: diagnostic criteria by fine-needle aspiration. *Arch Pathol Lab Med.* 1996;120:1039–1043.

94. Chow LT, Lee JC, Chow WH, et al. Cholesterol-rich thyroglossal cyst: report of a case diagnosed by fine needle aspiration. *Acta Cytol.* 1996;40:377–379.

95. Dedivitis RA, Guimaraes AV. Papillary thyroid carcinoma in thyroglossal duct cyst. *Int Surg.* 2000;85:198–201.

96. Chen F, Sheridan B, Nankervis J. Carcinoma of the thyroglossal duct: case reports and a literature review. *Aust N Z J Surg.* 1993;63:614–616.

97. Lustmann J, Benoliel R, Zeltser R. Squamous cell carcinoma arising in a thyroglossal duct cyst in the tongue. *J Oral Maxillofac Surg.* 1989;47:81–85.

98. Woods RH, Saunders JR Jr, Pearlman S, et al. Anaplastic carcinoma arising in a thyroglossal duct tract. *Otolaryngol Head Neck Surg.* 1993;109:945–949.

99. Fernandez JF, Ordonez NG, Schultz PN, et al. Thyroglossal duct carcinoma. *Surgery.* 1991;110:928–934; discussion 34–35.

100. Ferrer C, Ferrandez A, Dualde D, et al. Squamous cell carcinoma of the thyroglossal duct cyst: report of a new case and literature review. *J Otolaryngol.* 2000;29:311–314.

101. LiVolsi VA. *Surgical Pathology of the Thyroid.* Philadelphia, PA: WB Saunders; 1990.

102. Mehmood RK, Basha SI, Ghareeb E. A case of papillary carcinoma arising in ectopic thyroid tissue within a branchial cyst with neck node metastasis. *Ear Nose Throat J.* 2006;85:675–676.

103. Fumarola A, Trimboli P, Cavaliere R, et al. Thyroid papillary carcinoma arising in ectopic thyroid tissue within a neck branchial cyst. *World J Surg Oncol.* 2006;4:24.

104. Sidhu S, Lioe TF, Clements B. Thyroid papillary carcinoma in lateral neck cyst: missed primary tumour or ectopic thyroid carcinoma within a branchial cyst? *J Laryngol Otol.* 2000;114:716–718.

105. Matsumoto K, Watanabe Y, Asano G. Thyroid papillary carcinoma arising in ectopic thyroid tissue within a branchial cleft cyst. *Pathol Int.* 1999;49:444–446.

106. Balasubramaniam GS, Stillwell RG, Kennedy JT. Papillary carcinoma arising in ectopic thyroid tissue within a branchial cyst. *Pathology.* 1992;24:214–216.

107. Ford GR, Balakrishnan A, Evans JN, et al. Branchial cleft and pouch anomalies. *J Laryngol Otol.* 1992;106:137–143.

108. Williams ED, Toyn CE, Harach HR. The ultimobranchial gland and congenital thyroid abnormalities in man. *J Pathol.* 1989;159:135–141.

109. Hoyes AD, Kershaw DR. Anatomy and development of the thyroid gland. *Ear Nose Throat J.* 1985;64:318–333.

110. Butler JJ, Tulinius H, Ibanez ML, et al. Significance of thyroid tissue in lymph nodes associated with carcinoma of the head, neck or lung. *Cancer.* 1967;20:103–112.

111. Sampson RJ, Oka H, Key CR, et al. Metastases from occult thyroid carcinoma. An autopsy study from Hiroshima and Nagasaki, Japan. *Cancer.* 1970;25:803–811.

112. Kozol RA, Geelhoed GW, Flynn SD, et al. Management of ectopic thyroid nodules. *Surgery.* 1993;114:1103–1106; discussion 6–7.

113. Meyerowitz BR, Buchholz RB. Midline cervical ectopic thyroid tissue. *Surgery.* 1969;65:358–362.

114. Block MA, Wylie JH, Patton RB, et al. Does benign thyroid tissue occur in the lateral part of the neck? *Am J Surg.* 1966;112:476–481.

115. Gerard-Marchant R, Caillou B. Thyroid inclusions in cervical lymph nodes. *Clin Endocrinol Metab.* 1981;10:337–349.

116. Rosai J, Carcangiu ML, DeLellis RA. *Tumors of the Thyroid Gland.* Washington, DC: Armed Forces Institute of Pathology; 1992.

117. Kakudo K, Shan L, Nakamura Y, et al. Clonal analysis helps to differentiate aberrant thyroid tissue from thyroid carcinoma. *Hum Pathol.* 1998;29:187–190.

118. Saad AG, Biddinger PW, Lloyd RV, et al. Thyroid tissue within cervical lymph nodes: benign thyroid inclusions or metastasis from occult thyroid cancer? *Mod Pathol.* 2005;18:94A.

119. Zhu Z, Saad A, Nikiforov YE. Molecular alterations in the lymph node metastases of papillary thyroid carcinoma. *Mod Pathol.* 2006;19:99A.

120. Sisson JC, Schmidt RW, Beierwaltes WH. Sequestered nodular goiter. *N Engl J Med.* 1964;270:927–932.

121. Coutinho HB, King G, Robalinho TI, et al. Immunocytochemical demonstration of calcitonin in the Didelphis albiventris thyroid. *Mem Inst Oswaldo Cruz.* 1991;86:377–378.

122. Harach HR, Cabrera JA, Williams ED. Thyroid implants after surgery and blunt trauma. *Ann Diagn Pathol.* 2004;8:61–68.

123. Assi A, Sironi M, Di Bella C, et al. Parasitic nodule of the right carotid triangle. *Arch Otolaryngol Head Neck Surg.* 1996;122:1409–1411.

124. Shimizu M, Hirokawa M, Manabe T. Parasitic nodule of the thyroid in a patient with Graves' disease. *Virchows Arch.* 1999;434:241–244.

125. Hathaway BM. Innocuous accessory thyroid nodules. *Arch Surg.* 1965;90:222–227.

126. Roth LM, Talerman A. The enigma of struma ovarii. *Pathology.* 2007;39:139–146.

127. Tavassoli F, Devilee P, eds. *Pathology and Genetics of Tumours of the Breast and Female Genital Organs.* Lyon, France: International Agency for Research on Cancer; 2003.

128. Zhang X, Axiotis C. Thyroid-type carcinoma of struma ovarii. *Arch Pathol Lab Med.* 2010;134:786–791.

129. Roth LM, Miller AW III, Talerman A. Typical thyroid-type carcinoma arising in struma ovarii: a report of 4 cases and review of the literature. *Int J Gynecol Pathol.* 2008;27:496–506.

130. Robboy SJ, Shaco-Levy R, Peng RY, et al. Malignant struma ovarii: an analysis of 88 cases, including 27 with extraovarian spread. *Int J Gynecol Pathol.* 2009;28:405–422.

131. Garg K, Soslow RA, Rivera M, et al. Histologically bland "extremely well differentiated" thyroid carcinoma arising in struma ovarii can recur and metastasize. *Int J Gynecol Pathol.* 2009;28:222–230.

132. Roth LM, Karseladze AI. Highly differentiated follicular carcinoma arising from struma ovarii: a report of 3 cases, a review of the literature, and a reassessment of so-called peritoneal strumosis. *Int J Gynecol Pathol.* 2008;27:213–222.

133. Shaco-Levy R, Bean SM, Bentley RC, et al. Natural history of biologically malignant struma ovarii: analysis of 27 cases with extraovarian spread. *Int J Gynecol Pathol.* 2010;29:212–227.

134. Coyne C, Nikiforov YE. *RAS* mutation-positive follicular variant of papillary thyroid carcinoma arising in a struma ovarii. *Endocr Pathol.* 2010;21:144–147.

135. Celestino R, Magalhaes J, Castro P, et al. A follicular variant of papillary thyroid carcinoma in struma ovarii. Case report with unique molecular alterations. *Histopathology.* 2009;55:482–487.

136. Wolff EF, Hughes M, Merino MJ, et al. Expression of benign and malignant thyroid tissue in ovarian teratomas and the importance of multimodal management as illustrated by a *BRAF*-positive follicular variant of papillary thyroid cancer. *Thyroid.* 2010;20:981–987.

137. James A, Stewart C, Warrick P, et al. Branchial sinus of the piriform fossa: reappraisal of third and fourth branchial anomalies. *Laryngoscope.* 2007;117:1920–1924.

138. Thomas B, Shroff M, Forte V, et al. Revisiting imaging features and the embryologic basis of third and fourth branchial anomalies. *AJNR Am J Neuroradiol.* 2010;31:755–760.

139. Miyauchi A, Matsuzuka F, Kuma K, et al. Piriform sinus fistula and the ultimobranchial body. *Histopathology.* 1992;20:221–227.

140. Wang HK, Tiu CM, Chou YH, et al. Imaging studies of pyriform sinus fistula. *Pediatr Radiol.* 2003;33:328–333.

141. Sai Prasad TR, Chong CL, Mani A, et al. Acute suppurative thyroiditis in children secondary to pyriform sinus fistula. *Pediatr Surg Int.* 2007;23:779–783.

142. Beckner ME, Shultz JJ, Richardson T. Solid and cystic ultimobranchial body remnants in the thyroid. *Arch Pathol Lab Med.* 1990;114:1049–1052.

143. Park JY, Kim GY, Suh YL. Intrathyroidal branchial cleft-like cyst with heterotopic salivary gland-type tissue. *Pediatr Dev Pathol.* 2004;7:262–267.

144. Michal M, Mukensnabl P, Kazakov DV. Branchial-like cysts of the thyroid associated with solid cell nests. *Pathol Int.* 2006;56:150–153.

145. Ozaki T, Nagashima K, Kusakabe T, et al. Development of thyroid gland and ultimobranchial body cyst is independent of p63. *Lab Invest.* 2011;91:138–146.

Peter Kopp

Thyroid Physiology

THYROID HORMONE SYNTHESIS AND SECRETION

Thyroid hormones are essential for normal growth and development, particularly of the central nervous system, and they play a key role in regulating metabolism. The synthesis of thyroid hormones requires a normally developed thyroid gland, a functioning hypothalamic–thyroid axis, an adequate nutritional iodine intake, and a series of regulated biochemical steps within thyroid follicular cells. Thyroid hormone action occurs predominantly through regulating two specific nuclear transcription factors, thyroid hormone receptor α and β (TRα and TRβ), which alter the expression of numerous genes throughout the organism. Depending on the gene, this transcriptional regulation can be positive (e.g., myosin heavy chain α) or negative (e.g., TSH [thyroid-stimulating hormone]). In addition, thyroid hormones can also exert nongenomic effects.

The Hypothalamic–Thyroid Axis

The thyroid is controlled by a classic hypothalamic–pituitary axis (Fig. 3.1).[1] The hypothalamic tripeptide thyrotropin-releasing hormone (TRH) stimulates the production and secretion of the glycoprotein hormone TSH in the pituitary. TSH is formed of an α and a β subunit; the α subunit is common to the glycoproteins TSH, follicle-stimulating hormone, luteinizing hormone, and human chorionic gonadotropin.

On thyroid follicular cells, TSH binds to the TSH receptor, a G protein–coupled transmembrane receptor, which is expressed at the basolateral membrane (Fig. 3.2).[2] TSH binding results in stimulation of cell growth, cell differentiation, and thyroid hormone synthesis. Activation of the TSH receptor leads primarily to coupling with the stimulatory G protein Gs_α and subsequent activation of adenylyl cyclase. This, in turn, leads to an increase in intracellular cyclic AMP, phosphorylation of protein kinase A, and activation of numerous cytosolic and nuclear target proteins. At high doses of TSH, the TSH receptor also couples to $G_{q/11}$ and thereby activates the phospholipase C-dependent inositol phosphate Ca^{2+}/diacylglycerol pathway. This results in an increase in hydrogen peroxide (H_2O_2) generation and iodination.

After synthesis of the thyroid hormones, thyroxine (T4) and triiodothyronine (T3) (Fig. 3.3), a process that is discussed in more detail below, they are secreted into the bloodstream. In the serum, most T4 and T3 are protein bound to thyroxine-binding globulin (TBG), transthyretin (TTR), and albumin, and only a minute fraction is present as free hormone.[3] Thyroid hormones enter peripheral cells, a process that is at least partially mediated by amino acid channels.[4] In the cytosol, T4 is either 5'-deiodinated by deiodinase I or II, resulting in formation of the more active T3, or is inactivated to rT3 by deiodination of the inner ring (Fig. 3.3).[5] Thyroid hormone action is primarily mediated by two nuclear receptors, TRα and TRβ, which regulate the transcription of numerous genes.[6] In addition, several nongenomic actions are mediated by thyroid hormones. T3 exerts a negative feedback on TRH and TSH secretion (Fig. 3.1).

Thyroid Hormone Synthesis and Its Abnormalities

Thyroid hormone synthesis requires several biochemical steps within thyroid follicular cells and the follicular lumen, the functional unit of the thyroid.[7-9] Iodide is actively transported into thyroid follicular cells by the sodium-iodide symporter (NIS) at the basolateral membrane (Fig. 3.4).[10] This transport requires an electrochemical gradient, which is generated by the Na,K-ATPase. Iodide then reaches the apical membrane. At the apical membrane, iodide is released into the follicular lumen. This efflux occurs, at least in part, through the anion transporter pendrin (PDS/SLC26A4).[11] Once iodide reaches the follicular lumen, it is oxidized by the enzyme thyroperoxidase (TPO).[7] The oxidation of iodide by TPO requires the presence of H_2O_2. H_2O_2 production is catalyzed by the dual oxidase 2 (DUOX2), an enzyme that requires a specific maturation factor, DUOXA2, to reach the apical membrane.[12,13] The follicular lumen is filled with colloid, which consists largely of thyroglobulin (TG).[12] TG serves as matrix for the synthesis of T4 and T3. In a first step, TPO iodinates selected tyrosyl residues on TG, thereby generating monoiodotyrosine (MIT) and diiodotyrosine (DIT) (*organification reaction*). In a second step, iodotyrosines are coupled by TPO to form T4 and T3 (*coupling reaction*). To release thyroid hormones, TG is internalized into the follicular cell by micro- or macropinocytosis and digested in lysosomes. T4 (~80%) and T3 (~20%) are subsequently released into the blood stream, in part through the thyroid hormone–transporting channel monocarboxylate transporter 8 (MCT8).[13] To recycle iodide, which is a scarce micronutrient in many parts of the world,[14,15] MIT and DIT are deiodinated by a recently cloned iodotyrosine dehalogenase, DEHAL1.[16] After deiodination, the released iodide is recycled into the follicular lumen and reused for hormone synthesis (Fig. 3.4).

The Sodium-Iodide Symporter

Thyroid follicular cells concentrate iodide up to 40-fold compared with the serum iodide concentrations.[17] This active transport is mediated by NIS.[10,18] NIS transports two sodium ions and one iodide ion into the cell. This sodium-dependent transport requires a sodium gradient, which is generated by the Na^+/K^+-ATPase.[10,17,19]

The human NIS cDNA was cloned shortly after isolation of the rat NIS cDNA.[18,20] NIS belongs to the solute carrier family 5 (sodium/glucose cotransport family) and is also designated as SLC5A. The solute carriers of this family are dependent on an electrochemical sodium gradient as the driving force for solute transport. The human *NIS* gene is located on chromosome 19p13 and consists of 15 exons.[21] The encoded protein consists of 643 amino acids, is thought to have 13 transmembrane domains, and undergoes glycosylation.[22,23] The amino-terminus is located outside the cell and the carboxy-terminus inside the cytosol.[22,23]

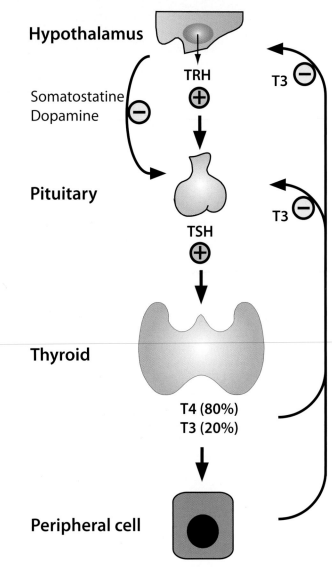

FIGURE 3.1. The hypothalamic–pituitary–thyroid axis. TRH, thyrotropin-releasing hormone; TSH, thyroid-stimulating hormone; T4, thyroxine; T3, triiodothyronine.

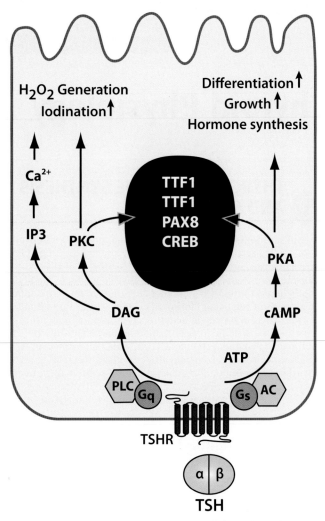

FIGURE 3.2. Signaling pathways in thyroid follicular cells. TSH, thyroid-stimulating hormone consisting of an α and a β subunit; TSHR, TSH receptor; AC, adenylyl cyclase; cAMP, cyclic AMP; PKA, protein kinase A; DAG, diacylglycerol; PKC, protein kinase C; PLC, phospholipase C; IP3, inositol triphosphate; PAX8, transcription factor PAX8; TTF1 (NKX2.1), thyroid transcription factor 1; TTF2 (FOXE2), thyroid transcription factor 2; CREB, cAMP response element binding protein.

NIS has a Km for iodide of ~36 μM.[18,24] Electrophysiologic studies revealed that NIS is electrogenic because of the influx of two sodium cations and one iodide anion.[25] NIS is blocked competitively by several anions, in particular perchlorate and thiocyanate.[26,27] Perchlorate is also actively transported by NIS,[28,29] but the transport is electroneutral.[25,29] Perchlorate has been used as an antithyroid drug in the treatment of hyperthyroidism in the past but is no longer used for this indication because it can rarely induce aplastic anemia. Although there is concern that contamination of water supplies with perchlorate may result in thyroid dysfunction, this does not seem to be common but may also depend on an adequate iodine intake.[30]

Perchlorate is also used diagnostically in the *perchlorate discharge test*. The perchlorate test is performed to determine the extent of iodide organification.[27] Under normal conditions, iodide is organified very rapidly on tyrosyl residues of TG after crossing the basolateral and the apical membrane (Fig. 3.4). Any intrathyroidal iodide that has not been incorporated into TG is released into the bloodstream, but as long as NIS is not blocked, it will again be transported into the cell. In contrast, all iodide that is released cannot be transported back into thyroid follicular cells if

NIS is inhibited by perchlorate. In the perchlorate test, radioactive iodide is administered to the patient and the counts accumulating in the thyroid are measured at frequent intervals (*uptake*). Then, 1 g of $KClO_4$ or $NaClO_4$ is administered, and the amount of intrathyroidal radioiodine is continually measured. In individuals with normal iodide organification, there is no decrease in intrathyroidal counts after the administration of perchlorate because the iodide has been organified into TG. In contrast, a loss of $\geq$ 10% of thyroidal counts indicates an organification defect. In a partial organification defect (PIOD), some of the iodide is organified. A PIOD can be associated with congenital defects with abnormal efflux of iodide into the follicular lumen such as in Pendred syndrome, defective H_2O_2 generation owing to DUOX and DUOXA2 defects, dysfunction of TPO, or a thyroiditis.[31–33] In the case of a total organification defect (TIOD), for example, in patients with complete inactivation of TPO, there is no meaningful organification and the radioiodine is completely released from the gland.

TSH stimulates iodide uptake in thyroid follicular cells through various mechanisms. It upregulates NIS mRNA and protein expression in vivo and in vitro[22,34–36] and prolongs the half-life of

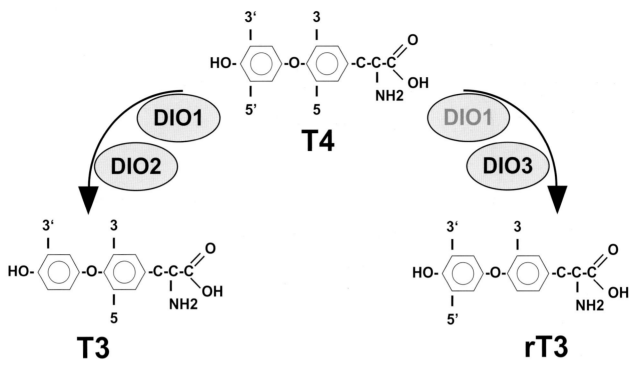

FIGURE 3.3. Thyroid hormone structure and modification by deiodinases. Structure of T4, T3, and rT3. T4 is activated to T3 by deiodinase 1 and 2. T4 is inactivated into rT3 by deiodinase 3 and to lesser extent by deiodinase 1.

NIS protein.[37] TSH also leads to increased insertion and retention of NIS in the plasma membrane.[10] Iodide accumulation and organification is also directly regulated by iodide.[38–40] NIS mRNA expression is decreased after exposure to moderate and high doses of iodide.[36,41] In addition, iodide may increase NIS protein turnover and induce a decrease in NIS activity.[41–44] High doses of iodide block thyroid hormone synthesis acutely through inhibition of the organification process (*Wolff–Chaikoff effect*).[38] This inhibition is transient and requires a high intracellular iodide concentration.[38,39] Because of the inhibition of NIS expression, the intracellular concentrations gradually decrease and the inhibitory effect dissipates.[45]

Inactivating homozygous or compound heterozygous mutations of the *NIS* gene have been identified in individuals with hypothyroidism associated with impaired iodide uptake.[10] Many of these patients have a diffuse or nodular goiter, a very low or no uptake of radioiodine, and a decreased saliva/serum radioiodine ratio.

Pendrin as Mediator of Iodide Efflux at the Apical Membrane

At the apical membrane, iodide is transported into the follicular lumen (Fig. 3.4). This is facilitated by an electrochemical gradient because the interior of the follicle is negatively charged. TSH rapidly stimulates iodide efflux into the follicular lumen, although leaving efflux in the basal direction unchanged.[46–48] On the basis of electrophysiologic studies performed with inverted plasma membrane vesicles, iodide efflux is thought to be mediated by two apical iodide channels with different affinities for the anion (Km ~70 μM and ~33 mM).[49] The demonstration of iodide transport by the anion channel PDS/SLC26A4, together with the clinical phenotype in patients with Pendred syndrome (see below), suggests that PDS/SLC26A4 could correspond to one of the channels.[11,50–53] Pendred syndrome is an autosomal recessive disorder caused by biallelic mutations in the *PDS/SLC26A* gene and defined by sensorineural deafness, goiter, and impaired iodide organification.[54–56]

The *PDS/SLC26A4* gene encompasses 21 exons and contains an open reading frame of 2,343 base pairs (bp).[50] The solute carrier family 26 contains several anion transporters and the motor protein of the outer hair cells, prestin (SLC26A5).[57–59] The genes encoding PDS/SLC26A4, DRA/SLC26A3 (downregulated in adenoma/congenital chloride diarrhea), and prestin (SCLC26A5) are located in proximity on chromosome 7q21-31 and have a very similar genomic structure suggesting a common ancestral gene. PDS/SLC26A4 is a hydrophobic membrane protein consisting of 780 amino acids with 12 putative transmembrane domains.[11,50,60] PDS/SLC26A4 contains a so-called STAS (sulfate transporter and anti-sigma factor antagonist) domain in its intracellular carboxy-terminus.[61] It has been suggested that the STAS domain of SLC26 members can interact with the regulatory domain of cystic fibrosis transmembrane conductance regulator in some epithelial cells,[62–64] but a clear functional role for this interaction has not been demonstrated.

PDS/SLC26A4 can mediate chloride and iodide uptake in *Xenopus* oocytes in a sodium-independent manner.[51] In thyroid cells, PDS/SLC26A4 is expressed at the apical membrane,[60,65] a finding suggesting that it could have a role in iodide transport into the follicle.[57,60] Functional studies in transfected cells confirmed that PDS/SLC26A4 can indeed mediate iodide efflux.[52,53] More definitive evidence for PDS/SLC26A4-mediated apical iodide efflux was obtained in a model system with polarized Madin–Darby canine kidney cells expressing NIS and PDS/SLC26A4.[11] Although TSH does not regulate the expression of PDS/SLC26A4, it rapidly upregulates membrane insertion, which results in increased efflux of iodide from thyroid cells.[66]

Naturally occurring mutations of PDS/SLC26A4 lead to a loss of function in iodide transport.[11,52,67] This observation is consistent with the PIOD observed in patients with Pendred syndrome.[50]

TG, the Matrix for Thyroid Hormone Synthesis

TG serves as the matrix for the synthesis of thyroxine (T4) and triiodothyronine (T3) and for the storage of thyroid hormone.[12]

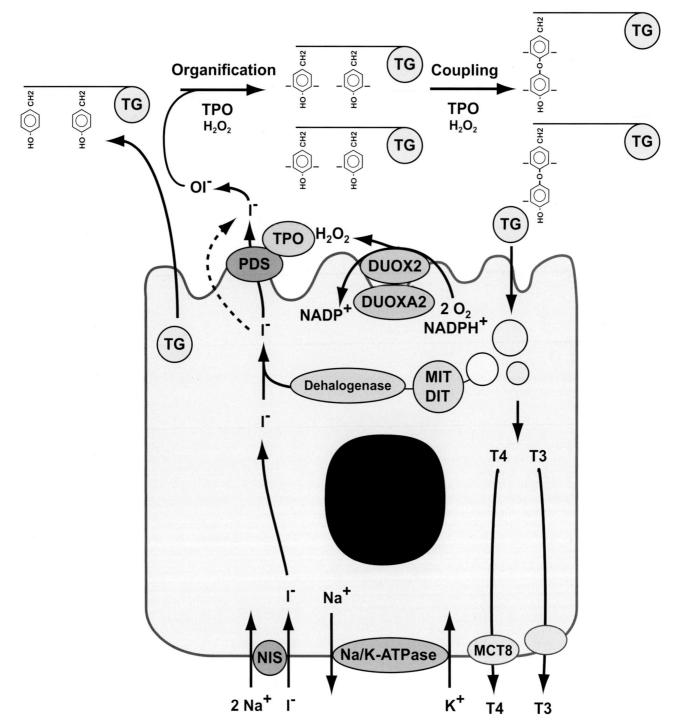

FIGURE 3.4. Thyroid hormone synthesis. NIS, sodium-iodide symporter; PDS, pendrin; TPO, thyroperoxidase; TG, thyroglobulin; DUOX2, dual oxidase 2; DUOXA2, DUOX2 maturation factor; MIT, monoiodotyrosine; DIT, diiodotyrosine; T4, thyroxine; T3, triiodothyronine; MCT8, monocarboxylate transporter 8. See text for details.

TG is encoded by a very large gene that consists of 48 exons.[68–70] It is located on chromosome 8q24.2-8q24.3.[71–73] The *TG* promoter is regulated by the transcription factors TTF1 (NKX2.1), TTF2 (FOXE2), and PAX8.[74,75] The open reading frame consists of 8,307 bp encoding a protein of 2,768 amino acids.[76,77] Alternative splicing generates various transcripts, and the *TG* gene contains numerous single-nucleotide polymorphisms.[78]

TG is secreted as dimer and is heavily glycosylated.[79–81] Other secondary modifications of TG include sulfation and

phosphorylation.[82–84] The TG protein has four major regions based on internal homology,[85–87] and the carboxy-terminal part of the TG monomer shares remarkable homology with acetylcholinesterase.[87,88] These structural characteristics suggest that the *TG* gene emerged from the fusion of two ancestral genes.[89]

Selected tyrosyl residues of TG located in the follicular colloid are iodinated (Fig. 3.4).[9] This *organification* reaction results in the generation of MIT and DIT.[7] A small fraction of these iodotyrosines are then fused in the *coupling* reaction to form tri-iodothyronine (T3) or thyroxine (T4).[7,90]

To secrete T4 and T3, TG is internalized predominantly by micropinocytosis.[91,92] After entering the cells, TG is digested in lysosomes and T4 (~80%) and T3 (~20%) are secreted into the blood stream (Fig. 3.4).[8] Intact TG is also transported from the apical to the basolateral membrane by transcytosis and released into the bloodstream.[91–94]

Biallelic mutations in the *TG* gene can lead to congenital goiter and, depending on the severity of the defect, can lead to hypothyroidism, subclinical hypothyroidism, or normal thyroid hormone levels.[95] The serum TG levels may be low, normal, or elevated. The radioiodine uptake is elevated. In many instances, the mutated TG protein is retained in the endoplasmic reticulum resulting in a classical endoplasmic reticulum storage disease.[96]

Clinically, the measurement of TG is used in the follow up of patients with well-differentiated thyroid cancer and serves as specific and sensitive tumor marker.[97] Endogenous antibodies against TG can interfere with these assays.[98]

Thyroperoxidase

To serve as an iodinating agent, iodide must be oxidized to a higher oxidation state. This oxidation of iodide is catalyzed by thyroperoxidase (TPO) and requires the presence of H_2O_2.[7,99] The human *TPO* gene consists of 17 exons and is located on chromosome 2pter-p12.[100–102] The full-length human TPO cDNA encodes a protein of 933 amino acids (TPO1).[101] In addition, there are several splice variants of uncertain biologic significance.[101]

TPO is a membrane-bound glycoprotein with a prosthetic heme group located in the follicular lumen. TPO catalyzes both the organification and the coupling reactions (Fig. 3.4).[7] The prosthetic heme group is distinct from the heme b (protoporphyrin IX) found in many other hemoproteins and is formed of a bis-hydroxylated heme b.[103] TPO displays a high degree of sequence similarity with myeloperoxidase and other mammalian peroxidases.[7]

Immunohistochemical studies localize TPO at the apical membrane,[104] but abundant immunopositivity is also found in the cytoplasm.[105] TSH rapidly increases insertion of TPO into the apical membrane through the secretory pathway, and it also increases enzymatic activity.[106,107]

TPO defects are among the more common causes of defective thyroid hormone synthesis.[108] Homozygosity or compound heterozygosity for mutations in the *TPO* gene has been reported in numerous individuals with a PIOD or TIOD.

The H_2O_2-Generating System

The presence of H_2O_2 is required for the oxidation of iodide and its organification, as well as the coupling reaction (Fig. 3.4).[109] It was known for many years that the H_2O_2-generating system contains a nicotinamide adenine dinucleotide phosphate (NADPH) oxidase that is using flavin adenine dinucleotide (FAD) as a cofactor,[7] but a more detailed characterization was only possible in recent years. Assuming a homology between the NADPH oxidase systems in thyroid follicular cells and neutrophil granulocytes, two cDNAs encoding thyroidal NADPH oxidases have been cloned.[110,111] These two oxidases are referred to as dual oxidases DUOX1 and DUOX2.[110,111] The name stems from the fact that these enzymes contain an NADPH oxidase and a peroxidase domain.[112]

The two *DUOX* genes both consist of 33 exons and are located in proximity on chromosome 15q15.[110,113] Human DUOX1 and DUOX2 have an open reading frame of 1,551 and 1,548 amino acids, respectively.[113] Secondary structure analyses predict seven putative transmembrane domains, two everted finger (EF) motifs in the first intracellular loop, four NADPH binding sites, and one FAD binding site.[110,111] These predictions are consistent with the previous biochemical characterization of the H_2O_2-generating

system. The DUOX proteins are glycosylated.[113] DUOX proteins are located at the apical membrane of thyroid follicular cells and colocalize with TPO.[111,114]

The DUOX proteins require specific maturation factors.[115] Using a data-mining approach analyzing tissue-specific transcripts, a gene product encoded by a gene arranged head-to-head and coexpressed with DUOX2 has been identified. This factor, named DUOX maturation factor DUOXA2, is required for transition of the protein from the endoplasmic reticulum to the Golgi apparatus and translocation to the plasma membrane. In the presence of DUOXA2, DUOX2 is able to generate H_2O_2. DUOX1 has a similar paralog, DUOXA1. Remarkably, the DUOX system shows a high degree of redundancy, and complex loss of DUOX2 can be partially compensated by DUOX1, which is expressed in thyrocytes, albeit at lower levels.[116,117]

Whether H_2O_2 is formed directly or through a process that includes the formation of O_2^- as an intermediate step remains unclear.[7] The successful reconstitution of a H_2O_2-generating system through coexpression of DUOX2 and DUOXA2 will allow clarifying this question.

Heterozygous loss of function mutations in the *DUOX2* gene results in mild transient or permanent congenital hypothyroidism; these patients appear to have *DUOX2* haploinsufficiency with manifestation often limited to the neonatal period when the requirement for thyroid hormone synthesis are particularly high.[118] In contrast, biallelic *DUOX2* mutations are usually associated with a severe phenotype.[32] Missense mutations in *DUOXA2* can also be associated with congenital hypothyroidism, demonstrating that this maturation factor is essential for H_2O_2 generation and thyroid hormone synthesis.[33]

Hormone Processing and Secretion

After completion of the *organification* and the *coupling* reactions, TG enters the thyrocytes through micropinocytosis (Fig. 3.4). This process can be initiated by nonselective fluid phase uptake and by receptor-mediated endocytosis.[91,119,120] The subsequent fusion of the TG-containing vesicles with lysosomes results in proteolytic breakdown of the TG and release of thyroid hormones or iodotyrosines.[8,81] After cleavage of TG by endopeptidases such as cathepsins,[121] it undergoes further degradation by several exopeptidases.[122,123] After degradation of TG carrying iodinated thyronines (T4 and T3) and tyrosines (DIT and MIT) in the lysosomal pathway, T4 and T3 are secreted into the bloodstream at the basolateral membrane.

Several transporters for thyroid hormones have been identified in the recent past.[13] The MCT8, which is encoded by a X-chromosomal gene located on human chromosome Xq13.2, has been particularly well studied. The *MCT8* gene contains six exons that encode a protein with 12 predicted transmembrane domains and intracellular amino- and carboxy-termini. Men with mutations in MCT8 display a complex neurologic phenotype referred to as Allan–Herndon–Dudley syndrome (mental retardation, severe hypotonia, spastic quadriplegia, dystonic movements).[124,125] Individuals with MCT8 mutations have low T4 and FT4, an elevated T3, a low rT3, and usually normal TSH levels. Heterozygous women usually do not have a neurologic phenotype. Among other cells, MCT8 is expressed at the basolateral membrane of thyroid follicular cells.[126] In mice with targeted disruption of the *Mct8* gene, the secretion of T4 from the thyroid is decreased, which explains, in part, the low T4 levels associated with MCT8 mutations. Other channels, which are not yet characterized, are likely to contribute to the secretion of T3 and T4 at the basolateral membrane of thyrocytes.

Dehalogenation of MIT and DIT

The iodotyrosines MIT and DIT, which are significantly more abundant in the TG molecule than in the T4 and T3, are only released in minute amounts into the circulation. The majority of these iodotyrosines are deiodinated by an thyroidal dehalogenase, and the iodide is recycled for hormone synthesis.[127,128] The gene encoding this dehalogenase, referred to as DEHAL1 or iodotyrosine deiodinase IYD, has been identified through serial analysis of gene expression based on its homology to nitroreductases.[129] The *DEHAL1* gene consists of five exons and is located on chromosome 6q25.1. Consistent with older biochemical data,[130] the peptide sequence also contains a flavin mononucleotide domain. Definitive evidence that DEHAL1 is the long-thought iodotyrosine deiodinase was obtained through the demonstration of biallelic mutations in several individuals with large goiters and hypothyroidism.[129] Remarkably, the phenotype is not necessarily apparent at birth, and therefore, the defect can be missed by neonatal screening. Serum diiodotyrosine levels are very high, and they loose large amounts of iodotyrosines in the urine.[129,131] Assessment of the enzymatic activity of the detected DEHAL1 mutations revealed absent or very major reduction in their ability to deiodinate iodotyrosines and an abolished or reduced induction in response to flavin mononucleotide.[129] The protein structure of murine DEHAL1/IYD, which is homologous to other proteins in the NADH oxidase/flavin reductase superfamily, has recently been solved.[132]

Thyroid Hormone Transport

Thyroid hormones circulate in the blood heavily bound to plasma proteins. Under physiologic conditions, only 0.03% of T4 and 0.3% of T3 circulate as free hormone.[133] The three major binding proteins are TBG, TTR, and albumin. Variations in these binding proteins can alter total thyroid hormone levels.[133,134] TTR variants are also associated with various forms of amyloidosis.

The prerequisite for the intracellular genomic actions of thyroid hormone is the translocation of the free hormone across the plasma membrane.[13,135,136] In contrast to the widely held concept that thyroid hormone could enter cells through diffusion, it has been shown that the uptake is saturable, energy dependent, and Na+ dependent, at least in certain cell types.[135] This led to the concept that specific transport proteins are responsible for the cellular uptake of thyroid hormones.[135] Recent studies have identified several transporters with affinity for thyroid hormones including, among others, MCT8, MCT10, and OATP1C1.[13] Whereas some of these transporters are highly specific for thyroid hormones, for example, MCT8, others are multifunicional. Functional characterization of rat MCT8 in *Xenopus laevis* oocytes revealed that it mediates uptake of the iodothyronines T4, T3, rT3, and 3,3-T2.[137] Subsequent studies of human MCT8 showed that its characteristics are highly similar to rat MCT8.[138] MCT8 is expressed in numerous tissues including the brain, heart, liver, kidney, adrenal gland and at the basolateral membrane of thyroid follicular cells (see above).[139,140] As discussed, MCT8 mutations lead to abnormal thyroid hormone profiles and a severe neurologic phenotype in affected men.[124,125]

MCT10 has a gene and protein structure that is similar to MCT8, and it has been shown to preferentially transport T3.[141] MCT10 is ubiquitously expressed. Its physiologic role in thyroid hormone transport needs further characterization. OATP1C1 belongs to the "organic anion-transporting polypeptide family," a large family of usually multifunctional transporters. OATP1C1 transports, among other ligands, T4 and rT3.[142,143] It is thought that OATP1C1 may play a particular role in thyroid hormone transport in the brain, but its exact physiologic role remains to be defined.[144] It is likely that the further characterization of these and other transporters will demonstrate that the uptake of thyroid hormone is regulated differentially in many tissues, thereby contributing to the complexity of thyroid hormone action at the cellular level.[13]

After entering the cell, T4 is metabolized into the more active compound T3, which binds to TRs with 10-fold higher affinity, by intracellular 5'-monodeiodination or into the inactive metabolite reverse T3 (rT3) by 5-monodeiodination (Fig. 3.3).[5] Because roughly 80% of T3 is generated by monodeiodination of T4, T4 is also considered a prohormone. Several enzymes with different tissue distributions are involved in monodeiodination (5'-monodeiodinase type I: liver, muscle, kidney, and skin; 5'-monodeiodinase type II: anterior pituitary, brain cortex, brown adipose tissue, thyroid; 5'-monodeiodinase type III: placenta—conversion from T4 to rT3).[5] The deiodinases are highly regulated enzymes that have a significant impact on tissue-specific thyroid hormone action by modulating T4 and T3 levels.[145,146]

Thyroid Hormone Action

At the level of a cell, thyroid hormone action is primarily mediated by TRs, ligand-regulated nuclear receptors modifying gene transcription.[6] TRs are encoded by two genes, *TRα* on chromosome 17 and *TRβ* on chromosome 3 (Fig. 3.5).[147–149] Both genes express various isoforms. Both receptors bind to thyroid hormones with high affinity, but they differ in some important properties including their developmental patterns of expression, tissue distributions, and patterns of splicing to create additional isoforms.[150] Depending on the target gene, T3 stimulates or inhibits gene expression.

TRs act in conjunction with thyroid receptor accessory proteins, for example, the nuclear receptor retinoic X receptor (RXR), corepressors, and coactivators (Fig. 3.6). The structure of the ligand-binding domain of TRβ has been solved.[151]

On positively regulated genes, the unliganded TRs repress transcription through the interaction with corepressors, which deacetylate histones (Fig. 3.6).[152,153] After binding of T3, the corepressor dissociates and the subsequent binding of coactivators, which leads to histone acetylation, leads to transcriptional activation through the recruitment of general transcription factors and RNA polymerase II.[6]

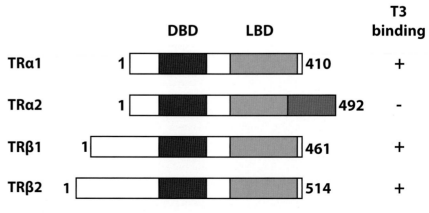

FIGURE 3.5. Thyroid hormone receptor (TR) structure. Schematic structure of the most abundant TR isoforms and their functional domains. The DBD consists of two zinc fingers. TRβ2 is most abundant in the pituitary gland and mediates negative regulation of thyroid-stimulating hormone. TRα2 does not bind to T3; its exact physiologic role is unknown. DBD, DNA-binding domain; LBD, ligand binding domain.

A

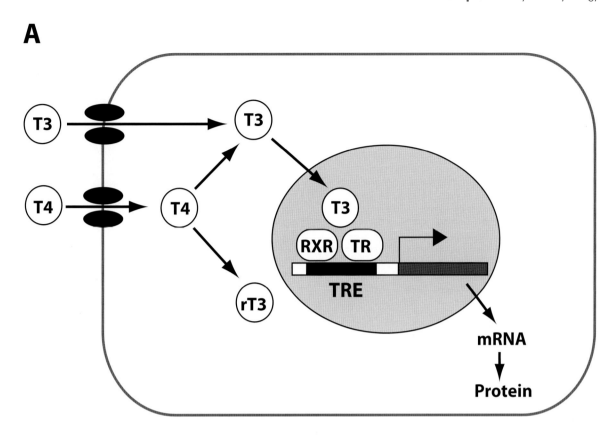

B

-T3
Gene silencing
Histone deacetylation

C

+T3
Transcriptional activation
Histone acetylation

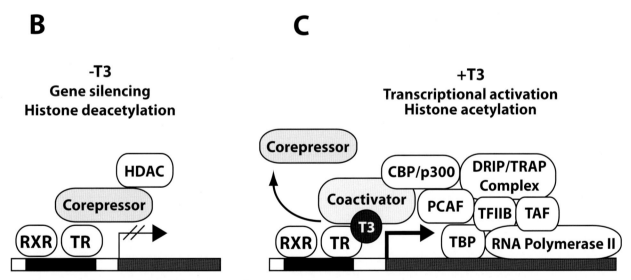

FIGURE 3.6. Mechanism of thyroid hormone action on a positively regulated gene. A: T4 and T3 enter the cell, in part by specific amino acid channels such as MCT8. T4 is converted by deiodinase 1 and 2 to T3 and then enters the nucleus where it binds to TRs. TRs form heterodimers with the nuclear receptor RXR and bind to thyroid hormone response elements in promoters of target genes. This interaction leads to changes in transcription and protein expression. **B:** In the absence of thyroid hormone, corepressors interact with TR homo- or heterodimers and silence transcription. Deacetylation of histones is associated with silenced transcription. **C:** Thyroid hormone relieves the interaction with corepressors, and after binding of coactivators and factors of the basal transcription apparatus, gene expression is started, a process that involves chromatin remodeling through histone acetylation. RXR, retinoic X receptor; TR, thyroid hormone receptor; TRE, thyroid hormone response element; HDAC, histone deacetylase; CBP, CREB binding protein; CREB, cAMP response element binding protein; HAT, histone acetylase; PCAF, p300/CBP-associated factor; DRIP/TRAP, vitamin D receptor interacting protein/TR associated protein; TBP, TATA binding protein; TAF, TBP-associated factors.

The mechanisms underlying negative regulation of a gene, for example, the TSH and TRH genes, are less well understood.[6,154]

Besides the genomic actions of thyroid hormone, nongenomic actions of physiologic relevance are increasingly recognized.[155,156] Nongenomic targets of thyroid hormone include the plasma membrane, cytoskeleton, sarcoplasmic reticulum, mitochondrial gene transcription, and alterations of contractile elements of the vascular smooth muscle cells.[155,156]

Resistance to thyroid hormone (RTH) is caused by monoallelic mutations in TRβ that exert a dominant negative effect on the normal allele.[157,158] RTH is characterized by decreased responsiveness to thyroid hormone in tissues that express predominantly TRβ and by increased transcriptional stimulation in tissues that express mainly TRα because of elevated T4 and T3 levels. Biochemically, the syndrome is defined by elevated free thyroid hormones and an inappropriately normal or elevated level of TSH. The clinical spectrum is highly variable and ranges from isolated biochemical abnormalities to a constellation of features that includes goiter, variable signs of hyper- and hypothyroidism, short stature, and delayed bone maturation. Familial cases of RTH without linkage to the TRβ locus have also been reported.[159]

PARAFOLLICULAR C CELLS AND CALCITONIN

The C cells secrete calcitonin. The human *CALCA* gene encoding calcitonin, also referred to as *calcitonin/calcitonin gene-related peptide (CT/CGRP)* gene, is located on chromosome 11p15.2-p15.1 and consists of six exons.[160,161] The cDNA encodes a precursor protein of 136 amino acids. Calcitonin, which consists of 32 amino acids, is generated by cleavage of the precursor protein. In addition to encoding the calcitonin precursor, the calcitonin gene generates a distinct transcript through alternative splicing, which encodes the CGRP.[162] Mature CGRP is found primarily in the nervous system. A highly homologous paralog gene, *CALCB*, is located in the same genomic region but does not seem to generate transcripts encoding calcitonin.[160]

The physiologic role of calcitonin remains controversial.[161] At supraphysiologic doses, calcitonin has a hypocalcemic effect but does not seem to be necessary for calcium homeostasis. Calcitonin may play a role as inhibitor of bone resorption during certain periods such as growth, pregnancy, and lactation.[161] Mice with ablation of the *CG/CGRP* gene have an increased bone loss during lactation and a decreased ability to respond to acute hypercalcemia.[163] More interestingly, bone mass is also increased in these mice because of enhanced bone formation. These observations are consistent with findings in mice with a monoallelic ablation of the calcitonin receptor[164] and suggest that calcitonin may have a physiologic role as a tonic inhibitor of bone formation.

The measurement of calcitonin is of great clinical importance in the surveillance of patients with medullary thyroid cancer because it serves as a sensitive and specific tumor marker.[165]

ACKNOWLEDGMENTS

This work has been partially supported by R03 HD061901 from NIH/NICHD.

REFERENCES

1. Skudlinski M, Kazlauskaite R, Weintraub B. Thyroid-stimulating hormone and regulation of the thyroid axis. In: DeGroot LJ, Jameson JL, eds. *Endocrinology*. 5th ed. Philadelphia, PA: Elsevier; 2006:1803–1822.
2. Kopp P. The TSH receptor and its role in thyroid disease. *Cell Mol Life Sci*. 2001;58:1301–1322.
3. Benvenga S. Thyroid hormone transport proteins and the physiology of hormone binding. In: Braverman L, Utiger R, eds. *Werner and Ingbar's the Thyroid: A Fundamental and Clinical Text*. 9th ed. Philadelphia, PA: Lippincott, Williams & Wilkins; 2005:97–108.
4. Jansen J, Friesema EC, Milici C, et al. Thyroid hormone transporters in health and disease. *Thyroid*. 2005;15:757–768.
5. Bianco AC, Salvatore D, Gereben B, et al. Biochemistry, cellular and molecular biology, and physiological roles of the iodothyronine selenodeiodinases. *Endocr Rev*. 2002;23:38–89.
6. Oetting A, Yen PM. New insights into thyroid hormone action. *Best Pract Res Clin Endocrinol Metab*. 2007;21:193–208.
7. Taurog A. Hormone synthesis: thyroid iodine metabolism. In: Braverman L, Utiger R, eds. *Werner and Ingbar's the Thyroid: A Fundamental and Clinical Text*. 8th ed. Philadelphia, PA: Lippincott, Williams & Wilkins; 2000:61–85.
8. Dunn J. Biosynthesis and secretion of thyroid hormones. In: De Groot L, Jameson J, eds. *Endocrinology*. Philadelphia, PA: WB Saunders; 2001:1290–1300.
9. Kopp P. Thyroid hormone synthesis: thyroid iodine metabolism. In: Braverman L, Utiger R, eds. *Werner and Ingbar's the Thyroid: A Fundamental and Clinical Text*. 9th ed. Philadelphia, PA: Lippincott, Williams & Wilkins; 2005:52–76.
10. Dohan O, De la Vieja A, Paroder V, et al. The sodium/iodide symporter (NIS): characterization, regulation, and medical significance. *Endocr Rev*. 2003;24:48–77.
11. Gillam MP, Sidhaye A, Lee EJ, et al. Functional characterization of pendrin in a polarized cell system: evidence for pendrin-mediated apical iodide efflux. *J Biol Chem*. 2004;279:13004–13010.
12. Arvan P, Di Jeso B. Thyroglobulin structure, function, and biosynthesis. In: Braverman L, Utiger R, eds. *Werner and Ingbar's the Thyroid: A Fundamental and Clinical Text*. 9th ed. Philadelphia, PA: Lippincott, Williams & Wilkins; 2005:77–95.
13. Visser WE, Friesema EC, Visser TJ. Minireview: thyroid hormone transporters: the knowns and the unknowns. *Mol Endocrinol*. 2011;25:1–14.
14. Zimmermann MB. Iodine deficiency. *Endocrine reviews*. 2009;30:376–408.
15. Zimmermann MB. Iodine deficiency in industrialized countries. *Clin Endocrinol (Oxf)*. 2011;75:287–288.
16. Moreno JC. Identification of novel genes involved in congenital hypothyroidism using serial analysis of gene expression. *Horm Res*. 2003;60:96–102.
17. Wolff J. Transport of iodide and other anions in the thyroid gland. *Physiol Rev*. 1964;44:45–90.
18. Dai G, Levy O, Carrasco N. Cloning and characterization of the thyroid iodide transporter. *Nature*. 1996;379:458–460.
19. De La Vieja A, Dohan O, Levy O, et al. Molecular analysis of the sodium/iodide symporter: impact on thyroid and extrathyroid pathophysiology. *Physiol Rev*. 2000;80:1083–1105.
20. Smanik PA, Liu Q, Furminger TL, et al. Cloning of the human sodium iodide symporter. *Biochem Biophys Res Commun*. 1996;226:339–345.
21. Smanik PA, Ryu KY, Theil KS, et al. Expression, exon-intron organization, and chromosome mapping of the human sodium iodide symporter. *Endocrinology*. 1997;138:3555–3558.
22. Levy O, Dai G, Riedel C, et al. Characterization of the thyroid Na$^+$/I$^-$ symporter with an anti-COOH terminus antibody. *Proc Natl Acad Sci U S A*. 1997;94:5568–5573.
23. Levy O, De la Vieja A, Ginter CS, et al. N-linked glycosylation of the thyroid Na$^+$/I$^-$ symporter (NIS). Implications for its secondary structure model. *J Biol Chem*. 1998;273:22657–22663.
24. Weiss SJ, Philp NJ, Grollman EF. Iodide transport in a continuous line of cultured cells from rat thyroid. *Endocrinology*. 1984;114:1090–1098.
25. Eskandari S, Loo DD, Dai G, et al. Thyroid Na$^+$/I$^-$ symporter. Mechanism, stoichiometry, and specificity. *J Biol Chem*. 1997;272:27230–27238.
26. Barker HM. The blood cyanates in the treatment of hypertension. *JAMA*. 1936;106:762–767.
27. Hilditch TE, Horton PW, McCruden DC, et al. Defects in intrathyroid binding of iodine and the perchlorate discharge test. *Acta Endocrinol (Copenh)*. 1982;100:237–244.
28. Van Sande J, Massart C, Beauwens R, et al. Anion selectivity by the sodium iodide symporter. *Endocrinology*. 2003;144:247–252.
29. Dohan O, Portulano C, Basquin C, et al. The Na+/I symporter (NIS) mediates electroneutral active transport of the environmental pollutant perchlorate. *Proc Natl Acad Sci U S A*. 2007;104:20250–20255.
30. Leung AM, Pearce EN, Braverman LE. Perchlorate, iodine and the thyroid. *Best Pract Res Clin Endocrinol Metab*. 2010;24:133–141.
31. Kopp P. Perspective: genetic defects in the etiology of congenital hypothyroidism. *Endocrinology*. 2002;143:2019–2024.
32. Moreno JC, Bikker H, Kempers MJ, et al. Inactivating mutations in the gene for thyroid oxidase 2 (THOX2) and congenital hypothyroidism. *N Engl J Med*. 2002;347:95–102.
33. Zamproni I, Grasberger H, Cortinovis F, et al. Biallelic Inactivation of the dual oxidase maturation factor 2 (DUOXA2) gene as a Novel Cause of Congenital Hypothyroidism. *J Clin Endocrinol Metab*. 2008;93:605–610.
34. Kogai T, Endo T, Saito T, et al. Regulation by thyroid-stimulating hormone of sodium/iodide symporter gene expression and protein levels in FRTL-5 cells. *Endocrinology*. 1997;138:2227–2232.
35. Saito T, Endo T, Kawaguchi A, et al. Increased expression of the Na$^+$/I$^-$ symporter in cultured human thyroid cells exposed to thyrotropin and in Graves' thyroid tissue. *J Clin Endocrinol Metab*. 1997;82:3331–3336.
36. Kogai T, Curcio F, Hyman S, et al. Induction of follicle formation in long-term cultured normal human thyroid cells treated with thyrotropin stimulates iodide uptake but not sodium/iodide symporter messenger RNA and protein expression. *J Endocrinol*. 2000;167:125–135.

37. Riedel C, Levy O, Carrasco N. Post-transcriptional regulation of the sodium/iodide symporter by thyrotropin. *J Biol Chem.* 2001;276:21458–21463.
38. Wolff J, Chaikoff I. Plasma inorganic iodide as homeostatic regulator of thyroid function. *J Biol Chem.* 1948;174:555–564.
39. Wolff J, Chaikoff I, Goldberg R, et al. The temporary nature of the inhibitory action of excess iodide on organic iodide synthesis in the normal thyroid. *Endocrinology.* 1949;45:504–513.
40. Grollman EF, Smolar A, Ommaya A, et al. Iodine suppression of iodide uptake in FRTL-5 thyroid cells. *Endocrinology.* 1986;118:2477–2482.
41. Uyttersprot N, Pelgrims N, Carrasco N, et al. Moderate doses of iodide in vivo inhibit cell proliferation and the expression of thyroperoxidase and Na$^+$/I$^-$ symporter mRNAs in dog thyroid. *Mol Cell Endocrinol.* 1997;131:195–203.
42. Spitzweg C, Joba W, Morris JC, et al. Regulation of sodium iodide symporter gene expression in FRTL-5 rat thyroid cells. *Thyroid.* 1999;9:821–830.
43. Eng PH, Cardona GR, Fang SL, et al. Escape from the acute Wolff-Chaikoff effect is associated with a decrease in thyroid sodium/iodide symporter messenger ribonucleic acid and protein. *Endocrinology.* 1999;140:3404–3410.
44. Eng PH, Cardona GR, Previti MC, et al. Regulation of the sodium iodide symporter by iodide in FRTL-5 cells. *Eur J Endocrinol.* 2001;144:139–144.
45. Braverman LE, Ingbar SH. Changes in thyroidal function during adaptation to large doses of iodide. *J Clin Invest.* 1963;42:1216 1231.
46. Weiss SJ, Philp NJ, Grollman EF. Effect of thyrotropin on iodide efflux in FRTL-5 cells mediated by Ca^{2+}. *Endocrinology.* 1984;114:1108–1113.
47. Nilsson M, Bjorkman U, Ekholm R, et al. Iodide transport in primary cultured thyroid follicle cells: evidence of a TSH-regulated channel mediating iodide efflux selectively across the apical domain of the plasma membrane. *Eur J Cell Biol.* 1990;52:270–281.
48. Nilsson M, Bjorkman U, Ekholm R, et al. Polarized efflux of iodide in porcine thyrocytes occurs via a cAMP-regulated iodide channel in the apical plasma membrane. *Acta Endocrinol (Copenh).* 1992;126:67–74.
49. Golstein P, Abramow M, Dumont JE, et al. The iodide channel of the thyroid: a plasma membrane vesicle study. *Am J Physiol.* 1992;263:C590–C597.
50. Everett LA, Glaser B, Beck JC, et al. Pendred syndrome is caused by mutations in a putative sulphate transporter gene (*PDS*). *Nature Genet.* 1997;17:411–422.
51. Scott DA, Wang R, Kreman TM, et al. The Pendred syndrome gene encodes a chloride-iodide transport protein. *Nature Genet.* 1999;21:440–443.
52. Taylor JP, Metcalfe RA, Watson PF, et al. Mutations of the *PDS* gene, encoding pendrin, are associated with protein mislocalization and loss of iodide efflux: implications for thyroid dysfunction in Pendred syndrome. *J Clin Endocrinol Metab.* 2002;87:1778–1784.
53. Yoshida A, Taniguchi S, Hisatome I, et al. Pendrin is an iodide-specific apical porter responsible for iodide efflux from thyroid cells. *J Clin Endocrinol Metab.* 2002;87:3356–3361.
54. Fraser GR, Morgans ME, Trotter WR. The syndrome of sporadic goitre and congenital deafness. *Q J Med.* 1960;29:279–295.
55. Medeiros-Neto G, Stanbury JB. Pendred's syndrome: association of congenital deafness with sporadic goiter. In: Medeiros-Neto G, Stanbury JB, eds. *Inherited Disorders of the Thyroid System.* Boca Raton, FL: CRC Press; 1994:81–105.
56. Kopp P. Pendred's syndrome and genetic defects in thyroid hormone synthesis. *Rev Endocr Metabol Dis.* 2000;1(1–2):109–121.
57. Everett LA, Green ED. A family of mammalian anion transporters and their involvement in human genetic diseases. *Hum Mol Genet.* 1999;8:1883–1891.
58. Zheng J, Shen W, He DZ, et al. Prestin is the motor protein of cochlear outer hair cells. *Nature.* 2000;405:149–155.
59. Liu XZ, Ouyang XM, Xia XJ, et al. Prestin, a cochlear motor protein, is defective in non-syndromic hearing loss. *Hum Mol Genet.* 2003;12:1155–1162.
60. Royaux IE, Suzuki K, Mori A, et al. Pendrin, the protein encoded by the Pendred syndrome gene (*PDS*), is an apical porter of iodide in the thyroid and is regulated by thyroglobulin in FRTL-5 cells. *Endocrinology.* 2000;141:839–845.
61. Aravind L, Koonin EV. The STAS domain—a link between anion transporters and antisigma-factor antagonists. *Curr Biol.* 2001;10:R53–R55.
62. Ko SB, Shcheynikov N, Choi JY, et al. A molecular mechanism for aberrant CFTR-dependent HCO(3)(–) transport in cystic fibrosis. *Embo J.* 2002;21:5662–5672.
63. Ko SB, Zeng W, Dorwart MR, et al. Gating of CFTR by the STAS domain of SLC26 transporters. *Nat Cell Biol.* 2004;6:343–350.
64. Shcheynikov N, Ko SB, Zeng W, et al. Regulatory interaction between CFTR and the SLC26 transporters. *Novartis Found Symp.* 2006;273:177–186; discussion 186–192, 261–264.
65. Bidart JM, Mian C, Lazar V, et al. Expression of pendrin and the Pendred syndrome (*PDS*) gene in human thyroid tissues. *J Clin Endocrinol Metab.* 2000;85:2028–2033.
66. Pesce L, Bizhanova A, Caraballo J, et al. TSH regulates pendrin membrane abundance and enhances iodide efflux in thyroid cells. Endocrinology. 2011; Nov 22. [Epub ahead of print].
67. Scott DA, Wang R, Kreman TM, et al. Functional differences of the *PDS* gene product are associated with phenotypic variation in patients with Pendred syndrome and non-syndromic hearing loss (DFNB4). *Hum Mol Genet.* 2000;9:1709–1715.
68. Mendive FM, Rivolta CM, Moya CM, et al. Genomic organization of the human thyroglobulin gene: the complete intron-exon structure. *Eur J Endocrinol.* 2001;145:485–496.
69. Mendive FM, Rivolta CM, Vassart G, et al. Genomic organization of the 3' region of the human thyroglobulin gene. *Thyroid.* 1999;9:903–912.
70. Moya CM, Mendive FM, Rivolta CM, et al. Genomic organization of the 5' region of the human thyroglobulin gene. *Eur J Endocrinol.* 2000;143:789–798.
71. Baas F, Bikker H, Geurts van Kessel A, et al. The human thyroglobulin gene: a polymorphic marker localized distal to C-MYC on chromosome 8 band q24. *Hum Genet.* 1985;69:138–143.
72. Rabin M, Barker PE, Ruddle FH, et al. Proximity of thyroglobulin and c-myc genes on human chromosome 8. *Somat Cell Mol Genet.* 1985;11:397–402.
73. Berge-Lefranc JL, Cartouzou G, Mattei MG, et al. Localization of the thyroglobulin gene by in situ hybridization to human chromosomes. *Hum Genet.* 1985;69:28–31.
74. Damante G, Di Lauro R. Thyroid-specific gene expression. *Biochim Biophys Acta.* 1994;1218:255–266.
75. Kambe F, Seo H. Thyroid-specific transcription factors. *Endocr J.* 1997;44:775–784.
76. Malthiery Y, Lissitzky S. Primary structure of human thyroglobulin deduced from the sequence of its 8448-base complementary DNA. *Eur J Biochem.* 1987;165:491–498.
77. van de Graaf SA, Pauws E, de Vijlder JJ, et al. The revised 8307 base pair coding sequence of human thyroglobulin transiently expressed in eukaryotic cells. *Eur J Endocrinol.* 1997;136:508–515.
78. van de Graaf SA, Ris-Stalpers C, Pauws E, et al. Up to date with human thyroglobulin. *J Endocrinol.* 2001;170:307–321.
79. Kim PS, Arvan P. Hormonal regulation of thyroglobulin export from the endoplasmic reticulum of cultured thyrocytes. *J Biol Chem.* 1993;268:4873–4879.
80. Arvan P, Kim PS, Kuliawat R, et al. Intracellular protein transport to the thyrocyte plasma membrane: potential implications for thyroid physiology. *Thyroid.* 1997;7:89–105.
81. Dunn JT, Dunn AD. Thyroglobulin: chemistry, biosynthesis, and proteolysis. In: Braverman LE, Utiger RD, eds. *Werner and Ingbar's the Thyroid: A Fundamental and Clinical Text.* 8th ed. Philadelphia, PA: Lippincott Williams & Wilkins; 2000:91–104.
82. Sakurai S, Fogelfeld L, Schneider AB. Anionic carbohydrate groups of human thyroglobulin containing both phosphate and sulfate. *Endocrinology.* 1991;129:915–920.
83. Blode H, Heinrich T, Diringer H. A quantitative assay for tyrosine sulfation and tyrosine phosphorylation in peptides. *Biol Chem Hoppe Seyler.* 1990;371:145–151.
84. Venot N, Nlend MC, Cauvi D, et al. The hormonogenic tyrosine 5 of porcine thyroglobulin is sulfated. *Biochem Biophys Res Commun.* 2002;298:193–197.
85. Molina F, Bouanani M, Pau B, et al. Characterization of the type-1 repeat from thyroglobulin, a cysteine-rich module found in proteins from different families. *Eur J Biochem.* 1996;240:125–133.
86. Yamashita M, Konagaya S. A novel cysteine protease inhibitor of the egg of chum salmon, containing a cysteine-rich thyroglobulin-like motif. *J Biol Chem.* 1996;271:1282–1284.
87. Mercken L, Simons MJ, De Martynoff G, et al. Presence of hormonogenic and repetitive domains in the first 930 amino acids of bovine thyroglobulin as deduced from the cDNA sequence. *Eur J Biochem.* 1985;147:59–64.
88. Swillens S, Ludgate M, Mercken L, et al. Analysis of sequence and structure homologies between thyroglobulin and acetylcholinesterase: possible functional and clinical significance. *Biochem Biophys Res Commun.* 1986;137:142–148.
89. Parma J, Christophe D, Pohl V, et al. Structural organization of the 5' region of the thyroglobulin gene. Evidence for intron loss and "exonization" during evolution. *J Mol Biol.* 1987;196:769–779.
90. Dunn AD, Corsi CM, Myers HE, et al. Tyrosine 130 is an important outer ring donor for thyroxine formation in thyroglobulin. *J Biol Chem.* 1998;273:25223–25229.
91. Marino M, McCluskey RT. Role of thyroglobulin endocytic pathways in the control of thyroid hormone release. *Am J Physiol Cell Physiol.* 2000;279:C1295–C1306.
92. Marino M, Pinchera A, McCluskey RT, et al. Megalin in thyroid physiology and pathology. *Thyroid.* 2001;11:47–56.
93. Herzog V. Transcytosis in thyroid follicle cells. *J Cell Biol.* 1983;97:607–617.
94. Druetta L, Bornet H, Sassolas G, et al. Identification of thyroid hormone residues on serum thyroglobulin: a clue to the source of circulating thyroglobulin in thyroid diseases. *Eur J Endocrinol.* 1999;140:457–467.
95. Vono-Toniolo J, Rivolta CM, Targovnik HM, et al. Naturally occurring mutations in the thyroglobulin gene. *Thyroid.* 2005;15:1021–1033.
96. Kim PS, Arvan P. Endocrinopathies in the family of endoplasmic reticulum (ER) storage diseases: disorders of protein trafficking and the role of ER molecular chaperones. *Endocr Rev.* 1998;19:173–202.
97. Baloch Z, Carayon P, Conte-Devolx B, et al. Laboratory medicine practice guidelines. Laboratory support for the diagnosis and monitoring of thyroid disease. *Thyroid.* 2003;13:3–126.
98. Spencer CA, Lopresti JS. Measuring thyroglobulin and thyroglobulin autoantibody in patients with differentiated thyroid cancer. *Nat Clin Pract Endocrinol Metab.* 2008;4:223–233.
99. Taurog A. Hormone synthesis: thyroid iodine metabolism. In: Braverman L, Utiger R, eds. *Werner and Ingbar's the Thyroid: A Fundamental and Clinical Text.* 7th ed. Philadelphia, PA: Lippincott-Raven; 1996:47–81.
100. Kimura S, Hong YS, Kotani T, et al. Structure of the human thyroid peroxidase gene: comparison and relationship to the human myeloperoxidase gene. *Biochemistry.* 1989;28:4481–4489.
101. Kimura S, Kotani T, McBride OW, et al. Human thyroid peroxidase: complete cDNA and protein sequence, chromosome mapping, and identification of two alternately spliced mRNAs. *Proc Natl Acad Sci U S A.* 1987;84:5555–5559.
102. de Vijlder JJ, Dinsart C, Libert F, et al. Regional localization of the gene for thyroid peroxidase to human chromosome 2pter-p12. *Cytogenet Cell Genet.* 1988;47:170–172.
103. Taurog A, Wall M. Proximal and distal histidines in thyroid peroxidase: relation to the alternatively spliced form, TPO-2. *Thyroid.* 1998;8:185–191.
104. Nilsson M, Molne J, Karlsson FA, et al. Immunoelectron microscopic studies on the cell surface location of the thyroid microsomal antigen. *Mol Cell Endocrinol.* 1987;53:177–186.

105. Pinchera A, Mariotti S, Chiovato L, et al. Cellular localization of the microsomal antigen and the thyroid peroxidase antigen. *Acta Endocrinol*. 1987;281:57–62.

106. Bjorkman U, Ekholm R, Ericson LE. Effects of thyrotropin on thyroglobulin exocytosis and iodination in the rat thyroid gland. *Endocrinology*. 1978;102:460–470.

107. Chiovato L, Vitti P, Lombardi A, et al. Expression of the microsomal antigen on the surface of continuously cultured rat thyroid cells is modulated by thyrotropin. *J Clin Endocrinol Metab*. 1985;61:12–16.

108. Bakker B, Bikker H, Vulsma T, et al. Two decades of screening for congenital hypothyroidism in The Netherlands: *TPO* gene mutations in total iodide organification defects (an update). *J Clin Endocrinol Metab*. 2000;85:3708–3712.

109. Corvilain B, van Sande J, Laurent E, et al. The H_2O_2-generating system modulates protein iodination and the activity of the pentose phosphate pathway in dog thyroid. *Endocrinology*. 1991;128:779–785.

110. Dupuy C, Ohayon R, Valent A, et al. Purification of a novel flavoprotein involved in the thyroid NADPH oxidase. Cloning of the porcine and human cDNAs. *J Biol Chem*. 1999;274:37265–37269.

111. De Deken X, Wang D, Many MC, et al. Cloning of two human thyroid cDNAs encoding new members of the NADPH oxidase family. *J Biol Chem*. 2000;275:23227–23233.

112. Edens WA, Sharling L, Cheng G, et al. Tyrosine cross-linking of extracellular matrix is catalyzed by Duox, a multidomain oxidase/peroxidase with homology to the phagocyte oxidase subunit gp91phox. *J Cell Biol*. 2001;154:879–891.

113. De Deken X, Wang D, Dumont JE, et al. Characterization of ThOX proteins as components of the thyroid H_2O_2-generating system. *Exp Cell Res*. 2002;273:187–196.

114. Caillou B, Dupuy C, Lacroix L, et al. Expression of reduced nicotinamide adenine dinucleotide phosphate oxidase (ThOX, LNOX, Duox) genes and proteins in human thyroid tissues. *J Clin Endocrinol Metab*. 2001;86:3351–3358.

115. Grasberger H, Refetoff S. Identification of the maturation factor for dual oxidase. Evolution of an eukaryotic operon equivalent. *J Biol Chem*. 2006;281:18269–18272.

116. Maruo Y, Takahashi H, Soeda I, et al. Transient congenital hypothyroidism caused by biallelic mutations of the dual oxidase 2 gene in Japanese patients detected by a neonatal screening program. *J Clin Endocrinol Metab*. 2008;93:4261–4267.

117. Hulur I, Hermanns P, Nestoris C, et al. A single copy of the recently identified dual oxidase maturation factor (*DUOXA*) 1 gene produces only mild transient hypothyroidism in a patient with a novel biallelic *DUOXA2* mutation and monoallelic *DUOXA1* deletion. *J Clin Endocrinol Metab*. 2011;96:E841–E845.

118. Grasberger H, Refetoff S. Genetic causes of congenital hypothyroidism due to dyshormonogenesis. *Current Opinion Peds*. 2011;23:421–428.

119. Bernier-Valentin F, Kostrouch Z, Rabilloud R, et al. Coated vesicles from thyroid cells carry iodinated thyroglobulin molecules. First indication for an internalization of the thyroid prohormone via a mechanism of receptor-mediated endocytosis. *J Biol Chem*. 1990;265:17373–17380.

120. Kostrouch Z, Bernier-Valentin F, Munari-Silem Y, et al. Thyroglobulin molecules internalized by thyrocytes are sorted in early endosomes and partially recycled back to the follicular lumen. *Endocrinology*. 1993;132:2645–2653.

121. Dunn AD, Crutchfield HE, Dunn JT. Proteolytic processing of thyroglobulin by extracts of thyroid lysosomes. *Endocrinology*. 1991;128:3073–3080.

122. Dunn AD, Crutchfield HE, Dunn JT. Thyroglobulin processing by thyroidal proteases. Major sites of cleavage by cathepsins B, D, and L. *J Biol Chem*. 1991;266:20198–20204.

123. Dunn AD, Myers HE, Dunn JT. The combined action of two thyroidal proteases releases T4 from the dominant hormone-forming site of thyroglobulin. *Endocrinology*. 1996;137:3279–3285.

124. Friesema EC, Grueters A, Biebermann H, et al. Association between mutations in a thyroid hormone transporter and severe X-linked psychomotor retardation. *Lancet*. 2004;364:1435–1437.

125. Dumitrescu AM, Liao XH, Best TB, et al. A novel syndrome combining thyroid and neurological abnormalities is associated with mutations in a monocarboxylate transporter gene. *Am J Hum Genet*. 2004;74:168–175.

126. Di Cosmo C, Liao XH, Dumitrescu AM, et al. Mice deficient in MCT8 reveal a mechanism regulating thyroid hormone secretion. *J Clin Invest*. 2010;120:3377–3388.

127. Roche J, Michel R, Michel O, et al. Sur la déshalgénation enzymatique des iodotyrosines par le corps thyroïde et sur son role physiologique. *Biochim Biophys Acta*. 1952;9:161–169.

128. Roche J, Michel O, Michel R, et al. Sur la déshalogénation enzymatique des iodotyrosines par le corps thyroïde et sur son role physiologique. II. *Biochim Biophys Acta*. 1953;12:570–576.

129. Moreno JC, Klootwijk W, van Toor H, et al. Mutations in the iodotyrosine deiodinase gene and hypothyroidism. *N Engl J Med*. 2008;358:1811–1818.

130. Goswami A, Rosenberg IN. Characterization of a flavoprotein iodotyrosine deiodinase from bovine thyroid. Flavin nucleotide binding and oxidation-reduction properties. *J Biol Chem*. 1979;254:12326–12330.

131. Stanbury JB, Kassenaar AA, Meijer JW, et al. The occurrence of mono- and di-iodotyrosine in the blood of a patient with congenital goiter. *J Clin Endocrinol Metab*. 1955;15:1216–1227.

132. Thomas SR, McTamney PM, Adler JM, et al. Crystal structure of iodotyrosine deiodinase, a novel flavoprotein responsible for iodide salvage in thyroid glands. *J Biol Chem*. 2009;284:19659–19667.

133. Bartalena L, Robbins J. Variations in thyroid hormone transport proteins and their clinical implications. *Thyroid*. 1992;2:237–245.

134. Kopp P. Genetic basis of thyroid disorders. In: Ganten D, Ruekpaul K, eds. *Genomics and Proteomics in Molecular Medicine*. 2nd ed. Berlin, Germany: Springer; 2006:1862–1867.

135. Hennemann G, Docter R, Friesema EC, et al. Plasma membrane transport of thyroid hormones and its role in thyroid hormone metabolism and bioavailability. *Endocr Rev*. 2001;22:451–476.

136. Visser W, Friesema E, Jansen J, et al. Thyroid hormone transport in and out of cells. *Trends Endocrinol Metab*. 2008;19:50–56.

137. Friesema EC, Ganguly S, Abdalla A, et al. Identification of monocarboxylate transporter 8 as a specific thyroid hormone transporter. *J Biol Chem*. 2003;278:40128–40135.

138. Friesema EC, Kuiper GG, Jansen J, et al. Thyroid hormone transport by the human monocarboxylate transporter 8 and its rate-limiting role in intracellular metabolism. *Mol Endocrinol*. 2006;20:2761–2772.

139. Price NT, Jackson VN, Halestrap AP. Cloning and sequencing of four new mammalian monocarboxylate transporter (MCT) homologues confirms the existence of a transporter family with an ancient past. *Biochem J*. 1998;329(pt 2):321–328.

140. Nishimura M, Naito S. Tissue-specific mRNA expression profiles of human solute carrier transporter superfamilies. *Drug Metab Pharmacokinet*. 2008;23:22–44.

141. Friesema EC, Jansen J, Jachtenberg JW, et al. Effective cellular uptake and efflux of thyroid hormone by human monocarboxylate transporter 10. *Mol Endocrinol*. 2008;22:1357–1369.

142. Hagenbuch B. Cellular entry of thyroid hormones by organic anion transporting polypeptides. *Best Pract Res Clin Endocrinol Metab*. 2007;21:209–221.

143. van der Deure WM, Hansen PS, Peeters RP, et al. Thyroid hormone transport and metabolism by organic anion transporter 1C1 and consequences of genetic variation. *Endocrinology*. 2008;149:5307–5314.

144. van der Deure WM, Appelhof BC, Peeters RP, et al. Polymorphisms in the brain-specific thyroid hormone transporter OATP1C1 are associated with fatigue and depression in hypothyroid patients. *Clin Endocrinol*. 2008;69:804–811.

145. Bianco AC. Minireview: cracking the metabolic code for thyroid hormone signaling. *Endocrinology*. 2011;152:3306–3311

146. Williams GR, Bassett JH. Deiodinases: the balance of thyroid hormone: local control of thyroid hormone action: role of type 2 deiodinase. *J Endocrinol*. 2011;209:261–272.

147. Sap J, Munoz A, Damm K, et al. The c-erb-A protein is a high-affinity receptor for thyroid hormone. *Nature*. 1986;324:635–640.

148. Weinberger C, Thompson CC, Ong ES, et al. The *c-erb-A* gene encodes a thyroid hormone receptor. *Nature*. 1986;324:641–646.

149. Zhang J, Lazar MA. The mechanism of action of thyroid hormones. *Annu Rev Physiol*. 2000;62:439–466.

150. Cheng SY, Leonard JL, Davis PJ. Molecular aspects of thyroid hormone actions. *Endocr Rev*. 2010;31:139–170.

151. Wagner RL, Apriletti JW, McGrath ME, et al. A structural role for hormone in the thyroid hormone receptor. *Nature*. 1995;378:690–697.

152. Horlein AJ, Naar AM, Heinzel T, et al. Ligand-independent repression by the thyroid hormone receptor mediated by a nuclear receptor co-repressor. *Nature*. 1995;377:397–404.

153. Chen JD, Evans RM. A transcriptional co-repressor that interacts with nuclear hormone receptors. *Nature*. 1995;377:454–457.

154. Ortiga-Carvalho TM, Shibusawa N, Nikrodhanond A, et al. Negative regulation by thyroid hormone receptor requires an intact coactivator-binding surface. *J Clin Invest*. 2005;115:2517–2523.

155. Davis PJ, Leonard JL, Davis FB. Mechanisms of nongenomic actions of thyroid hormone. *Front Neuroendocrinol*. 2008;29:211–218.

156. Davis PJ, Davis FB, Mousa SA, et al. Membrane receptor for thyroid hormone: physiologic and pharmacologic implications. *Annu Rev Pharmacol Toxicol*. 2011;51:99–115.

157. Refetoff S. Inherited thyroxine-binding globulin abnormalities in man. *Endocr Rev*. 1989;10:275–293.

158. Refetoff S, Weiss RE, Usala SJ. The syndromes of resistance to thyroid hormone. *Endocr Rev*. 1993;14:348–399.

159. Refetoff S, Dumitrescu AM. Syndromes of reduced sensitivity to thyroid hormone: genetic defects in hormone receptors, cell transporters and deiodination. *Best Pract Res Clin Endocrinol Metab*. 2007;21:277–305.

160. Steenbergh PH, Hoppener JW, Zandberg J, et al. Structure and expression of the human *calcitonin/CGRP* genes. *FEBS Lett*. 1986;209:97–103.

161. Martin T, Findlay D, Sexton P. Calcitonin. In: DeGroot LJ, Jameson JL, eds. *Endocrinology*. Philadelphia, PA: Elsevier; 2006:1419–1433.

162. Jacobs JW, Goodman RH, Chin WW, et al. Calcitonin messenger RNA encodes multiple polypeptides in a single precursor. *Science*. 1981;213:457–459.

163. Hoff AO, Catala-Lehnen P, Thomas PM, et al. Increased bone mass is an unexpected phenotype associated with deletion of the calcitonin gene. *J Clin Invest*. 2002;110:1849–1857.

164. Dacquin R, Davey RA, Laplace C, et al. Amylin inhibits bone resorption while the calcitonin receptor controls bone formation in vivo. *J Cell Biol*. 2004;164:509–514.

165. Brandi ML, Gagel RF, Angeli A, et al. Guidelines for diagnosis and therapy of MEN type 1 and type 2. *J Clin Endocrinol Metab*. 2001;86:5658–5671.

Thyroiditis

Thyroiditis encompasses a heterogeneous group of inflammatory diseases of the thyroid. The study of these inflammatory conditions can be challenging because of the different approaches to classification and various synonyms for a particular type of thyroiditis. Classification can be based on whether the clinical course is acute, subacute, chronic, or subclinical (Table 4.1). Other approaches to classification include the type of inflammatory response, the etiologic or pathogenic mechanism (e.g., autoimmune, infectious), or the effect on thyroid function.

This chapter is structured on the basis of predominant inflammatory cell type and utilizes the nomenclature for thyroiditis as shown in Table 4.1. The most common clinically significant form of thyroiditis is chronic lymphocytic thyroiditis, which describes histopathologically the autoimmune condition commonly called Hashimoto thyroiditis. In this chapter, chronic lymphocytic thyroiditis and Hashimoto thyroiditis are considered synonymous. Subacute forms of thyroiditis are divided according to the predominant inflammatory response (granulomatous or lymphocytic). The rare fibroinflammatory process known as *Riedel thyroiditis* is also included in this chapter. Diffuse toxic hyperplasia, or Graves disease, could qualify for consideration as an inflammatory disease of autoimmune etiology. However, it is covered in Chapter 5 as a hyperplastic disorder.

 ## ACUTE THYROIDITIS

Definition and Etiology

Acute thyroiditis is characterized by an inflammatory infiltration with a predominance of neutrophils. An alternate term is *suppurative thyroiditis*. This rare form of thyroiditis is usually caused by bacterial infection. Common infectious organisms include *Staphylococcus aureus, Streptococcus pyogenes, Streptococcus pneumoniae*, other streptococcal species, *Eikenella corrodens*, or a mixture of oropharyngeal flora.[1-6] Various other aerobic or anaerobic bacteria, mycobacteria, and parasites have also been reported as etiologic agents.[1,7-9] Fungi can cause thyroiditis with acute, chronic, and/or granulomatous inflammation, and fungal infections are discussed below in the section on granulomatous thyroiditis. Usually, the thyroid is secondarily involved either by an inflammatory process arising elsewhere in the neck or by a generalized septic process. Individuals with increased risk include those with preexisting thyroid disease such as carcinoma, chronic lymphocytic thyroiditis, or multinodular goiter; those with a pyriform sinus fistula; and immunocompromised or debilitated individuals.[10] Acute thyroiditis may be secondary to trauma or a rare complication of fine needle aspiration (FNA).[11-13]

In children, acute thyroiditis is usually associated with a pyriform sinus fistula.[5,14,15] Instances of acute thyroiditis owing to pyriform sinus fistula have also been reported in adults.[14-18] Pyriform sinus fistula is thought to be a developmental remnant of the thymopharyngeal duct (see Chapter 2).

The thymopharyngeal duct is a structure that forms as the thymus descends from the third pharyngeal pouch during fetal development. A persistent duct can result in a fistula, or more accurately a sinus tract, that typically extends in an antero-inferior direction from the pyriform sinus, ending blindly in the thyroid or perithyroidal tissue. Most cases occur on the left side.[5,15,19,20] Infections of the upper respiratory tract can be complicated by extension into a pyriform sinus fistula. These fistulae are usually demonstrated with a radiopaque fluid. A thyroglossal duct remnant is another potential means of a suppurative process reaching the thyroid.[21] Infections of thyroglossal duct cysts are relatively common, but the infectious process rarely involves the thyroid gland itself.[22,23]

Clinical Features

Common signs and symptoms of acute thyroiditis include fever, chills, sore throat, hoarseness, dysphagia, and neck pain. Neck pain is often unilateral and radiates to the jaw or ear. Acute thyroiditis is usually associated with a euthyroid state, but thyrotoxicosis has also been reported in some cases.[17,24-27]

Pathology

The size of an affected gland ranges from normal to mildly enlarged. Enlargement may be focal or diffuse, reflecting the extent of inflammation. Microscopic examination reveals a predominately neutrophilic infiltration (Fig. 4.1). The concentration of neutrophils can vary according to the causative agent and the immune status of the patient. Necrosis with microabscess formation is common in cases caused by pyogenic bacteria. Immunocompromised individuals may show minimal inflammatory response. FNA and culture are typically used to confirm a clinical diagnosis of acute thyroiditis. Aspiration yields evidence of acute inflammation, either overtly as purulent exudate or more subtly with a combination of cellular debris, fibrin strands, and neutrophils.[28]

Differential Diagnosis

Acute thyroiditis can present as a neck mass. The differential diagnosis of a painful anterior neck mass includes infected thyroglossal duct or branchial cleft cyst, lymphadenitis, cellulitis, and infected cystic hygroma.[4] Subacute granulomatous thyroiditis is typically associated with thyroid pain and fever, and although thyroid enlargement is usually diffuse, some cases present with localized, nodular enlargement (see Subacute Granulomatous Thyroiditis section below). Acute thyroiditis can also mimic a primary thyroid neoplasm, particularly anaplastic carcinoma if enlargement is rapid, or an extrathyroidal neoplasm with local extension.[29-32] Older adult age, history of dysphonia, right thyroid lobe involvement, large lesional size, sterile cultures of thyroid aspirates, and lack of improvement after antibiotic therapy favor neoplasia over acute thyroiditis.

Table 4.1

Thyroiditis Classification by Inflammatory Response and Clinical Course

Predominant Inflammatory Cell	Name	Synonyms	Subcategories	Clinical Course
Neutrophil	Acute thyroiditis	• Acute suppurative thyroiditis • Infectious thyroiditis	• Bacterial thyroiditis • Mycobacterial thyroiditis • Fungal thyroiditis • Parasitic thyroiditis	Acute
Macrophage/histiocyte	Subacute granulomatous thyroiditis	• de Quervain thyroiditis • Subacute thyroiditis • Painful subacute thyroiditis • Postviral thyroiditis • Giant cell thyroiditis • Subacute nonsuppurative thyroiditis • Pseudotuberculous thyroiditis • Struma granulomatosa		Subacute
	Infectious granulomatous thyroiditis	• Infectious thyroiditis	• Tuberculosis • Fungal thyroiditis	Subacute to chronic
	Sarcoidosis Granulomatous vasculitis Other granulomatous reactions		• Reaction to hemorrhage • Reaction to surgery • Foreign body reaction	Subacute to chronic to subclinical
	Palpation thyroiditis	• Multifocal granulomatous folliculitis		Subclinical
Lymphocyte	Chronic lymphocytic thyroiditis	• Hashimoto thyroiditis • Autoimmune thyroiditis • Struma lymphomatosum	• Classic • Fibrous variant • Atrophic or fibrous atrophy variant • Juvenile variant • Hashitoxicosis variant	Chronic
	Silent thyroiditis	• Sporadic thyroiditis • Painless thyroiditis • Painless sporadic thyroiditis • Painless thyroiditis with hyperthyroidism • Silent thyrotoxic thyroiditis • Subacute lymphocytic thyroiditis • Atypical subacute thyroiditis • Spontaneously resolving hyperthyroidism • Lymphocytic thyroiditis with spontaneously resolving hyperthyroidism		Subacute
	Postpartum thyroiditis	• Painless postpartum thyroiditis		
	Focal lymphocytic thyroiditis	• Nonspecific thyroiditis • Focal autoimmune thyroiditis		Subclinical
	Invasive fibrous thyroiditis	• Riedel thyroiditis • Fibrosing thyroiditis • Sclerosing thyroiditis		Chronic

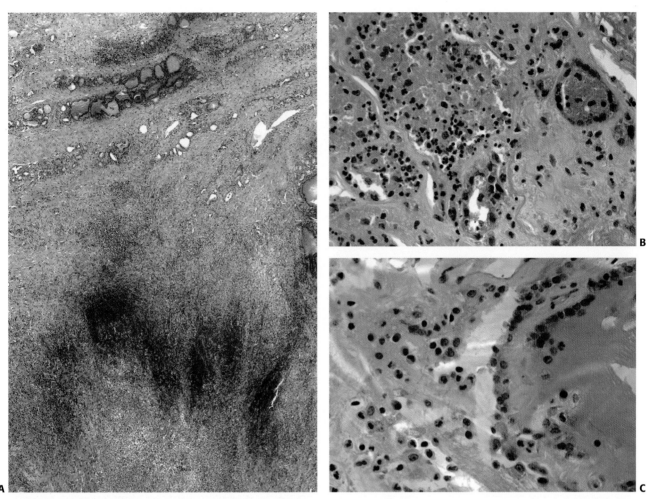

FIGURE 4.1. Acute thyroiditis secondary to a bacterial infection that initially affected extrathyroidal tissues. A: Low-power photomicrograph showing abscess **(lower)** with extension of inflammatory process into thyroid **(upper)**. **B and C:** Medium- and high-power photomicrographs showing abundant neutrophils associated with damaged and necrotic follicles.

GRANULOMATOUS THYROIDITIS

Subacute Granulomatous Thyroiditis (Subacute or de Quervain Thyroiditis)

Definition

Subacute granulomatous thyroiditis (SGT) is an inflammatory condition characterized by the presence of epithelioid macrophages and variable numbers of multinucleated giant cells. Alternate names include de Quervain thyroiditis, subacute thyroiditis, painful subacute thyroiditis, postviral thyroiditis, giant cell thyroiditis, subacute nonsuppurative thyroiditis, pseudotuberculous thyroiditis, struma granulomatosa, and other permutations of the preceding terms. This form of thyroiditis is known commonly as subacute thyroiditis, but the inclusion of granulomatous helps to distinguish it from subacute lymphocytic thyroiditis. Granulomatous inflammation of the thyroid may be the result of well-known causes of granulomatous inflammation such as tuberculosis, fungal infections, or sarcoidosis. Subacute granulomatous thyroiditis is a clinicopathologic entity that appears to be the sequela of a systemic illness.

Etiology

Viral infection is the most suspect etiology given the common prodromal signs and symptoms, and several studies offer support.[33-36]

The incidence is highest in the summer when the incidence of enteroviral infections is also highest.[37] One study of SGT demonstrated intrathyroidal activated T cytotoxic/suppressor cells and interferon γ (INF-γ) positive lymphocytes consistent with a viral infection.[38] Several viruses have been implicated as causative agents including coxsackievirus, adenovirus, mumps virus, Epstein–Barr virus, rubeola (measles), Varicella zoster (chicken pox), cytomegalovirus, influenza, rubella, and human foamy virus.[39] However, the etiologic association with viral infection is not conclusive because several studies have failed to find evidence of viral infection.[39-42]

Some cases of subacute granulomatous thyroiditis have been associated with antiviral therapy, particularly INF.[43-46] There have been recent reports of subacute granulomatous thyroiditis among individuals receiving etanercept, an antagonist of tumor necrosis factor α.[47,48] Certain individuals may have a genetic predisposition for this disease, including those with HLA-B35 haplotype.[49-54]

Clinical Features

Subacute granulomatous thyroiditis generally affects young to middle-aged adults.[55-59] Children are rarely affected.[60] Women are affected more commonly than men by a ratio ranging from 2 to 4:1.[57-59] Patients usually experience a prodrome of low-grade fever, myalgias, and fatigue, and present with fever and neck pain. Subacute granulomatous thyroiditis is the most common cause of a painful thyroid gland.[56,61] However, a significant number of patients do not experience pain or tenderness. C-reactive protein and erythrocyte sedimentation rate are usually elevated.[62] A minority of patients have significant elevation of antibodies to thyroglobulin (Tg) or thyroperoxidase (TPO), but these elevated titers are usually transient.[58,59,63–65]

Subacute granulomatous thyroiditis commonly presents with hyperthyroidism and, after a period of weeks to several months, passes through a euthyroid phase. Rarely, patients may present with thyroid storm.[66,67] The euthyroid stage is typically followed by a hypothyroid stage that may last for weeks to months before resumption of normal thyroid function.[10,64,68] Spontaneous return to euthyroidism occurs in most patients within 6 to 12 months, but between 2% and 15% of patients experience persistent hypothyroidism.[57,64,69–71] Recurrence has been reported in about 2% of cases after a latency that may exceed 10 years.[72,73] Conversion to chronic autoimmune thyroiditis or Graves disease has been reported.[74–78]

Pathology

The thyroid gland is enlarged, typically about twice its normal size. The enlargement is often asymmetric, even though the inflammatory process usually affects the entire gland. A small percentage of cases present as a solitary nodule.[79,80] Areas with more pronounced changes appear as tan to yellow-white, ill-defined nodules that are firm to palpation (Fig. 4.2).

Microscopic findings exhibit temporal variation. The early stage is characterized by follicular damage with loss of epithelium and colloid. Acute and chronic inflammatory cells fill the residual follicles and extend into the surrounding interfollicular areas. During the early stage, neutrophils are the predominant inflammatory cell and microabscesses may be present.

Over time, the inflammation attains a granulomatous and chronically inflamed appearance with epithelioid and nonepithelioid macrophages, multinucleated giant cells, lymphocytes, plasma cells, and variable degrees of fibrosis (Fig. 4.3).[81–83] Giant cells are typically associated with disrupted follicles and may encircle residual colloid. Distinct granulomata or lymphoid follicles are not characteristic of subacute granulomatous thyroiditis. Reparative changes become more apparent during the latter course of the disease as fibrous tissue replaces the areas of follicular destruction. With time, the fibrotic areas are partially or fully restored to follicular tissue. Zones of active inflammation can coexist with areas of fibrosis as the inflammatory process spreads to previously uninvolved thyroid parenchyma.

Controversy exists regarding the nature of multinucleated giant cells seen in subacute granulomatous thyroiditis. Some have thought that they represent altered follicular cells or macrophages surrounding extravasated colloid that collectively simulate giant cells (pseudogiant cells).[33,84] However, most consider them to be macrophages (histiocytes) that have fused into a single multinucleated cell comparable with those seen in other types of granulomatous inflammation. Immunohistochemical studies have found that most giant cells are positive for CD68, lysozyme, α1-antitrypsin, and vimentin although being typically negative for Tg, epithelial membrane antigen, and cytokeratin.[81,85] An ultrastructural study revealed that most multinucleated giant cells had structures identical with those of infiltrating macrophages.[85]

Cytopathology

Cases of subacute thyroiditis are rarely seen as resection specimens because most are diagnosed on the basis of clinical features and laboratory tests and are treated medically. Increased use of sonography and FNA have also decreased surgical procedures.[86] In the early stage of disease, fine needle aspirates contain neutrophils in addition to mononuclear inflammatory cells and

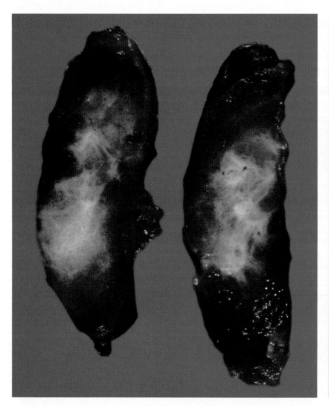
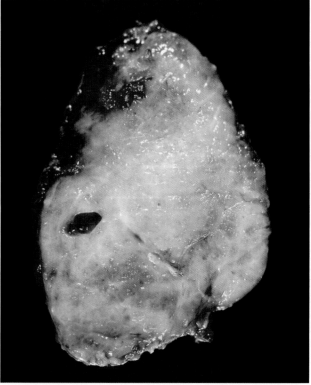

FIGURE 4.2. Cut surfaces of two different thyroids with subacute granulomatous thyroiditis. The inflammation and fibrosis in the thyroid pictured on the left resulted in a lesion clinically interpreted as a nodule.

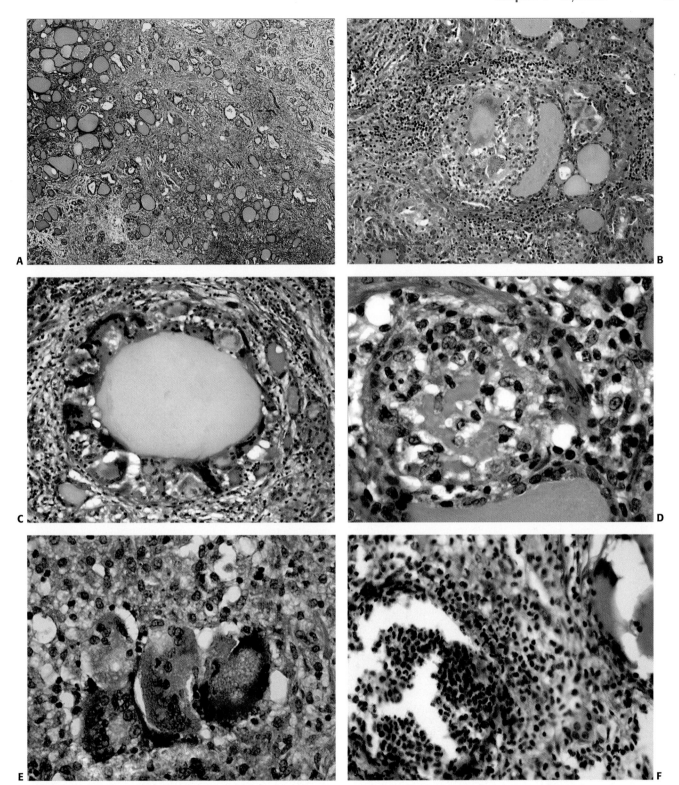

FIGURE 4.3. Subacute granulomatous thyroiditis. A: Low-power view showing decreased numbers of follicles. **B and C:** Medium-power views showing follicular damage with loss of epithelium and colloid and encirclement of follicle by multinucleated giant cells. **D and E:** High-power views showing granulomatous inflammation with predominance of macrophages and giant cells. **F:** High-power view showing mixture of acute and chronic inflammation with abundant neutrophils within an effaced follicle.

degenerated follicular cells.[82,83,87] Oncocytic follicular cells are absent. In the latter stages, characteristic findings include multinucleated giant cells, strands of fibrous tissue, and a mixture of

lymphocytes, macrophages, and possibly neutrophils.[88–90] Follicular cells are usually scant to absent, and granulomata are rarely seen.

Differential Diagnosis

The differential diagnosis of subacute granulomatous thyroiditis includes sarcoidosis, palpation thyroiditis, and other forms of granulomatous thyroiditis that are discussed in the next section.

Other Types of Granulomatous Thyroiditis

Palpation Thyroiditis

Palpation thyroiditis is a very common finding in surgically resected thyroid glands. As the name implies, it appears to be caused by pressure-induced damage and rupture of follicles by squeezing during manual examination.[91] Focally, palpation thyroiditis bears resemblance to subacute granulomatous thyroiditis, and an alternative name is multifocal granulomatous folliculitis. The damage associated with palpation thyroiditis is slight and not associated with clinical signs and symptoms, impairment of thyroid function, or significant release of Tg into the blood stream.[92]

Palpation thyroiditis is not evident grossly in most cases. Foci of hemorrhage are seen occasionally. Microscopic examination reveals focal damage limited to a single or small group of follicles. In the affected follicles, the epithelium is absent and a ring of multinucleated giant cells may encircle the residual colloid in its place (Fig. 4.4). The follicle may be totally effaced, with the colloid replaced by an infiltrate of macrophages, multinucleated giant cells, lymphocytes, and plasma cells. Palpation thyroiditis is distinguished from subacute granulomatous thyroiditis based on the very limited extent of changes. Typically, only single scattered follicles are affected, and there is absence of acute inflammatory cells and overt necrosis.

Tuberculosis

Tuberculosis of the thyroid is rare, and isolated tuberculosis is extremely rare because thyroid disease is usually associated with infection elsewhere in the body. Infection may occur through hematogenous dissemination or by direct extension from adjacent structures such as lymph nodes. The clinical presentation is variable. Normal thyroid function is usually maintained, and other thyroidal signs or symptoms may be absent, particularly if involvement represents miliary spread. Tuberculosis can also present as a nodule or abscess.[93-97] Diagnosis of tuberculosis in nodular lesions is typically a surprise discovery during the evaluation for neoplasia.

The pathologic manifestations of thyroid tuberculosis are similar to those found in the lungs and other extrapulmonary organs. The typical histologic finding is multiple coalescing granulomata with and without necrosis (caseation).[95,98] Abscess-like lesions can form when necrosis is abundant. Some lesions can exhibit marked fibrosis and therefore be particularly difficult to differentiate from subacute granulomatous thyroiditis. FNA plays an important role by allowing diagnosis without surgical resection. Tuberculosis should be included in the differential diagnosis when FNA reveals epithelioid granulomata, particularly when necrosis is also evident.[99-101] Diagnosis can be confirmed by the demonstration of *Mycobacterium tuberculosis* with an acid-fast stain, culture, and/or DNA polymerase chain reaction.[102]

Fungal Infection

Fungal infections of the thyroid can manifest with granulomatous inflammation, although a component of acute inflammation is often present and may predominate. Deep yeast infections such as histoplasmosis and coccidioidomycosis have been reported, but such cases are rare (Fig. 4.5).[103,104] *Aspergillus* species are the most common cause of fungal thyroiditis and are usually part of a disseminated infection affecting immunocompromised individuals.[8,105] The inflammatory response in these cases is not granulomatous but rather acute or absent (Fig. 4.6). The diagnosis of fungal thyroiditis rests on the demonstration of fungal yeast or hyphae, usually with the adjunct of specially stained sections.

Sarcoidosis

The thyroid may be involved in cases of sarcoidosis. Such instances seem to be rare, or at least rarely detected. Well-formed, nonnecrotizing granulomata, similar to those seen in other affected organs, are characteristic findings.[106,107] The granulomata are typically located in the stroma and do not center on follicles, in contrast to subacute granulomatous thyroiditis and palpation thyroiditis. Inflammatory changes in sarcoidosis range from minimal to foci with effacement of thyroid architecture. Special stains for acid-fast bacilli and fungi are indicated to help rule out an infectious etiology.

Definitive diagnosis of sarcoidosis is problematic because of its uncertain etiology and the need to eliminate other granulomatous diseases. Discovery of nonnecrotizing granulomata in the thyroid may be just the initial step if similar granulomata have not been demonstrated in other tissues. Additional studies will be necessary to yield a diagnosis of sarcoidosis with reasonable confidence.

Sarcoidosis can present as a cold nodule that mimics a neoplasm.[108,109] Coexistence of sarcoidosis and autoimmune thyroid

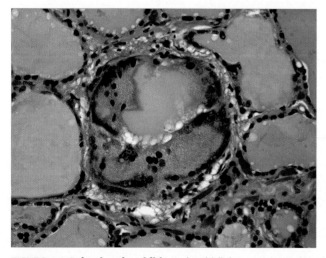
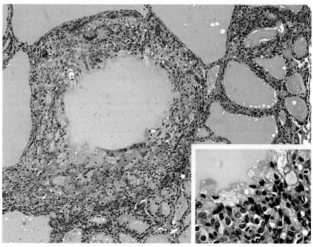

FIGURE 4.4. Palpation thyroiditis. Isolated follicle containing multinucleated giant cells **(left)**. Disruption of a single follicle with a more intense surrounding inflammatory response **(right)**. The high-power insert shows the predominance of macrophages.

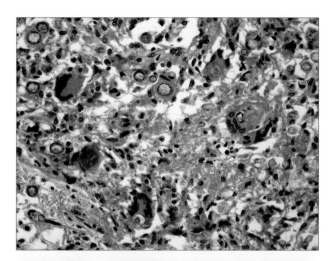

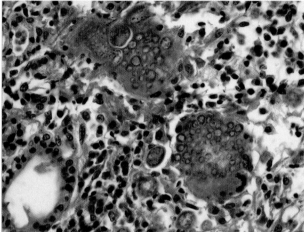

FIGURE 4.5. Coccidioidomycosis involving thyroid. An ill-defined granulomatous response is present focally **(top)** with scattered multinucleated giant cells. Overall, the inflammatory response in this case is predominately lymphoplasmacytic **(bottom)**. Variably sized spherules are shown along with endospores within large spherules.

diseases has been observed.[110–114] The most frequent coexisting disease is chronic lymphocytic (Hashimoto) thyroiditis. Although several cases of sarcoidosis with clinically overt chronic lymphocytic thyroiditis are relatively low, the incidence seems higher than by simple coincidence. The frequency of autoantibodies to Tg and/or TPO among individuals with sarcoidosis has been found to be as high[114] as 27%. Rare cases of sarcoidosis associated with hyperthyroidism have also been reported.[113,115–117]

 CHRONIC THYROIDITIS

General Overview

Any discussion of chronic thyroiditis, particularly thyroiditis with predominately lymphocytic infiltrates, is fraught with difficulty related to the wide spectrum of histologic and clinical features and the attendant nomenclature. Table 4.1 illustrates the various names and synonyms that comprise these potentially confusing and sometimes overlapping classifications. A unifying approach is to view the various types of lymphocytic thyroiditis as manifestations of autoimmune disease, sharing the common feature of circulating antibodies to thyroid antigens. The prevalence of thyroid autoantibodies is relatively high in the general population, but the range of manifestations is broad.[118] In many instances, autoimmunity is subclinical with no appreciable effect on thyroid function. The clinical course is variable because many cases remain subclinical for a prolonged time.[119] Development of overt hypothyroidism is common after periods of time ranging up to a decade or more, but progression to overt disease does not seem to be an inevitable event.

The associated pathologic changes in turn range from focal lymphocytic infiltrates with minimal follicular damage to dense lymphoplasmacytic infiltrates with germinal centers and metaplastic epithelial changes and to atrophic glands with marked fibrosis. The dividing lines between categories in the spectrum of lymphocytic thyroiditis are not drawn sharply. Classification can be problematic, particularly in cases with early or limited inflammatory changes, and definitive evaluation will likely require integration of pathologic, clinical, and other ancillary studies. These confounding factors make it difficult to determine precisely the incidence of lymphocytic thyroiditis and its forms. However, it appears to be a common condition. Focal lymphocytic aggregates are seen in 10% to 45% of adult thyroid glands at the time of autopsy.[120–122] Evidence of thyroiditis is more frequent among women, and in some groups of older women, >50% exhibit some degree of lymphocytic thyroiditis.

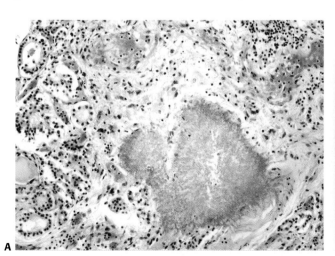

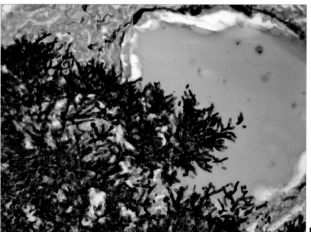

FIGURE 4.6. Fungal infection involving thyroid of an immunocompromised host. A: Medium-power photomicrograph showing aggregate of the fungus *Scedosporium prolificans* invading thyroid parenchyma with minimal inflammatory response (hematoxylin and eosin stain). **B:** High-power view showing fungal hyphae (Grocott methenamine silver stain).

Chronic Lymphocytic Thyroiditis (Hashimoto or Autoimmune Thyroiditis)

Definition

Chronic lymphocytic thyroiditis, alternatively known as Hashimoto thyroiditis or autoimmune thyroiditis, is an autoimmune disorder characterized by the destruction of follicular cells. The eponymous name recognizes Hakaru Hashimoto, who in 1912 described four cases for which he used the term *struma lymphomatosa*.[123] The major clinical manifestation of chronic lymphocytic thyroiditis is hypothyroidism because of immune-mediated loss of follicular cells.

Epidemiology

The disease has a peak incidence in the fifth decade of life, and affected individuals range from children to older adults.[10,124,125] Although adults are more commonly affected than children, chronic lymphocytic thyroiditis is the most common form of thyroiditis among children and adolescents.[124,126] Women are affected more commonly than men by a ratio ranging from 5 to 20:1.[10,125,127]

Some individuals have a genetic predisposition to develop chronic lymphocytic thyroiditis. The susceptibility genes appear to include the major histocompatibility gene *HLA-DR*, immune modifying genes including cytotoxic T-lymphocyte–associated factor 4 (*CTLA-4*), and thyroid-specific genes such as *Tg*.[128,129] Analysis of the HLA-DR peptide-binding pocket has revealed that certain amino acid sequences increase susceptibility to autoimmune thyroiditis. The sequences Tyr-26, Tyr-30, Gln-70, Lys-71, and Arg-74 have the highest predisposition, and Lys-71 shows the strongest individual association.[130]

Pathogenesis

The pathogenesis of chronic lymphocytic thyroiditis is an incompletely understood process that involves both cell-mediated and humoral mechanisms.[131] The initial event appears to be activation of CD4+ T helper lymphocytes. Activation of T helper cells is generally thought to result from a complex interaction of genes and environmental factors. Several environmental triggers have been implicated, and they include iodine intake, medications, infections, smoking, and environmental toxins.[132,133] The prevalence of chronic lymphocytic thyroiditis is highest in populations with the highest dietary intake of iodine.[134] Medications associated with an increased risk of autoimmune thyroiditis include INF-α and amiodarone. Various bacterial and viral infections have been implicated, but none conclusively. Hepatitis C virus infection appears to have the strongest association, and concomitant INF-α therapy may have a synergistic effect.[135,136]

Activated T helper cells in turn activate several mechanisms that damage follicular cells including production of cytokines, such as INF-γ, that recruit and activate macrophages and natural killer (NK) cells. T helper cells also stimulate B cells to secrete antibodies against various components of follicular cells. CD8+ cytotoxic T cells may play a role by their recognition of follicular cell antigens and destruction of these cells with perforin and other cytotoxic agents.

Potential mechanisms by which follicular cells become the target of immune injury include antigen mimicry and bystander activation of intrathyroidal lymphocytes. *Borrelia burgdorferi* and *Yersinia enterocolitica* have proteins that share homology with thyroid autoantigens and thus are suspects for antigen mimicry, although a direct causal effect remains unproven at this time.[137]

Several studies have provided evidence that autoimmune thyroiditis may be associated with a bystander mechanism in which release of cytokines owing to an infection or other stimulus activates autoreactive T cells.[138–140] These autoreactive T cells are present in the thyroid and are normally suppressed by regulatory T (Treg) cells or other tolerance mechanisms.[141] An environmental trigger such as a viral infection may cause release of cytokines and activation of normally dormant T cells.

CTLA-4 protein is a suppressor of T-cell activation, and decreased expression may contribute to excessive and prolonged T-cell activity. Autoimmune thyroiditis has been linked to the length of the AT repeat of the 3'UTP microsatellite of *CTLA-4*.[142] An increase in length is associated with decreased expression and consequent lower inhibitory activity. Other polymorphisms of *CTLA-4* may lead to diminished T-cell regulation and play a role in autoimmune thyroiditis.[143]

Apoptosis plays a significant role in follicular cell destruction. Increased numbers of apoptotic follicular cells are found in chronic lymphocytic thyroiditis, and the highest concentration of apoptotic cells correlates with proximity to lymphoid follicles.[144,145] Interaction between the Fas receptor (Fas, CD95, or APO-1) and its ligand (FasL or CD95L) has received considerable attention as having a major role in apoptosis. Although the Fas–FasL pathway appears to be operant in chronic lymphocytic thyroiditis, the details of the interaction are controversial. Follicular cells have been shown to express Fas, particularly when exposed to INF-γ and interleukin 1β (IL-1β).[146] Increased FasL expression has been observed in chronic lymphocytic thyroiditis along with low expression of the antiapoptotic protein Bcl-2, whereas infiltrating lymphocytes show low levels of Fas–FasL expression and relatively high levels of Bcl-2 expression.[147,148] These proportions of apoptotic and antiapoptotic factors appear to favor apoptosis of follicular cells and preservation of infiltrating lymphoid cells. Follicular cell expression of both Fas and FasL could result in lethal interactions among these cells.[147,149,150] However, expression of FasL by follicular cells in chronic lymphocytic thyroiditis has not been a universal observation, so the specifics of Fas–FasL interaction are unclear.[151,152] Further complicating the matter is the possible interplay of the soluble form of Fas, which appears to inhibit Fas–FasL interaction and prevent apoptosis of target cells.[153]

Autoantibodies against TPO and Tg are characteristically present in chronic lymphocytic thyroiditis.[154] Questions exist regarding the significance of these antibodies in the pathogenesis of chronic lymphocytic thyroiditis, particularly whether they play a primary or secondary role or are merely an epiphenomenon with limited importance beyond their role in diagnostic tests. Most individuals with measurable antibody levels are euthyroid. However, a subset of these euthyroid individuals will progress to a hypothyroid state.

TPO and Tg are sequestered antigens that do not normally interact with the immune system. These antigens can become exposed during follicular cell damage. The damage may be because of sublethal disruption of cell integrity by cytokines such as IL-1α, infiltration of the follicle by lymphocytes, or overt follicular necrosis by various mechanisms.[155] Follicular cell damage can expose TPO and Tg and can result in the stimulation of both T and B cells with subsequent formation of antibodies.[156] Antibodies to TPO, earlier known as antimicrosomal antibodies,[157] have the potential to damage follicular cells because of their ability to fix complement with subsequent cell lysis by antibody-dependent, cell-mediated cytotoxicity (ADCC).[158] TPO appears to be the major antigen involved in ADCC of the thyroid.[159] In ADCC, antibodies bind to target cells and then to NK cells, macrophages, and/or neutrophils through their Fc receptors. Antibodies binding to and blocking the thyroid-stimulating hormone receptor have also been described and may contribute to further impairment in thyroid function.

Some cases of chronic lymphocytic thyroiditis may be a manifestation of immunoglobulin G4–related sclerosing (or systemic) disease (IgG4-RSD).[160] IgG4-RSD was initially described in cases of sclerosing pancreatitis,[161] but elevated numbers of IgG4-positive plasma cells have since been described in fibroinflammatory disorders involving the thyroid, biliary tract, salivary gland, lacrimal gland, retroperitoneum, orbit, liver, lung, kidney, prostate gland, aorta, lymph node, breast, and other sites.[162] The basic pathologic features include lymphoplasmacytic infiltrates with significant numbers of IgG4-positive plasma cells and dense stromal fibrosis that may form a mass-like lesion. Correlation of these features with variants of chronic lymphocytic thyroiditis is discussed below.

The underlying pathogenic mechanisms of IgG4-RSD are in the process of elucidation. A study of IgG4-related sclerosing cholangitis found significant upregulation of T helper 2 cytokines IL-4, IL-5, and IL-13 and regulatory cytokines IL-10 and transforming growth factor β (TGF-β).[163] The investigators postulated that Treg cells might be responsible for the production of IL-10 and TGF-β

with subsequent IgG4 class switching and sclerosis. The study of IgG4-RSD is an area of active investigation, and the significance of IgG4-RSD and its relationship to other pathogenic mechanisms associated with chronic lymphocytic thyroiditis remain to be clarified.

Pathology

Thyroid glands with chronic lymphocytic thyroiditis typically show diffuse enlargement two to four times their normal size with an average weight around 40 g, although weights of 200 g or more have been reported.[86,127] The enlargement is usually symmetric, but some variation in the size of the lobes may be seen (Fig. 4.7). The central pyramidal lobe if present may be relatively prominent. The cut surfaces are usually paler than the normal red-brown color, in large part reflecting the infiltration

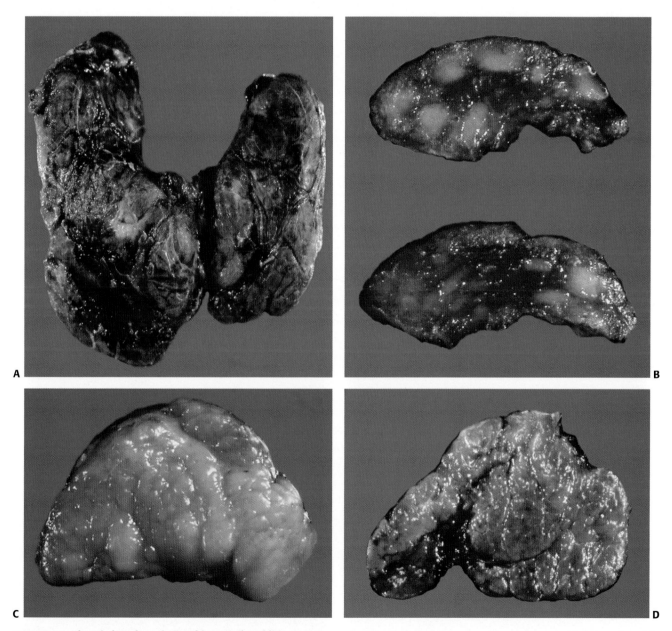

FIGURE 4.7. Chronic lymphocytic (Hashimoto) thyroiditis. A: Diffuse enlargement of gland. Enlargement is usually symmetric but can be mildly asymmetrical as shown with this gland's larger right lobe. Both lobes had comparable histopathologic features. Remnants of adhesions with the perithyroidal tissue are evident. **B–D:** Cut surfaces of three different glands showing accentuated lobulation and tissue paler than normal. The thyroid shown in **(B)** exhibits variegation with pale areas interspersed among the darker, more normal appearing tissue.

by lymphocytes and loss of follicular tissue. The cut surface may appear tan-yellow to pink-tan or yellowish gray and may show accentuated lobulation. The color can range from relatively homogeneous to variegated with pale areas interspersed among the darker, more normal appearing thyroid tissue.

Infiltration of the gland by lymphocytes and plasma cells is the most characteristic feature of chronic lymphocytic thyroiditis (Fig. 4.8). The lymphoplasmacytic infiltration is diffuse but variable in its intensity and effacement of the follicles. The lobules may be accentuated by increased fibrous tissue within the interlobular septa (Fig. 4.9). Histologic findings correlate with thyroid function. Individuals with the full spectrum of histopathologic changes associated with chronic lymphocytic thyroiditis, particularly diffuse lymphoplasmacytic infiltration and oncocytic metaplasia, usually have overt or latent hypothyroidism, whereas those with mild, more focal changes are likely to be euthyroid.[164]

Immunohistochemical stains reveal a mixed population of T and B lymphocytes. T cells predominate with both CD4+ helper cells and CD8+ suppressor/cytotoxic cells identifiable (Fig. 4.10).[165] The CD4+:CD8+ ratio is usually around 7:1.[166] Germinal center formation is also a characteristic of chronic lymphocytic thyroiditis. Similar to germinal centers within lymph nodes, B cells predominate. Plasma cells show polyclonality with staining for IgG, IgM, and IgA heavy chains, and κ and λ light chains.[167]

Some cases show an abundance of IgG4-positive plasma cells.[160] These cases have features associated with the fibrous variant of chronic lymphocytic thyroiditis and may represent IgG4-RSD involving the thyroid.

Some degree of fibrosis is common, and extensive fibrosis is the hallmark of the fibrous and fibrous atrophy variants. Lymphoepithelial lesions (LELs) are common (Fig. 4.11), and some degree of follicular atrophy and loss is seen in all cases. Follicular epithelium can be quite scant in areas of intense lymphoplasmacytic infiltration.

Follicular epithelial cells in the areas of inflammation may reveal prominent reactive changes with enlarged nuclei and clearing of chromatin, resembling the nuclear features of papillary carcinoma (Fig. 4.12). However, these changes in chronic lymphocytic thyroiditis are most prominent in the areas of active inflammation and gradually subside peripherally. Papillary carcinomas, in contrast, typically have a distinct border between the neoplastic and nonneoplastic cells.

Variable numbers of follicular epithelium exhibit enlargement and abundant, finely granular eosinophilic cytoplasm, variously known as oncocytic, oxyphilic, Hürthle cell, or Askanazy cell metaplasia (Fig. 4.13). The term *oncocytic* is preferable for usage in this context because of the trend away from eponymous terms and the international use of this term for tumors with comparable cytologic features.[168] Although the term *Hürthle cell* is deeply

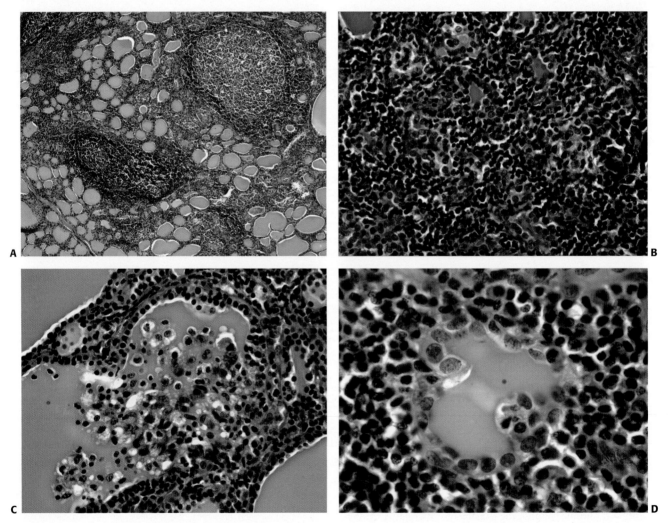

FIGURE 4.8. Chronic lymphocytic (Hashimoto) thyroiditis. A: Low-power view showing diffuse lymphoplasmacytic infiltration and germinal centers. **B:** Medium-power view showing dense lymphoplasmacytic infiltrate and loss of follicles. **C and D:** Medium- and high-power views showing follicular damage and extension of lymphocytes and macrophages into the central colloid region of follicles.

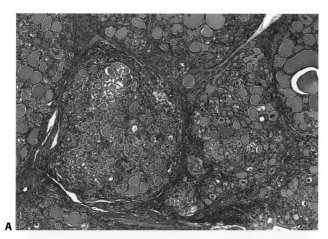

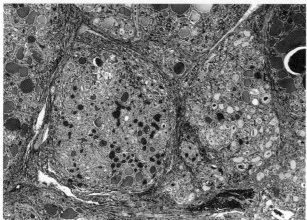

FIGURE 4.9. Chronic lymphocytic (Hashimoto) thyroiditis with lobular accentuation. A: Low-power photomicrograph showing lobular accentuation by increased interlobular fibrous tissue (hematoxylin and eosin stain). **B:** Low-power view of same region with fibrous tissue highlighted in blue by trichrome stain.

ingrained in common usage, it is problematic because Dr. Hürthle probably described C cells instead of follicular cells in his 1894 publication[169] (see Chapter 14).

The cytoplasmic granularity of oncocytic follicular cells correlates with the ultrastructural finding of numerous mitochondria and decreased numbers of other organelles. The mitochondria are abnormal with functional and molecular defects related to cytochrome c oxidase of the respiratory chain.[170] In addition to cytoplasmic enlargement, oncocytic follicular cells may also show nuclear enlargement and prominent nucleoli.

Squamous metaplasia also may be seen in chronic lymphocytic thyroiditis (Fig. 4.14A). Although squamous metaplasia can be present in the classical form of chronic lymphocytic thyroiditis, it is more common in the fibrous and fibrous atrophy variants. Rare cases with extreme degrees of squamous metaplasia that mimic squamous or mucoepidermoid carcinoma have been reported.[171] Occasionally, multinucleated giant cells are found in chronic lymphocytic thyroiditis, but they are few and should not cause confusion with subacute granulomatous thyroiditis (Fig. 4.14B). Most of these giant cells are derived from fusion of macrophages, although some may represent altered follicular cells.[167]

Cytologic Features
FNA yields cytologic findings reflective of the histologic features (Fig. 4.15). Aspirates tend to be cellular and populated with lymphocytes, plasma cells, and oncocytic follicular cells. Oncocytic cells exhibit more abundant cytoplasm with a subtle, fine granularity and nuclei that are larger and more variable in size compared with normal follicular cells. Extruded strings of nuclear chromatin are common because of the abundance of lymphocytes that are disrupted during the preparation of smears. Larger transformed lymphocytes and tingible body macrophages of germinal center derivation may be seen.

Perithyroidal Changes
Generally, the inflammatory process is confined to the thyroid gland but may sometimes extend into the perithyroidal tissues. The latter situation can manifest intraoperatively as the surgeon experiences difficultly dissecting the thyroid away from the adjacent tissues. However, adhesions are usually light and readily lysed in contrast to the dense confluence of the thyroid with perithyroidal tissues seen with invasive fibrous (Riedel) thyroiditis. Perithyroidal lymph nodes can exhibit reactive lymphadenopathy and raise concern of metastatic disease.

Associated Neoplasia

Individuals with chronic lymphocytic thyroiditis have an increased risk (~67-fold) of primary thyroid lymphoma.[172] Although the lymphoid population of chronic lymphocytic thyroiditis is polyclonal, a monoclonal population can emerge and progress to lymphoma.[165,173,174] Most lymphomas arising in the setting of chronic lymphocytic thyroiditis are either diffuse large B-cell lymphomas or low-grade B-cell mucosa-associated lymphoid tissue (MALT) lymphomas.[175] Thyroid lymphomas with T-cell phenotype are rare. Many of the diffuse large B-cell lymphomas appear to be transformations of low-grade MALT lymphomas, whereas evidence suggests that a subset of diffuse B-cell lymphomas arise de novo.[176] Features suggestive of low-grade MALT lymphoma include marked loss of follicular epithelium, predominance of B cells, and frequent B-cell LELs.[165] Monoclonality may be established by immunostains for κ and λ light chains or PCR for Ig heavy chain gene rearrangement.

Some studies suggest an association between chronic lymphocytic thyroiditis and papillary thyroid carcinoma. However, it is unclear whether chronic lymphocytic thyroiditis is a significant risk factor. This putative association is discussed in Chapter 11. Marked chronic lymphocytic thyroiditis may be seen in cases of *PTEN*-hamartoma tumor syndrome in association with nodular hyperplasia/multiple adenomatous nodules, papillary carcinoma, follicular carcinoma, and/or follicular adenomas.[177]

Variants of Chronic Lymphocytic Thyroiditis

Several variants of chronic lymphocytic thyroiditis exist including fibrous, fibrous atrophy, hashitoxicosis, and juvenile (Table 4.3).

Fibrous Variant
The classic form of chronic lymphocytic thyroiditis has slight to moderate fibrosis, which accentuates interlobular septa. The fibrous variant has marked deposition of dense fibrous tissue with effacement of the thyroid architecture and marked follicular atrophy (Figs. 4.16 and 4.17). The fibrosis is limited to the thyroid in contrast to the extrathyroidal fibrosis of invasive fibrous (Riedel) thyroiditis. Similar to classic chronic lymphocytic thyroiditis, the fibrous variant shows diffuse lymphoplasmacytic infiltrates, germinal centers, and oncocytic metaplasia. However, squamous metaplasia is more common and usually prominent. The fibrous variant is usually found in late middle-aged or elderly individuals with hypothyroidism who present with symptomatic goiter that

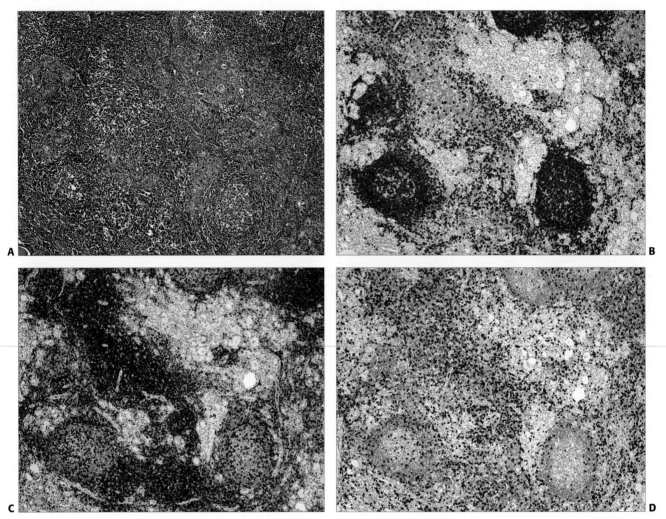

FIGURE 4.10. Chronic lymphocytic (Hashimoto) thyroiditis showing distribution and relative concentrations of B and T lymphocytes.
A: Hematoxylin and eosin–stained section. **B:** CD20-immunostained section showing highest concentration of B lymphocytes in germinal centers.
C: CD4-immunostained section highlighting T helper lymphocytes. **D:** CD8-immunostained section highlighting T suppressor/cytotoxic lymphocytes.

may require surgical removal to relieve problems caused by the enlargement.

Features of the fibrous variant have been associated with the presence of elevated numbers of IgG4-positive plasma cells.[160,162] A recent study divided cases of autoimmune thyroiditis into two groups using the criteria of >20 IgG4-positive plasma cells per high-power (400×) field plus >30% IgG4/IgG ratio.[160] The IgG4-positive plasma cell rich group exhibited a significantly higher degree of stromal fibrosis, lymphoplasmacytic infiltration, and follicular cell degeneration. Follicular cell degeneration was not explicitly defined but appears to encompass follicular atrophy and loss of colloid.

The IgG4-positive plasma cell rich group had a significant shorter disease duration period from the time of diagnosis to total thyroidectomy and had a relatively higher percentage of males, although females still outnumbered males in both groups. The significance of IgG4-positive plasma cell infiltrates and their degree of specificity for fibrous variant remain to be confirmed and clarified by additional investigation. However, the shorter duration of disease suggests that the fibrous variant is not simply the result of long-standing chronic lymphocytic thyroiditis.

Fibrous Atrophy Variant

The fibrous atrophy variant is histologically similar to the fibrous variant. The main difference between these two variants is the small size of glands with fibrous atrophy (Fig. 4.18). Individuals with fibrous atrophy variant are typically elderly with marked hypothyroidism. Whether most cases of fibrous atrophy variant are rich in IgG4-positive plasma cells is undetermined at this time. Also unclear at this time is whether the fibrous atrophy variant represents progression of the fibrous variant and/or classic form of chronic lymphocytic thyroiditis or has a distinct pathogenic mechanism. Few cases of chronic lymphocytic thyroiditis are followed on a histologic basis over time, but at least one study[178] showed similar histologic features in biopsies separated by an interval of 10 to 20 years. This suggests that fibrous atrophy may not be simply a matter of duration of disease.

Hashitoxicosis

Hashitoxicosis is a variant in which features of chronic lymphocytic (Hashimoto) thyroiditis coexist with diffuse toxic hyperplasia (Graves disease). Hashitoxicosis does not have uniform histologic features but instead is a variant with variations. The largest series with histologic correlation derived from the Mayo Clinic

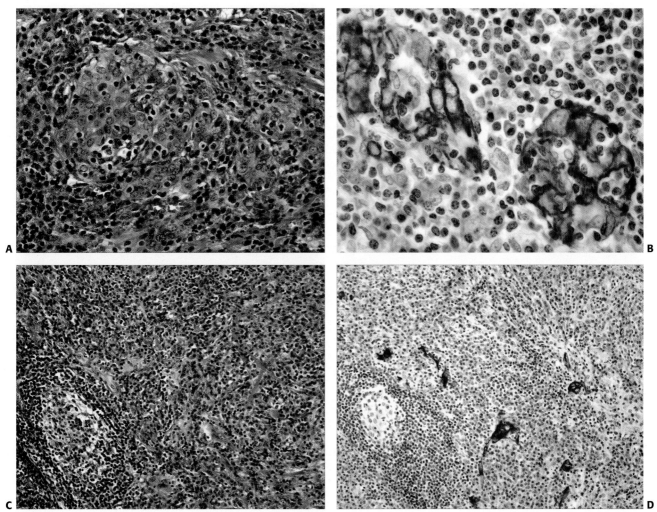

FIGURE 4.11. Chronic lymphocytic (Hashimoto) thyroiditis. A and B: LEL in which lymphocytes infiltrate altered follicular epithelium. **B:** Low molecular weight cytokeratin (CAM 5.2) immunostained section. **C and D:** Marked follicular loss with only small remnants of follicular epithelium demonstrable with cytokeratin immunostain (CAM 5.2).

in 1971.[179] The investigators found that some thyroids exhibited follicular epithelial hyperplasia in conjunction with the classical changes of chronic lymphocytic thyroiditis, whereas the other thyroids showed lymphocytic thyroiditis but more limited degrees of hyperplasia and/or oncocytic metaplasia.

Juvenile Variant

The juvenile variant is an ill-defined form of chronic lymphocytic thyroiditis that occurs in younger individuals and histologically shows little or no follicular atrophy.[127,180] Affected individuals may manifest thyroid function ranging from hyperthyroidism to hypothyroidism, and the clinical course is variable. Distinguishing this variant from silent thyroiditis or hashitoxicosis may be problematic. Further compounding the ill-defined nature of this variant is the broad clinical entity of juvenile autoimmune thyroiditis for which there is limited histopathologic correlation.

Postpartum Thyroiditis

Definition and Clinical Features

Postpartum thyroiditis is an autoimmune disease that occurs within the first year after delivery and results in temporary or permanent thyroid dysfunction. Thyroiditis may also occur after

a loss of pregnancy.[181] Classically, an initial hyperthyroid phase is followed by a hypothyroid phase.[182] The hyperthyroid phase usually occurs 1 to 6 months postpartum and lasts for 1 to 2 months. The hypothyroid phase usually manifests 3 to 8 months postpartum and lasts for 4 to 6 months.[10,170,183] However, one of the phases may not occur or be evident clinically as signs and symptoms tend to be mild. Although most patients return to a euthyroid state, the incidence of persistent or recurrent hypothyroidism is significant with reports ranging from 12% to 54%.[184–190] The prevalence of postpartum thyroiditis varies significantly among different studies, but in iodine-sufficient areas, it appears to be in the range of 5% to 8%.[170,186] Approximately 10% of postpartum women have detectable TPO antibodies, and about half of these experience postpartum thyroiditis.[170] Women with detectable TPO antibodies in early pregnancy have a 30% to 52% risk of developing postpartum thyroiditis. The degree of complement fixation by particular TPO antibodies may be an important factor in determining whether postpartum thyroiditis develops.[62]

Pathology

Most clinical studies of postpartum thyroiditis report mild enlargement of the thyroid.[182,185,191] Our knowledge regarding the histopathology of postpartum thyroiditis derives largely from the

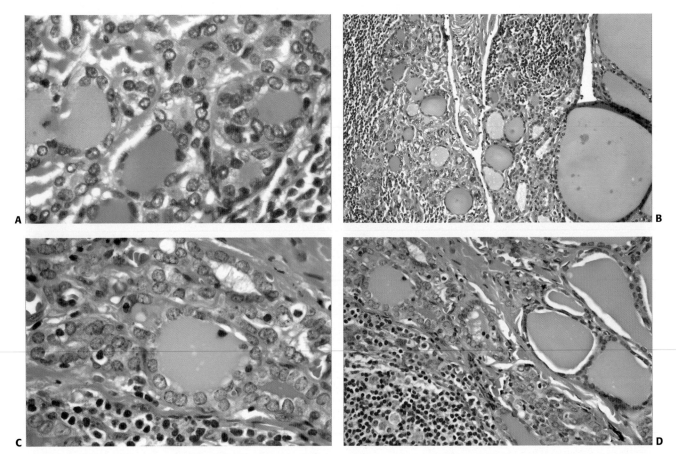

FIGURE 4.12. Photomicrographs of two cases of chronic lymphocytic (Hashimoto) thyroiditis (A and B) and (C and D) showing focal areas of follicular cell atypia mimicking papillary thyroid carcinoma. High-power views **(A and C)** show nuclear enlargement, crowding, and chromatin clearing. Lower-power views **(B and C)** show that the nuclear changes are present in ill-defined areas associated with lymphoid aggregates and that they subside with distance from the aggregates **(upper right)**.

report of Mizukami et al.,[192] who studied biopsies of 15 cases. Affected thyroids showed focal or diffuse lymphocytic infiltration comparable with that seen in silent thyroiditis. Follicular damage consisting of breakdown of follicles, infiltration of the follicle by degenerated, detached follicular epithelium, and dense infiltrates of lymphocytes around the follicles were commonly seen during the hypothyroid phase. Hyperplastic changes, defined as cuboidal or columnar epithelium and either irregularity of follicular shape or infolding of epithelium, were also common findings. During the recovery phase, follicular changes resolved and only

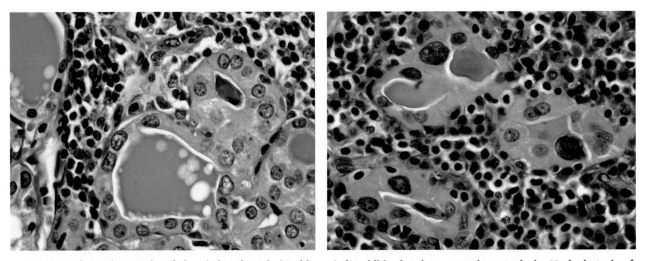

FIGURE 4.13. Photomicrographs of chronic lymphocytic (Hashimoto) thyroiditis showing oncocytic metaplasia. Marked atypia of metaplastic follicular epithelium is shown on the right.

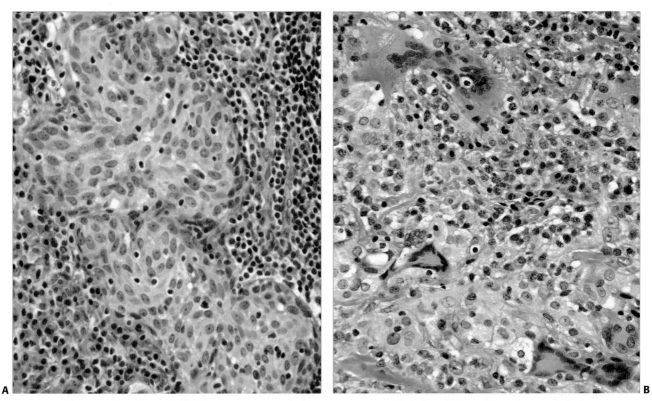

FIGURE 4.14. Chronic lymphocytic (Hashimoto) thyroiditis. A: Squamous metaplasia of follicular epithelium. **B:** Multinucleated giant cells admixed with follicular cells and lymphoplasmacytic infiltrate.

focal infiltration by lymphocytes was typically seen. Oncocytic metaplasia was absent or mild, and fibrosis was not present.

Clinical Course and Differential Diagnosis

The hyperthyroidism of postpartum thyroiditis appears to reflect disruption of follicles and release of thyroid hormone. This is supported by the low uptake of radioiodine during this phase.[192] The hypothyroid phase likely reflects sufficient follicular damage to impair hormone production, and the return to euthyroidism correlates with the resolution of follicular damage. The clinical course of transient hyperthyroidism followed by transient hypothyroidism is similar to subacute granulomatous thyroiditis. However, postpartum thyroiditis differs from subacute granulomatous thyroiditis in that the former lacks granulomatous inflammation, is painless, and seems to have a significantly higher rate of recurrent or permanent hypothyroidism. Postpartum thyroiditis differs from chronic lymphocytic thyroiditis by the absence of fibrosis, only mild or absent oncocytic metaplasia, and minimal to absent follicular atrophy. Clinically, postpartum thyroiditis differs from chronic lymphocytic thyroiditis by its frequent presentation as hyperthyroidism and spontaneous resolution in most cases.

Silent Thyroiditis

Definition and Clinical Features

Silent thyroiditis is also known as painless thyroiditis, painless thyroiditis with hyperthyroidism, sporadic thyroiditis, and various other combinations of silent, painless, sporadic, and hyperthyroidism (see Table 4.1). Silent thyroiditis has also been called chronic lymphocytic thyroiditis, leading to potential confusion

with the entity also known as Hashimoto thyroiditis. Silent thyroiditis is comparable with postpartum thyroiditis with the exception of antecedent pregnancy. Both types of thyroiditis represent subacute forms of autoimmune thyroiditis that classically have a transient period of hyperthyroidism followed by a period of hypothyroidism that spontaneously resolves. Resolution usually occurs within 2 to 5 months, and recurrence may occur but seems to be uncommon.[187,193] The etiology of silent thyroiditis is uncertain. Viral infection has been considered, but most studies have not yielded supporting evidence.[187] Various medications have been implicated including INF and lithium.[194–196]

Pathology

Analysis of silent thyroiditis is challenging given its various names and the limited number of histopathologic studies. Much of our knowledge regarding histopathologic changes derives from a study of biopsies by Mizukami et al.[197] Their series of 23 cases yielded findings similar to their study of postpartum thyroiditis (see above). All biopsies showed focal or diffuse lymphocytic infiltrates, with about even division between biopsies from the hyperthyroid or early recovery stage. Biopsies from the late stage of recovery only showed focal infiltrates. Most of the infiltrating lymphocytes marked as T cells, and the distribution of T and B cells was similar to that of chronic lymphocytic thyroiditis. About half of the biopsies contained lymphoid follicles. Follicular damage similar to that seen in postpartum thyroiditis was a characteristic feature in the earlier stages but was not a feature of the late recovery phase. Giant cells were visible in about two-thirds of the biopsies. Oncocytic metaplasia and fibrosis were usually absent or minimal. Similar histopathologic features were observed in other reports of cases with biopsy findings.[187,198-200]

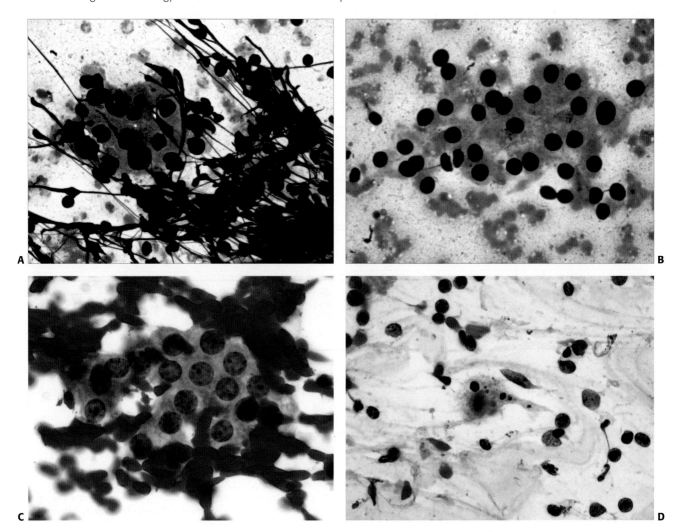

FIGURE 4.15. Fine needle aspirate cytologic features of chronic lymphocytic (Hashimoto) thyroiditis. A: Cluster of oncocytic follicular epithelium and numerous lymphocytes, many of which show crush artifact (Diff-Quik stain). **B:** Cluster of oncocytic follicular epithelium (Diff-Quik stain). **C:** Cluster of oncocytic follicular epithelium (Papanicolaou stain). **D:** Tingible body macrophage and surrounding lymphocytes (Papanicolaou stain).

Differential Diagnosis

Differentiation from subacute granulomatous thyroiditis, Graves disease, or chronic lymphocytic thyroiditis can be challenging. The absence of pain is a key clinical feature differentiating silent thyroiditis from subacute granulomatous thyroiditis. Histologically, silent thyroiditis may show some multinucleated giant cells in or around follicles, but it lacks the well-developed granulomatous inflammation of subacute granulomatous thyroiditis. In contrast to Graves disease, silent thyroiditis typically shows low uptake of radioactive iodine. This finding is consistent with the transient hyperthyroidism of silent thyroiditis being due to the release of thyroid hormone from damaged follicles as opposed to increased hormone production. Histologic features of silent thyroiditis overlap with chronic lymphocytic thyroiditis. The presence of oncocytic metaplasia, particularly if prominent, favors chronic lymphocytic thyroiditis. However, most cases will likely be distinguished on the basis of the clinical course.

Peritumoral Thyroiditis

Lymphocytic or lymphoplasmacytic infiltrates occur commonly around thyroid neoplasms, particularly papillary carcinoma.[201] The distinction between peritumoral thyroiditis and chronic

lymphocytic thyroiditis may be difficult with limited tissue sampling. However, in most cases, this is not a problem when non-neoplastic tissue away from the carcinoma can be evaluated for inflammatory features (Fig. 4.19). The significance of peritumoral thyroiditis is unclear in terms of pathogenesis, host response, and prognosis of thyroid neoplasia. Unfortunately, some studies of thyroiditis and thyroid carcinoma do not make a clear distinction between cases with peritumoral versus diffuse lymphocytic thyroiditis.

Focal Lymphocytic Thyroiditis

Definition and Clinical Features

Focal lymphocytic thyroiditis is a relatively common condition that is usually discovered incidentally in thyroid glands surgically resected for other reasons or those examined postmortem.[120–122] Alternate terms include *nonspecific thyroiditis* and *focal autoimmune thyroiditis*. The incidence is higher among women when compared with men, and among some population, it increases with age. One study found that about half of British women older than 70 years of age showed focal lymphocytic thyroiditis.[121] Whether focal lymphocytic thyroiditis represents an early or mild form of autoimmune thyroiditis is unclear. Making this determination for a lesion that is usually found incidentally at autopsy

Table 4.2

Characteristics of Different Types of Thyroiditis

	Acute Thyroiditis	Subacute Granulomatous (de Quervain) Thyroiditis	Palpation Thyroiditis	Chronic Lymphocytic (Hashimoto) Thyroiditis	Postpartum Thyroiditis	Silent (Painless and/or Sporadic) Thyroiditis	Focal Lymphocytic Thyroiditis	Invasive Fibrous (Riedel) Thyroiditis
Gross pathologic features	• Normal size to mild thyroid enlargement • May be associated with pyriform sinus fistula	• Mild to moderate thyroid enlargement, often asymmetric	• Not evident grossly • Any gross abnormality reflects concurrent disease	• Moderate thyroid enlargement • Enlargement usually symmetric	• Normal to mild thyroid enlargement	• Slight to mild thyroid enlargement	• Usually normal thyroid size	• Extremely firm fibrosis involving all or part of thyroid • Fibrosis contiguous with adjacent extrathyroidal tissues
Microscopic features	• Neutrophils predominant • Necrosis	• Granulomatous inflammation • Neutrophils may predominant early	• Focal granulomatous inflammation limited to single follicles • Effacement of follicle by multinucleated giant cells and macrophages • Absence of acute inflammation or necrosis	• Diffuse lymphoplasmacytic infiltration • Germinal centers • Oncocytic metaplasia • Follicular damage and loss • Variable degree of fibrosis	• Focal to diffuse lymphocytic infiltration • Follicular damage and hyperplastic changes in early stage	• Focal to diffuse lymphocytic infiltration • Follicular damage and hyperplastic changes in early stage	• Focal collections of lymphocytes • Absence of follicular damage or appreciable loss • Rare presence of germinal centers and oncocytic metaplasia	• Marked fibrosis with extension beyond capsule • Diffuse lymphocytic infiltration • Vasculitis of small to medium sized veins
Etiology/ pathogenic mechanism	• Infection	• Uncertain • Postinfection possibly	• Mechanical disruption	• Autoimmune	• Autoimmune	• Autoimmune	• Autoimmune possibly	• Uncertain, may be a form of IgG4-RSD
Antibodies (anti-TPO and/or anti-Tg)	• Absent	• Usually absent • Usually transient if present	• Absent (or present if concomitant autoimmune thyroiditis)	• Present	• Present	• Present	• Present	• Usually present

(continued)

Table 4.2

Characteristics of Different Types of Thyroiditis (continued)

	Acute Thyroiditis	Subacute Granulomatous (de Quervain) Thyroiditis	Palpation Thyroiditis	Chronic Lymphocytic (Hashimoto) Thyroiditis	Postpartum Thyroiditis	Silent (Painless and/or Sporadic) Thyroiditis	Focal Lymphocytic Thyroiditis	Invasive Fibrous (Riedel) Thyroiditis
Thyroid function	• Usually euthyroid	• Initial hyperthyroidism followed by hypothyroidism • Usual return to euthyroidism	• Euthyroid	• Hypothyroidism • Occasional hyperthyroidism	• Initial hyperthyroidism followed by hypothyroidism • Usual return to euthyroidism	• Initial hyperthyroidism followed by hypothyroidism • Usual return to euthyroidism	• Euthyroid	• Usually euthyroid • About one-third hypothyroidism
Painful vs. painless	• Painful	• Painful	• Painless	• Painless	• Painless	• Painless	• Painless	• Painless
Age at onset	• Broad range from young children to older adults	• Young to middle aged adults	• Any age	• Usually 30–50 years of age	• Childbearing	• Usually 30–40 years of age	• Adolescence to young adults	• Middle aged adults
Gender ratio (F:M)	• 1:1	• 3–6:1	• Not applicable	• 5–20:1	—	• 2:1	• 2–3:1	• 3–5:1
Clinical course	• Usually dependent on underlying disorder and effectiveness of treatment	• Usually resolves within several months • Minority experience persistent hypothyroidism, recurrence, or development of chronic thyroiditis	• Clinically inapparent	• Euthyroid or hypothyroidism at time of diagnosis • Steady progression to hypothyroidism	• Usually resolves within postpartum year • 12%–30% experience persistent or recurrent hypothyroidism	• Usually resolves within 2–5 months • ~20% experience persistent or recurrent hypothyroidism	• Clinically inapparent	• Hypothyroidism in up to 40% • Usually self-limited • May require surgical therapy for tracheal or esophageal obstruction

Table 4.3

Variants of Chronic Lymphocytic (Hashimoto) Thyroiditis

	Classic	Fibrous	Fibrous Atrophy	Hashitoxicosis	Juvenile
Gross pathologic features	• Moderate thyroid enlargement • Enlargement usually symmetric	• Moderate to marked thyroid enlargement	• Small thyroid	• Moderate thyroid enlargement • Variable symmetry	• Usually normal thyroid size
Microscopic features	• Diffuse lymphoplasmacytic infiltration • Germinal centers • Oncocytic metaplasia • Follicular damage and atrophy • Variable degree of fibrosis • Occasional squamous metaplasia	• Marked fibrosis • Marked follicular loss • Diffuse lymphoplasmacytic infiltration • Germinal centers • Oncocytic metaplasia • Prominent squamous metaplasia	• Marked fibrosis • Marked follicular loss • Diffuse lymphoplasmacytic infiltration • Germinal centers • Oncocytic metaplasia • Prominent squamous metaplasia	• Diffuse lymphoplasmacytic infiltration • Germinal centers • Variable oncocytic metaplasia • Variable follicular epithelial hyperplasia • Variable atrophy, fibrosis • Squamous metaplasia occasional or absent	• Diffuse lymphoplasmacytic infiltration • Germinal centers • Oncocytic metaplasia • Minimal follicular loss • Variable degree of fibrosis • Occasional squamous metaplasia
Thyroid function	• Hypothyroidism	• Hypothyroidism	• Hypothyroidism	• Hyperthyroidism	• Variable
Age at onset	• Usually 30–50 years of age	• Late middle age to elderly	• Elderly	• Children to older adults	• Children to young adults
Clinical course	• Presentation with hypothyroidism or steady progression to hypothyroidism	• Present with hypothyroidism • Thyroid enlargement may be symptomatic and treated with surgical resection	• Severe hypothyroidism	• Hyperthyroidism ranges from mild to severe	• Variable, ranging from hyperthyroidism to hypothyroidism
Comment		• May be a manifestation of IgG4-RSD		• Variable combination of features of classic chronic lymphocytic thyroiditis (CLT) and diffuse toxic hyperplasia (Graves disease)	• Ill-defined entity with limited histologic correlation

or after surgical resection is problematic. Although the etiology and pathogenesis of focal lymphocytic thyroiditis are debatable, these incidentally found lesions appear to have little or no clinical significance.

Pathology

Affected glands are grossly unremarkable or show pathologic changes aside from focal lymphocytic thyroiditis. Microscopically, the thyroid tissue contains focal interfollicular collections of lymphocytes. Lymphocytes are not characteristically seen within follicles by light microscopy, although they may be observed ultrastructurally.[202] The follicles are typically intact without appreciable atrophy or oncocytic metaplasia. Germinal centers are rarely seen. These focal lymphocytic collections are usually small and can be seen in conjunction with hyperplastic and neoplastic lesions.

Invasive Fibrous Thyroiditis (Riedel Thyroiditis)

Definition and Clinical Features

Invasive fibrous thyroiditis, alternatively known as Riedel thyroiditis, fibrosing thyroiditis, or sclerosing thyroiditis, is a rare disease of uncertain etiology characterized by progressive fibrosis of the thyroid. The eponymous name recognizes the initial description by Riedel in 1896.[203] Patients with invasive fibrous thyroiditis are usually euthyroid at the time of diagnosis; however, about 25% to 35% are hypothyroid at the time of diagnosis, and up to 40% develop hypothyroidism as the thyroid parenchyma is replaced by fibrous tissue.[204–207] About one-third of patients either present with or develop another fibroinflammatory disorder within 10 years.[208] These disorders include mediastinal or retroperitoneal fibrosis, sclerosing cholangitis, and orbital

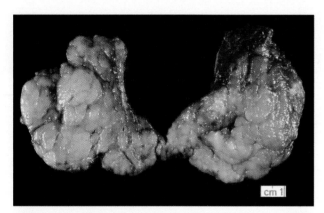

FIGURE 4.16. Fibrous variant of chronic lymphocytic (Hashimoto) thyroiditis showing abnormally pale cut surfaces with accentuated lobulation.

pseudotumor. Invasive fibrous thyroiditis may be a manifestation of IgG4-RSD.

The average age at onset is about 50 years and may occur as early as the third decade. Women are three to five times more frequently affected than men. Signs and symptoms are usually

related to tracheal or esophageal compression. Other local effects include hoarseness because of recurrent laryngeal nerve compromise, restriction of blood flow because of compression of large veins, and Horner syndrome secondary to the involvement of the cervical sympathetic nerve trunk. Parathyroid function may be compromised with subsequent hypocalcemia and related symptoms of cramping and paresthesia. Serum antibodies to TPO and/or Tg are seen in about half to two-thirds of cases.[205,208,209] Titers are usually low.

Pathogenesis

Several hypotheses have been proposed regarding etiology and pathogenesis. The systemic autoimmune hypothesis seems to have the most support. This hypothesis basically views invasive fibrous thyroiditis as a manifestation of disordered fibroblastic proliferation owing to a hypersensitivity reaction and consequent release of stimulating growth factors.[210] The initiating event is unknown, but vascular injury is thought to be a possible mechanism.

Pathology

Affected glands are extremely firm and fixed to the surrounding tissues. The consistency has been compared to wood. The gland may

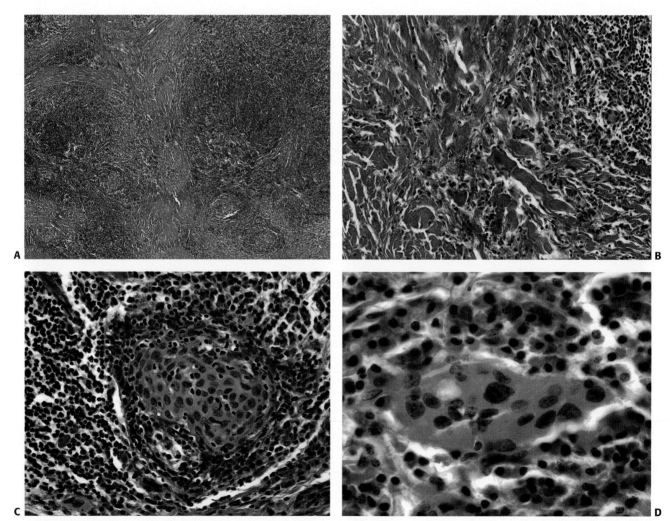

FIGURE 4.17. Fibrous variant of chronic lymphocytic (Hashimoto) thyroiditis. A: Low-power view showing diffuse lymphoplasmacytic infiltrate, marked fibrosis, and absence of follicles. **B:** Medium-power view showing dense, keloid-like fibrosis. **C:** Medium-power view showing squamous metaplasia. **D:** High-power view showing small residual focus of follicular epithelium with oncocytic metaplasia.

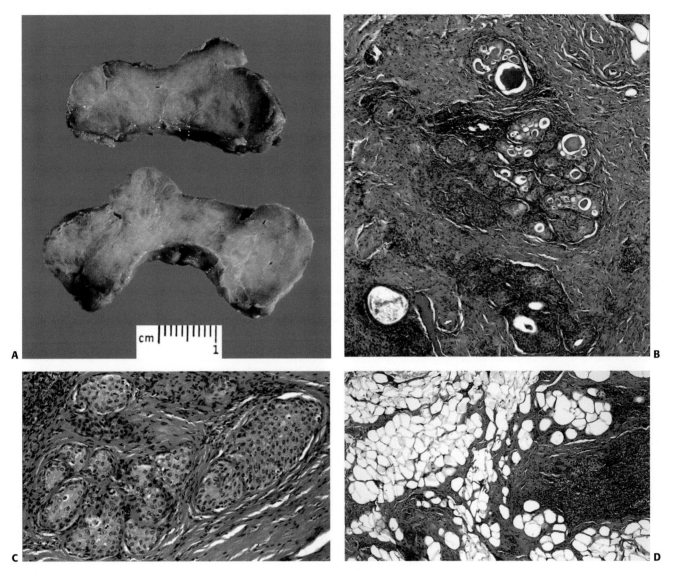

FIGURE 4.18. Fibrous atrophy variant of chronic lymphocytic (Hashimoto) thyroiditis. A: Gross photograph of thyroid gland that weighed 4 g at the time of autopsy. **B:** Low-power view of surgically resected thyroid showing marked fibrosis, follicular atrophy, and squamous metaplasia. **C:** Squamous metaplasia. **D:** Follicular atrophy and focal replacement by adipose tissue.

be involved partially or in its entirety. Cut surfaces generally have a relatively homogeneous tan-white or tan-gray appearance and lack lobulation or other findings characteristic of normal thyroid (Fig. 4.20). The principal histologic feature is effacement of the thyroid parenchyma by chronic inflammation and fibrosis with extension of the process beyond the thyroid capsule into the adjacent tissues including skeletal muscle (Fig. 4.21). Lymphocytes and plasma cells constitute most of the inflammatory cells, but eosinophils and neutrophils may be seen. Immunohistochemical staining for T and B lymphocytes reveals both types in ratio similar to that seen in chronic lymphocytic thyroiditis. Granulomatous inflammation is absent, but an occasional giant cell may be present. Small- to medium-sized veins may exhibit occlusive vasculitis with infiltration of their walls by lymphocytes and plasma cells. This vasculitis seems to be distinctive for invasive fibrous thyroiditis. Follicles are usually absent in affected areas, and residual ones are typically atrophic and difficult to recognize. FNA typically yields acellular or paucicellular specimens and thus is almost always nondiagnostic.

A recent study of three cases of invasive fibrous thyroiditis revealed IgG4-positive plasma cells ranging from 8 to 53 per high-power (400×) field and an IgG4/IgG ratio ranging from 0.2 to 0.8.[211] One patient had a similar concurrent fibroinflammatory process in a lung and obstructive biliary disease, whereas the other two only had thyroid disease. The number of IgG4-positive plasma cells for two cases was below the criterion used in a study of chronic lymphocytic thyroiditis (see above), but their presence does suggest that this form of thyroiditis may be a manifestation of IgG4-RSD. Appreciation of the full spectrum of IgG4-RSD is still emerging, and additional studies are anticipated that will clarify its role in thyroid disorders.

Differential Diagnosis

The differential diagnosis includes fibrous variant of chronic lymphocytic thyroiditis and multiple neoplastic lesions. Features distinguishing invasive fibrous (Riedel) thyroiditis from fibrous variant of chronic lymphocytic thyroiditis are (1) extrathyroidal

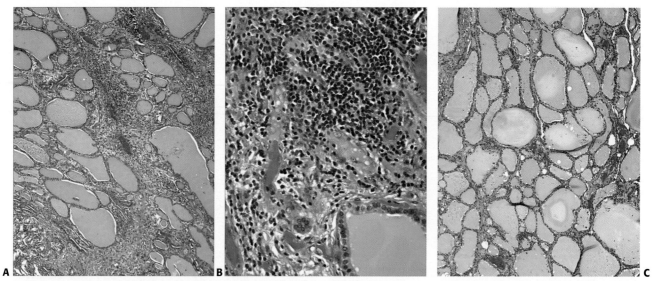

FIGURE 4.19. Peritumoral fibrosis. A: Low-power photomicrograph of peritumoral region of thyroid with chronic inflammation (small amount of papillary carcinoma just present in lower left corner). **B:** High-power photomicrograph of peritumoral region showing dense focus of lymphocytes, loss of follicles, and fibrosis. **C:** Representative low-power photomicrograph of thyroid tissue more distant from tumor showing absence of inflammation.

fibrosis, (2) loss of thyroid lobularity, (3) absence or rarity of lymphoid follicles, (4) absence of appreciable oncocytic metaplasia,

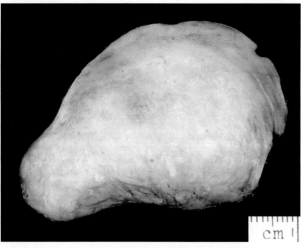

FIGURE 4.20. Invasive fibrous (Riedel) thyroiditis showing homogeneous tan-white tissue without lobulation or other features characteristic of normal thyroid.

and (5) occlusive vasculitis. Concurrent instances of invasive fibrous thyroiditis and chronic lymphocytic thyroiditis have been reported, but these are generally considered separate pathologic processes and their association coincidental. However, some of these cases may prove to be linked as manifestations of IgG4-RSD.

Neoplastic lesions in the differential diagnosis include anaplastic thyroid carcinoma, diffuse sclerosing variant of papillary carcinoma, nodular sclerosis type of Hodgkin disease, solitary fibrous tumor, and various types of spindle cell sarcoma. Most of these neoplasms can be identified with adequate sampling, consideration of the possibility, and use of appropriate immunostains.

Clinical Course

Surgical therapy may be necessary if compressive signs and symptoms become intolerable. Resection may be quite challenging if there is extensive extrathyroidal disease and involvement of the parathyroid glands and/or recurrent laryngeal nerves. Corticosteroid therapy has been used with some success.[212] Although invasive fibrous thyroiditis is fortunately a rare disease, its rarity has precluded clinical trials of various treatment options.

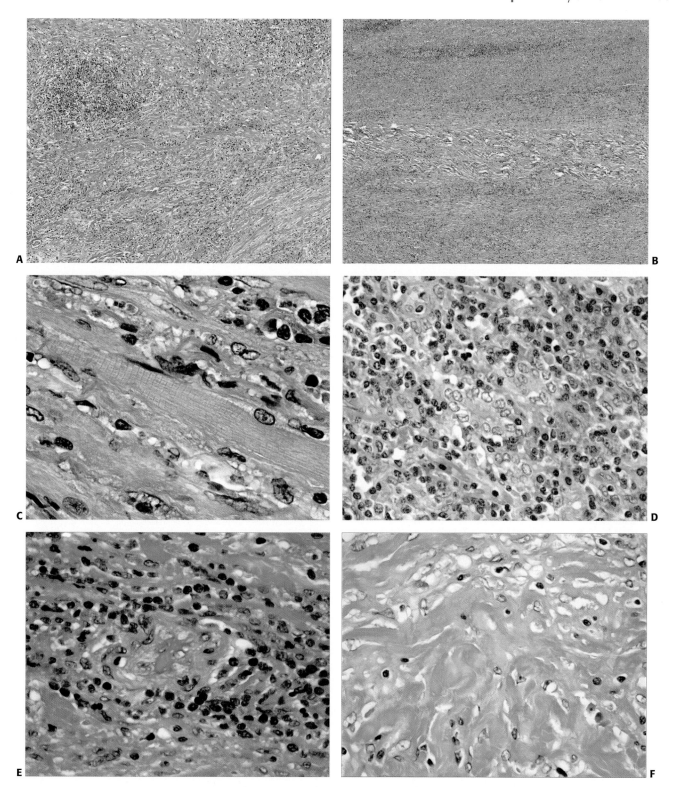

FIGURE 4.21. Invasive fibrous (Riedel) thyroiditis. A: Low-power view showing effacement of thyroid parenchyma by diffuse fibrosis and chronic inflammation. **B:** Low-power view showing extension of fibroinflammatory changes into perithyroidal tissue. The remnant of the thyroid capsule, barely visible, is located horizontally in the midportion of the field. **C:** High-power view showing fibroinflammatory process engulfing skeletal muscle adjacent to the thyroid. **D:** Atrophic follicular remnants surrounded by lymphoplasmacytic infiltrates. **E:** Lymphoplasmacytic infiltration of the wall of small vein. **F:** Keloid-like fibrosis.

REFERENCES

1. Brook I. Microbiology and management of acute suppurative thyroiditis in children. *Int J Pediatr Otorhinolaryngol.* 2003;67:447–451.
2. Chang P, Tsai WY, Lee PI, et al. Clinical characteristics and management of acute suppurative thyroiditis in children. *J Formos Med Assoc.* 2002;101:468–471.
3. Lambert MJ III, Johns ME, Mentzer R. Acute suppurative thyroiditis. *Am Surg.* 1980;46:461–463.
4. Farwell AP, Braverman LE. Inflammatory thyroid disorders. *Otolaryngol Clin North Am.* 1996;29:541–556.
5. Chi H, Lee YJ, Chiu NC, et al. Acute suppurative thyroiditis in children. *Pediatr Infect Dis J.* 2002;21:384–387.
6. Pahlavan S, Haque W, Pereira K, et al. Microbiology of third and fourth branchial pouch cysts. *Laryngoscope.* 2010;120:458–462.
7. Jeng LB, Lin JD, Chen MF. Acute suppurative thyroiditis: a ten-year review in a Taiwanese hospital. *Scand J Infect Dis.* 1994;26:297–300.
8. Berger SA, Zonszein J, Villamena P, et al. Infectious diseases of the thyroid gland. *Rev Infect Dis.* 1983;5:108–122.
9. Guttler R, Singer PA, Axline SG, et al. *Pneumocystis carinii* thyroiditis. Report of three cases and review of the literature. *Arch Intern Med.* 1993;153:393–396.
10. Pearce EN, Farwell AP, Braverman LE. Thyroiditis. *N Engl J Med.* 2003;348:2646–2655.
11. Nishihara E, Miyauchi A, Matsuzuka F, et al. Acute suppurative thyroiditis after fine-needle aspiration causing thyrotoxicosis. *Thyroid.* 2005;15:1183–1187.
12. Tien KJ, Chen TC, Hsieh MC, et al. Acute suppurative thyroiditis with deep neck infection: a case report. *Thyroid.* 2007;17:467–469.
13. Yung BC, Loke TK, Fan WC, et al. Acute suppurative thyroiditis due to foreign body-induced retropharyngeal abscess presented as thyrotoxicosis. *Clin Nucl Med.* 2000;25:249–252.
14. Miyauchi A, Matsuzuka F, Kuma K, et al. Piriform sinus fistula: an underlying abnormality common in patients with acute suppurative thyroiditis. *World J Surg.* 1990;14:400–405.
15. Seki N, Himi T. Retrospective review of 13 cases of pyriform sinus fistula. *Am J Otolaryngol.* 2007;28:55–58.
16. Cases JA, Wenig BM, Silver CE, et al. Recurrent acute suppurative thyroiditis in an adult due to a fourth branchial pouch fistula. *J Clin Endocrinol Metab.* 2000;85:953–956.
17. Fukata S, Miyauchi A, Kuma K, et al. Acute suppurative thyroiditis caused by an infected piriform sinus fistula with thyrotoxicosis. *Thyroid.* 2002;12:175–178.
18. Gopan T, Strome M, Hoschar A, et al. Recurrent acute suppurative thyroiditis attributable to a piriform sinus fistula in an adult. *Endocr Pract.* 2007;13:662–666.
19. Miyauchi A, Matsuzuka F, Kuma K, et al. Piriform sinus fistula and the ultimobranchial body. *Histopathology.* 1992;20:221–227.
20. Sai Prasad TR, Chong CL, Mani A, et al. Acute suppurative thyroiditis in children secondary to pyriform sinus fistula. *Pediatr Surg Int.* 2007;23:779–783.
21. Kawanaka M, Sugimoto Y, Suehiro M, et al. Thyroid imaging in a typical case of acute suppurative thyroiditis with abscess formation due to infection from a persistent thyroglossal duct. *Ann Nucl Med.* 1994;8:159–162.
22. Kaselas Ch, Tsikopoulos G, Chortis C, et al. Thyroglossal duct cyst's inflammation. When do we operate? *Pediatr Surg Int.* 2005;21:991–993.
23. Ostlie DJ, Burjonrappa SC, Snyder CL, et al. Thyroglossal duct infections and surgical outcomes. *J Pediatr Surg.* 2004;39:396–9; discussion 396.
24. Abe K, Taguchi T, Okuno A, et al. Acute suppurative thyroiditis in children. *J Pediatr.* 1979;94:912–914.
25. McLaughlin SA, Smith SL, Meek SE. Acute suppurative thyroiditis caused by *Pasteurella multocida* and associated with thyrotoxicosis. *Thyroid.* 2006;16:307–310.
26. Sicilia V, Mezitis S. A case of acute suppurative thyroiditis complicated by thyrotoxicosis. *J Endocrinol Invest.* 2006;29:997–1000.
27. Li CC, Wang CH, Tsan KW. Graves' disease and diabetes mellitus associated with acute suppurative thyroiditis: a case report. *Zhonghua Yi Xue Za Zhi (Taipei).* 1997;59:59–64.
28. Singh SK, Agrawal JK, Kumar M, et al. Fine needle aspiration cytology in the management of acute suppurative thyroiditis. *Ear Nose Throat J.* 1994;73:415–417.
29. Lin KD, Lin JD, Huang MJ, et al. Acute suppurative thyroiditis and aggressive malignant thyroid tumors: differences in clinical presentation. *J Surg Oncol.* 1998;67:28–32.
30. Yamashita J, Ogawa M, Yamashita S, et al. Acute suppurative thyroiditis in an asymptomatic woman: an atypical presentation simulating thyroid carcinoma. *Clin Endocrinol (Oxf).* 1994;40:145–149; discussion 149–150.
31. Kodama T, Ito Y, Obara T, et al. Acute suppurative thyroiditis in appearance of unusual neck mass. *Endocrinol Jpn.* 1987;34:427–430.
32. Walfish PG, Chan JY, Ing HD, et al. Esophageal carcinoma masquerading as recurrent acute suppurative thyroiditis. *Arch Intern Med.* 1985;145:346–347.
33. Volpé R. The pathology of thyroiditis. *Hum Pathol.* 1978;9:429–438.
34. Eylan E, Zmucky R, Sheba C. Mumps virus and subacute thyroiditis; evidence of a causal association. *Lancet.* 1957;272:1062–1063.
35. McArthur AM. Subacute giant cell thyroiditis associated with mumps. *Med J Aust.* 1964;1:116–117.
36. Volta C, Carano N, Street ME, et al. Atypical subacute thyroiditis caused by Epstein-Barr virus infection in a three-year-old girl. *Thyroid.* 2005;15:1189–1191.
37. Martino E, Buratti L, Bartalena L, et al. High prevalence of subacute thyroiditis during summer season in Italy. *J Endocrinol Invest.* 1987;10:321–323.
38. Karlsson FA, Tötterman TH, Jansson R. Subacute thyroiditis: activated HLA-DR and interferon-gamma expressing T cytotoxic/suppressor cells in thyroid tissue and peripheral blood. *Clin Endocrinol (Oxf).* 1986;25:487–493.
39. Desailloud R, Hober D. Viruses and thyroiditis: an update. *Virol J.* 2009;6:5.
40. Luotola K, Hyöty H, Salmi J, et al. Evaluation of infectious etiology in subacute thyroiditis—lack of association with coxsackievirus infection. *APMIS.* 1998;106:500–504.
41. Mori K, Yoshida K, Funato T, et al. Failure in detection of Epstein-Barr virus and cytomegalovirus in specimen obtained by fine needle aspiration biopsy of thyroid in patients with subacute thyroiditis. *Tohoku J Exp Med.* 1998;186:13–17.
42. Oksa H, Järvenpää P, Metsähonkala L, et al. No seasonal distribution in subacute de Quervain's thyroiditis in Finland. *J Endocrinol Invest.* 1989;12:495.
43. Paraná R, Cruz M, Lyra L, et al. Subacute thyroiditis during treatment with combination therapy (interferon plus ribavirin) for hepatitis C virus. *J Viral Hepat.* 2000;7:393–395.
44. Omür O, Daglýöz G, Akarca U, et al. Subacute thyroiditis during interferon therapy for chronic hepatitis B infection. *Clin Nucl Med.* 2003;28:864–865.
45. Shen L, Bui C, Mansberg R, et al. Thyroid dysfunction during interferon alpha therapy for chronic hepatitis C. *Clin Nucl Med.* 2005;30:546–547.
46. Falaschi P, Martocchia A, D'Urso R, et al. Subacute thyroiditis during interferon-alpha therapy for chronic hepatitis C. *J Endocrinol Invest.* 1997;20:24–28.
47. Cañas CA, Tobón GJ, Arango LG, et al. Developing of granulomatous thyroiditis during etanercept therapy. *Clin Rheumatol.* 2009;28(suppl 1):S17–S19.
48. Vassilopoulos D, Sialevris K, Malahtari S, et al. Subacute thyroiditis presenting as fever of unknown origin in a patient with rheumatoid arthritis under etanercept treatment. *J Clin Rheumatol.* 2010;16:88–89.
49. Hamaguchi E, Nishimura Y, Kaneko S, et al. Subacute thyroiditis developed in identical twins two years apart. *Endocr J.* 2005;52:559–562.
50. Kramer AB, Roozendaal C, Dullaart RP. Familial occurrence of subacute thyroiditis associated with human leukocyte antigen-B35. *Thyroid.* 2004;14:544–547.
51. Ohsako N, Tamai H, Sudo T, et al. Clinical characteristics of subacute thyroiditis classified according to human leukocyte antigen typing. *J Clin Endocrinol Metab.* 1995;80:3653–3656.
52. Rubin RA, Guay AT. Susceptibility to subacute thyroiditis is genetically influenced: familial occurrence in identical twins. *Thyroid.* 1991;1:157–161.
53. Peretianu D, Balmes E, Gudovan E, et al. The diagnostic and prognostic value of HLA B 35 antigen in viral subacute thyroiditis. *Endocrinologie.* 1990;28:63–66.
54. Nyulassy S, Hnilica P, Buc M, et al. Subacute (de Quervain's) thyroiditis: association with HLA-Bw35 antigen and abnormalities of the complement system, immunoglobulins and other serum proteins. *J Clin Endocrinol Metab.* 1977;45:270–274.
55. Woolner LB, McConahey WM, Beahrs OH. Granulomatous thyroiditis (De Quervain's thyroiditis). *J Clin Endocrinol Metab.* 1957;17:1202–1221.
56. Sniezek JC, Francis TB. Inflammatory thyroid disorders. *Otolaryngol Clin North Am.* 2003;36:55–71.
57. Fatourechi V, Aniszewski JP, Fatourechi GZ, et al. Clinical features and outcome of subacute thyroiditis in an incidence cohort: Olmsted County, Minnesota, study. *J Clin Endocrinol Metab.* 2003;88:2100–2105.
58. Erdem N, Erdogan M, Ozbek M, et al. Demographic and clinical features of patients with subacute thyroiditis: results of 169 patients from a single university center in Turkey. *J Endocrinol Invest.* 2007;30:546–550.
59. Benbassat CA, Olchovsky D, Tsvetov G, et al. Subacute thyroiditis: clinical characteristics and treatment outcome in fifty-six consecutive patients diagnosed between 1999 and 2005. *J Endocrinol Invest.* 2007;30:631–635.
60. Ogawa E, Katsushima Y, Fujiwara I, et al. Subacute thyroiditis in children: patient report and review of the literature. *J Pediatr Endocrinol Metab.* 2003;16:897–900.
61. Greene JN. Subacute thyroiditis. *Am J Med.* 1971;51:97–108.
62. Pearce EN, Bogazzi F, Martino E, et al. The prevalence of elevated serum C-reactive protein levels in inflammatory and noninflammatory thyroid disease. *Thyroid.* 2003;13:643–648.
63. Volpé R, Row VV, Ezrin C. Circulating viral and thyroid antibodies in subacute thyroiditis. *J Clin Endocrinol Metab.* 1967;27:1275–1284.
64. Lio S, Pontecorvi A, Caruso M, et al. Transitory subclinical and permanent hypothyroidism in the course of subacute thyroiditis (de Quervain). *Acta Endocrinol.* 1984;106:67–70.
65. Weetman AP, Smallridge RC, Nutman TB, et al. Persistent thyroid autoimmunity after subacute thyroiditis. *J Clin Lab Immunol.* 1987;23:1–6.
66. Swinburne JL, Kreisman SH. A rare case of subacute thyroiditis causing thyroid storm. *Thyroid.* 2007;17:73–76.
67. Sherman SI, Ladenson PW. Subacute thyroiditis causing thyroid storm. *Thyroid.* 2007;17:283.
68. Teixeira VL, Romaldini JH, Rodrigues HF, et al. Thyroid function during the spontaneous course of subacute thyroiditis. *J Nucl Med.* 1985;26:457–460.
69. Bogazzi F, Dell'Unto E, Tanda ML, et al. Long-term outcome of thyroid function after amiodarone-induced thyrotoxicosis, as compared to subacute thyroiditis. *J Endocrinol Invest.* 2006;29:694–699.
70. Kitchener MI, Chapman IM. Subacute thyroiditis: a review of 105 cases. *Clin Nucl Med.* 1989;14:439–442.
71. Carlé A, Laurberg P, Pedersen IB, et al. Epidemiology of subtypes of hypothyroidism in Denmark. *Eur J Endocrinol.* 2006;154:21–28.
72. Iitaka M, Momotani N, Ishii J, et al. Incidence of subacute thyroiditis recurrences after a prolonged latency: 24-year survey. *J Clin Endocrinol Metab.* 1996;81:466–469.
73. Yamamoto M, Saito S, Sakurada T, et al. Recurrence of subacute thyroiditis over 10 years after the first attack in three cases. *Endocrinol Jpn.* 1988;35:833–839.
74. Iitaka M, Kakinuma S, Yamanaka K, et al. Induction of autoimmune hypothyroidism and subsequent hyperthyroidism by TSH receptor antibodies following subacute thyroiditis: a case report. *Endocr J.* 2001;48:139–142.
75. Iitaka M, Momotani N, Hisaoka T, et al. TSH receptor antibody-associated thyroid dysfunction following subacute thyroiditis. *Clin Endocrinol (Oxf).* 1998;48:445–453.

76. Bartalena L, Bogazzi F, Pecori F, et al. Graves' disease occurring after subacute thyroiditis: report of a case and review of the literature. *Thyroid.* 1996;6:345–348.
77. Fukata S, Matsuzuka F, Kobayashi A, et al. Development of Graves' disease after subacute thyroiditis: two unusual cases. *Acta Endocrinol.* 1992;126:495–496.
78. Wartofsky L, Schaaf M. Graves' disease with thyrotoxicosis following subacute thyroiditis. *Am J Med.* 1987;83:761–764.
79. Hardoff R, Baron E, Sheinfeld M, et al. Localized manifestations of subacute thyroiditis presenting as solitary transient cold thyroid nodules. A report of 11 patients. *Clin Nucl Med.* 1995;20:981–984.
80. Bartels PC, Boer RO. Subacute thyroiditis (de Quervain) presenting as a painless "cold" nodule. *J Nucl Med.* 1987;28:1488–1490.
81. Kojima M, Nakamura S, Oyama T, et al. Cellular composition of subacute thyroiditis. an immunohistochemical study of six cases. *Pathol Res Pract.* 2002;198:833–837.
82. Lu CP, Chang TC, Wang CY, et al. Serial changes in ultrasound-guided fine needle aspiration cytology in subacute thyroiditis. *Acta Cytol.* 1997;41:238–243.
83. García Solano J, Giménez Bascuñana A, Sola Pérez J, et al. Fine-needle aspiration of subacute granulomatous thyroiditis (De Quervain's thyroiditis): a clinico-cytologic review of 36 cases. *Diagn Cytopathol.* 1997;16:214–220.
84. Satoh M. Ultrastructure of the giant cell in de Quervain's subacute thyroiditis. *Acta Pathol Jpn.* 1976;26:133–137.
85. Mizukami Y, Michigishi T, Kawato M, et al. Immunohistochemical and ultrastructural study of subacute thyroiditis, with special reference to multinucleated giant cells. *Hum Pathol.* 1987;18:929–935.
86. Duininck TM, van Heerden JA, Fatourechi V, et al. de Quervain's thyroiditis: surgical experience. *Endocr Pract.* 2002;8:255–258.
87. Thompson LD, Heffess CS. Subacute (de Quervain's) thyroiditis. *Ear Nose Throat J.* 2002;81:623.
88. Shabb NS, Salti I. Subacute thyroiditis: fine-needle aspiration cytology of 14 cases presenting with thyroid nodules. *Diagn Cytopathol.* 2006;34:18–23.
89. Shabb NS, Tawil A, Gergeos F, et al. Multinucleated giant cells in fine-needle aspiration of thyroid nodules: their diagnostic significance. *Diagn Cytopathol.* 1999;21:307–312.
90. Jayaram G, Marwaha RK, Gupta RK, et al. Cytomorphologic aspects of thyroiditis. A study of 51 cases with functional, immunologic and ultrasonographic data. *Acta Cytol.* 1987;31:687–693.
91. Carney JA, Moore SB, Northcutt RC, et al. Palpation thyroiditis (multifocal granulomatour folliculitis). *Am J Clin Pathol.* 1975;64:639–647.
92. Buergi U, Gebel F, Maier E, et al. Serum thyroglobulin before and after palpation of the thyroid. *N Engl J Med.* 1983;308:777.
93. Goldfarb H, Schifrin D, Graig FA. Thyroiditis caused by tuberculous abscess of the thyroid gland. Case report and review of the literature. *Am J Med.* 1965;38:825–828.
94. Crompton GK, Cameron SJ. Tuberculosis of the thyroid gland mimicking carcinoma. *Tubercle.* 1969;50:61–64.
95. Marwaha RK, Sankar R, Magdum M, et al. Clinical, biochemical and cytomorphological observations in juvenile chronic lymphocytic thyroiditis. *Indian Pediatr.* 1998;35:967–973.
96. Takami H, Kozakai M. Tuberculous thyroiditis: report of a case with a review of the literature. *Endocr J.* 1994;41:743–747.
97. Bulbuloglu E, Ciralik H, Okur E, et al. Tuberculosis of the thyroid gland: review of the literature. *World J Surg.* 2006;30:149–155.
98. Ozekinci S, Mizrak B, Saruhan G, et al. Histopathologic diagnosis of thyroid tuberculosis. *Thyroid.* 2009;19:983–986.
99. Das DK, Pant CS, Chachra KL, et al. Fine needle aspiration cytology diagnosis of tuberculous thyroiditis. A report of eight cases. *Acta Cytol.* 1992;36:517–522.
100. Orlandi F, Fiorini S, Gonzatto I, et al. Tubercular involvement of the thyroid gland: a report of two cases. *Horm Res.* 1999;52:291–294.
101. Ghosh A, Saha S, Bhattacharya B, et al. Primary tuberculosis of thyroid gland: a rare case report. *Am J Otolaryngol.* 2007;28:267–270.
102. Gupta N, Sharma K, Barwad A, et al. Thyroid tuberculosis—role of PCR in diagnosis of a rare entity. *Cytopathology.* 2010;22:392–396.
103. Goldani LZ, Klock C, Diehl A, et al. Histoplasmosis of the thyroid. *J Clin Microbiol.* 2000;38:3890–3891.
104. Smilack JD, Argueta R. Coccidioidal infection of the thyroid. *Arch Intern Med.* 1998;158:89–92.
105. Goldani LZ, Zavascki AP, Maia AL. Fungal thyroiditis: an overview. *Mycopathologia.* 2006;161:129–139.
106. Harach HR, Williams ED. The pathology of granulomatous diseases of the thyroid gland. *Sarcoidosis.* 1990;7:19–27.
107. Vailati A, Marena C, Aristia L, et al. Sarcoidosis of the thyroid: report of a case and a review of the literature. *Sarcoidosis.* 1993;10:66–68.
108. Ozkan Z, Oncel M, Kurt N, et al. Sarcoidosis presenting as cold thyroid nodules: report of two cases. *Surg Today.* 2005;35:770–773.
109. Mizukami Y, Nonomura A, Michigishi T, et al. Sarcoidosis of the thyroid gland manifested initially as thyroid tumor. *Pathol Res Pract.* 1994;190:1201–1205; discussion 1206–1207.
110. Sasaki H, Harada T, Eimoto T, et al. Concomitant association of thyroid sarcoidosis and Hashimoto's thyroiditis. *Am J Med Sci.* 1987;294:441–443.
111. Karlish AJ, MacGregor GA. Sarcoidosis, thyroiditis, and Addison's disease. *Lancet.* 1970;2:330–333.
112. Rubinstein I, Baum GL, Hiss Y, et al. Sarcoidosis and Hashimoto's thyroiditis—a chance occurrence? *Respiration.* 1985;48:136–139.
113. Papadopoulos KI, Hörnblad Y, Liljebladh H, et al. High frequency of endocrine autoimmunity in patients with sarcoidosis. *Eur J Endocrinol.* 1996;134:331–336.
114. Nakamura H, Genma R, Mikami T, et al. High incidence of positive autoantibodies against thyroid peroxidase and thyroglobulin in patients with sarcoidosis. *Clin Endocrinol (Oxf).* 1997;46:467–472.
115. Yarman S, Kahraman H, Tanakol R, et al. Concomitant association of thyroid sarcoidosis and Graves' disease. *Horm Res.* 2003;59:43–46.
116. Hancock BW, Millard LG. Sarcoidosis and thyrotoxicosis: a study of five patients. *Br J Dis Chest.* 1976;70:129–133.
117. Thompson WD, McGrouther DA, Stockdill G. Thyrotoxicosis with sarcoid-like granulomata. *J Pathol.* 1973;111:289–291.
118. Hollowell JG, Staehling NW, Flanders WD, et al. Serum TSH, T(4), and thyroid antibodies in the United States population (1988 to 1994): National Health and Nutrition Examination Survey (NHANES III). *J Clin Endocrinol Metab.* 2002;87:489–499.
119. Huber G, Staub JJ, Meier C, et al. Prospective study of the spontaneous course of subclinical hypothyroidism: prognostic value of thyrotropin, thyroid reserve, and thyroid antibodies. *J Clin Endocrinol Metab.* 2002;87:3221–3226.
120. Williams ED, Doniach I. The post-mortem incidence of focal thyroiditis. *J Pathol Bacteriol.* 1962;83:255–264.
121. Okayasu I, Hatakeyama S, Tanaka Y, et al. Is focal chronic autoimmune thyroiditis an age-related disease? Differences in incidence and severity between Japanese and British. *J Pathol.* 1991;163:257–264.
122. Okayasu I, Hara Y, Nakamura K, et al. Racial and age-related differences in incidence and severity of focal autoimmune thyroiditis. *Am J Clin Pathol.* 1994;101:698–702.
123. Hashimoto H. Zur Kenntnis der lymphomatösen Veränderung der Schilddrüse (Struma lymphomatosum). *Arch Klin Chir.* 1912;97:219–248.
124. Lorini R, Gastaldi R, Traggiai C, et al. Hashimoto's thyroiditis. *Pediatr Endocrinol Rev.* 2003;1(suppl 2):205–211; discussion 211.
125. Dayan CM, Daniels GH. Chronic autoimmune thyroiditis. *N Engl J Med.* 1996;335:99–107.
126. Rallison ML, Dobyns BM, Meikle AW, et al. Natural history of thyroid abnormalities: prevalence, incidence, and regression of thyroid diseases in adolescents and young adults. *Am J Med.* 1991;91:363–370.
127. LiVolsi VA. *Surgical Pathology of the Thyroid.* Philadelphia, PA: WB Saunders; 1990.
128. Golden B, Levin L, Ban Y, et al. Genetic analysis of families with autoimmune diabetes and thyroiditis: evidence for common and unique genes. *J Clin Endocrinol Metab.* 2005;90:4904–4911.
129. Jacobson EM, Tomer Y. The CD40, CTLA-4, thyroglobulin, TSH receptor, and PTPN22 gene quintet and its contribution to thyroid autoimmunity: back to the future. *J Autoimmun.* 2007;28:85–98.
130. Menconi F, Monti MC, Greenberg DA, et al. Molecular amino acid signatures in the MHC class II peptide-binding pocket predispose to autoimmune thyroiditis in humans and in mice. *Proc Natl Acad Sci U S A.* 2008;105:14034–14039.
131. Caturegli P, Kuppers RC, Mariotti S, et al. IgG subclass distribution of thyroglobulin antibodies in patients with thyroid disease. *Clin Exp Immunol.* 1994;98:464–469.
132. Eschler DC, Hasham A, Tomer Y. Cutting edge: the etiology of autoimmune thyroid diseases. *Clin Rev Allergy Immunol.* 2011;41:190–197.
133. Tanda ML, Piantanida E, Lai A, et al. Thyroid autoimmunity and environment. *Horm Metab Res.* 2009;41:436–442.
134. Laurberg P, Cerqueira C, Ovesen L, et al. Iodine intake as a determinant of thyroid disorders in populations. *Best Pract Res Clin Endocrinol Metab.* 2010;24:13–27.
135. Menconi F, Hasham A, Tomer Y. Environmental triggers of thyroiditis: hepatitis C and interferon-alpha. *J Endocrinol Invest.* 2011;34:78–84.
136. Mori K, Yoshida K. Viral infection in induction of Hashimoto's thyroiditis: a key player or just a bystander? *Curr Opin Endocrinol Diabetes Obes.* 2010;17:418–424.
137. Benvenga S, Santarpia L, Trimarchi F, et al. Human thyroid autoantigens and proteins of *Yersinia* and *Borrelia* share amino acid sequence homology that includes binding motifs to HLA-DR molecules and T-cell receptor. *Thyroid.* 2006;16:225–236.
138. Arata N, Ando T, Unger P, et al. By-stander activation in autoimmune thyroiditis: studies on experimental autoimmune thyroiditis in the GFP+ fluorescent mouse. *Clin Immunol.* 2006;121:108–117.
139. Akeno N, Blackard JT, Tomer Y. HCV E2 protein binds directly to thyroid cells and induces IL-8 production: a new mechanism for HCV induced thyroid autoimmunity. *J Autoimmun.* 2008;31:339–344.
140. Akeno N, Smith EP, Stefan M, et al. IFN-a mediates the development of autoimmunity both by direct tissue toxicity and through immune cell recruitment mechanisms. *J Immunol.* 2011;186:4693–4706.
141. Fournié GJ, Mas M, Cautain B, et al. Induction of autoimmunity through bystander effects. Lessons from immunological disorders induced by heavy metals. *J Autoimmun.* 2001;16:319–326.
142. Jacobson EM, Tomer Y. The CD40, CTLA-4, thyroglobulin, TSH receptor, and PTPN22 gene quintet and its contribution to thyroid autoimmunity: back to the future. *J Autoimmun.* 2007;28:85–98.
143. Ueda H, Howson JM, Esposito L, et al. Association of the T-cell regulatory gene CTLA4 with susceptibility to autoimmune disease. *Nature.* 2003;423:506–511.
144. Kotani T, Aratake Y, Hirai K, et al. Apoptosis in thyroid tissue from patients with Hashimoto's thyroiditis. *Autoimmunity.* 1995;20:231–236.
145. Banga JP, Mirakian R, Hammond L, et al. Characterization of monoclonal antibodies directed towards the microsomal/microvillar thyroid autoantigen recognized by Hashimoto autoantibodies. *Clin Exp Immunol.* 1986;64:544–554.
146. Mezosi E, Wang SH, Utsugi S, et al. Induction and regulation of Fas-mediated apoptosis in human thyroid epithelial cells. *Mol Endocrinol.* 2005;19:804–811.
147. Giordano C, Richiusa P, Bagnasco M, et al. Differential regulation of Fas-mediated apoptosis in both thyrocyte and lymphocyte cellular compartments correlates with opposite phenotypic manifestations of autoimmune thyroid disease. *Thyroid.* 2001;11:233–244.

148. Xu WC, Chen SR, Huang JX, et al. Expression and distribution of S-100 protein, CD83 and apoptosis-related proteins (Fas, FasL and Bcl-2) in thyroid tissues of autoimmune thyroid diseases. *Eur J Histochem*. 2007;51:291–300.

149. Stassi G, Todaro M, Bucchieri F, et al. Fas/Fas ligand-driven T cell apoptosis as a consequence of ineffective thyroid immunoprivilege in Hashimoto's thyroiditis. *J Immunol*. 1999;162:263–267.

150. Bossowski A, Czarnocka B, Bardadin K, et al. Identification of apoptotic proteins in thyroid gland from patients with Graves' disease and Hashimoto's thyroiditis. *Autoimmunity*. 2008;41:163–173.

151. Arscott PL, Baker JR Jr. Apoptosis and thyroiditis. *Clin Immunol Immunopathol*. 1998;87:207–217.

152. Weetman AP. Cellular immune responses in autoimmune thyroid disease. *Clin Endocrinol (Oxf)*. 2004;61:405–413.

153. Cheng J, Zhou T, Liu C, et al. Protection from Fas-mediated apoptosis by a soluble form of the Fas molecule. *Science*. 1994;263:1759–1762.

154. Mariotti S, Caturegli P, Piccolo P, et al. Antithyroid peroxidase autoantibodies in thyroid diseases. *J Clin Endocrinol Metab*. 1990;71:661–669.

155. Nilsson M, Husmark J, Björkman U, et al. Cytokines and thyroid epithelial integrity: interleukin-1alpha induces dissociation of the junctional complex and paracellular leakage in filter-cultured human thyrocytes. *J Clin Endocrinol Metab*. 1998;83:945–952.

156. Iitaka M, Miura S, Yamanaka K, et al. Increased serum vascular endothelial growth factor levels and intrathyroidal vascular area in patients with Graves' disease and Hashimoto's thyroiditis. *J Clin Endocrinol Metab*. 1998;83:3908–3912.

157. Ruf J, Czarnocka B, De Micco C, et al. Thyroid peroxidase is the organ-specific "microsomal" autoantigen involved in thyroid autoimmunity. *Acta Endocrinol Suppl (Copenh)*. 1987;281:49–56.

158. Chiovato L, Bassi P, Santini F, et al. Antibodies producing complement-mediated thyroid cytotoxicity in patients with atrophic or goitrous autoimmune thyroiditis. *J Clin Endocrinol Metab*. 1993;77:1700–1705.

159. Rodien P, Madec AM, Ruf J, et al. Antibody-dependent cell-mediated cytotoxicity in autoimmune thyroid disease: relationship to antithyroperoxidase antibodies. *J Clin Endocrinol Metab*. 1996;81:2595–2600.

160. Li Y, Nishihara E, Hirokawa M, et al. Distinct clinical, serological, and sonographic characteristics of Hashimoto's thyroiditis based with and without IgG4-positive plasma cells. *J Clin Endocrinol Metab*. 2010;95:1309–1317.

161. Hamano H, Kawa S, Horiuchi A, et al. High serum IgG4 concentrations in patients with sclerosing pancreatitis. *N Engl J Med*. 2001;344:732–738.

162. Kakudo K, Li Y, Hirokawa M, et al. Diagnosis of Hashimoto's thyroiditis and IgG4-related sclerosing disease. *Pathol Int*. 2011;61:175–183.

163. Zen Y, Fujii T, Harada K, et al. Th2 and regulatory immune reactions are increased in immunoglobin G4-related sclerosing pancreatitis and cholangitis. *Hepatology*. 2007;45:1538–1546.

164. Mizukami Y, Michigishi T, Kawato M, et al. Chronic thyroiditis: thyroid function and histologic correlations in 601 cases. *Hum Pathol*. 1992;23:980–988.

165. Hsi ED, Singleton TP, Svoboda SM, et al. Characterization of the lymphoid infiltrate in Hashimoto thyroiditis by immunohistochemistry and polymerase chain reaction for immunoglobulin heavy chain gene rearrangement. *Am J Clin Pathol*. 1998;110:327–333.

166. Jansson R, Karlsson A, Forsum U. Intrathyroidal HLA-DR expression and T lymphocyte phenotypes in Graves' thyrotoxicosis, Hashimoto's thyroiditis and nodular colloid goitre. *Clin Exp Immunol*. 1984;58:264–272.

167. Knecht H, Saremaslani P, Hedinger C. Immunohistological findings in Hashimoto's thyroiditis, focal lymphocytic thyroiditis and thyroiditis de Quervain. Comparative study. *Virchows Arch A Pathol Anat Histol*. 1981;393:215–231.

168. DeLellis RA, Lloyd RV, Heitz PU, et al, eds. *Pathology and Genetics of Tumours of Endocrine Organs (IARC WHO Classification of Tumours)*. Lyon, France: IARC Press; 2004.

169. Hürthle K. Beiträge zur kenntniss des secretions vorgangs in der schilddrüse. *Arch Gesammte Physiol*. 1894;56:1–44.

170. Müller-Höcker J. Expression of bcl-2, Bax and Fas in oxyphil cells of Hashimoto thyroiditis. *Virchows Arch*. 2000;436:602–607.

171. Ryska A, Ludvíková M, Rydlová M, et al. Massive squamous metaplasia of the thyroid gland—report of three cases. *Pathol Res Pract*. 2006;202:99–106.

172. Holm LE, Blomgren H, Löwhagen T. Cancer risks in patients with chronic lymphocytic thyroiditis. *N Engl J Med*. 1985;312:601–604.

173. Ben-Ezra J, Wu A, Sheibani K. Hashimoto's thyroiditis lacks detectable clonal immunoglobulin and T cell receptor gene rearrangements. *Hum Pathol*. 1988;19:1444–1448.

174. Saxena A, Alport EC, Moshynska O, et al. Clonal B cell populations in a minority of patients with Hashimoto's thyroiditis. *J Clin Pathol*. 2004;57:1258–1263.

175. Pedersen RK, Pedersen NT. Primary non-Hodgkin's lymphoma of the thyroid gland: a population based study. *Histopathology*. 1996;28:25–32.

176. Sato Y, Nakamura N, Nakamura S, et al. Deviated VH4 immunoglobulin gene usage is found among thyroid mucosa-associated lymphoid tissue lymphomas, similar to the usage at other sites, but is not found in thyroid diffuse large B-cell lymphomas. *Mod Pathol*. 2006;19:1578–1584.

177. Nosé V. Familial thyroid cancer: a review. *Mod Pathol*. 2011;24(suppl 2):S19–S33.

178. Hayashi Y, Tamai H, Fukata S, et al. A long term clinical, immunological, and histological follow-up study of patients with goitrous chronic lymphocytic thyroiditis. *J Clin Endocrinol Metab*. 1985;61:1172–1178.

179. Fatourechi V, McConahey WM, Woolner LB. Hyperthyroidism associated with histologic Hashimoto's thyroiditis. *Mayo Clin Proc*. 1971;46:682–689.

180. Gopalakrishnan S, Marwaha RK. Juvenile autoimmune thyroiditis. *J Pediatr Endocrinol Metab*. 2007;20:961–970.

181. Marqusee E, Hill JA, Mandel SJ. Thyroiditis after pregnancy loss. *J Clin Endocrinol Metab*. 1997;82:2455–2457.

182. Ginsberg J, Walfish PG. Post-partum transient thyrotoxicosis with painless thyroiditis. *Lancet*. 1977;1:1125–1128.

183. Minelli R, Girasole G, Pedrazzoni M, et al. Lack of increased serum interleukin-6 and soluble IL-6 receptor concentrations in patients with thyroid diseases following recombinant human interferon alpha therapy. *J Investig Med*. 1996;44:370–374.

184. Othman S, Phillips DI, Parkes AB, et al. A long-term follow-up of postpartum thyroiditis. *Clin Endocrinol (Oxf)*. 1990;32:559–564.

185. Lucas A, Pizarro E, Granada ML, et al. Postpartum thyroiditis: epidemiology and clinical evolution in a nonselected population. *Thyroid*. 2000;10:71–77.

186. Stagnaro-Green A. Postpartum thyroiditis. *Best Pract Res Clin Endocrinol Metab*. 2004;18:303–316.

187. Nikolai TF, Brosseau J, Kettrick MA, et al. Lymphocytic thyroiditis with spontaneously resolving hyperthyroidism (silent thyroiditis). *Arch Intern Med*. 1980;140:478–482.

188. Tachi J, Amino N, Tamaki H, et al. Long term follow-up and HLA association in patients with postpartum hypothyroidism. *J Clin Endocrinol Metab*. 1988;66:480–484.

189. Stuckey BG, Kent GN, Ward LC, et al. Postpartum thyroid dysfunction and the long-term risk of hypothyroidism: results from a 12-year follow-up study of women with and without postpartum thyroid dysfunction. *Clin Endocrinol (Oxf)*. 2010;73:389–395.

190. Stagnaro-Green A, Schwartz A, Gismondi R, et al. High rate of persistent hypothyroidism in a large-scale prospective study of postpartum thyroiditis in southern Italy. *J Clin Endocrinol Metab*. 2011;96:652–657.

191. Amino N, Mori H, Iwatani Y, et al. High prevalence of transient post-partum thyrotoxicosis and hypothyroidism. *N Engl J Med*. 1982;306:849–852.

192. Mizukami Y, Michigishi T, Nonomura A, et al. Postpartum thyroiditis. A clinical, histologic, and immunopathologic study of 15 cases. *Am J Clin Pathol*. 1993;100:200–205.

193. Mittra ES, McDougall IR. Recurrent silent thyroiditis: a report of four patients and review of the literature. *Thyroid*. 2007;17:671–675.

194. Larson SD, Jackson LN, Riall TS, et al. Increased incidence of well-differentiated thyroid cancer associated with Hashimoto thyroiditis and the role of the PI3k/Akt pathway. *J Am Coll Surg*. 2007;204:764–773; discussion 773–765.

195. Kamikubo K, Takami R, Suwa T, et al. Case report: silent thyroiditis developed during alpha-interferon therapy. *Am J Med Sci*. 1993;306:174–176.

196. Miller KK, Daniels GH. Association between lithium use and thyrotoxicosis caused by silent thyroiditis. *Clin Endocrinol (Oxf)*. 2001;55:501–508.

197. Mizukami Y, Michigishi T, Hashimoto T, et al. Silent thyroiditis: a histologic and immunohistochemical study. *Hum Pathol*. 1988;19:423–431.

198. Gluck FB, Nusynowitz ML, Plymate S. Chronic lymphocytic thyroiditis, thyrotoxicosis, and low radioactive iodine uptake. Report of four cases. *N Engl J Med*. 1975;293:624–628.

199. Inada M, Nishikawa M, Naito K, et al. Reversible changes of the histological abnormalities of the thyroid in patients with painless thyroiditis. *J Clin Endocrinol Metab*. 1981;52:431–435.

200. Gorman CA, Duick DS, Woolner LB, et al. Transient hyperthyroidism in patients with lymphocytic thyroiditis. *Mayo Clin Proc*. 1978;53:359–365.

201. LiVolsi VA. The pathology of autoimmune thyroid disease: a review. *Thyroid*. 1994;4:333–339.

202. Bay BH, Sit KH, Pang AS. Lymphocytic infiltration in focal thyroiditis: an ultrastructural case study. *Immunobiology*. 1994;190:290–294.

203. Riedel BM. Die chronische, sur bildung elsenharter tumoren führende entzündung der schilddrüse. *Verh Dtsch Ges Chir*. 1896;25:101–105.

204. de Lange WE, Freling NJ, Molenaar WM, et al. Invasive fibrous thyroiditis (Riedel's struma): a manifestation of multifocal fibrosclerosis? A case report with review of the literature. *Q J Med*. 1989;72:709–717.

205. Schwaegerle SM, Bauer TW, Esselstyn CB Jr. Riedel's thyroiditis. *Am J Clin Pathol*. 1988;90:715–722.

206. Beahrs OH, McConahey WM, Woolner LB. Invasive fibrous thyroiditis (Riedel's struma). *J Clin Endocrinol Metab*. 1957;17:201–220.

207. Papi G, LiVolsi VA. Current concepts on Riedel thyroiditis. *Am J Clin Pathol*. 2004;121(suppl):S50–S63.

208. Hay ID. Thyroiditis: a clinical update. *Mayo Clin Proc*. 1985;60:836–843.

209. Papi G, Corrado S, Carapezzi C, et al. Riedel's thyroiditis and fibrous variant of Hashimoto's thyroiditis: a clinicopathological and immunohistochemical study. *J Endocrinol Invest*. 2003;26:444–449.

210. Heufelder AE, Goellner JR, Bahn RS, et al. Tissue eosinophilia and eosinophil degranulation in Riedel's invasive fibrous thyroiditis. *J Clin Endocrinol Metab*. 1996;81:977–984.

211. Dahlgren M, Khosroshahi A, Nielsen GP, et al. Riedel's thyroiditis and multifocal fibrosclerosis are part of the IgG4-related systemic disease spectrum. *Arthritis Care Res (Hoboken)*. 2010;62:1312–1318.

212. Bagnasco M, Passalacqua G, Pronzato C, et al. Fibrous invasive (Riedel's) thyroiditis with critical response to steroid treatment. *J Endocrinol Invest*. 1995;18:305–307.

Diffuse and Nodular Hyperplasia

 ## GRAVES DISEASE (DIFFUSE TOXIC HYPERPLASIA)

Definition

Graves disease, also known as diffuse toxic hyperplasia or diffuse toxic goiter, is an autoimmune disorder characterized by excessive production of thyroid hormone and diffuse hyperplasia with enlargement of the thyroid. In addition to generalized manifestations of hyperthyroidism, Graves disease is associated with distinct extrathyroidal lesions including inflammation of the orbital tissues, known as Graves ophthalmopathy, and excessive accumulation of glycosaminoglycans in the skin. The latter most often occurs in the anterior region of the leg and is known as pretibial myxedema.

Historical Comments

The commonly used eponymous term *Graves disease* recognizes the Irish physician Robert Graves. In 1835, he published lectures describing several cases of cardiac palpitations associated with enlargement of the thyroid and, in one case, exophthalmos.[1] Karl Adolph von Basedow published his description of the triad of goiter, palpitations, and exophthalmos in 1840, and his name is also linked eponymously to this disease, particularly in Europe.[2] Caleb Parry predated Graves and von Basedow with his description of the signs and symptoms of hyperthyroidism in association with goiter in an 1825 posthumous publication.[3] Several other apparent descriptions consistent with Graves disease preceded all of the above, some dating back into antiquity, and it seems quite probable that there were other reports now lost or very difficult to access.

Appreciation of thyroid hyperfunction as the principal explanation for clinical features evolved over time. Parry and Graves considered the disease to be primarily a disorder of the heart, whereas others considered it a disease of the nervous system. In 1884, Ludwig Rehn reported cure of toxic signs and symptoms with thyroidectomy, and in an 1886 publication, Paul Möbius gave support to thyroid hyperfunction as the prime abnormality.[4,5] By the early 20th century, the disease was well established as a thyroid disorder.

Several important events occurred in the middle of the 20th century. Antithyroid drugs were developed and used in cases of Graves disease as was radioactive iodine.[6,7] Adams and Purves identified long-acting thyroid stimulator (LATS) in 1956, and subsequent studies revealed that it was an immunoglobulin directed against thyroid-stimulating hormone receptor (TSHR).[8,9] Building on these key pieces in the puzzle, our knowledge of Graves disease has grown considerably over the past half century.

Epidemiology

Graves disease is one of the most common autoimmune diseases with an estimated prevalence of approximately 0.4% to 1% in the US population.[10–12] Prevalence and incidence data of various studies are difficult to compare because of differences in diagnostic criteria and the changes in analytic technology over time. Some studies do not differentiate Graves disease from other causes of hyperthyroidism such as toxic multinodular goiter and toxic adenoma. The annual incidence of Graves disease in iodine-sufficient regions usually falls in the range of 20 to 25 per 100,000.[12] The disease can affect all ages but is rare before adolescence and has a peak incidence in the fourth to sixth decades.[10,13,14] Women are three to eight times more commonly affected than men.[10,11,13–16]

Etiologic Factors

Both environmental and genetic risk factors play roles in the development of Graves disease.[17,18] The precise etiology is unknown, but the disease appears to develop in the setting of genetic susceptibility combined with one or more environmental triggers that precipitate an autoimmune response. Female gender is a major risk factor, similar to most other autoimmune diseases. Explanations tend to involve immune modulation, but much remains uncertain.

Iodine supplementation of previously deficient populations is associated with an increased incidence of hyperthyroidism (Jod-Basedow phenomenon).[19] Most cases are due to toxic multinodular goiter; however, subclinical cases of Graves disease may be unmasked when increased iodine intake permits increased thyroid hormone production. In a comparative study of genetically similar populations in regions with high- and low-dietary iodine, the annual incidence of Graves disease was greater in the region with high intake.[20] However, the total annual incidence of thyrotoxicosis owing to all causes was higher in the region with low-dietary iodine. The relationship of iodine intake to Graves disease seems in large part an unmasking of the underlying autoimmune process, but a more direct role may exist. Iodine may be capable of follicular cell injury by production of autoreactive thyroid epitopes or generation of reactive metabolites.[17,21]

Stress is suspected as a significant etiologic factor. An increase in the incidence of Graves disease has been observed after stressful life events and in regions affected by war.[17,22,23] Although attempts to link stress with Graves disease may be problematic in terms of methodology, stress is generally accepted as having significant effects on the immune system, and such effects may potentiate an autoimmune process.[24]

Women have about a 6-fold increase in risk of Graves disease during the first year postpartum.[25] During pregnancy, many autoimmune disorders decrease in severity, apparently reflecting increased immune tolerance important for the health of the fetus. Inflammation and autoantibody titers typically decrease. Post partum, a rebound of immunologic activity including production of antibodies to thyroid stimulating hormone (TSH) receptors, can manifest as the initial presentation or relapse of Graves disease.[26] Another possible reason pregnancy is a risk factor is the accumulation of fetal cells in the maternal thyroid (fetal microchimerism) with consequent development of an autoimmune response.[27]

Smoking is associated with about a 2- to 3-fold increased risk of Graves disease, and the risk of ophthalmopathy among smokers is four to five times that for nonsmokers.[28,29] The risk increases with higher pack-years of smoking, and cessation results in a progressive decline over time. The mechanisms of increased risk are uncertain at this time, but considerations include tissue damage because of increased generation of reactive oxygen species, increased production of autoantibodies, and increased concentration of soluble adhesion molecules.[30]

Infectious microorganisms have been implicated as etiologic agents because of antigen mimicry or other mechanisms resulting in autoimmunity. *Yersinia enterocolitica* is high on the list of suspects for causing Graves disease. It possesses one or more outer membrane proteins that have homology with TSHR and studies have revealed significantly higher levels of antibodies to *Y. enterocolitica* among patients with Graves disease.[17] However, most individuals with *Y. enterocolitica* infection do not develop thyroid disease, and a definitive link to it or other infectious agents has not been established at this time.

Graves disease has genetic risk factors, but no single gene has been identified as causative or necessary. The concordance rate for monozygotic twins is 20% to 35%, whereas the concordance rate for dizygotic twins is <5%.[12] This not only supports a genetic role but also indicates the involvement of other factors. The human leukocyte antigen (HLA) gene *HLA-DR3* has been identified as a major susceptibility gene and is discussed below. Individuals with *HLA-DR3*, typically of European origin, have a relative risk in the range of 3 to 4.[18]

Pathogenesis and Molecular Genetics

Hyperthyroidism of Graves disease is due to the production of autoantibodies to the TSHR on follicular cells. The autoantibodies activate the receptor and stimulate thyroid hormone synthesis and secretion in addition to diffuse proliferation of the follicular epithelium. Before recognition as autoantibodies, they were called LATS. This term derived from the observation that sera of patients with Graves disease stimulated the thyroids of test animals for a longer time than TSH.[8] Further studies revealed that the long-acting stimulator was an immunoglobulin (thyroid-stimulating immunoglobulin) that binds to the extracellular domain of TSHR. TSHR is a member of the superfamily of G protein–coupled receptors. The gene coding for the protein was cloned in 1989 and maps to chromosome 14q31.[31-33] TSHR is composed of three domains, one extracellular, one intracellular, and a connecting seven-loop transmembrane domain. The extracellular domain is relatively large, accounting for approximately half of the molecular size of the receptor, and serves as the binding site for TSH.[34] The binding of TSH to TSHR results in stimulation of second messenger pathways predominately through cyclic AMP (cAMP) with eventual effect on the gene expression of follicular cells (see Chapter 8, Fig. 8.2).

Antibodies to TSHR attach to epitopes in the region of the TSH-binding pocket of the extracellular domain and can have stimulatory, blocking, or neutral effects on thyroid function.[35-37] Stimulatory antibodies are specific for Graves disease, and these antibodies are detectable in almost all cases using modern assays. Blocking antibodies are more typically found in chronic lymphocytic (Hashimoto) thyroiditis and can contribute to hypothyroidism by preventing the binding of TSH. Both stimulatory and blocking antibodies may be detected in some cases of Graves disease. These stimulatory and blocking antibodies share comparable features of low serum concentration, high affinity, and similar binding epitopes on TSHR.[38]

A relatively unique aspect of TSHR is the phenomenon of molecular cleavage with shedding of the α subunit. This subunit constitutes the majority of the extracellular domain, and shedding exposes epitopes in the TSHR region to antibodies that may be partially hindered sterically when the receptor is attached to the follicular cell membrane.[39] The shedding of the α subunit may play a role in the initiation or amplification of the autoimmune response. Follicular cells may also contribute to increased vascularity of the thyroid by secreting vascular endothelial growth factor in response to stimulation by TSHR autoantibodies.[40]

A complex interaction of T and B lymphocytes and thyroid follicular cells underlies the pathogenic autoantibody response.[41] Our knowledge of the extent and specifics of the various immunologic mechanisms is incomplete, but it seems clear that T lymphocytes play an important role in the pathogenesis. Thyroids with Graves disease contain CD8+ and CD4+ T cells including CD4+ T_h1, CD4+ T_h2, and CD4+ T_{reg} (CD25+) subsets. The main functions of CD4+ T_h1 cells are related to cell-mediated immune responses, whereas CD4+ T_h2 cells are involved predominately in antibody production. Graves disease is primarily a T_h2 type of autoimmune disease because of the role of autoantibodies to TSHR. Stimulation of either the T_h1 or the T_h2 pathway results in reciprocal inhibition of the other. The CD4+ CD25+ T_{reg} cells have an inhibitory effect on both T_h1 and T_h2 cells.

During pregnancy, the immune system is shifted toward a T_h2 response with consequent decrease in T_h1, a seemingly paradoxical finding given that women with Graves disease frequently experience a decrease in severity. This suggests that immunomodulation mechanisms are more complex than a simple shift in the $T_h1:T_h2$ ratio and that much remains to be clarified in regard to the autoimmune mechanisms associated with Graves disease. However, it does seem clear that perturbation of the balance of immune response and inhibition with the net loss of self-tolerance is a basic feature of autoimmunity, and these lymphocytes appear to have prime roles in Graves disease.

Thyroid follicular cells also appear to play an active role in the autoimmune process. They are capable of major histocompatibility complex (MHC) class II (HLA-DR) expression owing to various stimuli, and one of the prime inducers is interferon γ (IFN-γ).[42] Expression of HLA-DR antigens could result from cytokines produced by infection (e.g., viral-induced IFN production) or other environmental factors with the subsequent initiation of an autoimmune response.

HLA genes of the MHC located on chromosome 6p21 are associated with Graves disease, particularly *HLA-DR3 (HLA-DRB1*03)*.[43] Increased risk of Graves disease is particularly associated with an arginine residue at position 74 of the DR β-1 chain.[44] The three-dimensional configuration of the peptide-binding pocket is different with the presence of a positively charged arginine residue compared with a neutral alanine or glutamine residue. A recent study of an ethnic Han Chinese population revealed Graves disease–associated HLA alleles different from those associated with Caucasian populations, with *HLA-DPB1*05:01* identified as the major susceptibility gene.[45]

The risk of Graves disease also developing in an HLA-matched sibling is lower than that of a monozygotic twin, supporting the concept that genes other than HLA alleles are involved.[46] *CTLA-4* is a non-HLA gene whose product downregulates T-cell–mediated immune response and is important for maintaining self-tolerance. Polymorphisms of this gene have been associated with autoimmune diseases including Graves disease.[47] Other immune regulatory genes have been implicated in the pathogenesis of Graves disease including *CD40* and protein tyrosine phosphatase-2 (*PTPN2*).[43] The *CD40* gene, located on chromosome 20q, has also been linked to Graves disease. CD40 is a member of the tumor necrosis factor receptor superfamily and is expressed on B lymphocytes and antigen presenting cells. It functions as a co-stimulatory protein that is involved in various immune responses, and a polymorphism that results in increased CD40 expression could augment the development of autoimmunity.[48] *PTPN2* codes for a lymphoid tyrosine phosphatase that is an inhibitor of T-cell activation. A single-nucleotide polymorphism at codon 620 in which tryptophan is substituted for arginine has been found to be linked to Graves disease and other autoimmune disorders.[48,49] Several other genes have shown association with Graves disease in some populations, and it is highly likely that others will be identified with the broader application of newer molecular pathology techniques.

Ophthalmopathy

Ophthalmopathy is the most frequent and significant extrathyroidal manifestation of Graves disease.[50] The extraocular muscles become inflamed and edematous, and the orbital fibroadipose tissue and lacrimal glands increase in volume. The extraocular muscles and fibroadipose tissue are infiltrated by lymphocytes, predominately T cells, and the tissues accumulate excessive amounts of hydrophilic glycosaminoglycans that derive from fibroblasts. Over time, the extraocular muscles can become atrophic and surrounded by fibrotic tissue.

The basic pathogenic mechanism appears to be autoantibodies directed at orbital tissues.[51] Orbital preadipocyte fibroblasts express TSHR, and stimulation by autoantibodies results in the generation of increased adipose tissue. Autoantibodies to insulin-like growth factor receptor have also been implicated. Stimulation of this receptor causes glycosaminoglycans production along with T-cell recruitment and activation.

Clinical Presentation and Imaging

Presenting signs and symptoms of Graves disease parallel those of increased sympathetic nervous system activity. Common symptoms include nervousness, anxiety, fatigue, heat hypersensitivity, increased perspiration, palpitations, and increased appetite but with loss of weight. Physical examination typically reveals warm moist skin, tremor, tachycardia, hypertension, muscle weakness, lid lag and stare, and mild to moderate goiter. A personal or family history of autoimmune disease is common. Scintigraphic imaging studies with radioiodine reveal diffusely elevated uptake (Fig. 5.1).

Laboratory Tests

Thyroid function tests reveal elevated free T_4 in most cases of Graves disease. However, a normal free T_4 concentration can be found in a small percentage of cases, and thus, measurement of free T_3 may be necessary to demonstrate elevated hormone production. TSH is abnormally low or undetectable and is particularly useful in the evaluation of hyperthyroidism.

Antibodies to TSH receptors are detectable in almost all untreated cases and are highly specific with few false positive results using modern techniques. Two assays are used to detect TSHR antibodies, one measuring TSH-binding inhibitory immunoglobulins (TBII) and the other thyroid-stimulating antibodies. The two assays do not yield totally comparable results because TSHR autoantibodies are heterogeneous and can have agonistic, antagonistic, or neutral effects on the receptor.[35] Both stimulating and blocking antibodies are detected by the TBII assay, and blocking antibodies can interfere with the detection of stimulating antibodies.

The TBII test is an immunoassay that measures inhibition of TSH binding to TSH receptors. Current methodology uses

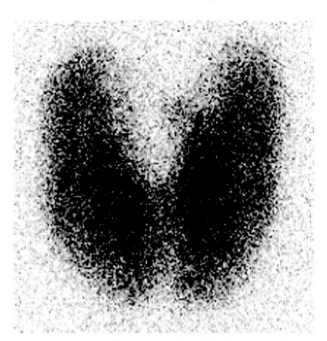

FIGURE 5.1. Radioiodine scan of thyroid with Graves disease showing high uptake throughout gland.

solubilized TSH receptors and an enzymatic detection system. Alternative names for the TBII test include thyroid receptor antibody and LATS.

Stimulating antibodies are detected by a bioassay measuring the release of cAMP from thyroid membranes or cell lines transfected with the TSH receptor. This test is often known by the acronym TSI (thyroid-stimulating immunoglobulin) or TSAb (thyroid-stimulating antibody). This same basic bioassay can be utilized to detect thyroid-blocking antibodies by adding TSH to both patient and control sera and then comparing the relative release of cAMP. The presence of blocking antibodies results in reduced detection of cAMP.

After therapy with radioiodine, the frequency of TSHR antibody detection decreases over the following decade, although there may be an initial transient increase.[52] Antibodies to thyroperoxidase (TPO) are found in most cases, and about half have antibodies to thyroglobulin (TG). However, antibodies to TPO and TG are relatively nonspecific and of limited utility in the evaluation of Graves disease.

Pathology
Gross Features

Thyroid glands show mild to moderate diffuse symmetrical enlargement with a weight usually in the 50 to 150 g range (Fig. 5.2). The color of the cut surface can range from red to reddish brown or tan to a pinkish gray appearance, the variation in color reflective of differing degrees of vascularity. Untreated cases have high vascularity and a dark red appearance, whereas treated cases appear lighter and more similar to normal thyroid because of decreased vascularity and the accumulation of colloid. The consistency ranges from spongy to firm. Various culinary adjectives such as succulent, meaty, or beefy have been used in descriptions, and untreated thyroids bear resemblance to skeletal muscle. Vague nodularity may be seen, but fibrous septa are absent or inconspicuous.

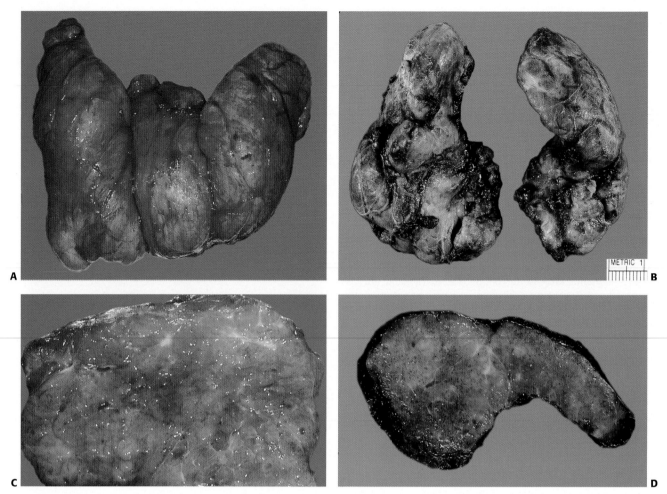

FIGURE 5.2. Two examples of Graves disease **(A and B)** with respective cut surfaces shown below **(C and D)**. One specimen **(A)** shows enlargement of the isthmus and pyramidal lobe in addition to the lateral lobes. Specimen **(B)** has separated lobes because of excision by a minimally invasive surgical technique.

Histologic Features

Diffuse hyperplasia of follicular epithelium is the characteristic histologic finding. The follicles are lined by tall columnar cells that exhibit papillary infolding within the lumina. The papillae are generally simple and nonbranching with limited projection into the central space. In cases with florid hyperplasia, such as those with little or no treatment, papillae may be more prominent and occupy a large portion of the lumen (Fig. 5.3).

Untreated cases contain very little colloid; however, some form of therapy precedes the resection of most cases, and colloid is usually seen. The amount of colloid can vary in different areas depending on the degree of epithelial hyperplasia (Fig. 5.4). Although some variability in the degree of hyperplasia and amount of colloid is typically seen from area to area, the hyperplastic change is diffuse and identifiable in all sections obtained from one or both lobes.

Colloid usually stains lighter and may appear quite pale compared with that in normal thyroids. Scalloping is seen at the interface of the colloid with the follicular cells, particularly in areas with hyperplastic papillae. Cytoplasm of follicular cells can be eosinophilic, amphophilic, microvacuolated, or even clear because of lipid or glycogen accumulation (Fig. 5.5).

Follicular cells contain round to oval, basally located nuclei with finely granular chromatin. Small nucleoli can be seen in some cells. Most nuclei are normochromatic and mildly increased in size. Only mild variation in nuclear size and shape is typically seen. The prime exception is nuclear atypia after radioiodine therapy (Fig. 5.6). Some nuclei may appear hyperchromatic or hypochromatic, and the latter can cause concern for papillary carcinoma. However, the degree of hypochromasia is usually less than that seen in papillary carcinoma, and the nuclei lack other features characteristic of malignancy.

Lymphocytes are commonly seen in the interfollicular stroma. The distribution and total quantity is variable in a given thyroid, ranging from scant or absent to focally dense with germinal centers. Fibrous tissue is usually absent or scant with the exception of some long-standing cases or those treated with radioactive iodine.

Immunohistochemistry

Immunostains have limited diagnostic applicability in Graves disease. Cells typically reveal proliferative activity below 5% as measured by Ki-67 labeling and retain p27 immunoreactivity in most nuclei.[53] Focal lesions questionable for neoplasia can be analyzed with appropriate stains (see Chapter 11). Most lymphocytes infiltrating the thyroid are T lymphocytes with both CD4+ and CD8+ cells demonstrable. Overall, CD8+ lymphocytes tend to outnumber CD4+ lymphocytes, and the cells infiltrating the follicular epithelium are predominately CD8+.[54–56]

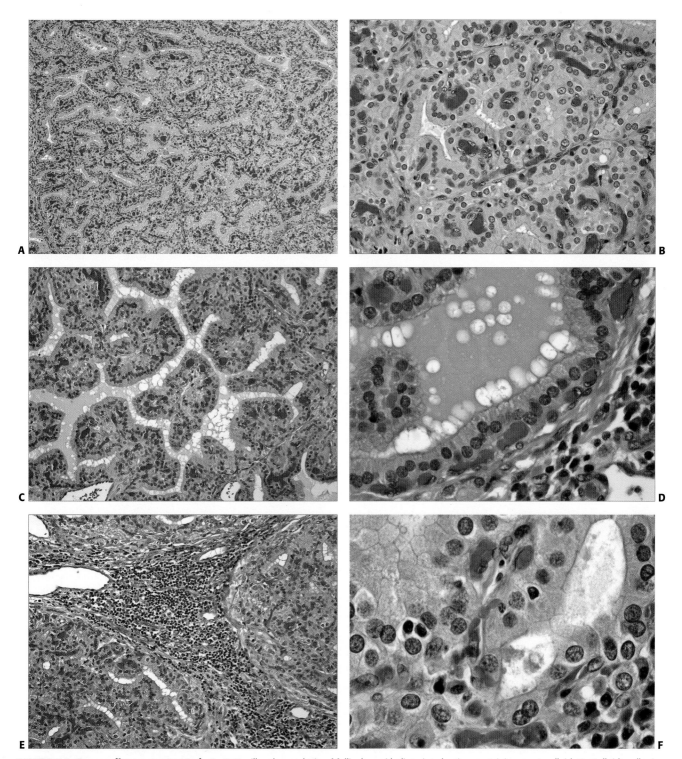

FIGURE 5.3. Graves disease, untreated. A–C: Papillary hyperplasia of follicular epithelium into lumina containing scant colloid. **D:** Colloid scalloping at the periphery of lumen. **E:** Stromal collection of lymphocytes. **F:** Lymphocytes infiltrating between follicular cells.

CD4+ lymphocytes predominate in the interfollicular stroma.[57] CD20+ B cells comprise the majority of lymphocytes in germinal centers. The perifollicular regions contain a mixture of CD4+ and CD8+ T lymphocytes with the latter more frequent. Expression of HLA-DR can be demonstrated in both lymphocytes and follicular cells.[58]

Effects of Therapy

Most surgically resected thyroid glands have been subject to prior treatment with antithyroid drugs or radioactive iodine. Rarely does a surgical pathologist examine an untreated gland. Methimazole and propylthiouracil are common antithyroid drugs that act primarily by blocking hormone synthesis through

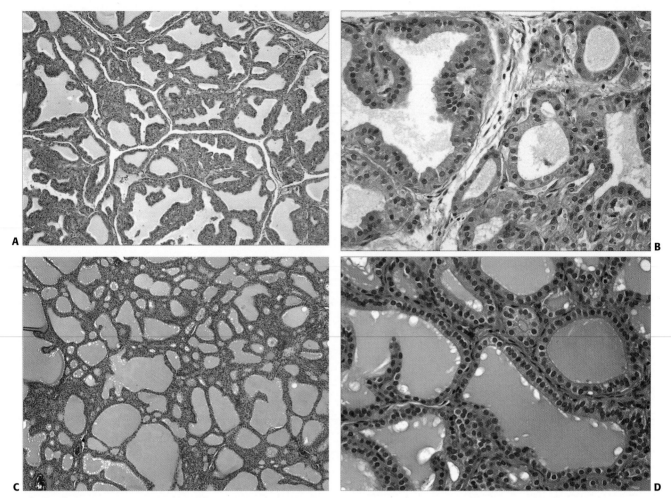

FIGURE 5.4. Graves disease, treated. Two cases treated with antithyroid drugs before resection (A and B) and (C and D). Both cases contain more colloid and less papillary hyperplasia compared to the untreated case shown in Fig. 5.3.

interference with peroxidase-mediated iodination of tyrosyl residues. Thyroid glands may show regression of hyperplastic changes, but the regression is typically incomplete with focal areas of follicular hyperplasia still present. β-Adrenergic blockers such as propranolol do not induce appreciable morphologic changes in the thyroid.[59] Nonradioactive iodine therapy was common in the past but unusual today as a first-line or sole medication. Iodine inhibits release of thyroid hormones and peripheral conversion of T_4 to T_3, the biologically active form of thyroid hormone. Nonradioactive iodine reduces thyroid vascularity, increases colloid stores, and promotes involution of the follicular epithelium. Owing to its reduction of vascularity,

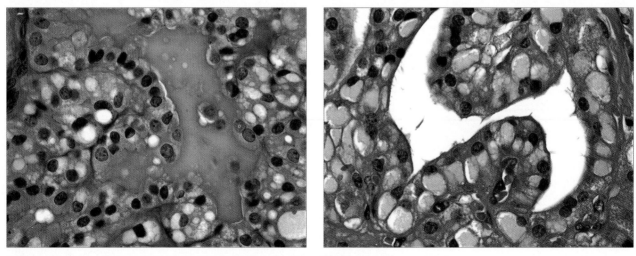

FIGURE 5.5. Graves disease: two cases with focal vacuolization of follicular cells.

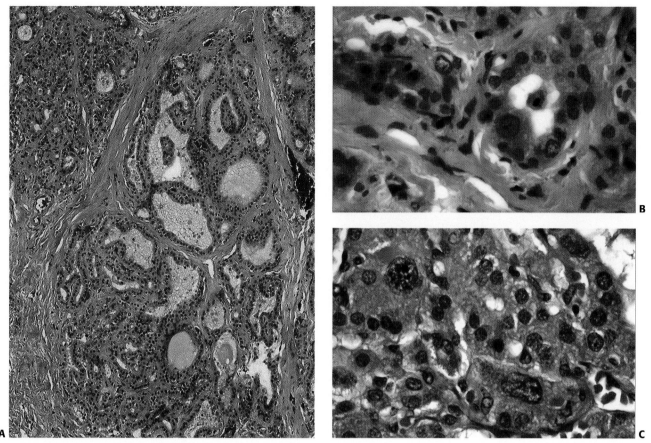

FIGURE 5.6. Graves disease treated with ¹³¹I about 1 year before resection. A: Low-power view showing extensive interstitial fibrosis and marked reduction of hyperplasia. **B and C:** High-power views showing foci of cytologic atypia.

nonradioactive iodine is commonly administered before surgical resection.

Radioactive iodine therapy is associated with various histopathologic features. The range of findings includes follicular atrophy, fibrosis, oncocytic metaplasia, nuclear atypia, formation of hyperplastic nodules, and persistence of lymphocytic infiltrates.[60,61] A diagnosis of nodular hyperplasia or chronic lymphocytic (Hashimoto) thyroiditis may be considered by a pathologist unaware of the clinical diagnosis and prior treatment.

Nodules

Nodular lesions are found in 10% to 25% of thyroids with Graves disease, and most are benign with features of follicular hyperplasia or colloid nodule. However, about 10% to 20% of nodules are found to have carcinoma.[62–65] The overwhelming majority of carcinomas are papillary thyroid carcinoma, and many are incidental microcarcinomas. The overall incidence of carcinoma in Graves disease is 1% to 9% with large, more recent studies yielding results in the range of 1% to 4%.[62–65] Lymphoma rarely occurs in association with Graves disease.

Cytologic Features

Fine needle aspiration (FNA) usually yields scant material that appears bloody. Microscopic examination of smears typically shows low to moderate cellularity with collections of follicular cells admixed with blood. Colloid is scant or difficult to recognize because of its thin, pale appearance, particularly in Papanicolaou-stained slides. Follicular cells are usually arranged in flat sheets or microfollicles, and papillae are typically few or absent.

The cytoplasm of follicular cells is increased and usually has a pale finely granular appearance. Clusters of cells may exhibit marginal vacuolization of their cytoplasm. These vacuoles are clear in Papanicolaou-stained slides but have a pink granular appearance in Diff-Quik–stained preparations (Fig. 5.7). These vacuolated cells are known as flame, fire, or flare cells. Although initially described as distinctive for Graves disease, these cells can be seen in cases of nodular hyperplasia, follicular neoplasia, and papillary carcinoma.[66]

Nuclei are generally round and mildly enlarged. Variation in size may be seen with some nuclei having a diameter several times that of a normal follicular cell. Small nucleoli are common. Lymphocytes and/or oncocytic cells are seen in about 40% to 50% of aspirates.[67] Less frequently, multinucleated giant cells and clusters of epithelioid macrophages may be present. Aspirates of glands after treatment with antithyroid drugs or radioiodine may show cytologic atypia suggestive of malignancy, particularly papillary thyroid carcinoma.[68,69]

Cases of Graves disease are seldom aspirated because the diagnosis is usually based on clinical findings and confirmatory laboratory tests. Aspiration is typically performed when a nodular lesion is detected, and thus, the cytologic findings are likely to be those of another thyroid lesion such as nodular hyperplasia, papillary carcinoma, or follicular neoplasia. Features of Graves disease may be absent or only evident in a minority of the cell population.

Differential Diagnosis

The clinical differential diagnosis of thyrotoxicosis comprises various conditions including those caused by hyperactivity of the

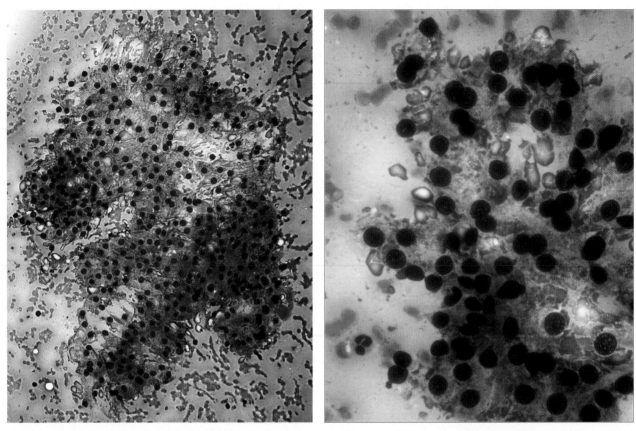

FIGURE 5.7. Cytologic aspirate of Graves disease showing collections of flare/fire/flame cells (Diff-Quik stain). This finding is characteristic but not specific for Graves disease and can be seen in other hyperplastic or neoplastic thyroid disorders. Thin, pale colloid surrounds the cells.

thyroid gland (hyperthyroidism) and those caused by extrathyroidal abnormalities (Table 5.1). Morphologically, the differential diagnosis includes thyroid neoplasia, particularly papillary carcinoma, chronic lymphocytic thyroiditis with hyperthyroidism (hashitoxicosis), and toxic nodular hyperplasia. Acquisition of clinical history and laboratory test results is an important step in the evaluation of these thyroids. The effects of treatment may transform a diffusely hyperplastic thyroid to one with features similar to other conditions.

On a purely histologic basis, differentiation from papillary carcinoma poses the greatest challenge because of the presence of papillae and, in some cases, hypochromatic nuclei (Fig. 5.8 and Table 5.2). Even psammoma bodies have been reported in Graves disease, although this seems to be a rare observation.[70] The absence of both well-developed fibrovascular cores in hyperplastic papillae and the broader range of nuclear features characteristic of papillary thyroid carcinoma combined with the diffuse nature of hyperplastic changes are the key features for excluding a neoplastic process. Immunostaining for p27 may be of help because it shows positivity in most nuclei in Graves disease, whereas it is frequently lost in nuclei of papillary carcinoma cells.[53] Distinct nodular lesions require more scrutiny, and immunostains such as galectin-3 and HBME-1 may be helpful (see Chapter 11).

Hashitoxicosis exhibits follicular hyperplasia that can mimic Graves disease, but generally, it has more pronounced oncocytic metaplasia, lymphocytic infiltrates, and germinal centers. Areas of follicular atrophy and fibrosis also favor hashitoxicosis. Differentiation of Graves disease from toxic multinodular goiter is usually not a problem because a grossly multinodular appearance is not a characteristic of Graves disease. Although one or more nodules of nodular hyperplasia may show hyperplastic changes

comparable with Graves disease, most show follicles in a resting state with abundant colloid.

Treatment and Prognosis

Treatment options for Graves disease include antithyroid medications, radioactive iodine, and surgery, and they have particular advantages and disadvantages.[71] As discussed above, numerous medications are used to treat Graves disease. β-Adrenergic blockers such as propranolol are used for relief of cardiovascular and neurologic symptoms. Antithyroid medications such as methimazole, carbimazole (metabolized to methimazole), and propylthiouracil inhibit synthesis of thyroid hormones and lead to a reduction of levels over a period of weeks to months. Treatment with antithyroid medications induces euthyroidism for a majority of patients, but a significant percentage experience relapse following withdrawal of therapy.

Radioactive iodine therapy with ^{131}I is very common and effective. It ablates the thyroid and eliminates the signs and symptoms of hyperthyroidism over a period of weeks to months. Most patients treated with radioiodine eventually become hypothyroid and require T_4 replacement.

The surgical option is bilateral subtotal or near-total thyroidectomy. This approach is generally reserved for patients who need very rapid amelioration of hyperthyroidism, those for whom nonsurgical therapies are ineffective or unacceptable, or children or young adults because of higher potential risk of radiation-induced thyroid carcinoma associated with ^{131}I therapy. A nodule suspicious or confirmed for malignancy is another indication for surgical resection. Surgical resection carries a low risk of recurrent hyperthyroidism and a low to moderate risk of hypothyroidism.

Table 5.1

Causes of Thyrotoxicosis

Condition	Relative Etiologic Frequency
Hyperplasia	
• Diffuse toxic hyperplasia (Graves disease)	Very common
• Toxic nodular hyperplasia	Common
Neoplasia	
• Toxic (hyperfunctioning) follicular adenoma	Common
• Trophoblastic (human chorionic gonadotropin secreting) neoplasms	Rare
	Rare
• Struma ovarii	Rare
• Pituitary adenoma	Rare
• Metastatic thyroid carcinoma	Rare
Thyroiditis	
• Subacute granulomatous (de Quervain) thyroiditis	Uncommon
• Chronic lymphocytic (Hashimoto) thyroiditis	Uncommon
• Postpartum thyroiditis	Common
• Silent thyroiditis	Common
• Acute thyroiditis	Uncommon
Drug induced	
• Iatrogenic hormone administration	Common
• Exogenous thyroid hormone ingestion	Rare
• Iodine (Jod-Basedow phenomenon)	Rare
• Amiodarone	Uncommon
Hereditary/genetic	
• McCune–Albright syndrome	Rare
• Pituitary resistance to T4	Rare
Miscellaneous	
• Surgical manipulation	Uncommon
• Pregnancy and hCG effect	Uncommon

 # NODULAR HYPERPLASIA

Nodular hyperplasia is the general histopathologic description of changes clinically known as goiter. *Goiter* is a nonspecific term meaning enlargement of the thyroid. The different types of goiter include multinodular, endemic, dyshormonogenetic, toxic multinodular, and amyloid goiter. Amyloid goiter, although characterized by thyroid enlargement, is not associated with follicular hyperplasia, and this entity is covered in Chapter 6. The other forms of goiter are characterized by follicular hyperplasia, and they are discussed below.

Multinodular Goiter

Definition

Multinodular goiter is a common condition characterized clinically by enlargement of the thyroid gland with variable amounts

of nodularity. Synonyms include nodular or multinodular hyperplasia, nodular goiter, nontoxic goiter, colloid goiter, colloid nodule, adenomatoid nodule, adenomatous hyperplasia, and other combinations of these terms. The term *nodular* or *multinodular hyperplasia* reflects histopathologic changes seen in this condition and is more appropriate for usage in pathologic description and diagnosis as compared with goiter, although the latter is also used commonly.

The term *simple goiter* or *diffuse nontoxic goiter* is applicable to euthyroid cases of diffuse thyroid hyperplasia without nodularity. Over time, almost all simple goiters develop nodularity. Cases of hyperplasia associated with hyperthyroidism are prefaced by the term *toxic*.

Multinodular goiters occur on a sporadic or endemic basis, and their pathologic features are comparable. Endemic goiter is usually due to dietary iodine deficiency, and its specific aspects are discussed in a separate section below.

Epidemiology

Prevalence and incidence of multinodular goiter are difficult to ascertain given differences in definition, diagnostic methodology, and dietary iodine. The prevalence of multinodular goiter in iodine-deficient regions is higher compared with those with adequate dietary intake. The Whickham Survey of an iodine-sufficient population in England revealed a prevalence of goiter of 23% for women and 5% for men.[72] The prevalence among the same group 20 years later was 10% women and 2% men, suggesting either a decrease in frequency with age or change in the diagnostic criteria. Multinodular goiter is about 5 to 10 times more frequent among women.[73]

Etiologic Factors

Sporadic multinodular goiter accounts for fewer cases worldwide compared with endemic goiter, and in most instances, a single etiologic factor is not identifiable. Some cases represent either individual deficiency of dietary iodine or excessive ingestion of goitrogenic foods. Smoking increases the risk of nodular hyperplasia, particularly in iodine-deficient regions.[74] The mechanism appears to be through the action of thiocyanate, which is a component of cigarette smoke. Multiple medications cause or contribute to nodular hyperplasia because of their interference with thyroid hormone synthesis and/or release. These include lithium, thionamides, thalidomide, perchlorate, iodine, amiodarone, and other iodine-containing compounds. Heritable defects in the pathways of thyroid hormone synthesis and release can result in hypothyroidism and a form of goiter known as dyshormonogenetic goiter (see below). Genetic defects with lesser impairment of hormone synthesis and release may contribute to the development of euthyroid nodular hyperplasia.

Although cases of sporadic multinodular goiter may reflect increased TSH secretion, a large percentage have no appreciable TSH stimulation.[75] Most cases of sporadic multinodular goiter are likely due to intrinsic characteristics of follicular cells coupled with environmental and genetic factors. Studies of multinodular goiter among twins in endemic and nonendemic regions have revealed significantly higher concordance rates for monozygotic compared with dizygotic pairs.[76,77] These findings support a multifactorial etiology of multinodular goiter with both genetic and environmental factors playing roles. In the study of a nonendemic region, genetic factors appeared to play the dominant role.

Pathogenesis and Molecular Genetics

Follicular cells are heterogeneous in their capacity to produce thyroid hormone, having variable ability to transport iodine into

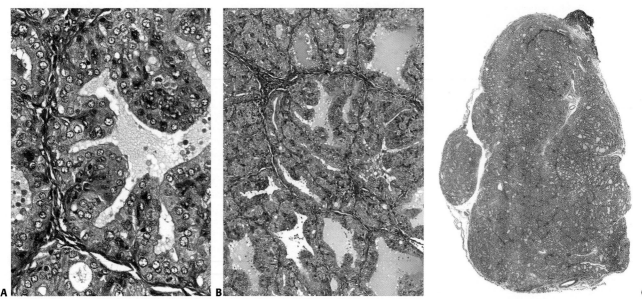

FIGURE 5.8. Graves disease mimicking papillary thyroid carcinoma. A: High-power photomicrograph showing papillary infoldings along with nuclear enlargement, focal overlapping, and chromatin clearing. **B and C:** Progressive lower power photomicrographs showing diffuse nature of changes.

the cell and iodinate TG.[78] Follicular cells also have variable growth potential.[79,80] Some possess relatively high proliferative potential both in response to TSH stimulation and autonomously when TSH levels are low.

Hyperplasia of follicular cells at one or more foci is the basis of nodule formation. The increased number of follicular cells results in an increased number of follicles and an increased size of some follicles. The formation of nodules can be explained by several mechanisms. The different rates of proliferation of different follicular cell subpopulations are likely to lead to

expanding foci that become ever more apparent microscopically, and eventually macroscopically. Nodules also can be accentuated by fibrous tissue secondary to focal hemorrhage and necrosis. The heterogeneous qualities of follicular cells correlate with the histologic features of nodular hyperplasia. Follicular cells with a high production rate of TG and colloid but low rate of endocytosis and hormone release are associated with large follicles with abundant colloid.

The search for genes involved in predisposition to or development of multinodular goiter is an active process with most

Table 5.2

Features Helpful in Distinguishing Graves Disease from Papillary Thyroid Carcinoma

Feature	Graves Disease	Papillary Thyroid Carcinoma
Thyroid function	Hyperthyroid	Euthyroid
Distribution of papillary architecture	Diffuse	Limited to tumor
Papillae	Simple, nonbranching infoldings; no well-developed fibrovascular cores	Complex papillae with distinct fibrovascular cores
Follicular cells		
Nuclear location	Basal region	Not polarized
Nuclear size	Mildly enlarged	Distinctly enlarged
Other nuclear features characteristic of papillary carcinoma (hypochromasia, overlapping, irregular contours, grooves, pseudoinclusions)	Absent or partially developed	Present
Cytoplasm	Vacuolated	Not vacuolated
Psammoma bodies	Absent	Common
Colloid	Pale; often exhibits scalloping	Intensely eosinophilic; absence of scalloping
p27 Nuclear immunostaining	Usually positive	Usually negative
Galectin-3 and HBME-1 immunostaining	Negative	Positive
Mutational testing	No mutations	Frequent *BRAF* mutation[a]; may have *RET/PTC*

[a]Owing to tall cell appearance, most common differential diagnosis includes tall cell variant of papillary thyroid carcinoma, which frequently has *BRAF* V600E mutation.

candidate genes being those involved in thyroid growth and hormone synthesis such as *TG, TPO*, sodium-iodide symporter, and *TSHR*. Linkage analyses and entire genomic scans have been used in attempts to identify loci. Studies of two families with numerous members affected by euthyroid multinodular goiter identified a locus on chromosome 14q31 that has been named *MNG1*.[81,82] *TSHR* is also located on 14q, but it is outside the region of *MNG1*. A study of another pedigree of familial euthyroid multinodular goiter revealed linkage to chromosome *Xp22*.[83] However, subsequent studies of other families suggest that *MNG1* and *Xp22* are unlikely to play a general role in multinodular goiter.[84] Studies of additional euthyroid goiter families have found candidate loci on chromosomes 3p, 2q, 7q, and 8p.[85] Other candidate genes such as transforming growth factor β have emerged, and the evaluation of others continues.[73,86] Most cases of multinodular goiter appear to be the result of complex interaction between multiple genes and various environmental factors. Even for cases of familial multinodular goiter, the etiologic factors appear to be multiple and indicative of genetic heterogeneity.

An exception to the general multifactorial concept is *PTEN*-hamartoma tumor syndrome (PHTS). PHTS is a rare disorder that encompasses both Cowden and Bannayan–Riley–Ruvalcaba syndromes, and multiple hyperplastic/adenomatous nodules may be seen in association with chronic lymphocytic thyroiditis, papillary carcinoma, follicular carcinoma, and/or follicular adenomas.[87,88] PHTS is caused by a germ line mutation of the *PTEN* tumor suppressor gene that maps to chromosome 10q23 and negatively regulates the prosurvival PI3K/Akt/mTOR pathway. PHTS accounts for a small proportion of multinodular goiters, reflective of the rarity of the syndrome.

Studies have identified *TSHR* genetic mutations in some nodules of multinodular goiter.[73] TSHR has a relatively high degree of susceptibility to constitutive activation, which is receptor signaling in the absence of ligand binding, and activating mutations in the *TSHR* gene have been identified. The net result is follicular cell growth and division autonomous from the stimulation of TSH. In some cases, constitutive activation leads to not only growth but also excessive hormone production. Somatic mutations conferring a higher proliferative rate can be transmitted to subsequent generations and allow for the emergence of a clonal population.

Oxidative injury caused by H_2O_2 is a potential explanation for somatic mutations of *TSHR* leading to constitutive activation of follicular cells.[73,86,89] H_2O_2 is necessary along with TPO for the oxidation of iodine before attachment to tyrosyl residues on TG. When iodine is deficient or TPO activity impaired, H_2O_2 may accumulate to toxic concentrations in follicular cells.[90,91] Consequent oxidative damage of DNA could result in somatic mutations that affect cellular growth and function.

Clonal analysis of nodules by molecular methods that assess random versus nonrandom inactivation of X chromosomes has shown that a significant proportion of discrete nodules in glands affected by multinodular goiter have identical patterns of inactivation.[73] An identical pattern of inactivation is interpreted as evidence of monoclonality, and monoclonality is generally regarded as a feature of neoplasia. Caution has been raised regarding clonality of thyroid nodules because the patch size of normal human thyroid tissue is large (see Chapter 20).[92,93] Multiple clones of similar genotype can form a single patch. Therefore, a large normal patch size combined with limited sampling of a hyperplastic nodule may yield monoclonal findings that, in fact, may represent normal thyroid clonality.[94]

Cytogenetically, most goiters show a normal karyotype, whereas some reveal small clones with various numerical and/or structural chromosomal aberrations, the most common of which is trisomy or tetrasomy 7.[95,96] These data, together with clonality

studies based on X chromosome inactivation, suggest that some discrete nodules in multinodular goiter are likely of monoclonal origin.

Should multinodular goiter be considered a neoplastic disorder? Numerous experts in the field support the concept that nodular hyperplasia is fundamentally a neoplastic process.[73,75] These lesions show autonomous growth and, arguably, monoclonality, features generally considered characteristic of neoplasia. Attempts to divide what may be a spectrum of proliferative lesions into one of two categories are problematic. At this time, it remains unclear whether discrete nodules within multinodular goiter represent hyperplasia or neoplasia. As our understanding of the molecular biology of these nodules becomes more complete, we will likely resolve this issue and achieve consensus in classification. Meanwhile, pathologists are faced with the practical issues of evaluating nodular lesions in a manner that is clinically relevant, timely, and cost-effective. Continued use of standard criteria (see Pathology and Differential Diagnosis sections below and Chapter 8) for the differentiation of multinodular goiter from follicular adenoma seems advisable for the present time.

Clinical Presentation and Imaging

Patients usually seek medical attention because of problems associated with thyroid enlargement. In addition to cosmetic disfigurement, the enlarged thyroid may cause stridor owing to tracheal compression or dysphagia owing to interference with swallowing. Occasionally, multinodular goiter extends into the mediastinum and is associated with stridor or superior vena cava syndrome. The onset of signs and symptoms is usually gradual. Rapid enlargement or sudden discomfort may result from intrathyroidal hemorrhage.

Most affected individuals are euthyroid. A minority manifest signs and symptoms of hyperthyroidism. Generally, these are elderly individuals with long-standing disease. Scintigraphic imaging studies with radioiodine usually reveal focal uptake scattered throughout the gland (Fig. 5.9). In a minority of cases, uptake is limited to one or only a few nodules.

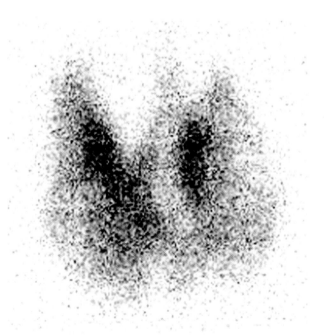

FIGURE 5.9. Radioiodine scan of thyroid with multinodular goiter showing patchy uptake in different areas of the gland.

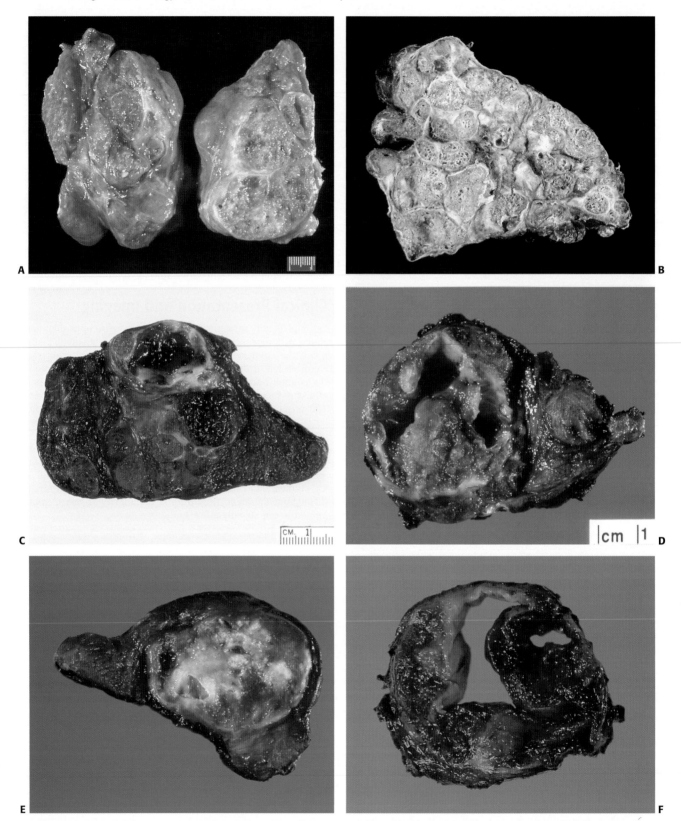

FIGURE 5.10. A–D: Multinodular goiters. **(A)** and **(B)** show marked thyroid enlargement and multinodularity. Distinct fibrous septa separate many of the nodules. **(C)** and **(D)** have nodules with hemorrhage and cystic degeneration. **E:** Dominant hyperplastic nodule that appears almost entirely encapsulated. The nodule has a heterogeneous appearance and, microscopically, exhibited variable cellularity and colloid content, fibrosis, and evidence of past hemorrhage. The surrounding thyroid tissue exhibited mild hyperplastic changes microscopically. **F:** Multinodular goiter showing area of marked cystic degeneration.

Laboratory Tests

Most individuals with multinodular goiter are euthyroid and thus have TSH and free T_4 levels within normal ranges. Periodic testing for TSH is commonly performed to screen for the development of toxic multinodular goiter.[97,98] A low TSH level warrants the determination of free T_4 and the determination of free T_3 if free T_4 is not elevated.

Pathology

Gross Features

Multinodular goiter is characterized by thyroid enlargement that can range from mild to massive. Enlarged thyroids may achieve weights of more than 1,000 g, and most cases of extreme thyroid enlargement are due to multinodular goiter. The full potential of thyroid enlargement is rarely attained in modern developed countries, and weights of thyroids resected for multinodular goiter are usually <200 g.

Most cases have multiple nodules evident grossly (Fig. 5.10). Early cases may lack distinct nodularity, and some cases have only a single macroscopic nodule (Fig. 5.10E). However, microscopic examination typically shows similar changes in the thyroid tissue surrounding the dominant nodule.

The nodules exhibit variable size. Distortion of the normal thyroid size and shape correlates with the number and size of nodules, and thyroid enlargement may be symmetric or asymmetric. Small nodules may be attached to the main portion of the gland by thin fibrous strands or located nearby but separately (parasitic nodule; see Chapter 2).

The sectioned surfaces typically have a nodular, heterogeneous appearance. Portions may look glistening and semitranslucent because of abundant colloid. Numerous secondary changes are common including foci of hemorrhage, fibrosis, cystic degeneration, and calcification (Fig. 5.10). Nodules may appear partially encapsulated by fibrous tissue.

Histologic Features

Microscopic pathologic changes parallel the macroscopic appearance. Follicles exhibit variable size and shape. They range from small with minimal colloid to very large colloid lakes (Fig. 5.11). The large follicles are typically lined by flattened epithelium, whereas the smaller follicles are composed of cuboidal or columnar epithelial cells. Some refer to a nodule with high cellularity associated with a microfollicular or solid growth pattern and scant colloid as an *adenomatous nodule*, whereas the term *colloid nodule* is applied to those with abundant colloid and a low density of follicular cells. Areas can contain follicular epithelium with oncocytic or clear cell features (Fig. 5.12). Rounded clusters of small follicles known as Sanderson polsters can be seen in large follicles, extending from the periphery into the colloid (Fig. 5.12). Follicles can also show papillary infolding of epithelium and complex mixtures of follicles that form papillary-like structures (Fig. 5.13). An unusual finding is widespread presence of follicular cells with large signet-ring–like vacuoles (Fig. 5.14).

Larger nodules may compress surrounding thyroid tissue. Nodules commonly show partial encapsulation by fibrous tissue of varying thickness. Some may be surrounded entirely by

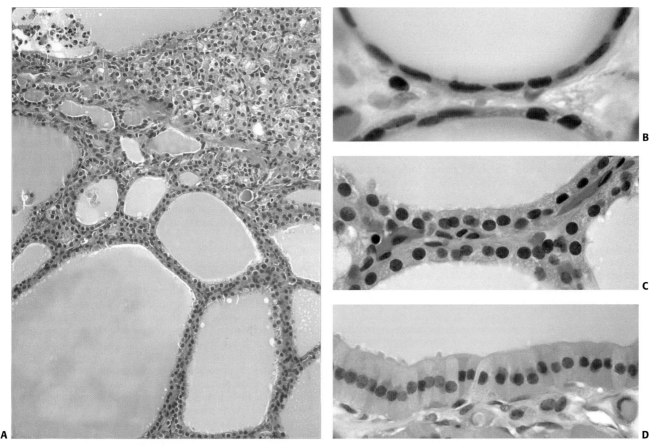

FIGURE 5.11. Multinodular goiter. A: Variation in follicular size with small follicles **(upper region)** and large follicles with abundant colloid. **B–D:** High-power views showing range of follicular epithelium. **B:** Flat. **C:** Cuboidal. **D:** Columnar.

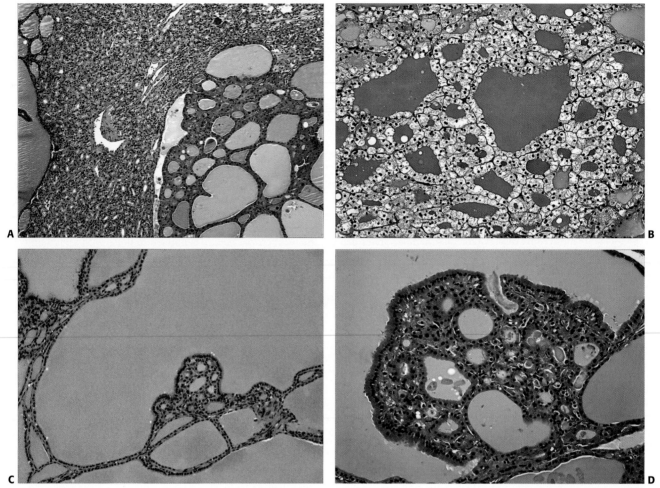

FIGURE 5.12. Various microscopic findings in multinodular goiter. A: Ill-defined nodule with oncocytic follicular epithelium **(lower right side).** **B:** Focal area of clear cell change. **C and D:** Sanderson polsters.

a fibrous rim and raise the question of a follicular adenoma or carcinoma. Various secondary changes can be seen including hemorrhage and fibrosis. The hemorrhage may be fresh or old, with areas of past hemorrhage marked by the presence of hemosiderin-laden macrophages, foamy macrophages, cholesterol crystals, and accentuated fibrosis (Fig. 5.15). Dystrophic calcification also can be present because of past hemorrhage and necrosis.

Reactive endothelial hyperplasia may be seen in multinodular goiter. This appears to be a rare but possibly underreported or underappreciated finding that has similarities to intravascular papillary endothelial hyperplasia.[99–101] Reactive endothelial hyperplasia is found within thyroid hematomas and represents an organizational process. Histologically, it appears as irregular vascular channels or papillary structures lined by plump endothelial cells within a background of fibrinous or hemorrhagic material (Fig. 5.16). Reactive endothelial hyperplasia may also resemble a hemangioma. These lesions are typically identified in thyroids previously sampled by FNA or biopsy, and this may be the underlying cause. Reactive endothelial hyperplasia has the potential to be misdiagnosed as anaplastic thyroid carcinoma or angiosarcoma. The endothelial nature of the cells can be confirmed with immunostains for factor VIII–related antigen, CD34, or CD31. Distinction from angiosarcoma relies on appreciating the ambient multinodular goiter and the specific setting of an organizing hematoma.

Metaplastic changes involving nonepithelial components can be seen. Osseous metaplasia may occur, particularly in areas of dystrophic calcification, and the stroma can undergo adipose metaplasia (Fig. 5.17). Inflammation may accompany nodular hyperplasia. Focal or diffuse lymphocytic infiltrates can be present and may represent coincidental autoimmune thyroiditis. Focal granulomatous inflammation may be seen secondary to rupture of follicles.

Cytologic Features

Multinodular goiters are examined commonly by FNA. Grossly, the specimen ranges from abundant to scant, from thin to viscous, and from red (bloody) to brown to translucent yellow in color. Typical microscopic findings include colloid, foamy macrophages, hemosiderin-laden macrophages, cell debris, and variable numbers of follicular cells (Fig. 5.18).

Aspirates from nodules with abundant colloid may coat the slide with a proteinaeous film that has a cracked, mosaic-like appearance after drying. The presence of abundant colloid favors multinodular goiter over neoplasia.

Follicular cells can be present in monolayer sheets, microfollicular clusters, and/or singly. Aspirates from cellular hyperplastic nodules may show flame/fire/flare cells similar to those seen in Graves disease. Oncocytic cells and multinucleated giant cells may be seen as well as small numbers of lymphocytes or neutrophils.

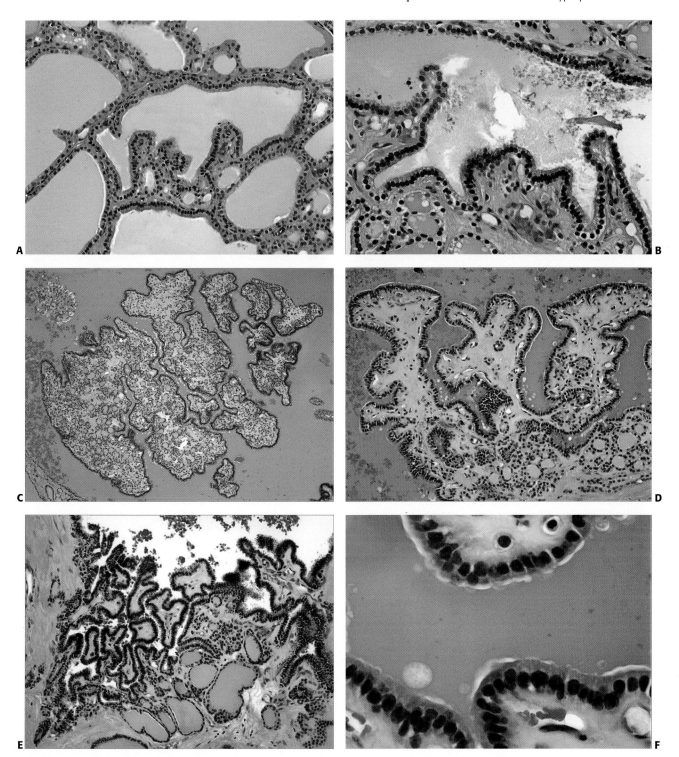

FIGURE 5.13. Multinodular goiter. A–F: Photomicrographs showing variable patterns and degrees of papillary infolding of follicular epithelium. High-power view **(F)** shows nuclei that are basally located with dark uniform chromatin.

Differential Diagnosis

The most common diagnostic challenge associated with multi-nodular goiter is distinguishing a dominant nodule from a follicular adenoma. In most cases that have multiple vaguely defined nodules, this is not a problem. Features of a nodule favoring hyperplasia over a follicular neoplasm include being one of multiple

nodules, encapsulation absent or partial, variable cellularity and growth patterns within the nodule, similar histologic features in the adjacent thyroid tissue, abundant colloid, and little, if any, compression of adjacent thyroid tissue (see Chapter 8, Table 8.1).

As discussed above, some consider multinodular goiter a neoplastic process, and they may consider this exercise moot. However, standard pathology practice still attempts to differentiate

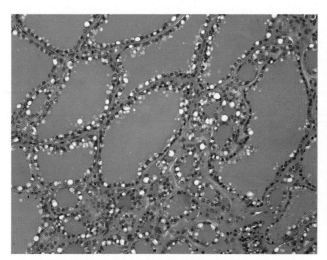 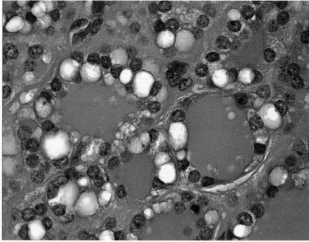

FIGURE 5.14. Multinodular goiter with diffuse signet-ring–like vacuolization of follicular epithelium.

hyperplastic nodules from follicular adenomas on a morphologic basis. One must acknowledge that the features of a given nodule may not line up entirely on one side of the ledger and that the diagnosis is based on the preponderance of findings. In addition, a morphologically convincing adenoma may coexist with multinodular goiter.

Another relatively frequent diagnostic challenge is whether a case of multinodular goiter also contains papillary carcinoma. Follicular cells of multinodular goiter can exhibit hypochromatic nuclei that suggest carcinoma, and papillary-like structures may also raise concerns of malignancy. Careful evaluation for the spectrum of nuclear features characteristic of papillary carcinoma is essential. Adjunct immunohistochemical studies for galectin-3 and HBME-1 expression and molecular analysis for *BRAF* and other mutations may also help in borderline cases (see Chapter 11).

Dyshormonogenetic goiter is grossly indistinguishable from multinodular goiter, and their microscopic features can overlap. Although there are features suggestive of dyshormonogenetic goiter over multinodular goiter, definitive diagnosis is dependent on correlation with clinical and other ancillary information. Dyshormonogenetic goiter is discussed in a section below.

Treatment and Prognosis

Patients with multinodular goiters that have minimal signs or symptoms may not require specific treatment other than periodic physical evaluation. Treatment is usually indicated for cases that show significant growth with compression of neck or mediastinal structures, progressive growth of a particular nodule, hyperthyroidism, or marked disfigurement owing to size. Treatment options include bilateral subtotal thyroidectomy, T_4 therapy, or subtotal ablation with radioiodine.[97,98]

Surgery permits rapid treatment of compressive symptoms, is more effective in treating large goiters, and allows pathologic examination of the thyroid. Multinodular goiter can recur in some cases. Radioiodine therapy is effective, but reduction of size may be slow and never reach normal. In addition, a significant number of patients eventually develop hypothyroidism after several years. T_4 therapy is an option for small goiters but may have minimal effect on large goiters, and long-term therapy may be problematic for the patient.

Endemic Goiter

Definition

The term *endemic goiter* is applied to thyroid enlargement that occurs in a significant portion of a region or population. A commonly applied criterion is when 5% or more of children aged 6 to 12 have thyroid enlargement.[102] The vast majority of endemic goiters are caused by iodine deficiency. The severity of iodine deficiency in a region can be rated mild, moderate, or severe based on the prevalence of goiter or median urinary iodine concentration in individuals age 6 or older (Table 5.3).[103] The pathologic features of endemic goiter are comparable with those of multinodular goiter.

Epidemiology

In iodine deficient regions, thyroid ultrasonography reveals prevalence as high as 30% to 40% among women and 20% to 30% among men.[73] An estimated 31% of the world population, or almost two billion people, have insufficient iodine intake (Table 5.4).[103] Regional risk factors include low levels of iodine in soil and water, mountainous terrain, river plains, far distance from sea, and a staple diet of cassava. Deficient intake of iodine and other micronutrients is more likely to affect poorer populations in endemic regions because of food shortages and lack of dietary diversity. Fortunately, iodination of salt can be achieved with relative ease technologically and economically.

Etiology and Pathophysiology

The most frequent cause of endemic goiter is iodine deficiency.[104] Dietary deficiency with consequent impairment of thyroid hormone production triggers increased TSH release through the hypothalamic–pituitary axis. TSH stimulates the thyroid to increase in size, although TSH stimulation alone does not seem to account for the extent of goitrous changes. Goiter may represent a maladaptive response to iodine deficiency that affects multiple aspects of thyroid growth and metabolism.[105] The thyroid may become nodular by some of the same mechanisms described in the preceding section on multinodular goiter.

Endemic goiter can be caused by other dietary or environmental factors that interfere with thyroid hormone synthesis and metabolism in a direct or indirect manner. Various foods including cassava, cauliflower, Brussels sprouts, cabbage, turnips, and other members of the Brassicaceae (or Cruciferae) family contain goitrogenic compounds such as thiocyanates and others similar to propylthiouracil. Cassava, also known as manioc, is a member of the Euphorbiaceae family, and metabolism of its edible root generates thiocyanate, which interferes with iodine uptake and organification.[106] Cassava is the staple food of certain populations and for this reason has a relatively frequent association with endemic goiter, particularly in iodine-deficient regions.

Selenium deficiency may play a contributing role in the development of endemic goiter in iodine-deficient areas.[107] A potential mechanism of selenium deficiency is reduced intracellular

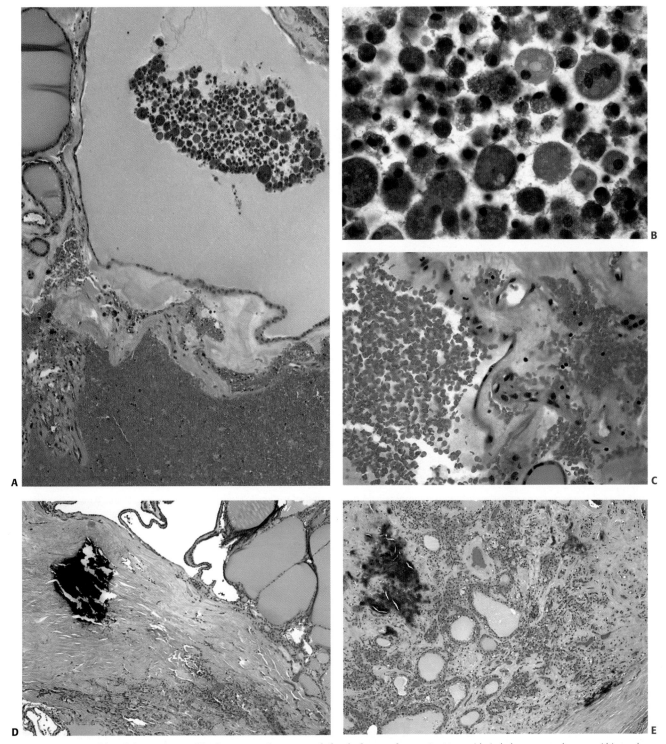

FIGURE 5.15. Multinodular goiter with features of past and fresh hemorrhage. A: Hemosiderin-laden macrophages within a large follicle and extravasated erythrocytes in perifollicular stroma. **B:** High-power view of hemosiderin-laden macrophages. **C:** Focus of fresh hemorrhage. **D and E:** Areas of fibrosis and focal calcification.

glutathione peroxidase with subsequent increased H_2O_2 accumulation and oxidative cell injury.[108] Selenium deficiency by itself does not appear to cause endemic goiter.[109]

Clinical Presentation

Endemic goiter is a component of iodine deficiency disorder that can affect humans across the entire range of life. Problems associated with iodine deficiency include increased risk of stillbirth,

spontaneous abortion, congenital anomalies, and perinatal mortality.[103] Endemic goiter and hypothyroidism can occur in neonates, children, and adults and can be associated with impaired neurologic development and cognitive functioning.

Pathology

The gross and microscopic pathologic findings are the same as those of multinodular goiter as described in the preceding section.

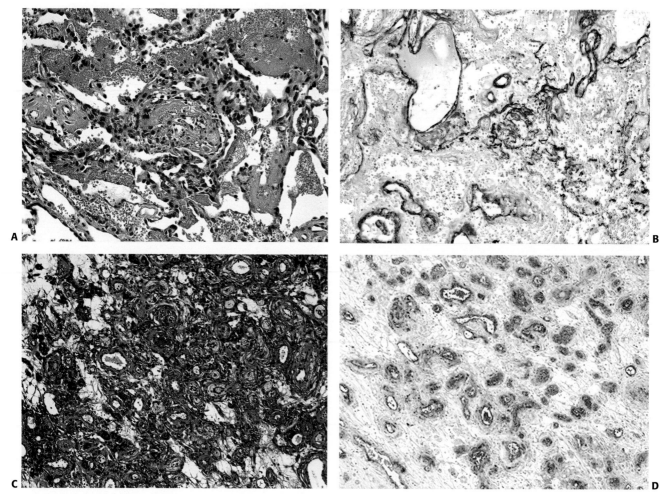

FIGURE 5.16. Intranodular reactive endothelial hyperplasia in multinodular goiter. Two cases (**A** and **B**) and (**C** and **D**) with hematoxylin and eosin (left side) and corresponding factor VIII–related antigen immunostained sections (right side). (Images courtesy of Marco Volante and Mauro Papotti, University of Turin, Italy.)

Dyshormonogenetic Goiter

Definition

Dyshormonogenetic goiter is thyroid enlargement because of a hereditary defect in thyroid hormone synthesis.

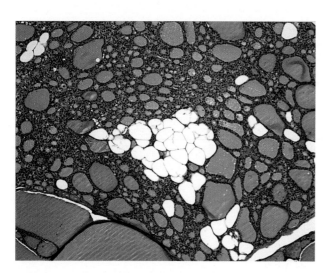

FIGURE 5.17. Multinodular goiter with focus of adipose metaplasia.

Epidemiology

Dyshormonogenetic goiters compose one of the groups of thyroid disorders responsible for permanent congenital hypothyroidism. Congenital hypothyroidism occurs at a rate of 1 in 3,000 to 4,000 births, and approximately 15% of cases are because of dyshormonogenetic goiter, whereas the remainder are because of the group of conditions collectively known as thyroid dysgenesis (see Chapter 2).[110,111] Most cases manifest before the age of 25.[112,113] Most dyshormonogenetic goiters exhibit autosomal recessive inheritance.[110,111]

Pathogenesis and Molecular Pathology

A genetic defect in one of the steps of thyroid hormone synthesis is the underlying pathogenic mechanism. The physiology and genetics of thyroid hormone synthesis are covered in detail in Chapter 3. The congenital mutations associated with dyshormonogenetic goiter are found in those genes involved in TG synthesis, iodine transport, iodide oxidation and organification, coupling of MIT (monoiodotyrosine) and DIT (diiodotyrosine), proteolytic breakdown of TG, and iodide recycling (Table 5.5). Deficiency in TPO activity is the most frequent cause of dyshormonogenetic goiter.[111] Thyroid enlargement is due to insufficient hormone production that results in continuous TSH stimulation.

Pathology

Thyroids are grossly multinodular and enlarged with the degree of enlargement varying from mild to marked. Weights are usually

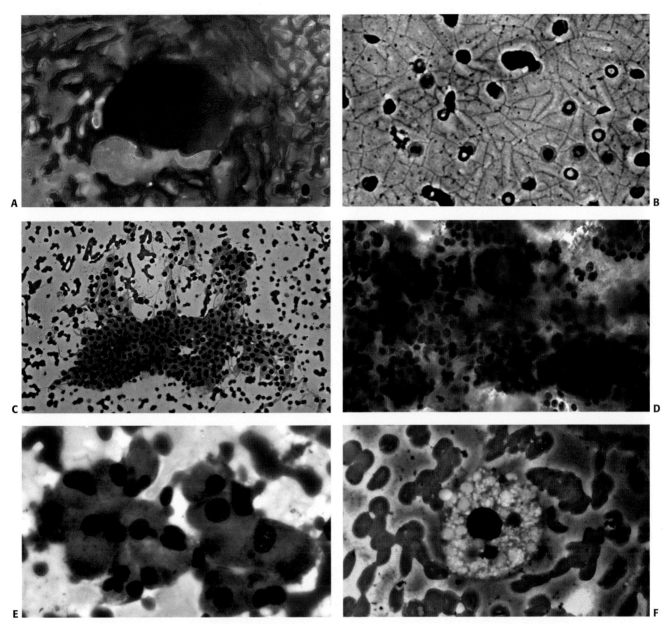

FIGURE 5.18. Cytologic features of aspirates of multinodular goiter. A: Dense colloid retaining spherical shape of follicle **(center)** surrounded by watery colloid and erythrocytes. **B:** Colloid film showing mosaic cracking. **C:** Follicular cells arranged in large, flat monolayer. **D:** Follicular cells forming microfollicles. **E:** Follicular cells showing oncocytic change. **F:** Foamy macrophage. **A–C, E, and F:** Diff-Quik stain; **D:** Papanicolaou stain.

within the range of 50 to 250 g, but they can exceed 500 g.[112,113] The nodules and entire thyroid parenchyma (internodular parenchyma) in dyshormonogenetic goiter usually exhibit marked cellularity with a predominately solid or microfollicular pattern (Fig. 5.19).[113] A trabecular or insular pattern may also be seen. Nodules frequently show marked nuclear atypia with enlarged hyperchromatic nuclei that may also have significant irregularity of contours. Although nuclear atypia is more pronounced within discrete nodules, intervening thyroid parenchyma also shows some degree of nuclear atypia in many cases. In most cases, virtually no colloid is seen within the entire gland. When present, colloid is usually minimal and may be more evident in the better defined nodules.

Differential Diagnosis

The differential diagnosis includes multinodular or endemic goiter, thyroid carcinoma, and iatrogenic goiter caused by

antithyroidal drugs (Table 5.6). Colloid is minimal in contrast to multinodular or endemic goiter in which some or most follicles usually contain abundant colloid. Dyshormonogenetic goiter exhibits pronounced hyperplasia throughout the entire gland, not just the nodules. Also dyshormonogenetic goiter usually shows little, if any, secondary degenerative changes (hemorrhage, foamy and hemosiderin-laden macrophages, fibrosis, and dystrophic calcification). Iatrogenic goiter caused by antithyroidal drugs may be indistinguishable on a histologic basis.

The marked hypercellularity and atypia characteristic of dyshormonogenetic goiter may raise concern of malignancy because areas bear resemblance to one or more types of thyroid cancer. In most cases, follicular carcinoma is suspected. Irregular perinodular fibrosis can simulate capsular invasion. Appreciation of the range and widespread distribution of histopathologic findings seen in dyshormonogenetic goiter, as well as the absence of vascular invasion or clear cut invasion through a thick capsule,

Table 5.3

World Health Organization Epidemiological Criteria for Assessing Iodine Nutrition

Population Group	Median Urinary Iodine (µg/L)	Iodine Intake	Iodine Status
Children ≥6 years and adults	<20	Insufficient	Severe deficiency
	20–49	Insufficient	Moderate deficiency
	50–99	Insufficient	Mild deficiency
	100–199	Adequate	Adequate nutrition
	200–299	Above requirements	Slight risk of adverse consequences
	>300	Excessive	Risk of adverse consequences
Pregnant and lactating women	<150	Insufficient	
	150–249	Adequate	
	250–499	Above requirements	
	>500	Excessive	

Table 5.4

Prevalence of Insufficient Iodine Intake[a] in World Health Organization (WHO) Regions, 1994 to 2006

WHO Region	Number (Millions)	% of Total Regional Population	% of Households with Access to Iodized Salt
Africa	313	42	67
United States	99	11	87
Eastern Mediterranean	259	47	47
Europe	460	52	49
Southeast Asia	504	30	61
Western Pacific	375	21	90
Total	**1,901**	**31**	**70**

[a]On the basis of median urinary iodine <100 µg per L.
From de Benoist B, Burrow G, Delange F, et al. *Assessment of Iodine Deficiency Disorders and Monitoring Their Elimination: A Guide for Programme Managers*. 3rd ed. Geneva, Switzerland: World Health Organization; 2007.

Table 5.5

Synthetic Defects Associated with Dyshormonogenetic Goiter

Step in Thyroid Hormone Synthesis	Related Genes
Thyroglobulin (TG) synthesis	Thyroglobulin (*TG*)
Iodine transport into follicular cell	Sodium-iodide symporter (*NIS*)
Iodine transport into lumen	Pendrin (*PDS*)
	Thyroperoxidase (*TPO*)
Oxidation of iodine	Dual or thyroid oxidase 1 (*DUOX1* or *THOX1*)
	Dual or thyroid oxidase 2 (*DUOX2* or *THOX2*)
Organification of TG	*TPO*
Coupling of MIT and DIT	*TPO*
Proteolytic breakdown of TG	Various lysosomal endopeptidases and exopeptidases
Dehalogenation of MIT and DIT	Dehalogenase 1 (*DEHAL1*)

is important to making the distinction from follicular carcinoma. These pathologic changes in a child or young adult should raise suspicion for dyshormonogenetic goiter; however, a definitive diagnosis will depend on integration of pathologic findings with clinical information, laboratory test results, and other ancillary studies.

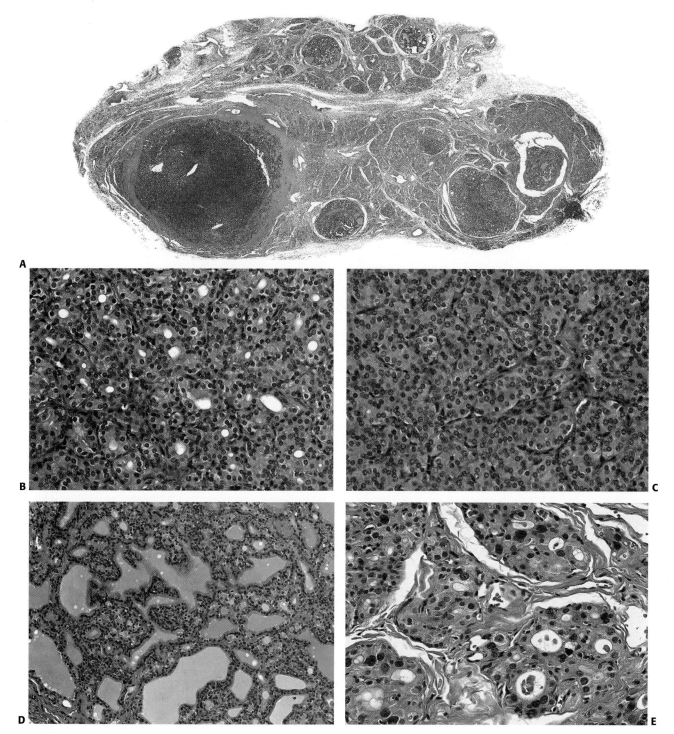

FIGURE 5.19. Dyshormonogenetic goiter. A: Low-power photomicrograph showing pronounced nodularity, fibrosis, and minimal colloid. **B:** Microfollicular pattern. **C:** Insular pattern. **D:** Focal papillary proliferations in a nodule with significant colloid accumulation. **E:** Nodules with marked nuclear atypia and surrounding fibrosis.

Toxic (Hyperfunctioning) Multinodular Goiter

Definition

Toxic multinodular goiter is a multinodular goiter associated with hyperthyroidism. Synonyms include the various

alternative names for multinodular goiter preceded by the word toxic. Toxic multinodular goiter is also known as Plummer disease, named in honor of Dr. Henry Plummer of the Mayo Clinic, who distinguished toxic multinodular goiter from Graves disease in 1913.[114] A hyperfunctioning nodule may be a component of multinodular goiter or a distinct follicular adenoma. Toxic (hyperfunctioning) adenoma is described in detail in Chapter 8.

Table 5.6

Differential Diagnosis of Dyshormonogenetic Goiter

Morphologic Features	Dyshormonogenetic Goiter	Multinodular Goiter	Endemic Goiter	Iatrogenic Goiter Because of Antithyroidal Drugs	Follicular Carcinoma
Follicular hyperplasia	Diffuse, both in nodules and internodular areas	Focal or multifocal	Focal or multifocal	Morphologic features of thyroids after treatment with drugs interfering with synthetic pathway may be indistinguishable from dyshormonogenetic goiter	Usually high cellularity
Colloid content	Minimal	Usually abundant	Usually abundant		Usually minimal (microfollicular or solid pattern)
Secondary degenerative changes	Little if any	Common	Common		Variable; may be present because of FNA
Nodularity	Multinodular	Multinodular	Multinodular		Distinct nodule distinct from adjacent thyroid
Perinodular fibrosis	Variable, may be partial or complete and simulate capsule	Partial or absent	Partial or absent		Complete encapsulation
Transcapsular or vascular invasion	Absent	Absent	Absent		One or both identifiable

Pathogenesis and Molecular Genetics

Toxic multinodular goiter is a complication of multinodular goiter in which one or more nodular collections of follicular cells develop hypersecretion of thyroid hormone. Individuals with multinodular goiter on the basis of iodine deficiency can develop hyperthyroidism when given supplemental iodine, known as Jod-Basedow phenomenon.[19] Other cases represent the development of autonomous hyperfunction. Studies attempting to identify the pathogenic mechanism have yielded mixed results, in particular variable rates of TSHR constitutive activation.[73] Although *TSHR* mutations seem to account for some, or even most cases, they do not account for all. $G_s\alpha$ mutations account for only a very small percentage. Other aberrations, possibly involving the intracellular signaling pathway proteins or extracellular growth factors, may also play a pathogenic role.

Clinical Presentation and Imaging

Toxic multinodular goiter arises in a significant proportion of multinodular goiters. One study found a 10% incidence of hyperthyroidism over a 5-year mean follow-up period.[115] Studies generating incidence data are limited, and whether hyperthyroidism is caused by a hyperfunctioning nodule or adenoma is not always clear.

The typical patient is an elderly individual with long-standing goiter. The signs and symptoms of thyroid excess tend to manifest slowly and are comparable with those seen in other types of thyrotoxicosis as described in the earlier section on Graves disease. However, unlike Graves disease, ophthalmopathy is absent. Because individuals with toxic multinodular goiter tend to be older than those with Graves disease, cardiovascular abnormalities

may be more apparent and life-threatening. Scintigraphic imaging studies with radioiodine reveal increased uptake in one or more nodules with the remainder of the gland showing minimal uptake.

Pathology

Affected glands are grossly comparable with nontoxic multinodular goiter. Microscopically, one or more nodules show features of cell hyperfunction including the tall shape of follicular cells, formation of delicate papillary infoldings, and scant, watery colloid with peripheral scalloping. The hyperfunctioning nodules are often surrounded by fibrous tissue and may appear encapsulated. The rest of the thyroid parenchyma typically shows features of decreased functional status with follicles filled with dense colloid and lined by flattened epithelial cells (Fig. 5.20). However, in some cases, the histologic features of toxic multinodular goiter described above may not be well developed and overlap with those of nontoxic multinodular goiter, so clinical and laboratory findings of hyperthyroidism are necessary to establish the diagnosis definitively.

Differential Diagnosis

The differential diagnosis includes toxic follicular neoplasms and Graves disease. Most hyperfunctional tumors are follicular adenomas. The pathologic features of toxic (hyperfunctioning) follicular adenomas are presented in Chapter 8. Toxic follicular carcinomas are exceedingly rare.

Long-standing cases of Graves disease can develop nodules. Hyperplastic follicular epithelium with histologic features of hyperfunction limited to one or a few nodules with the remainder

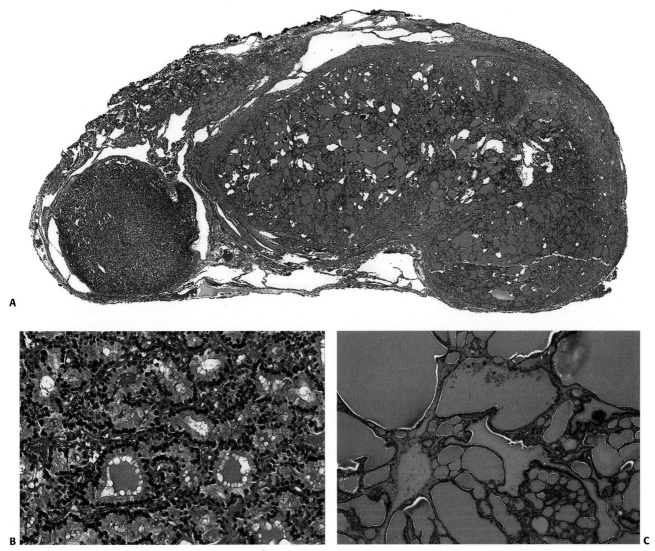

FIGURE 5.20. Toxic multinodular goiter. A: Low-power photomicrograph showing well-defined toxic nodule **(left)**. **B:** High-power view of toxic nodule showing hyperplastic features of high cellularity, columnar follicular epithelium, and relatively scant colloid with peripheral scalloping. **C:** Representative high-power view of remainder of thyroid with inactive features of abundant colloid and low cuboidal follicular epithelium.

of the gland appearing relatively inactive favors toxic multinodular goiter. Graves disease should show diffuse hyperplastic changes, although this may be subtle in some treated cases. The presence of stimulatory autoantibodies to TSHR supports the diagnosis of Graves disease as does the presence of ophthalmopathy.

Treatment and Prognosis

Most cases of toxic multinodular goiter are treated successfully with radioiodine ablation. Patients may experience a transient period of increased hyperthyroidism owing to release of thyroid hormone from damaged follicles but most eventually become euthyroid or hypothyroid. As with nontoxic multinodular goiters, radioiodine therapy reduces the size of toxic multinodular goiters, but a normal size may not be achieved, particularly for large goiters. Subtotal thyroidectomy is an effective alternative therapy, particularly for those who need rapid reduction of hyperthyroidism, have a lesion suspicious for malignancy, or have a large, disfiguring goiter.

REFERENCES

1. Graves RJ. Newly observed affection of the thyroid gland in females. *London Med Surg J.* 1835;7:516–517.
2. von Basedow KA. Exophthalmus durch Hypertrophie des Zellgewebes in der Augenhöhle. *Wochenschr Ges Heilk Berl.* 1840;6:197–220.
3. Parry CH. *Collections from the Unpublished Medical Writings of the Late Caleb Hillier Parry.* London, England: Underwood; 1825.
4. Rehn L. Über die Estirpation des Kropfs bei Morbus basedowii. *Berlin Klin Wochenschr.* 1884;21:163.
5. Möbius PJ. *Basedowsche Krankheit.* Vienna, Austria: Alfred Holder; 1886.
6. Astwood EB. Treatment of hyperthyroidism with thiourea and thiouracil. *JAMA.* 1943;122:78.
7. Hertz S, Roberts A. Application of radioactive iodine in therapy of Graves' disease [abstract]. *J Clin Invest.* 1942;21:624.
8. Adams DD, Purves HD. Abnormal responses in the assay of thyrotropin. *Proc Univ Otago Med Sch.* 1956;34:11–12.
9. Kriss JP, Pleshakov V, Chien JR. Isolation and identification of the long-acting thyroid stimulator and its relation to hyperthyroidism and circumscribed pretibial myxedema. *J Clin Endocrinol Metab.* 1964;24:1005–1028.
10. Furszyfer J, Kurland LT, McConahey WM, et al. Epidemiologic aspects of Hashimoto's thyroiditis and Graves' disease in Rochester, Minnesota (1935–1967), with special reference to temporal trends. *Metab Clin Exp.* 1972;21:197–204.
11. Jacobson DL, Gange SJ, Rose NR, et al. Epidemiology and estimated population burden of selected autoimmune diseases in the United States. *Clin Immunol Immunopathol.* 1997;84:223–243.

12. Tomer Y, Davies TF. Searching for the autoimmune thyroid disease susceptibility genes: from gene mapping to gene function. *Endocr Rev*. 2003;24:694–717.
13. Cox SP, Phillips DI, Osmond C. Does infection initiate Graves disease? A population based 10 year study. *Autoimmunity*. 1989;4:43–49.
14. Phillips DI, Barker DJ, Rees Smith B, et al. The geographical distribution of thyrotoxicosis in England according to the presence or absence of TSH-receptor antibodies. *Clin Endocrinol (Oxf)*. 1985;23:283–287.
15. Berglund J, Christensen SB, Hallengren B. Total and age-specific incidence of Graves' thyrotoxicosis, toxic nodular goitre and solitary toxic adenoma in Malmo 1970-74. *J Intern Med*. 1990;227:137–141.
16. Brownlie BE, Wells JE. The epidemiology of thyrotoxicosis in New Zealand: incidence and geographical distribution in north Canterbury, 1983–1985. *Clin Endocrinol (Oxf)*. 1990;33:249–259.
17. Prummel MF, Strieder T, Wiersinga WM. The environment and autoimmune thyroid diseases. *Eur J Endocrinol*. 2004;150:605–618.
18. Jacobson EM, Huber A, Tomer Y. The HLA gene complex in thyroid autoimmunity: from epidemiology to etiology. *J Autoimmun*. 2008;30:58–62.
19. Stanbury JB, Ermans AE, Bourdoux P, et al. Iodine-induced hyperthyroidism: occurrence and epidemiology. *Thyroid*. 1998;8:83–100.
20. Laurberg P, Pedersen KM, Vestergaard H, et al. High incidence of multinodular toxic goitre in the elderly population in a low iodine intake area vs. high incidence of Graves' disease in the young in a high iodine intake area: comparative surveys of thyrotoxicosis epidemiology in East-Jutland Denmark and Iceland. *J Intern Med*. 1991;229:415–420.
21. Brown TR, Zhao G, Palmer KC, et al. Thyroid injury, autoantigen availability, and the initiation of autoimmune thyroiditis. *Autoimmunity*. 1998;27:1–12.
22. Winsa B, Adami HO, Bergström R, et al. Stressful life events and Graves' disease. *Lancet*. 1991;338:1475–1479.
23. Matos-Santos A, Nobre EL, Costa JG, et al. Relationship between the number and impact of stressful life events and the onset of Graves' disease and toxic nodular goitre. *Clin Endocrinol (Oxf)*. 2001;55:15–19.
24. Elenkov IJ, Chrousos GP. Stress hormones, proinflammatory and antiinflammatory cytokines, and autoimmunity. *Ann N Y Acad Sci*. 2002;966:290–303.
25. Jansson R, Dahlberg PA, Winsa B, et al. The postpartum period constitutes an important risk for the development of clinical Graves' disease in young women. *Acta Endocrinol*. 1987;116:321–325.
26. Lazarus JH. Thyroid disorders associated with pregnancy: etiology, diagnosis, and management. *Treat Endocrinol*. 2005;4:31–41.
27. Ando T, Imaizumi M, Graves PN, et al. Intrathyroidal fetal microchimerism in Graves' disease. *J Clin Endocrinol Metab*. 2002;87:3315–3320.
28. Vestergaard P. Smoking and thyroid disorders—a meta-analysis. *Eur J Endocrinol*. 2002;146:153–161.
29. Holm IA, Manson JE, Michels KB, et al. Smoking and other lifestyle factors and the risk of Graves' hyperthyroidism. *Arch Intern Med*. 2005;165:1606–1611.
30. Costenbader KH, Karlson EW. Cigarette smoking and autoimmune disease: what can we learn from epidemiology? *Lupus*. 2006;15:737–745.
31. Parmentier M, Libert F, Maenhaut C, et al. Molecular cloning of the thyrotropin receptor. *Science*. 1989;246:1620–1622.
32. Nagayama Y, Kaufman KD, Seto P, et al. Molecular cloning, sequence and functional expression of the cDNA for the human thyrotropin receptor. *Biochem Biophys Res Commun*. 1989;165:1184–1190.
33. Libert F, Passage E, Lefort A, et al. Localization of human thyrotropin receptor gene to chromosome region 14q3 by in situ hybridization. *Cytogenet Cell Genet*. 1990;54:82–83.
34. Szkudlinski MW, Fremont V, Ronin C, et al. Thyroid-stimulating hormone and thyroid-stimulating hormone receptor structure-function relationships. *Physiol Rev*. 2002;82:473–502.
35. Watanabe Y, Tahara K, Hirai A, et al. Subtypes of anti-TSH receptor antibodies classified by various assays using CHO cells expressing wild-type or chimeric human TSH receptor. *Thyroid*. 1997;7:13–19.
36. Smith BR, Sanders J, Furmaniak J. TSH receptor antibodies. *Thyroid*. 2007;17:923–938.
37. Jeffreys J, Depraetere H, Sanders J, et al. Characterization of the thyrotropin binding pocket. *Thyroid*. 2002;12:1051–1061.
38. Morgenthaler NG, Ho SC, Minich WB. Stimulating and blocking thyroid-stimulating hormone (TSH) receptor autoantibodies from patients with Graves' disease and autoimmune hypothyroidism have very similar concentration, TSH receptor affinity, and binding sites. *J Clin Endocrinol Metab*. 2007;92:1058–1065.
39. Rapoport B, McLachlan SM. The thyrotropin receptor in Graves' disease. *Thyroid*. 2007;17:911–922.
40. Sato K, Yamazaki K, Shizume K, et al. Stimulation by thyroid-stimulating hormone and Grave's immunoglobulin G of vascular endothelial growth factor mRNA expression in human thyroid follicles *in vitro* and flt mRNA expression in the rat thyroid in vivo. *J Clin Invest*. 1995;96:1295–1302.
41. Weetman AP. Cellular immune responses in autoimmune thyroid disease. *Clin Endocrinol (Oxf)*. 2004;61:405–413.
42. Bottazzo GF, Pujol-Borrell R, Hanafusa T, et al. Role of aberrant HLA-DR expression and antigen presentation in induction of endocrine autoimmunity. *Lancet*. 1983;2:1115–1119.
43. Tomer Y. Genetic susceptibility to autoimmune thyroid disease: past, present, and future. *Thyroid*. 2010;20:715–725.
44. Ban Y, Davies TF, Greenberg DA, et al. Arginine at position 74 of the HLA-DR beta1 chain is associated with Graves' disease. *Genes Immun*. 2004;5:203–208.
45. Chen PL, Fann CS, Chu CC, et al. Comprehensive genotyping in two homogeneous Graves' disease samples reveals major and novel HLA association alleles. *PLoS ONE*. 2011;6:e16635.
46. Brix TH, Kyvik KO, Hegedüs L. What is the evidence of genetic factors in the etiology of Graves' disease? A brief review. *Thyroid*. 1998;8:727–734.
47. Guarneri F, Benvenga S. Environmental factors and genetic background that interact to cause autoimmune thyroid disease. *Curr Opin Endocrinol Diabetes Obes*. 2007;14:398–409.
48. Jacobson EM, Tomer Y. The *CD40, CTLA-4*, thyroglobulin, TSH receptor, and *PTPN22* gene quintet and its contribution to thyroid autoimmunity: back to the future. *J Autoimmun*. 2007;28:85–98.
49. Velaga MR, Wilson V, Jennings CE, et al. The codon 620 tryptophan allele of the lymphoid tyrosine phosphatase (LYP) gene is a major determinant of Graves' disease. *J Clin Endocrinol Metab*. 2004;89:5862–5865.
50. Heufelder AE. Pathogenesis of ophthalmopathy in autoimmune thyroid disease. *Rev Endocr Metab Disord*. 2000;1:87–95.
51. Khoo TK, Bahn RS. Pathogenesis of Graves' ophthalmopathy: the role of autoantibodies. *Thyroid*. 2007;17:1013–1018.
52. Aizawa Y, Yoshida K, Kaise N, et al. Long-term effects of radioiodine on thyrotrophin receptor antibodies in Graves' disease. *Clin Endocrinol (Oxf)*. 1995;42:517–522.
53. Erickson LA. p27(kip1) and other cell-cycle protein expression in normal and neoplastic endocrine tissues. *Endocr Pathol*. 2000;11:109–122.
54. Misaki T, Konishi J, Nakashima T, et al. Immunohistological phenotyping of thyroid infiltrating lymphocytes in Graves' disease and Hashimoto's thyroiditis. *Clin Exp Immunol*. 1985;60:104–110.
55. Bene MC, Derennes V, Faure G, et al. Graves' disease: in situ localization of lymphoid T cell subpopulations. *Clin Exp Immunol*. 1983;52:311–316.
56. Warford A, McLachlan SM, Malcolm AJ, et al. Characterization of lymphoid cells in the thyroid of patients with Graves' disease. *Clin Exp Immunol*. 1984;57:626–632.
57. Margolick JB, Hsu SM, Volkman DJ, et al. Immunohistochemical characterization of intrathyroid lymphocytes in Graves' disease. Interstitial and intraepithelial populations. *Am J Med*. 1984;76:815–821.
58. Lloyd RV, Johnson TL, Blaivas M, et al. Detection of HLA-DR antigens in paraffin-embedded thyroid epithelial cells with a monoclonal antibody. *Am J Pathol*. 1985;120:106–111.
59. Lee KS, Kim K, Hur KB, et al. The role of propranolol in the preoperative preparation of patients with Graves' disease. *Surg Gynecol Obstet*. 1986;162:365–369.
60. Mizukami Y, Michigishi T, Nonomura A, et al. Histologic changes in Graves' thyroid gland after 131I therapy for hyperthyroidism. *Acta Pathol Jpn*. 1992;42:419–426.
61. Friedman NB, Catz B. The reactions of euthyroid and hyperthyroid glands to radioactive iodine. *Arch Pathol Lab Med*. 1996;120:660–661.
62. Carnell NE, Valente WA. Thyroid nodules in Graves' disease: classification, characterization, and response to treatment. *Thyroid*. 1998;8:571–576.
63. Kraimps JL, Bouin-Pineau MH, Mathonnet M, et al. Multicentre study of thyroid nodules in patients with Graves' disease. *Br J Surg*. 2000;87:1111–1113.
64. Stocker DJ, Burch HB. Thyroid cancer yield in patients with Graves' disease. *Minerva Endocrinol*. 2003;28:205–212.
65. Phitayakorn R, McHenry CR. Incidental thyroid carcinoma in patients with Graves' disease. *Am J Surg*. 2008;195:292–7; discussion 297.
66. Das DK. Marginal vacuoles (fire-flare appearance) in fine needle aspiration smears of thyroid lesions: does it represent diffusing out of thyroid hormones at the base of follicular cells? *Diagn Cytopathol*. 2006;34:277–283.
67. Jayaram G, Singh B, Marwaha RK. Grave's disease. Appearance in cytologic smears from fine needle aspirates of the thyroid gland. *Acta Cytol*. 1989;33:36–40.
68. Centeno BA, Szyfelbein WM, Daniels GH, et al. Fine needle aspiration biopsy of the thyroid gland in patients with prior Graves' disease treated with radioactive iodine. Morphologic findings and potential pitfalls. *Acta Cytol*. 1996;40:1189–1197.
69. Oz F, Urgancioglu I, Uslu I, et al. Cytologic changes induced by 131I in the thyroid glands of patients with hyperthyroidism; results of fine needle aspiration cytology. *Cytopathology*. 1994;5:154–163.
70. Patchefsky AS, Hoch WS. Psammoma bodies in diffuse toxic goiter. *Am J Clin Pathol*. 1972;57:551–556.
71. Cooper DS. Hyperthyroidism. *Lancet*. 2003;362:459–468.
72. Vanderpump MP, Tunbridge WM, French JM, et al. The incidence of thyroid disorders in the community: a twenty-year follow-up of the Whickham Survey. *Clin Endocrinol (Oxf)*. 1995;43:55–68.
73. Krohn K, Führer D, Bayer Y, et al. Molecular pathogenesis of euthyroid and toxic multinodular goiter. *Endocr Rev*. 2005;26:504–524.
74. Knudsen N, Bülow I, Laurberg P, et al. High occurrence of thyroid multinodularity and low occurrence of subclinical hypothyroidism among tobacco smokers in a large population study. *J Endocrinol*. 2002;175:571–576.
75. Derwahl M, Studer H. Hyperplasia versus adenoma in endocrine tissues: are they different? *Trends Endocrinol Metab*. 2002;13:23–28.
76. Malamos B, Koutras DA, Kostamis P, et al. Endemic goitre in Greece: a study of 379 twin pairs. *J Med Genet*. 1967;4:16–18.
77. Brix TH, Kyvik KO, Hegedüs L. Major role of genes in the etiology of simple goiter in females: a population-based twin study. *J Clin Endocrinol Metab*. 1999;84:3071–3075.
78. Jhiang SM, Cho JY, Ryu KY, et al. An immunohistochemical study of Na+/I− symporter in human thyroid tissues and salivary gland tissues. *Endocrinology*. 1998;139:4416–4419.
79. Peter HJ, Studer H, Forster R, et al. The pathogenesis of "hot" and "cold" follicles in multinodular goiters. *J Clin Endocrinol Metab*. 1982;55:941–946.
80. Peter HJ, Gerber H, Studer H, et al. Pathogenesis of heterogeneity in human multinodular goiter. A study on growth and function of thyroid tissue transplanted onto nude mice. *J Clin Invest*. 1985;76:1992–2002.
81. Neumann S, Willgerodt H, Ackermann F, et al. Linkage of familial euthyroid goiter to the multinodular goiter-1 locus and exclusion of the candidate genes thyroglobulin, thyroperoxidase, and Na+/I− symporter. *J Clin Endocrinol Metab*. 1999;84:3750–3756.

82. Bignell GR, Canzian F, Shayeghi M, et al. Familial nontoxic multinodular thyroid goiter locus maps to chromosome 14q but does not account for familial nonmedullary thyroid cancer. *Am J Hum Genet*. 1997;61:1123–1130.

83. Capon F, Tacconelli A, Giardina E, et al. Mapping a dominant form of multinodular goiter to chromosome Xp22. *Am J Hum Genet*. 2000;67:1004–1007.

84. Neumann S, Bayer Y, Reske A, et al. Further indications for genetic heterogeneity of euthyroid familial goiter. *J Mol Med*. 2003;81:736–745.

85. Bayer Y, Neumann S, Meyer B, et al. Genome-wide linkage analysis reveals evidence for four new susceptibility loci for familial euthyroid goiter. *J Clin Endocrinol Metab*. 2004;89:4044–4052.

86. Paschke R. Molecular pathogenesis of nodular goiter. *Langenbecks Arch Surg*. 2011;396:1127–1136.

87. Blumenthal GM, Dennis PA. PTEN hamartoma tumor syndromes. *Eur J Hum Genet*. 2008;16:1289–1300.

88. Nosé V. Familial thyroid cancer: a review. *Mod Pathol*. 2011;24(suppl 2):S19–S33.

89. Poncin S, Van Eeckoudt S, Humblet K, et al. Oxidative stress: a required condition for thyroid cell proliferation. *Am J Pathol*. 2010;176:1355–1363.

90. Maier J, van Steeg H, van Oostrom C, et al. Iodine deficiency activates antioxidant genes and causes DNA damage in the thyroid gland of rats and mice. *Biochim Biophys Acta*. 2007;1773:990–999.

91. Poncin S, Gérard AC, Boucquey M, et al. Oxidative stress in the thyroid gland: from harmlessness to hazard depending on the iodine content. *Endocrinology*. 2008;149:424–433.

92. Novelli M, Cossu A, Oukrif D, et al. X-inactivation patch size in human female tissue confounds the assessment of tumor clonality. *Proc Natl Acad Sci USA*. 2003;100:3311–3314.

93. Jovanovic L, Delahunt B, McIver B, et al. Thyroid gland clonality revisited: the embryonal patch size of the normal human thyroid gland is very large, suggesting X-chromosome inactivation tumor clonality studies of thyroid tumors have to be interpreted with caution. *J Clin Endocrinol Metab*. 2003;88:3284–3291.

94. Levy A. Monoclonality of endocrine tumours: what does it mean? *Trends Endocrinol Metab*. 2001;12:301–307.

95. Belge G, Thode B, Rippe V, et al. A characteristic sequence of trisomies starting with trisomy 7 in benign thyroid tumors. *Hum Genet*. 1994;94:198–202.

96. Iliszko M, Kuzniacka A, Lachinski A, et al. Karyotypic characterization of 64 nonmalignant thyroid goiters. *Cancer Genet Cytogenet*. 2005;161:178–180.

97. Bonnema SJ, Bennedbaek FN, Ladenson PW, et al. Management of the nontoxic multinodular goiter: a North American survey. *J Clin Endocrinol Metab*. 2002;87:112–117.

98. Bonnema SJ, Bennedbaek FN, Wiersinga WM, et al. Management of the nontoxic multinodular goitre: a European questionnaire study. *Clin Endocrinol (Oxf)*. 2000;53:5–12.

99. Sapino A, Papotti M, Macrì L, et al. Intranodular reactive endothelial hyperplasia in adenomatous goitre. *Histopathology*. 1995;26:457–462.

100. Aulicino MR, Kaneko M, Uinger PD. Excessive endothelial cell proliferation occurring in an organizing thyroid hematoma: report of a case and review of the literature. *Endocr Pathol*. 1995;6:153–158.

101. Winkler A, Mueller B, Diem P. Masson's papillary endothelial hyperplasia mimicking a poorly differentiated thyroid carcinoma: a case report. *Eur J Endocrinol*. 2001;145:667–668.

102. Allen L, de Benoist B, Dary O, et al, eds. *Guidelines on Food Fortification with Micronutrients*. Geneva, Switzerland: World Health Organization; 2006.

103. de Benoist B, Burrow G, Delange F, et al. *Assessment of Iodine Deficiency Disorders and Monitoring Their Elimination: A Guide for Programme Managers*. 3rd ed. Geneva, Switzerland: World Health Organization; 2007.

104. Delange F. The disorders induced by iodine deficiency. *Thyroid*. 1994;4:107–128.

105. Dumont JE, Ermans AM, Maenhaut C, et al. Large goitre as a maladaptation to iodine deficiency. *Clin Endocrinol (Oxf)*. 1995;43:1–10.

106. Delange F. Cassava and the thyroid. In: Gaitan E, ed. *Environmental Goitrogenesis*. Boca Raton, FL: CRC Press; 1989:173–194.

107. Vanderpas JB, Contempré B, Duale NL, et al. Iodine and selenium deficiency associated with cretinism in northern Zaire. *Am J Clin Nutr*. 1990;52:1087–1093.

108. Corvilain B, Contempré B, Longombé AO, et al. Selenium and the thyroid: how the relationship was established. *Am J Clin Nutr*. 1993;57(suppl):244S–248S.

109. Ma T, Guo J, Wang F. The epidemiology of iodine-deficiency diseases in China. *Am J Clin Nutr*. 1993;57(suppl):264S–266S.

110. De Felice M, Di Lauro R. Thyroid development and its disorders: genetics and molecular mechanisms. *Endocr Rev*. 2004;25:722–746.

111. Park SM, Chatterjee VK. Genetics of congenital hypothyroidism. *J Med Genet*. 2005;42:379–389.

112. Kennedy JS. The pathology of dyshormonogenetic goitre. *J Pathol*. 1969;99:251–264.

113. Ghossein RA, Rosai J, Heffess C. Dyshormonogenetic goiter: a clinicopathologic study of 56 cases. *Endocr Pathol*. 1997;8:283–292.

114. Plummer HS. The clinical and pathologic relationship of simple and exophthalmic goitre. *Trans Assoc Am Physicians*. 1913;28:587–594.

115. Elte JW, Bussemaker JK, Haak A. The natural history of euthyroid multinodular goitre. *Postgrad Med J*. 1990;66:186–190.

Other Nonneoplastic Disorders

AMIODARONE-INDUCED THYROID DISEASE

Amiodarone is an iodinated drug used for the treatment of cardiac arrhythmias. Although an effective drug for arrhythmias, amiodarone can produce side effects in various organs including the thyroid. The effects range from subclinical abnormalities of thyroid function tests to overt thyroid hypofunction or hyperfunction.[1,2] Most patients receiving amiodarone remain euthyroid. The reported incidence of amiodarone-induced hypothyroidism (AIH) usually ranges from 10% to 20%, whereas the incidence of amiodarone-induced thyrotoxicosis (AIT) ranges from 5% to 10%.[2]

Pharmacology

Amiodarone is a benzofuran derivative with two atoms of iodine per molecule, and its structure bears resemblance to thyroid hormones (Fig. 6.1). Iodine constitutes 37.5% of the molecular weight of amiodarone. Metabolism releases free iodine from about 10% of the bodily content of amiodarone per day. Typical maintenance

Amiodarone

Thyroxine (T₄)

3,5,3'-Triiodothyronine (T₃)

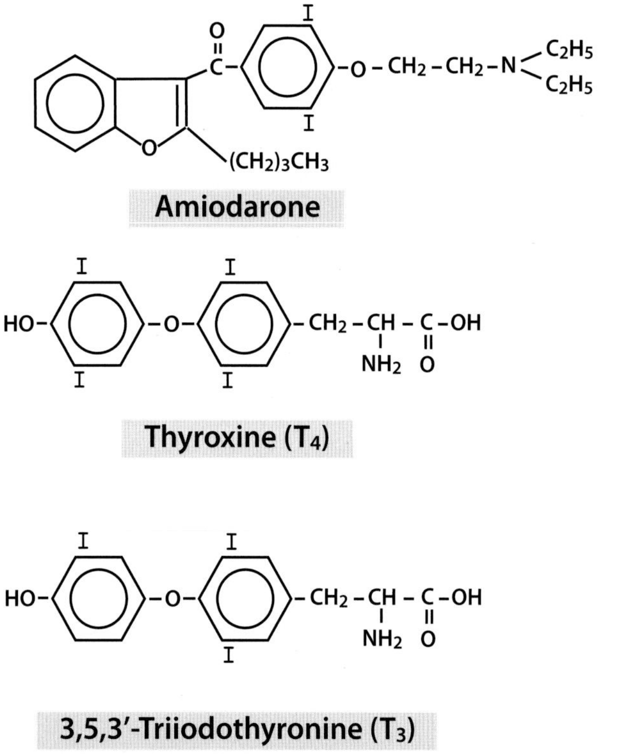

FIGURE 6.1. Structures of amiodarone, thyroxine (T4), and triiodothyronine (T3).

doses in the 200 to 400 mg range thus yield about 7 to 15 mg of iodine per day, far in excess of the World Health Organization's recommended daily adult intake of 0.15 mg.[3]

Amiodarone is amphiphilic and distributes widely in the body. Its high lipid solubility results in storage in various sites including adipose tissue, liver, lung, myocardium, skeletal muscle, kidney, thyroid, and brain. Amiodarone is slowly released with a half-life in the range of 1 to 3 months and thus can have effects long after therapy is discontinued.[1,4,5]

Effect on Thyroid Follicular Cells and Hormone Synthesis

The release of excessive iodine results in reduction of iodine oxidation by the thyroid and decreased thyroid hormone synthesis, an adaptive phenomenon known as the Wolff–Chaikoff effect.[6] Generally, the thyroid escapes from this inhibition within a couple of weeks.[7] Amiodarone and its main metabolite, desethylamiodarone, appear to have a direct toxic effect on follicular cells, although the release of excessive iodine may be a significant factor.[8] A potential indirect mechanism of amiodarone injury is the promotion of thyroid autoimmunity. However, most studies have shown that amiodarone is unlikely to be associated with an increase in thyroid autoantibodies if the individual lacked them before therapy.[1]

Effect on Thyroid Hormone Metabolism

Amiodarone decreases the peripheral conversion of thyroxine (T4) to 3,5,3'-triiodothyronine (T3) and 3,3',5'-triiodothyronine (rT3) to 3,3'-diiodothyronine (T2) because of its inhibition of 5'-deiodinase (5'-D).[9,10] Amiodarone also inhibits uptake of T4, T3, and rT3 by peripheral tissues.[11] This results in the elevation of serum T4 and rT3 and the decrease of serum T3 in patients receiving amiodarone, although these levels may still remain within the normal range. Serum thyroid-stimulating hormone (TSH) may be elevated during the early months of therapy, but it generally returns to normal.[12]

Amiodarone-Induced Hypothyroidism

AIH is more prevalent in areas with high dietary iodine intake.[1,2,13] Studies tend to show a slight female predominance with a ratio of 1.5:1.[1,2] About two-thirds of patients have preexisting thyroid disease, whereas the remaining one-third start with apparently normal glands (Table 6.1).[1] The preexisting thyroid disease is usually autoimmune (Hashimoto) thyroiditis. Patients with preexisting thyroperoxidase (TPO) and/or thyroglobulin antibodies are at higher risk to develop AIH when treated with amiodarone.[1,14,15] AIH may be transient or persistent. Although 10% to 20% of patients develop AIH in the short term, the prevalence appears to decrease to 5% to 10% after a year of therapy.[2] Persistence is usually associated with an underlying disease such as autoimmune thyroiditis.[16]

Several pathogenic mechanisms appear to be involved in AIH. One is failure to escape from the Wolff–Chaikoff effect. This effect is usually transient, but those with AIH may have a defect in hormonogenesis

Table 6.1

Comparison of AIH and AIT

	AIH	AIT	
		Type 1	Type 2
Underlying thyroid abnormally	Yes (~2/3) • Hashimoto thyroiditis • Multinodular goiter	Yes • Multinodular goiter • Graves disease	No
Basic pathogenic abnormality	Impaired hormone synthesis	Excessive hormone synthesis	Destructive thyroiditis with excessive hormone release
Predominant histopathologic changes	• Preexisting thyroid disease (minimal published data available)	• Preexisting thyroid disease	• Focal destruction of follicles • Collections of foamy macrophages • Focal fibrosis
Therapy	• Oral thyroxine supplementation	• Thioamide suppression of hormone synthesis • Perchlorate inhibition of iodine uptake	• Glucocorticosteroids

that prevents escape.[15] The defect in hormonogenesis may be related to preexisting thyroid disease, particularly autoimmune thyroiditis. Direct and indirect cytotoxic mechanisms may also be involved. However, at this time, the pathogenic mechanisms remain unclear, particularly for those individuals lacking preexisting thyroid disease.

Pathology

The pathologic findings of AIH are not well documented in the medical literature. Preexisting thyroid disease is probably the predominant finding in most cases. Extrapolation from animal studies suggests that most cases would show various ultrastructural changes of the follicular cells such as increased lysosomes, lysosomal inclusion bodies, evidence of necrosis and apoptosis, lipofuscin production, and markedly dilated endoplasmic reticulum.[17]

Amiodarone-Induced Thyrotoxicosis

AIT is more prevalent in areas with low dietary iodine intake.[1] AIT tends to have a higher frequency among men.[2,16] Two forms of thyrotoxicosis are associated with amiodarone therapy (Table 6.1). Type 1 is caused by excessive production and release of thyroid hormone and is usually associated with an underlying thyroid disease such as multinodular goiter or Graves disease (diffuse toxic hyperplasia).[1,2] Type 1 AIT is a manifestation of the Jod-Basedow phenomenon characterized by hyperthyroidism because of an increased supply of iodine.[2,18] Type 2 AIT is caused by a destructive thyroiditis that develops in thyroid glands without preexisting disease.[1,2] Type 2 AIT currently appears to be the more common of the forms.[2,19] Ultrasonic assessment typically shows elevated color Doppler flow in type 1 AIT, whereas it shows decreased color Doppler flow in type 2 AIT.[20] The differentiation of the two types of AIT can be challenging because there are cases with mixed or indefinite features.[2,21] Differentiating whether a case is "pure" type 1 AIT or a mixture of both types can be difficult.

Pathology

The pathologic changes associated with type 1 AIT are predominantly those of the underlying thyroid disease. Type 2 AIT is characterized by involution features in most of the thyroid parenchyma with scattered foci of follicular destruction.[22,23]

Grossly, the cut surfaces have a homogenous dark red to reddish-brown gelatinous appearance, reflective of abundant colloid (Fig. 6.2). The disrupted follicles contain detached follicular cells, foamy macrophages, and lymphocytes (Fig. 6.3). Sometimes all that remains of a damaged follicle is a solid collection of macrophages. Multinucleated giant cells also may be present in areas of follicular disruption. Fibrosis may be associated with the areas of follicular damage. The intact follicles are lined predominantly by flat epithelial cells and contain abundant thick colloid, consistent with involution because of low plasma TSH. Some follicular cells exhibit cytoplasmic vacuolization.

Treatment and Prognosis

Treatment of AIH is supplementation with oral thyroxine if amiodarone is necessary for the control of the cardiac arrhythmia. If amiodarone therapy can be discontinued, most patients will return to a euthyroid state, particularly if they did not have a preexisting thyroid disorder. Those patients with autoimmune thyroiditis are less likely to achieve normal thyroid function.

Treatment of AIT can be challenging. Therapy for type 1 AIT is directed at blocking the synthesis of thyroid hormones and decreasing the uptake of iodine by the thyroid.[1] Methimazole or

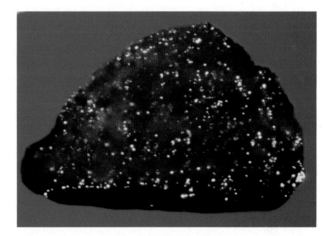

FIGURE 6.2. Cross-section of thyroid with AIT, type 2. The gland has a gelatinous appearance because of abundant colloid.

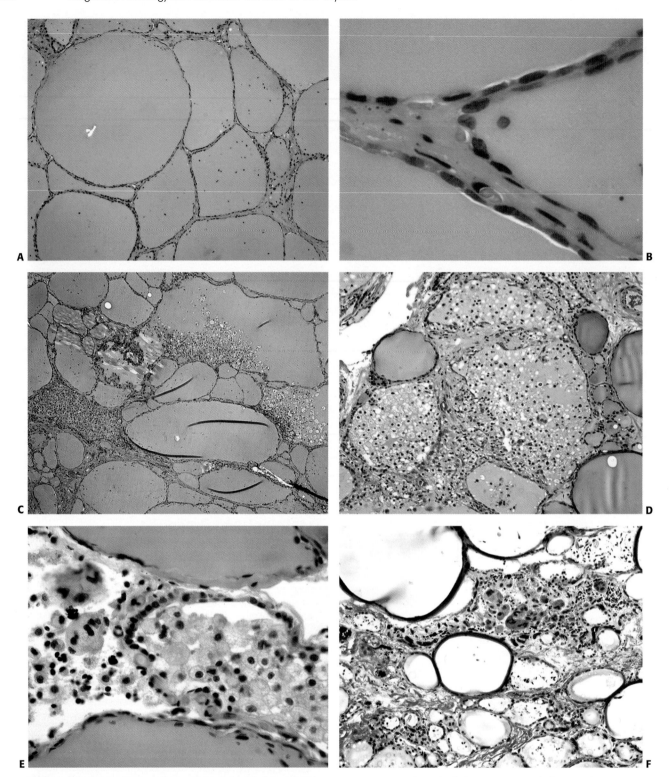

FIGURE 6.3. Representative photomicrographs of thyroid with AIT, type 2. Most thyroid follicles are intact and show involution features **(A and B)**. Focal follicular disruption with infiltration and replacement of colloid by foamy macrophages is shown in images **(C–F)**. A high-power view of focal follicular disruption is shown in image **(E)** with multinucleated giant cells admixed with the macrophages. Focal fibrosis in the region of damaged follicles is shown in image **(F)** (trichrome stain).

another thioamide is generally used to diminish hormone synthesis, whereas potassium perchlorate is used to decrease iodine uptake. In contrast, glucocorticosteroid therapy is used for type 2 AIT. The anti-inflammatory effects of steroids are often effective in ameliorating the destructive thyroiditis characteristic of type 2 AIT.

Definitive treatment of type 1 AIT is directed at the underlying thyroid disorder, which may require radioablation or thyroidectomy. Cessation of amiodarone therapy will eventually allow most type 2 AIT patients to return to a euthyroid state, but this may not be a satisfactory option for individuals with life-threatening arrhythmias refractory to other medications. Thyroidectomy is a consideration if amiodarone must be continued and medical control of thyrotoxicosis is unsuccessful.

MINOCYCLINE-ASSOCIATED CHANGES ("BLACK THYROID")

Dark brown to black pigment can accumulate in the thyroid after long-term use of minocycline, a long-acting antibiotic of the tetracycline group. The degree of pigmentation can be sufficient to give the thyroid a diffusely black gross appearance.

Pathogenesis

The composition of the pigment and mechanism of formation are not entirely clear, but numerous studies indicate that the pigment derives from oxidation of minocycline by TPO.[24-26] The pigment appears to be a unique polymeric product with many properties similar to melanin and lipofuscin. The pigment accumulates within the lysosomes of the follicular cells.[27,28]

In vitro studies have shown minocycline to be an inhibitor of TPO-catalyzed iodination.[26,29] The mechanism is consistent with substrate inhibition of TPO-catalyzed iodination of tyrosyl residues in thyroglobulin.[29] The reaction may also generate a reactive intermediate metabolite, and thus, there is the possibility of associated damage to follicular cells and impaired thyroid function. However, the potential for clinically significant toxicity appears to be very low given the scarcity of cases with abnormal thyroid function. A study in which human volunteers were given high doses of minocycline for up to 85 days failed to reveal abnormal pigmentation in thyroid biopsies.[24] This suggests that one or more other factors may be involved in the pathogenesis of pigment formation.

Clinical Presentation

Most cases are discovered coincidentally when a thyroid lesion is excised surgically because of a nodular lesion or the thyroid is examined at the time of autopsy. The incidence of minocycline-associated thyroid pigmentation is unknown, but it appears to be quite low given the small number of reported cases and the large number of individuals who have received the drug since its introduction in 1967. However, cases may go unrecognized because of normal thyroid function and absence of gross distortion, and individual cases may no longer gain publication in contemporary medical literature.

Almost all published cases either report normal thyroid function or do not note abnormal function. A case associated with hypothyroidism has been reported.[27] Other cases have been associated with nodular hyperplasia or follicular derived neoplasms, but no clear association with these processes has been made.

Pathology
Gross Features

The external and cut surfaces of the thyroid have a diffuse dark brown to black appearance (Fig. 6.4). Most affected thyroid glands are of normal size. The cut surfaces usually are otherwise unremarkable unless a coincidental neoplasm is present. Coincidental neoplasms such as papillary carcinomas usually lack appreciable pigmentation, resulting in a marked contrast between tan-white tumors and the surrounding black nonneoplastic tissue. Cases of black follicular adenomas have been reported.[30-32]

Histologic Features

The characteristic finding is coarsely granular dark brown to black pigment within the apical cytoplasm of follicular cells (Fig. 6.5). Pigment is also commonly seen within the colloid and macrophages. Otherwise, the thyroid parenchyma is typically unremarkable. A case with chronic inflammation and fibrosis has been reported, but this may be unique and possibly because of coincidental and etiologically unrelated chronic thyroiditis.[27]

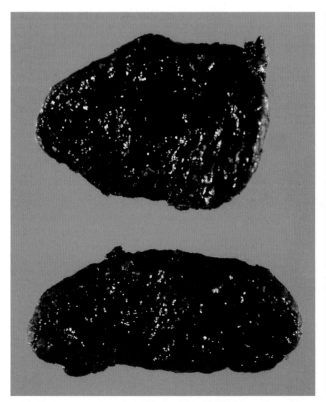
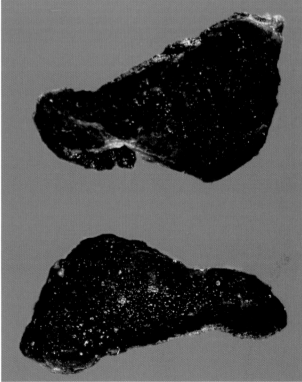

FIGURE 6.4. Two separate cases of black pigmentation of thyroid associated with minocycline therapy.

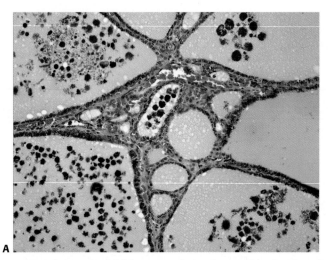
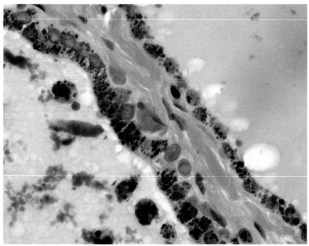

FIGURE 6.5. Low- and high-power photomicrographs showing pigment deposition because of minocycline therapy (A and B). The coarsely granular dark brown to black pigment is present within the cytoplasm of follicular cells **(B)** and colloid. Some of the intracolloidal pigment is located within macrophages.

The pigment is highlighted by the Schmorl and Fontana-Masson stains and is bleached by the potassium permanganate/oxalic acid method, similar to melanin.[24,27,28,33] The pigment is usually positive with the periodic acid-Schiff (PAS) and PAS-diastase stains.[33] Immunohistochemical stains do not have particular diagnostic utility. Ultrastructural examination shows electron-dense material within the lysosomes of follicular cells.[27,28]

Cytologic Features

Fine needle aspiration (FNA) may yield follicular cells with intra-cytoplasmic pigmented granules, particularly if the thyroid contains a pigmented hyperplastic nodule or follicular neoplasm.[32,34] The pigment granules have a finely granular appearance and have a more uniform size and shape compared with hemosiderin. The granules appear dark brown in Papanicolaou-stained preparations, whereas they are dark blue in those stained with Diff-Quik.[35] Follicular epithelial cells may exhibit nuclear hyperchromasia and chromatin clumping that raise suspicion for neoplasia.[34]

Differential Diagnosis

The differential diagnosis includes deposition of hemosiderin, lipofuscin, or melanin. Iron is found commonly in thyroids secondary to hemorrhage, particularly in cases of multinodular goiter or in areas sampled by FNA. Diffuse iron deposition can be seen in cases of primary hemochromatosis or marked secondary hemosiderosis. Hemosiderin has a more refractile, golden-brown appearance and is highlighted with iron stains (e.g., Prussian blue stain).

Lipofuscin, or lipochrome pigment, can be found in the thyroid as a yellow-brown pigment. It is an insoluble polymeric material derived from the peroxidation of lipids and subcellular membranes. Lipofuscin has properties similar to minocycline-associated pigment. Both are highlighted with the Schmorl, Ziehl–Neelsen, and Sudan IV stains.[24] In addition, energy dispersive X-ray analysis reveals similar elemental spectra.[24] However, lipofuscin's yellow-brown pigmentation in hematoxylin and eosin–stained sections and more finely granular appearance are generally sufficient to distinguish it from the dark brown-black pigment of minocycline-associated pigment. Also lipofuscin accumulation does not yield a black gross appearance.

Melanin per se may be difficult to distinguish from minocycline-associated pigment given their similar appearance and staining characteristics. Of importance is the context in which the pigmentation is seen, as intrathyroidal melanin is almost always because of a neoplastic process. Usually, this is metastatic malignant melanoma but very rarely may be because of the melanin-producing variant of medullary carcinoma (see Chapter 14).

Deposition of dark pigment because of alkaptonuria/ochronosis is at least a theoretic consideration. Individuals with alkaptonuria/ochronosis have a genetic defect with resultant incomplete metabolism of homogentisic acid, tyrosine, and phenylalanine. Deposition of black pigment can be seen in this disease, particularly in collagen-rich tissues. Thus far, no formal reports of a thyroid with appreciable ochronotic pigment have appeared in the medical literature.

Treatment and Prognosis

Owing to the potential for follicular cell injury, some have advocated monitoring thyroid function of individuals receiving long-term minocycline therapy. However, those treated with minocycline seem to have a low incidence of pigment accumulation, and clinical evidence of thyroid dysfunction is rare.

 # POSTRADIATION CHANGES

The thyroid is subject to radiation exposure in various medical situations, both diagnostic and therapeutic, and through accidental environment exposure. Postradiation changes of the thyroid vary by radiation dose and source. In general, postradiation changes can be approached on the basis of acute, or early, changes and chronic, or late, changes, and the latter can be further subdivided into nonneoplastic and neoplastic.[36] Certain thyroid neoplasms, papillary carcinoma in particular, have a strong link to radiation exposure (Chapter 11). This section focuses on the nonneoplastic changes associated with radiation of the thyroid.

Acute/Early Changes

Acute changes in the thyroid caused by radiation injury manifest within days to weeks after exposure. The changes are dose dependent and manifest sooner with increasing amounts of irradiation. Early changes include cytoplasmic vacuolization, nuclear pyknosis, and stromal edema (Table 6.2). Follicular disruption, focal necrosis, hemorrhage, and influx of macrophages are typically seen, particularly with ablative doses[37] of [131]I. Minimal acute

Table 6.2

Postradiation Changes of the Thyroid

	Acute/Early	Chronic/Late
Cellular changes	• Cytoplasmic vacuolization • Nuclear pyknosis • Single cell and confluent necrosis	• Follicular atrophy • Nuclear atypia • Compensatory hyperplasia (focal, nodular) • Oncocytic metaplasia
Vascular changes	• Endothelial swelling • Thrombosis • Fibrinoid necrosis • Focal hemorrhage	• Vascular sclerosis and stenosis
Stromal changes	• Edema • Macrophage infiltration • Minimal acute inflammation	• Fibrosis • Lymphocytic infiltration
Neoplasia		• Benign • Malignant

inflammation is seen unless the radiation dose is sufficient to cause widespread necrosis of follicular epithelium. Microvascular injury is common with small-caliber blood vessels exhibiting endothelial swelling. Foci of fibrinoid necrosis and thrombosis may be evident with higher doses.

Chronic/Late Changes

Chronic changes manifest months to years after exposure. These changes can be separated into two general groups. One group is composed of nonneoplastic changes at the tissue and cellular level.

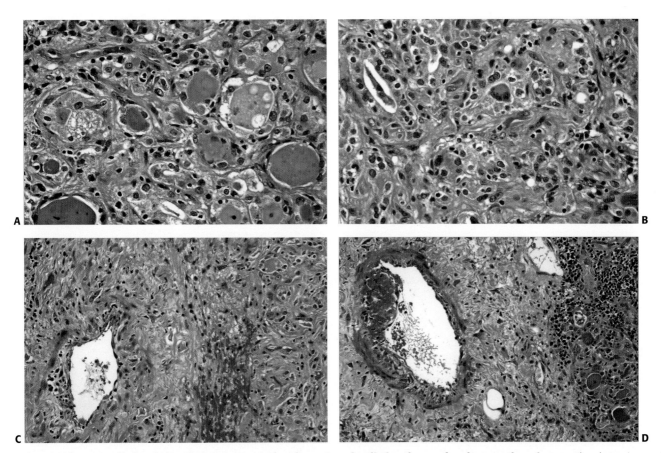

FIGURE 6.6. Subacute radiation-induced changes 3 months after external radiation therapy for pharyngeal carcinoma. The photomicrographs show variable loss of follicles, from the areas in which they are readily identifiable **(A)** to the areas in which they have no colloid **(B)** and to the areas in which they have been replaced by fibrous tissue **(C and D)**. Vacuolation of follicular epithelium is seen **(A)** as well as follicular damage and infiltration by mononuclear inflammatory cells **(B)**. Focal hemorrhage and vascular intimal proliferation are present **(C)** as well as an occasional organizing thrombus **(D)**.

These changes include interstitial fibrosis, follicular atrophy, vascular sclerosis, nuclear atypia, lymphocytic infiltrates, and oncocytic metaplasia (Table 6.2).[36,38] The other general group is composed of proliferative changes resulting in hyperplastic nodules or neoplasms.

Interstitial fibrosis develops frequently in irradiated thyroids (Fig. 6.6).[36] Internally deposited ^{131}I seems to be more fibrogenic compared with external beam radiation.[39] Follicular atrophy is often seen in association with interstitial fibrosis, and it too seems more common when the radiation source is [131]I. Irradiated follicular cells often exhibit pleomorphic features including variation in nuclear and overall cell size and large hyperchromatic nuclei (Figs. 6.7 and 6.8). Oncocytic change of follicular cells has also been reported as a late effect of radiation.[37–39]

Segmental sclerosis of arterioles and small- to medium-sized arteries is a common late manifestation of radiation in most tissues, and the thyroid is no exception. The vessel walls appear thickened and often hyalinized (Fig. 6.9). The affected vessels are seen both within the thyroid and the perithyroidal soft tissues. Elastic stains often show focal reduplication, fragmentation, and calcification of the internal elastic lamina.[36] Intimal proliferation and fibrosis with focal marked stenosis may be seen.

Areas of follicular hyperplasia may be present, ranging from microscopic foci to clinically palpable nodules.[36,38,40,41] These hyperplastic nodules may be multiple or single, and they often exhibit cystic degenerative changes. Diffuse hyperplasia, characterized by small follicles, diminished colloid, and aggregates of lymphocytes similar to Graves disease may be seen.[38] Other proliferative lesions secondary to radiation include neoplasms derived from follicular epithelium, notably papillary carcinoma, follicular adenoma, and follicular carcinoma.

AMYLOIDOSIS

The most frequent cause of amyloid deposition in the thyroid is medullary carcinoma. Amyloid can also accumulate in association with either primary or secondary systemic amyloidosis. Amyloid deposits that are only identifiable microscopically and have no clinically significant effect on the thyroid are commonly seen in thyroids of individuals with systemic amyloidosis either because of plasma cell dyscrasias or because of chronic inflammatory conditions.[42] Amyloid goiter is a rare condition defined by clinically apparent thyroid enlargement due to amyloid deposition.

Pathogenesis

The specific mechanisms that cause amyloid accumulation sufficient to result in goiter are unknown. The most common underlying condition of amyloid goiter is secondary amyloidosis because of a chronic inflammatory condition.[43,44] Secondary amyloidosis is also known as reactive systemic amyloidosis. The AA form of amyloid, a nonimmunoglobulin protein synthesized by the liver, accumulates in this condition. This same form of amyloid is associated with familial Mediterranean fever.

Amyloid goiter may also occur in association with primary systemic amyloidosis, the form of amyloidosis associated with plasma cell dyscrasias. The AL form of amyloid, which derives from immunoglobulin light chains, is deposited in primary systemic amyloidosis. Amyloid goiter is a very rare complication of this form of amyloidosis.[45]

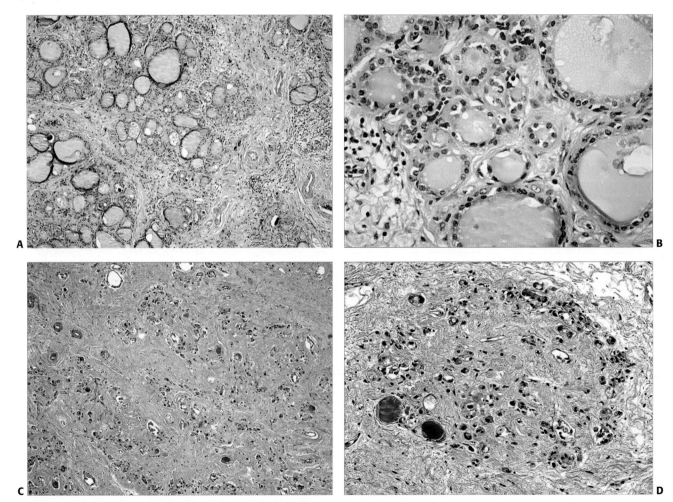

FIGURE 6.7. Radiation-induced fibrosis and follicular atrophy. Two cases, **(A and B)** and **(C and D),** of thyroids treated remotely with radioiodine. The case shown in panels **(C)** and **(D)** exhibits extreme follicular atrophy.

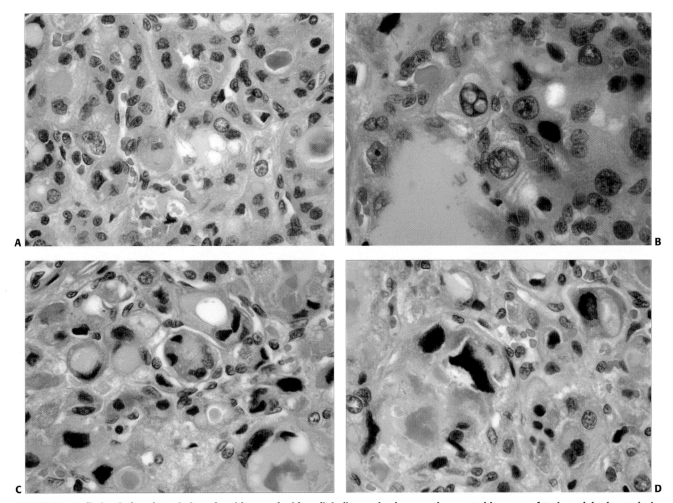

FIGURE 6.8. Radiation-induced atypia in a thyroid treated with radioiodine and subsequently resected because of toxic nodular hyperplasia. The nuclei exhibit atypia ranging from mild enlargement to markedly enlarged and from vacuolated to markedly hyperchromatic and bizarrely shaped.

Clinical Presentation and Imaging

Amyloid goiter is defined by clinically detectable enlargement of the thyroid. Such enlargement may result in a mass lesion with localized pressure symptoms such as dysphagia, dyspnea, or hoarseness. The enlargement may be rapid and raise concern for malignant neoplasia such as lymphoma or anaplastic carcinoma.[43] Most affected individuals are middle-aged to older adults, but cases in younger individuals have also been reported.[46]

Most affected individuals are clinically euthyroid.[43] Thyroid function tests may show abnormalities in the absence of clinical dysfunction, and both overt hypothyroidism and hyperthyroidism have been reported.[42,47,48] Scintigraphic scanning with Tc-99m pyrophosphate shows diffuse uptake because of affinity for amyloid.[49] However, the uptake is not specific for amyloid.

Pathology

Gross Features

Most cases of amyloidosis involving the thyroid because of systemic amyloidosis do not exhibit gross abnormalities. The small fraction that qualify as amyloid goiter show variable enlargement, with weights ranging from about twice normal[43,50] to >300 g. The thyroid has a rubbery to firm consistency, and the cut surfaces have a white, tan, or light pink appearance. These features are usually diffuse but may be nodular. Cases with abundant adipose tissue may appear yellow.

Histologic Features

In cases of nongoitrous amyloidosis, amyloid is typically seen within the walls of small blood vessels. The normal follicular architecture is intact, and no appreciable amount of adipose tissue is present. In contrast, histologic examination of amyloid goiter shows effacement of the normal thyroid architecture (Fig. 6.10). Several follicles are reduced, usually markedly, and the residual follicles are surrounded by amyloid stroma.[44] Colloid may be quite scant. An appreciable amount of stromal adipose tissue is typically present, and it is the predominant finding in some cases.[44,51]

The diagnosis of amyloid can be confirmed with histochemical stains, Congo red being the most popular (Fig. 6.11). Congo red–stained foci of amyloid exhibit light green birefringence when viewed with polarizing filters. Loss of Congo red staining by pretreatment with potassium permanganate will distinguish AA protein from the other amyloid proteins. Immunostains for the various amyloid proteins may be of diagnostic utility.

Differential Diagnosis

The most important differential diagnosis is medullary thyroid carcinoma. Medullary carcinomas with abundant amyloid stroma may have a subtle cellular component, particularly with limited sampling. Because medullary carcinoma is statistically more likely than amyloid goiter, this neoplastic possibility should be considered whenever encountering amyloid in the thyroid. Immunostaining for calcitonin can help identify the neoplastic C cells in challenging cases.

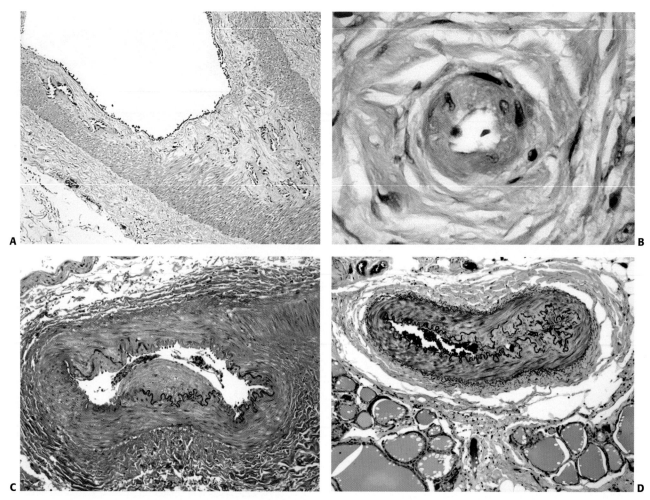

FIGURE 6.9. Radiation-induced vascular changes. A and B: Changes in a thyroid after external beam radiation therapy for laryngeal carcinoma. A medium-sized perithyroidal artery shows focal intimal proliferation and calcification of the internal elastic lamina **(A)**. Small intrathyroidal blood vessels with thickened, hyalinized wall are seen in **(B)**. **C and D:** Vascular changes in perithyroidal arteries of a 14-year-old child **(C)** and 7-year-old child **(D)** associated with accidental exposure to radiation after the Chernobyl accident. Medium-sized arteries show intimal thickening and marked calcification and fragmentation of the internal elastic lamina. **D:** Trichrome-elastic stain.

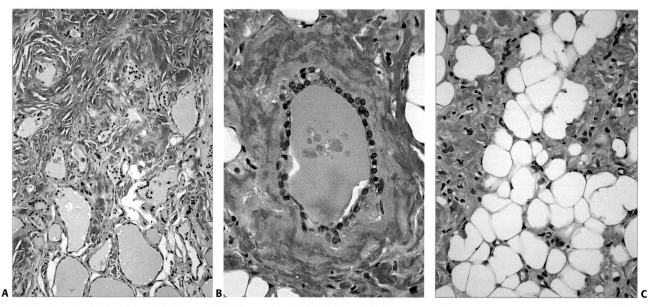

FIGURE 6.10. Amyloid goiter showing partial effacement of follicular architecture (A) by amyloid that encircles residual follicles (B). Stromal adipose tissue is shown in **(C)**.

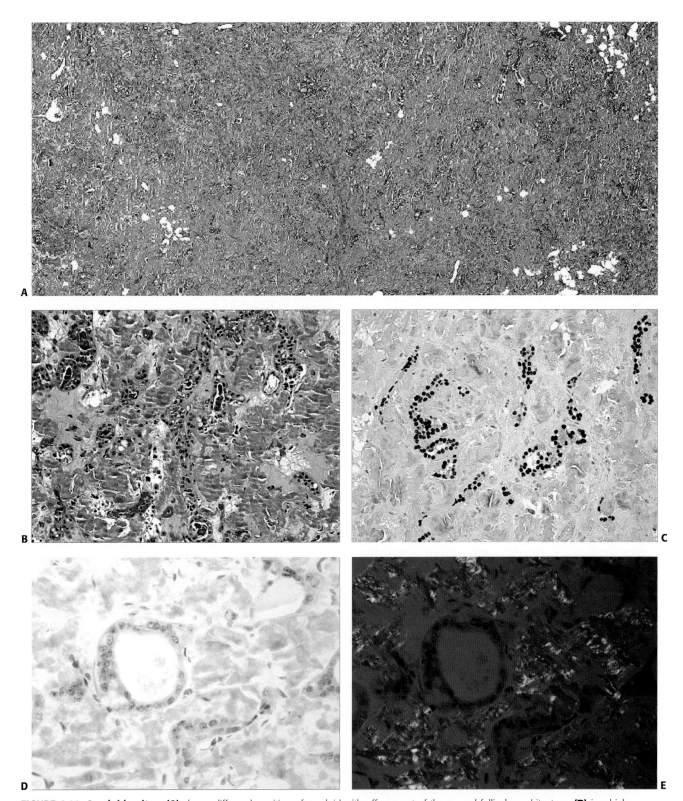

FIGURE 6.11. Amyloid goiter. (A) shows diffuse deposition of amyloid with effacement of the normal follicular architecture. **(B)** is a higher power view showing replacement of most of the thyroid parenchyma by amyloid. **(C)** is the same area immunostained for TTF1, which highlights the nuclei of residual follicular cells. The Congo red stain demonstrates amyloid surrounding the follicles **(D)** and light green birefringence is evident when the Congo red–stained section is viewed with polarizing filters **(E)**.

Hyalinizing trabecular tumor may be another consideration because of the hyalinized stroma. However, the stroma of hyalinizing trabecular tumor is negative for amyloid, and the trabecular growth pattern is usually distinctive compared with the residual follicles of amyloid goiter.

Treatment and Prognosis

Treatment for amyloid goiter is not necessary unless the size causes symptoms or significant disfigurement or a rapid increase in size is worrisome for a malignant neoplasm. The overall prognosis reflects the underlying disease responsible for the amyloid deposition.

ALTERATIONS FOLLOWING FNA OF THE THYROID

FNA biopsy is a very common diagnostic procedure for evaluation of thyroid lesions. The procedure can induce reactive and reparative changes that may cause concern, and possibly misdiagnosis. LiVolsi and Merino[52] coined the term *worrisome histologic alterations following FNA of the thyroid*, or WHAFFT. The alterations that most commonly cause concern are lesions that mimic true capsular or vascular invasion, exuberant vascular proliferation, spindle cell proliferation, reactive follicular epithelial atypia, and infarction. These alterations are less frequent when a nonaspirational FNA technique is used and are less pronounced with decreasing size of the needle.[53]

Invasion versus Pseudoinvasion

Distinction between true capsular and pseudoinvasion secondary to FNA can be challenging. True capsular invasion is characterized by neoplastic cells traversing the capsule and extending into the surrounding thyroid parenchyma, often in a mushroom or hook-like manner. Capsules of follicular carcinomas tend to be relative thick compared with those of adenomas, and hyalinization and myxoid changes of the capsule may be seen in the area of invasion.[54]

A focus of capsular pseudoinvasion because of prior FNA typically has a linear shape (Fig. 6.12). The capsule may be distorted by the needle tract, and neoplastic cells may be present in and peripheral to the capsule. Features that help recognize pseudoinvasion include recent or old hemorrhage, inflammation, and/or reparative changes in the area immediately adjacent to the capsular lesion. The relative amounts of inflammation and fibroblastic proliferation vary with the time between FNA and surgical resection.

Vascular Proliferation

FNA can cause reactive endothelial hyperplasia because of organization of intrathyroidal hematomas as discussed in Chapter 5

(see Fig. 5.16). The endothelial cells may exhibit significant cytologic atypia and a proliferative pattern that resembles angiosarcoma. The endothelial proliferation also can exhibit papillary architecture that superficially mimics papillary thyroid carcinoma.

Vascular proliferation within and adjacent to the capsule can mimic true vascular invasion either by its intrinsic architecture and degree of cellularity or by the incorporation of neoplastic thyroid tissue into the area of vascular proliferation. Strict adherence to criteria for vascular invasion (see Chapter 10) is critical to prevent misinterpretation of pseudoinvasion as true invasion. Immunostains for endothelial markers may also prove helpful in assessing these lesions.

Spindle Cell Proliferation

Spindle cell proliferation similar to that described in the lower genitourinary tract may occur in the thyroid following FNA.[55] These proliferations have a nodular appearance and usually range from several millimeters up to a centimeter in diameter. The nodules have ill-defined borders and tend to be located within the central area of the aspirated lesion but may be more peripheral and near the thyroid capsule.

Histologic examination reveals irregular bundles of plump spindle cells with vesicular nuclei, inconspicuous nucleoli, and interspersed macrophages and lymphocytes (Fig. 6.13A–C). These reparative lesions may be exuberant to the point of raising concern for an anaplastic carcinoma or sarcoma. Hemosiderin-laden macrophages are typically present at least focally, and these support a reparative response to needle trauma with hemorrhage. Mitotic figures are rarely seen, in contrast to the genitourinary spindle cell proliferations.

Immunohistochemical staining of the spindle cells shows features consistent with myofibroblastic differentiation. The cells are positive for smooth muscle actin and negative for pankeratin. Endothelial markers highlight the small caliber blood vessels interspersed among the spindle cells.

Reactive Follicular Epithelial Atypia

Follicular epithelium adjacent to needle tracks can show nuclear enlargement and chromatin clearing, raising suspicion for

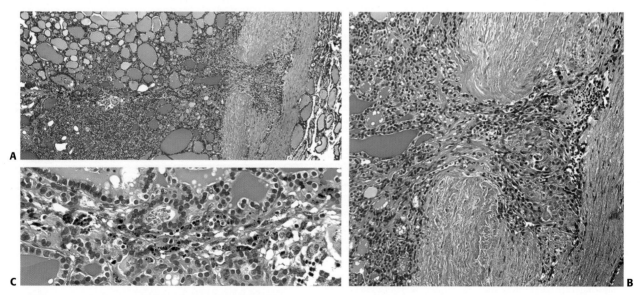

FIGURE 6.12. Capsular pseudoinvasion at site of FNA biopsy. A: Low-power photomicrograph shows linear needle tract within a follicular adenoma. **B:** High-power view shows fibroblastic proliferation and inflammation in capsule. **C:** High-power view shows linear accumulation of hemosiderin along deeper portion of tract.

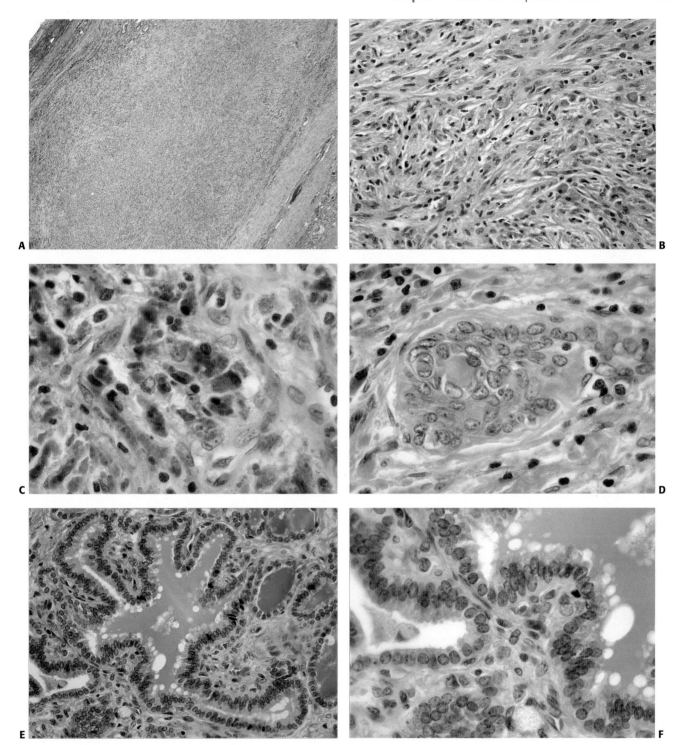

FIGURE 6.13. Spindle cell proliferation secondary to FNA biopsy. Low-power photomicrograph **(A)** shows effacement of thyroid follicular tissue. High-power views show spindle cells **(B)** and hemosiderin-laden macrophages **(C)**. Images **(D–F)** show adjacent reactive epithelial changes. The nuclear enlargement and crowding, hypochromasia, and pseudopapillary architecture shown in **(E)** and **(F)** mimic papillary carcinoma. However, these changes were only present in proximity to the reparative changes. The full spectrum of nuclear changes characteristic of papillary carcinoma is absent.

papillary carcinoma (Fig. 6.13D–F). However, other nuclear features of papillary carcinoma such as irregular nuclear contours, grooves, and inclusions are absent. Important diagnostic clues are the restriction of the nuclear atypia to the region immediately adjacent to the needle tract and the associated reparative changes.

Infarction

Infarction of nodular thyroid lesions may occur following FNA. Oncocytic neoplasms seem to be particularly vulnerable to this complication (Fig. 6.14).[56,57] The infarction may be total or near total resulting in a rim of granulation tissue or residual capsule

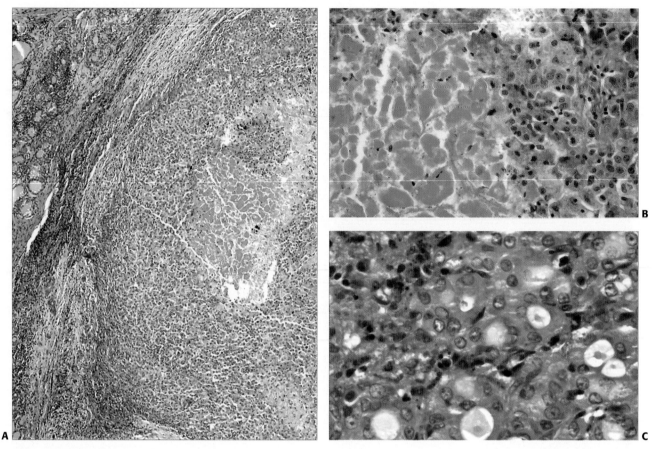

FIGURE 6.14. Infarction secondary to FNA biopsy. Photomicrographs of an oncocytic adenoma resected 2 months after FNA. **A:** Low-power view showing area of infarction within adenoma. **B:** Medium-power view of infracted tumor **(left)** and pigment-laden macrophages **(right)**. **(C)** High-power view of peripheral rim of viable oncocytic adenoma.

surrounding necrotic debris. Reparative spindle cell proliferation as described above may be evident. The diagnosis of the lesion can be made if sufficient viable tissue is present. In the absence of viable lesional tissue, diagnosis will depend on the FNA findings.

REFERENCES

1. Martino E, Bartalena L, Bogazzi F, et al. The effects of amiodarone on the thyroid. *Endocr Rev*. 2001;22:240–254.
2. Cohen-Lehman J, Dahl P, Danzi S, et al. Effects of amiodarone therapy on thyroid function. *Nat Rev Endocrinol*. 2010;6:34–41.
3. World Health Organization, Food and Agriculture Organization of the United Nations. *Vitamin and Mineral Requirements in Human Nutrition, Second Edition*. Geneva, Switzerland: WHO & FAO; 2004.
4. Holt DW, Tucker GT, Jackson PR, et al. Amiodarone pharmacokinetics. *Am Heart J*. 1983;106:840–847.
5. Pollak PT, Bouillon T, Shafer SL. Population pharmacokinetics of long-term oral amiodarone therapy. *Clin Pharmacol Ther*. 2000;67:642–652.
6. Wolff J, Chaikoff I. Plasma inorganic iodide as a homeostatic regulator of thyroid function. *J Biol Chem*. 1948;174:555–564.
7. Loh KC. Amiodarone-induced thyroid disorders: a clinical review. *Postgrad Med J*. 2000;76:133–140.
8. Chiovato L, Martino E, Tonacchera M, et al. Studies on the in vitro cytotoxic effect of amiodarone. *Endocrinology*. 1994;134:2277–2282.
9. Sogol PB, Hershman JM, Reed AW, et al. The effects of amiodarone on serum thyroid hormones and hepatic thyroxine 5'-monodeiodination in rats. *Endocrinology*. 1983;113:1464–1469.
10. Kannan R, Ookhtens M, Chopra IJ, et al. Effects of chronic administration of amiodarone on kinetics of metabolism of iodothyronines. *Endocrinology*. 1984;115:1710–1716.
11. Krenning EP, Docter R, Bernard B, et al. Decreased transport of thyroxine (T4), 3,3',5-triiodothyronine (T3) and 3,3',5'-triiodothyronine (rT3) into rat hepatocytes in primary culture due to a decrease of cellular ATP content and various drugs. *FEBS Lett*. 1982;140:229–233.
12. Burger A, Dinichert D, Nicod P, et al. Effect of amiodarone on serum triiodothyronine, reverse triiodothyronine, thyroxin, and thyrotropin. A drug influencing peripheral metabolism of thyroid hormones. *J Clin Invest*. 1976;58:255–259.
13. Martino E, Safran M, Aghini-Lombardi F, et al. Environmental iodine intake and thyroid dysfunction during chronic amiodarone therapy. *Ann Intern Med*. 1984;101:28–34.
14. Trip MD, Wiersinga W, Plomp TA. Incidence, predictability, and pathogenesis of amiodarone-induced thyrotoxicosis and hypothyroidism. *Am J Med*. 1991;91:507–511.
15. Martino E, Aghini-Lombardi F, Mariotti S, et al. Amiodarone iodine-induced hypothyroidism: risk factors and follow-up in 28 cases. *Clin Endocrinol (Oxf)*. 1987;26:227–237.
16. Harjai KJ, Licata AA. Effects of amiodarone on thyroid function. *Ann Intern Med*. 1997;126:63–73.
17. Pitsiavas V, Smerdely P, Li M, et al. Amiodarone induces a different pattern of ultrastructural change in the thyroid to iodine excess alone in both the BB/W rat and the Wistar rat. *Eur J Endocrinol*. 1997;137:89–98.
18. Stanbury JB, Ermans AE, Bourdoux P, et al. Iodine-induced hyperthyroidism: occurrence and epidemiology. *Thyroid*. 1998;8:83–100.
19. Bogazzi F, Bartalena L, Dell'Unto E, et al. Proportion of type 1 and type 2 amiodarone-induced thyrotoxicosis has changed over a 27-year period in Italy. *Clin Endocrinol (Oxf)*. 2007;67:533–537.
20. Eaton SE, Euinton HA, Newman CM, et al. Clinical experience of amiodarone-induced thyrotoxicosis over a 3-year period: role of colour-flow Doppler sonography. *Clin Endocrinol (Oxf)*. 2002;56:33–38.
21. Bogazzi F, Bartalena L, Martino E. Approach to the patient with amiodarone-induced thyrotoxicosis. *J Clin Endocrinol Metab*. 2010;95:2529–2535.
22. Smyrk TC, Goellner JR, Brennan MD, et al. Pathology of the thyroid in amiodarone-associated thyrotoxicosis. *Am J Surg Pathol*. 1987;11:197–204.
23. Saad A, Falciglia M, Steward DL, et al. Amiodarone-induced thyrotoxicosis and thyroid cancer: clinical, immunohistochemical, and molecular genetic studies of a case and review of the literature. *Arch Pathol Lab Med*. 2004;128:807–810.
24. Gordon G, Sparano BM, Kramer AW, et al. Thyroid gland pigmentation and minocycline therapy. *Am J Pathol*. 1984;117:98–109.
25. Enochs WS, Nilges MJ, Swartz HM. The minocycline-induced thyroid pigment and several synthetic models: identification and characterization by electron paramagnetic resonance spectroscopy. *J Pharmacol Exp Ther*. 1993;266:1164–1176.
26. Taurog A, Dorris ML, Doerge DR. Minocycline and the thyroid: antithyroid effects of the drug, and the role of thyroid peroxidase in minocycline-induced black pigmentation of the gland. *Thyroid*. 1996;6:211–219.

27. Alexander CB, Herrera GA, Jaffe K, et al. Black thyroid: clinical manifestations, ultrastructural findings, and possible mechanisms. *Hum Pathol*. 1985;16:72–78.
28. Bell CD, Kovacs K, Horvath E, et al. Histologic, immunohistochemical, and ultrastructural findings in a case of minocycline-associated "black thyroid". *Endocr Pathol*. 2001;12:443–451.
29. Doerge DR, Divi RL, Deck J, et al. Mechanism for the anti-thyroid action of minocycline. *Chem Res Toxicol*. 1997;10:49–58.
30. Reid JD. The black thyroid associated with minocycline therapy. A local manifestation of a drug-induced lysosome/substrate disorder. *Am J Clin Pathol*. 1983;79:738–746.
31. Koren R, Bernheim J, Schachter P, et al. Black thyroid adenoma. Clinical, histochemical, and ultrastructural features. *Appl Immunohistochem Mol Morphol*. 2000;8:80–84.
32. Wajda KJ, Wilson MS, Lucas J, et al. Fine needle aspiration cytologic findings in the black thyroid syndrome. *Acta Cytol*. 1988;32:862–865.
33. Pastolero GC, Asa SL. Drug-related pigmentation of the thyroid associated with papillary carcinoma. *Arch Pathol Lab Med*. 1994;118:79–83.
34. Keyhani-Rofagha S, Kooner DS, Landas SK, et al. Black thyroid: a pitfall for aspiration cytology. *Diagn Cytopathol*. 1991;7:640–643.
35. Hall AH, Bean SM. Minocycline-induced black thyroid. *Diagn Cytopathol*. 2010;38:579 580.
36. Nikiforov YE, Gnepp DR. Pathomorphology of thyroid gland lesions associated with radiation exposure: the Chernobyl experience and review of the literature. *Adv Anat Pathol*. 1999;6:78–91.
37. Kennedy JS, Thomson JA. The changes in the thyroid gland after irradiation with ^{131}I or partial thyroidectomy for thyrotoxicosis. *J Pathol*. 1974;112:65–81.
38. Nikiforov YE, Heffess CS, Korzenko AV, et al. Characteristics of follicular tumors and nonneoplastic thyroid lesions in children and adolescents exposed to radiation as a result of the Chernobyl disaster. *Cancer*. 1995;76:900–909.
39. Lindsay S, Dailey ME, Jones MD. Histologic effects of various types of ionizing radiation on normal and hyperplastic human thyroid glands. *J Clin Endocrinol Metab*. 1954;14:1179–1218.
40. Lindsay S, Chaikoff IL. The Effects of Irradiation on the thyroid gland with particular reference to the induction of thyroid neoplasms. *Cancer Res*. 1964;24:1099–1107.
41. Carr RF, LiVolsi VA. Morphologic changes in the thyroid after irradiation for Hodgkin's and non-Hodgkin's lymphoma. *Cancer*. 1989;64:825–829.
42. Arean VM, Klein RE. Amyloid goiter. Review of the literature and report of a case. *Am J Clin Pathol*. 1961;36:341–355.
43. Hamed G, Heffess CS, Shmookler BM, et al. Amyloid goiter. A clinicopathologic study of 14 cases and review of the literature. *Am J Clin Pathol*. 1995;104:306–312.
44. Villa F, Dionigi G, Tanda ML, et al. Amyloid goiter. *Int J Surg*. 2008;6(suppl 1):S16–S18.
45. Siddiqui MA, Gertz M, Dean D. Amyloid goiter as a manifestation of primary systemic amyloidosis. *Thyroid*. 2007;17:77–80.
46. Villamil CF, Massimi G, D'Avella J, et al. Amyloid goiter with parathyroid involvement: a case report and review of the literature. *Arch Pathol Lab Med*. 2000;124:281–283.
47. Duhra P, Cassar J. Thyroid function tests in amyloid goitre. *Postgrad Med J*. 1990;66:304–306.
48. Kanoh T, Shimada H, Uchino H, et al. Amyloid goiter with hypothyroidism. *Arch Pathol Lab Med*. 1989;113:542–544.
49. Lee VW, Rubinow A, Pehrson J, et al. Amyloid goiter: preoperative scintigraphic diagnosis using Tc-99m pyrophosphate. *J Nucl Med*. 1984;25:468–471.
50. Goldsmith JD, Lai ML, Daniele GM, et al. Amyloid goiter: report of two cases and review of the literature. *Endocr Pract*. 2000;6:318–323.
51. Himmetoglu C, Yamak S, Tezel GG. Diffuse fatty infiltration in amyloid goiter. *Pathol Int*. 2007;57:449–453.
52. LiVolsi VA, Merino MJ. Worrisome histologic alterations following fine-needle aspiration of the thyroid (WHAFFT). *Pathol Annu*. 1994;29(pt 2):99–120.
53. Sharma C, Krishnanand G. Histologic analysis and comparison of techniques in fine needle aspiration-induced alterations in thyroid. *Acta Cytol*. 2008;52:56–64.
54. Baloch ZW, LiVolsi VA. Post fine-needle aspiration histologic alterations of thyroid revisited. *Am J Clin Pathol*. 1999;112:311–316.
55. Baloch ZW, Wu H, LiVolsi VA. Post-fine-needle aspiration spindle cell nodules of the thyroid (PSCNT). *Am J Clin Pathol*. 1999;111:70–74.
56. Keyhani-Rofagha S, Kooner DS, Keyhani M, et al. Necrosis of a Hurthle cell tumor of the thyroid following fine needle aspiration. Case report and literature review. *Acta Cytol*. 1990;34:805–808.
57. Kini SR. Post-fine-needle biopsy infarction of thyroid neoplasms: a review of 28 cases. *Diagn Cytopathol*. 1996;15:211–220.

CHAPTER 7

Yuri E. Nikiforov

Thyroid Tumors: Classification, Staging, and General Considerations

CLASSIFICATION

A histologic classification of thyroid tumors is shown in Table 7.1. It incorporates main principles of the current World Health Organization (WHO) classification of thyroid tumors.[1] Thyroid tumors can be broadly subdivided into primary and secondary or metastatic tumors. Metastatic thyroid tumors are rare. Most primary thyroid tumors are epithelial tumors that originate from thyroid follicular cells. This group encompasses the most common types of thyroid neoplasms, that is, benign follicular adenoma and malignant well-differentiated papillary and follicular carcinomas. Poorly differentiated and anaplastic carcinomas also originate from follicular cells, and many of them are believed to develop as a result of dedifferentiation of a well-differentiated papillary or follicular carcinoma (Fig. 7.1). It is likely that some follicular carcinomas arise as a result of malignant transformation of pre-existing follicular adenomas, whereas others may bypass this premalignant stage. Medullary carcinomas originate from thyroid parafollicular or C cells.

Current thyroid tumor classifications encounter several controversial issues. One is related to the placement of thyroid oncocytic (Hürthle cell) adenomas and carcinomas. These tumors display several basic histologic features that are similar to those of conventional follicular tumors (i.e., follicular growth pattern, encapsulation) but are different in other microscopic features, in certain clinical characteristics, and possibly in some molecular alterations. Oncocytic adenomas and carcinomas are considered by some as separate types of thyroid tumors and by others as a variant of follicular adenoma and follicular carcinoma. The current WHO classification designates them as a variant of follicular tumors.[1] This may change in the future as new molecular studies characterizing these tumors emerge.

Poorly differentiated thyroid carcinoma is a distinct type of thyroid cancer. However, the diagnostic criteria for this tumor have not been universally accepted. On the basis of the characteristic growth pattern, many of these tumors are being designated as insular carcinomas. This term, however, places emphasis on the growth pattern rather than the cytologic features of tumor cells, and its use should be discouraged. The consensus diagnostic criteria for poorly differentiated carcinoma have been proposed based on the results of an international conference held in Turin, Italy in 2006.[2] When diagnosed based on these criteria, this tumor falls into a distinctly intermediate prognostic category between indolent well-differentiated papillary and follicular carcinomas and almost always lethal anaplastic carcinoma.

The placement of hyalinizing trabecular tumor represents another problematic issue for the classification of thyroid tumors. This rare tumor had been originally described as hyalinizing trabecular adenoma and typically has a benign course, despite sharing several histologic features with papillary carcinoma.[3] More recent studies suggest that this tumor may harbor molecular alterations characteristic of papillary carcinomas.[4,5] Although, currently, there is no sufficient evidence to reclassify this tumor

as a variant of papillary carcinoma, it deserves placement into a separate classification group.

Owing to the difficulty in diagnosing the encapsulated follicular variant of papillary carcinoma and the uncertainty in the malignant behavior of tumors with only partially developed nuclear features of papillary carcinoma, attempts have been made to introduce a different terminology for these tumors, such as "well-differentiated tumor of uncertain malignant potential."[6] This terminology, however, is not widely accepted, in part because of the lack of information on the implication of this diagnosis for clinical management of these patients.

INCIDENCE AND EPIDEMIOLOGY

Thyroid cancer is the most common type of endocrine malignancy. It constitutes 3% of all newly diagnosed cancer cases in the United States[7] and 1.7% of all newly diagnosed cancer cases worldwide.[8] The incidence of thyroid cancer is about three times higher among females than males in the United States and most of other countries.[7,8] For example, in the United States, the age-adjusted incidence of thyroid cancer in 2008 was 6.47 per 100,000 men and 19.39 per 100,000 women based on the Surveillance, Epidemiology, and End Results (SEER) national cancer data registry.[9] Worldwide, the incidence varies in different geographic regions and is overall higher in more economically developed countries. The highest rates are observed in South Korea, Northern America, Australia, and the several countries of Europe and Middle East (Fig. 7.2).[8] The incidence varies between different ethnic groups. In the United States, thyroid cancer is about twice more common in whites than in blacks.[10,11]

Thyroid cancer is rare in children, but its incidence begins to rise sharply in the second decade of life and peaks during the fifth and sixth decades of life (Fig. 7.3A). This age distribution reflects the incidence of the three most common types of thyroid cancer, namely, papillary carcinoma that constitutes ~80% of all thyroid cancer cases, follicular carcinoma (15%), and medullary carcinoma (3%).[10,12] Anaplastic carcinoma, which accounts for <2% of thyroid tumors, typically occurs in the older age group and its incidence continues to rise with age.

The incidence of thyroid cancer has been steadily rising over the past three decades, and particularly since the mid-1990s, in many countries around the world.[13–15] On the basis of the SEER data, the incidence in the United States practically tripled since 1973, growing at a rate of 2.4% per year in 1980 to 1997 and 6.5% per year since 1997 (Fig. 7.3B).[9] In fact, thyroid cancer is currently the fastest-increasing cancer in the United States in both men and women and has become the fifth most common type of cancer in women.[7] Mortality from thyroid cancer remains low (Fig. 7.3B), although it has been rising since 1992 at a rate of 0.6% per year.[7]

The increase in incidence is almost entirely attributed to papillary carcinoma, whereas the rates of follicular, medullary, and

---

Table 7.1

Histologic Classification of Thyroid Tumors

I. Primary   **II. Secondary (Metastatic)**

1. **Epithelial**   2. **Nonepithelial**

  A. *Follicular cell origin*   - Primary lymphoma and plasmacytoma

  A.1. Benign   - Angiosarcoma

    - Follicular adenoma   - Teratoma

      a. Conventional type   - Smooth muscle tumors

      b. Oncocytic type   - Peripheral nerve sheath tumors

  A.2. Uncertain malignant potential   - Paraganglioma

    - Hyalinizing trabecular tumor   - Solitary fibrous tumor

  A.3. Malignant   - Follicular dendritic cell tumor

    - Papillary carcinoma   - Langerhans cell histiocytosis

    - Follicular carcinoma   - Rosai–Dorfman disease

      a. Conventional type   - Granular cell tumor

      b. Oncocytic type

    - Poorly differentiated carcinoma

    - Anaplastic (undifferentiated) carcinoma

  B. *C-cell origin*

    - Medullary carcinoma

  C. *Mixed follicular and C-cell origin*

    - Mixed medullary and follicular carcinoma

    - Mixed medullary and papillary carcinoma

  D. *Epithelial tumors of different or uncertain cell origin*

    - Mucoepidermoid carcinoma

    - Sclerosing mucoepidermoid carcinoma with eosinophilia

    - Squamous cell carcinoma

    - Mucinous carcinoma

    - Spindle cell tumor with thymus-like differentiation (SETTLE)

    - Carcinoma showing thymus-like differentiation (CASTLE)

    - Ectopic thymoma

---

anaplastic cancer did not change significantly (Fig. 7.4).[14,16,17] The increase affects both classic papillary carcinoma and the follicular variant of papillary carcinoma and is more pronounced for tumors of 1 cm or less in size.[18] However, the incidence of tumors >1 cm and even >4 to 5 cm in size is also on the rise.[17,19,20] Although exact reasons for the rising incidence of thyroid cancer are not entirely clear, several factors are likely to play a role. First, it may be in part because of improved cancer detection by ultrasonography and thyroid fine needle aspiration (FNA).[21,22] Thyroid ultrasound has been used increasingly since the 1980s and can detect thyroid nodules as small as 0.2 cm in size. Under ultrasound guidance, even very small nodules can be biopsied using FNA technique and examined cytologically. These advances in health care are likely to have resulted in the increased detection of small asymptomatic cancer nodules, which are highly prevalent in the general population and rarely progress to a

clinically relevant disease.[23] Second, the increase may reflect a better recognition of the follicular variant of papillary carcinoma. In the past, many of the tumors currently diagnosed as the follicular variant of papillary carcinoma were interpreted as follicular carcinomas. In addition, owing to a progressive decrease in the stringency of microscopic criteria for the diagnosis of the follicular variant of papillary carcinoma during the 1990s, tumors with partially developed nuclear features of papillary carcinoma, which had been diagnosed as benign lesions in the past, are now more likely to be interpreted as malignant.[24] However, it is unlikely that these factors are responsible for the entire increase in thyroid cancer incidence. In fact, recent studies suggest that the proportion of papillary carcinoma carrying a *BRAF* mutation, which is a marker of more aggressive cancer, has been constant or even increasing during the last decades.[25,26] The growing incidence of *BRAF*-positive tumors and tumors >1 cm argues against

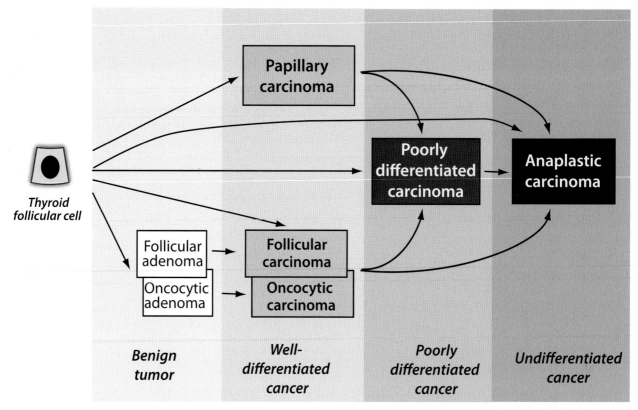

FIGURE 7.1. Scheme of putative progression and dedifferentiation of follicular cell-derived thyroid tumors.

the possibility that thyroid cancer increase is solely because of better medical surveillance and detection of small, clinically irrelevant, nonprogressive thyroid cancers.

 ## GENETIC SUSCEPTIBILITY AND OTHER RISK FACTORS

The development of thyroid tumors is likely to involve the interaction between the genetic predisposition, the endogenous hormonal factors, and the environmental risk factors (Table 7.2). The role of genetic predisposition is best established for medullary carcinoma. Approximately 25% of these tumors occur as part of one of the multiple endocrine neoplasia (MEN) syndromes, MEN type 2A, MEN type 2B, and familial medullary thyroid carcinoma (FMTC). The disease is caused by a germline mutation in the *RET* gene and has an autosomal dominant inheritance with almost complete penetrance but variable expressivity.

Approximately 5% of thyroid cancers of follicular cell origin show familial occurrence. Those are either associated with well-defined hereditary cancer syndromes or inherited through yet unidentified genetic mechanisms.[27] Overall, the risk of thyroid cancer in the first-degree relatives of patients with follicular cell-derived thyroid cancer is 4- to 10-folds higher than that in the general population.[28,29] One of the known genetic syndromes is familial adenomatous polyposis (FAP), which is caused by a germline mutation of the adenomatous polyposis coli (*APC*) gene on 5q21. Thyroid tumors in these patients typically manifest during the third decade of life and affect predominantly females.[30] Most

of the FAP-associated thyroid tumors are papillary carcinomas, and they exhibit distinct histologic features.[31] Thyroid tumors are found in patients affected by *PTEN*-hamartoma tumor syndrome, which encompass Cowden syndrome and other rare syndromes caused by a germline mutation of the *PTEN* gene on 10q23.31. Most of these tumors are follicular carcinomas, although papillary carcinomas may also be seen in these patients.[32] Thyroid neoplasms may also present as a rare manifestation of the Carney complex, Werner syndrome, Peutz–Jeghers syndrome, and MEN syndromes. Most familial follicular cell-derived thyroid cancers, however, are not part of the known inherited syndromes. These tumors are also known as familial nonmedullary thyroid cancer. Most of these tumors (~90%) are papillary carcinomas, and they are presumed to have an autosomal dominant inheritance with reduced penetrance.[33,34] The inherited nature of these tumors is established with certainty when three or more first-degree relatives are diagnosed with thyroid cancer.[35,36] Genetic linkage studies have mapped susceptibility loci to chromosomes 19p13.2, 1q21, and 2q21, although no specific susceptibility genes have been identified in these regions yet.[33]

Exposure to ionizing radiation during childhood is a well-established risk factor for thyroid cancer. Both external radiation (X-ray and γ-radiation) and internal exposure to radioiodine ^{131}I result in the increased risk, although the risk from exposure to radioiodine ^{131}I is clearly established only after accidental exposure during childhood. The risk has strong inverse correlation with age at exposure and is linear for thyroid doses in the range of 0.1 to 2 Gy received by children <15 years old.[37,38] The minimal latent period for thyroid cancer development is 4 years after exposure, and the risk remains elevated for >40 years.[39–41] Most radiation-induced cancers are papillary

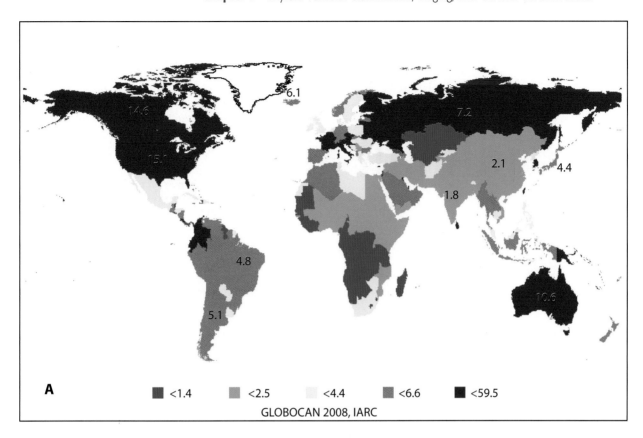

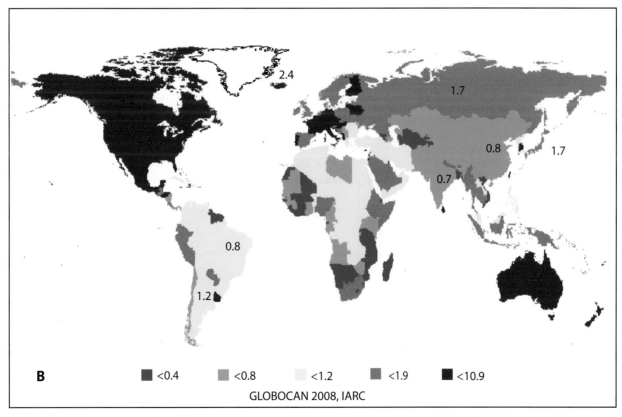

FIGURE 7.2. Age-standardized incidence of thyroid cancer per 100,000 in females (A) and in males (B). The shown age-standardized rates are per 100,000 population per year. (From Ferlay J, Shin HR, Bray F, et al. Estimates of worldwide burden of cancer in 2008: GLOBOCAN 2008. *Int J Cancer*. 2010;127:2893–2917.)

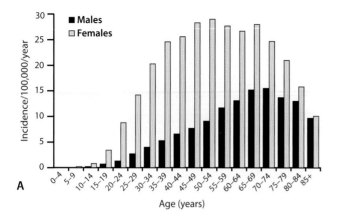

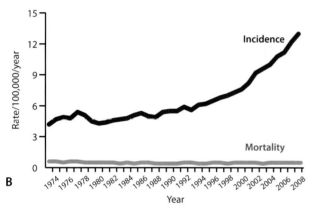

carcinomas, many of which show a solid growth pattern and are diagnosed as the solid variant of papillary carcinoma.[42] The risk of developing follicular cancer and benign nodules after radiation exposure is overall less pronounced, and these lesions may develop after a longer latency. Molecular mechanisms of radiation-associated papillary carcinogenesis primarily involve the generation of chromosomal rearrangements, such as *RET/PTC*, whereas point mutations of *BRAF* and other genes are much less common in these tumors.[43–45] The most recent outbreak of radiation-induced thyroid cancer has been registered in the populations of children and young adults exposed to radiation after the Chernobyl nuclear accident. In other regions of the world, therapeutic radiation for cancers of other locations is the leading source of exposure. In the United States, a history of prior exposure to radiation is found in ~5% of patients with thyroid cancer.[12]

A history of preexisting benign thyroid nodule/adenoma or multinodular goiter is another strong risk factor for thyroid cancer. Benign thyroid nodules/adenomas appear to confer a higher risk than nontoxic goiter does. The risk of cancer is higher during the first 10 years after diagnosis of a benign thyroid disease and remains elevated >10 years later.[46,47] The risk is comparable for papillary and follicular cancer in individuals diagnosed with goiter and may be slightly higher for follicular carcinoma in those diagnosed with a benign nodule/adenoma. The risk of anaplastic carcinoma cannot be calculated in case-control studies because of the low incidence of this disease, although many patients with anaplastic carcinoma have a history of long-standing goiter. In the United States, a history of benign goiter/nodular thyroid disease is found in about 15% of patients with differentiated thyroid cancer and in about 25% of patients diagnosed with anaplastic carcinoma.[48] The molecular mechanisms underlying the association between preexisting benign thyroid disease and cancer are not well understood. The transition from adenoma to carcinoma may involve somatic mutations of the *RAS* genes, which are about equally prevalent in follicular adenomas and carcinomas. These mutations are

FIGURE 7.3. A: Age-specific incidence of thyroid cancer in men and women. **B:** Thyroid cancer incidence and mortality, SEER 1973 to 2008. (From Howlader N, Noone AM, Krapcho M, et al. SEER cancer statistics review, 1975–2008. National Cancer Institute. SEER web site. http://seer.cancer.gov/csr/1975_2008/.)

FIGURE 7.4. Trends in the incidence of the four major types of thyroid cancer in the United States, SEER 1973 to 2008. From Howlader N, Noone AM, Krapcho M, et al. SEER cancer statistics review, 1975–2008. National Cancer Institute. SEER web site. http://seer.cancer.gov/csr/1975_2008/.

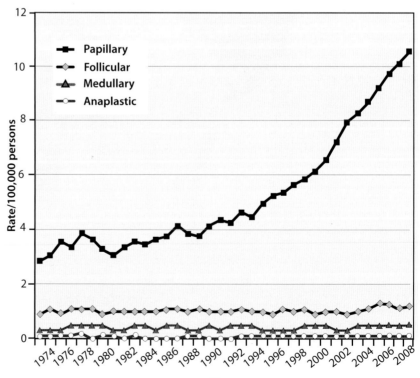

Table 7.2

Risk Factors for Thyroid Tumors and Their Genetic Basis

Genetic predisposition

a. MEN2A, MEN2B, FMTC syndromes: *medullary carcinoma* — *RET* germline mutation

b. FAP: *papillary carcinoma* — *APC* germline mutation

c. *PTEN*-hamartoma tumor syndrome (Cowden syndrome): *follicular carcinoma, occasionally papillary carcinoma* — *PTEN* germline mutation

d. Familial follicular cell-derived thyroid cancer: *papillary carcinoma* — Loci on 19p13.2, 1q21, 2q21

Ionizing radiation

a. External X-ray or γ-radiation, therapeutic or accidental exposure: *papillary carcinoma* — *RET/PTC* and other chromosomal rearrangements

b. Accidental exposure to ^{131}I during childhood: *papillary carcinoma* — *RET/PTC* and other chromosomal rearrangements

Preexisting benign thyroid disease

a. Thyroid nodule/adenoma, multinodular goiter: *follicular carcinoma, papillary carcinoma* — Genetics not clear, possibly somatic *RAS* mutations, TSH stimulation

b. Hashimoto thyroiditis: *primary thyroid lymphoma* — Genetics not clear

c. Graves disease: *risk for thyroid carcinoma controversial*

Iodine intake — Genetics not clear

a. Iodine deficiency: *follicular carcinoma, anaplastic carcinoma*

b. Iodine sufficiency/excess: *papillary carcinoma*

Hormonal and reproductive factors

a. Female gender, particularly during reproductive age; role of specific hormonal factors remains unknown: *papillary carcinoma, follicular carcinoma* — Genetics not clear

---

FMTC, familial medullary thyroid carcinoma.

also found in some papillary carcinomas. *RAS* mutations occur early in the process of tumor formation and may predispose to malignant transformation.[49,50] Another possible mechanism may involve a cooperation between oncogenic mutations and thyroid cell proliferation in benign nodules, particularly in patients with higher levels of thyroid-stimulating hormone (TSH). Several epidemiologic studies have showed the association between higher serum TSH levels and risk of thyroid cancer in patients with thyroid nodules.[51–53] The risk of cancer increased incrementally with the higher levels of TSH, even within the normal range. In addition, experimental evidence has been offered indicating that expression of mutant *BRAF* at physiologic levels requires simultaneous TSH stimulation to transform thyroid cells and to initiate papillary carcinoma development in transgenic mice.[54]

The association between thyroid carcinoma and Graves disease or chronic lymphocytic (Hashimoto) thyroiditis remains controversial. Several studies have reported a higher than expected frequency of thyroid cancer in patients with surgically treated Graves disease and Hashimoto thyroiditis.[55,56] However, case-control studies have not found the association between these conditions and increased risk of thyroid carcinoma, in contrast to a 67-fold higher risk of thyroid lymphoma found in patients with Hashimoto thyroiditis.[57,58]

A higher incidence of thyroid follicular and anaplastic carcinomas was observed in areas of dietary iodine deficiency, particularly among those individuals who lived in these regions

for at least 20 years or during childhood.[59,60] On the contrary, in the areas of high iodine intake, such as Iceland and the Pacific islands, the relative frequency of papillary carcinoma appears to be higher.[61,62] In the geographic areas with severe iodine deficiency, iodine supplementation coincided with a significant reduction in the incidence of follicular and anaplastic cancer and the increase in the proportion of papillary carcinomas.[61,63] It is unclear, however, whether the increase in papillary carcinoma was caused by an iodine-rich diet or whether it reflected the decrease in the proportion of other thyroid tumor types or coincided with the increase in the incidence of papillary cancer observed in many countries.

The role of endogenous hormonal factors is supported by a significantly higher incidence of all main types of thyroid cancer in women than in men. The gender difference is most pronounced during the female reproductive age, and the rate of cancer in women steadily decreases after menopause. However, a search for specific hormonal risk factors has been mostly unsuccessful. Some, but not all, studies have found a slightly increased cancer risk associated with the use of estrogen-containing preparations, including oral contraceptives, miscarriage of the first pregnancy, artificially induced menopause, several pregnancies, and late age at first birth.[61,64–66]

The link between thyroid cancer risk and obesity has been found in several, but not all, case-control and prospective cohort studies.[66–69] The elevated risk was seen more often in women and appeared to be stronger in postmenopausal women.[68]

CLINICAL PRESENTATION AND MANAGEMENT

Thyroid tumors typically present as a lump in the neck incidentally discovered by a patient or felt by a health care provider during clinical exam. The mass is typically asymptomatic or may have associated symptoms of hoarseness or dysphasia. Rarely, thyroid cancer manifests as a metastatic nodules in the neck, pulmonary nodules, or a pathologic fracture of a bone.

Most common diagnostic modalities in the evaluation of thyroid nodules include ultrasonography, FNA biopsy, and radionuclide scanning.[70-72] Cytologic evaluation of thyroid FNA biopsy is the most reliable diagnostic approach which establishes a definitive diagnosis of benign or malignant disease in 70-80% of cases. Other aspirates either do not yield sufficient cells for evaluation or are diagnosed as indeterminate. The indeterminate group primarily encompasses the follicular-pattern lesions, that is, cellular hyperplasic nodule, follicular adenoma, follicular carcinoma, and the follicular variant of papillary carcinoma, where the definitive diagnosis cannot be reliably established based on cytology. The FNA procedure can be performed with palpation or ultrasound guidance. Thyroid ultrasound is particularly useful to guide the FNA biopsy of small thyroid nodules. It is helpful to determine whether nodules are solid or cystic, as cancer is rare in nodules lacking substantial solid component, and to identify other suspicious sonographic features. Radionuclide scan (with ^{123}I or Tc-99m) usually demonstrates that malignant tumor nodules are hypofunctioning or "cold" (i.e., have tracer uptake lower than surrounding normal thyroid tissue). CT and MRI can be used to better evaluate lymph node involvement or tumor extension to the adjacent neck structures.

The preferred surgical treatment for most patients with the established diagnosis of thyroid cancer is total or near-total thyroidectomy. Lymph node dissection may be performed in patients with evidence of nodal disease and with medullary thyroid carcinoma. Thyroid lobectomy is a typical initial approach for nodules with indeterminate cytology. If a malignant diagnosis is established in the lobectomy specimen during intraoperative evaluation of frozen sections or postoperatively, completion thyroidectomy is usually performed.

Postoperative ^{131}I therapy is typically administered for differentiated carcinomas of follicular cell origin that are at least 1 cm in size, are multicentric, or reveal extrathyroidal extension.[70,73,74] It allows to eliminate residual microscopic or metastatic disease and to ablate residual nonneoplastic thyroid tissue to facilitate postoperative disease monitoring. Adjuvant external beam radiotherapy may be used in patients with extensive extrathyroidal extension of the tumor and when the tumor cannot be fully excised by surgery. Long-term monitoring of differentiated thyroid cancer of follicular cell origin is achieved by ultrasound and measuring serum levels of thyroglobulin. Most disease-free patients have undetectable serum thyroglobulin and its increase serves as a sensitive marker of tumor recurrence. Medullary carcinomas can be monitored by measuring serum concentrations of calcitonin and carcinoembryonic antigen.

Anaplastic carcinoma usually presents with widely invasive local disease and frequent distant metastases. Unless confined to the thyroid, surgery does not prolong survival and treatment is generally palliative, typically using external beam radiotherapy.

More recent therapeutic approaches are based on the use of tyrosine kinase inhibitors that block molecular pathways activated by cancer-specific mutations. Although still in early stages of its clinical use, several agents have shown therapeutic efficacy for treating anaplastic thyroid carcinoma and advanced well-differentiated thyroid cancer.[75-78]

SURVIVAL, PROGNOSTIC FACTORS, AND STAGING

Overall mortality from thyroid cancer is low (Fig. 7.3B). Despite a sharply growing incidence, mortality from thyroid has a small but significant increase at a rate of 0.6% per year.[7] In the United States, the age-adjusted death rate is close to 0.5 per 100,000 people and is similar for both genders and all ethnic groups.[7] In 2008, the 5-year survival rate for patients with all types of thyroid cancer in the United States was 97%.[7] However, the mortality rate varies significantly by age at diagnosis, tumor stage, and cancer type. The 5-year survival rate for all tumors progressively decreases from 99.5% for patients younger than 45 years to 82.2% for those 75 years and older at the time of diagnosis.[7] By tumor stage, the survival rate is 99.8% for localized disease, 96.9% for regional disease dissemination, and 56.4% for distant spread.[7] Survival rates also vary significantly between specific tumor types and are sharply different between all well-differentiated carcinomas and anaplastic carcinoma. In 1985 to 1995, the 10-year survival rate in the United States was 93% for papillary carcinoma, 85% for follicular carcinoma, 76% for oncocytic follicular carcinoma, 75% for medullary carcinoma, and 14% for anaplastic carcinoma.[12]

Several prognostic systems are used for thyroid cancer. The TNM-based staging system, recommended by the American Joint Commission on Cancer (AJCC) and International Union Against Cancer (Union Internationale Conrole le Cancer), takes into account the known risk factors such as specific tumor type, age at diagnosis, tumor size, extrathyroidal tumor extension, and distant metastasis (Table 7.3).[79] In this system, papillary and follicular carcinomas are staged similarly and separately from medullary carcinoma and anaplastic carcinoma. In addition, separate stage groupings are applied to papillary and follicular carcinomas in patients younger than 45 years and those 45 years and older. The most recent, seventh edition of AJCC staging[79] contains several differences when compared with previous editions. T1 lesions, which are intrathyroidal tumors up to 2 cm, are now subdivided into T1a (≤1 cm) and T1b (>1 to 2 cm). As in the previous, sixth edition, extrathyroidal extension is subdivided into minimal (tumor invasion into immediate perithyroidal soft tissues or sternothyroid muscle), which corresponds to T3, and extensive (tumor invasion into subcutaneous soft tissues, larynx, trachea, esophagus, or recurrent laryngeal nerve), which is T4.

In addition to the TNM-based staging system, which serves as a good predictor of survival,[12,73,80] several other prognostic schemes have been developed. Their main purpose is to better stratify patients with well-differentiated follicular-cell derived cancer who are at higher risk for tumor recurrence and disease-specific mortality (Table 7.4).[81-87] These schemes use a different combination of various prognostic factors, such as age, sex, tumor type, extrathyroidal extension, tumor size, and distant metastases, which are weighted differently in each scoring system. Most of these systems allow accurate identification of the majority of low-risk patients who can be treated less aggressively as compared with the patients falling into the high-risk group.[70,88,89]

Table 7.3

AJCC/UICC TNM-Based Staging of Thyroid Cancer

Papillary or follicular carcinoma (age younger than 45 years)

Stage I	Any T	Any N	M0
Stage II	Any T	Any N	M1

Papillary or follicular carcinoma (age 45 years and older)

Stage I	T1	N0	M0
Stage II	T2	N0	M0
Stage III	T3	N0	M0
	T1–T3	N1a	M0
Stage IVA	T4a	N0	M0
	T4a	N1a	M0
	T1–T4a	N1b	M0
Stage IVB	T4b	Any N	M0
Stage IVC	Any T	Any N	M1

Medullary carcinoma

Stage I	T1	N0	M0
Stage II	T2, T3	N0	M0
Stage III	T1–T3	N1a	M0
Stage IVA	T4a	N0	M0
	T4a	N1a	M0
	T1–T4a	N1b	M0
Stage IVB	T4b	Any N	M0
Stage IVC	Any T	Any N	M1

Anaplastic carcinoma

Stage IVA	T4a	Any N	M0
Stage IVB	T4b	Any N	M0
Stage IVC	Any T	Any N	M1

Definition of TNM

Primary tumor (T)

TX = Primary tumor cannot be assessed

T0 = No evidence of primary tumor

T1 = Tumor 2 cm or less in greatest dimension, limited to the thyroid

  T1a = Tumor 1 cm or less in greatest dimension, limited to the thyroid

  T2b = Tumor >1 cm but not >2 cm in greatest dimension, limited to the thyroid

T2 = Tumor >2 cm but not >4 cm in greatest dimension, limited to the thyroid

T3 = Tumor >4 cm in greatest dimension, limited to the thyroid or any tumor with minimal extrathyroid extension (e.g., extension to sternothyroid muscle or perithyroid soft tissues)

T4a = Moderately advanced disease

Tumor of any size extending beyond the thyroid capsule to invade subcutaneous soft tissues, larynx, trachea, esophagus, or recurrent laryngeal nerve

T4b = Very advanced disease

Tumor invades prevertebral fascia or encases carotid artery or mediastinal vessels

All anaplastic carcinomas are considered T4 tumors

T4a = Intrathyroidal anaplastic carcinoma

T4b = Extrathyroidal anaplastic carcinoma with gross extrathyroidal extension

Table 7.3

AJCC/UICC TNM-Based Staging of Thyroid Cancer   *(continued)*

Regional lymph nodes (N)	NX = Regional lymph nodes cannot be assessed
	N0 = No regional lymph node metastasis
	N1 = Regional lymph node metastasis
	N1a = Metastasis to Level VI (pretracheal, paratracheal, and prelaryngeal/Delphian lymph nodes)
	N1b = Metastasis to unilateral, bilateral, or contralateral cervical lymph nodes (Levels I, II, III, IV, or V) or to superior mediastinal lymph nodes (Level VII)
Distant metastasis (M)	M0 = No distant metastasis
	M1 = Distant metastasis

UICC, Union Internationale Conrole le Cancer.

Reproduced with the permission from American Joint Committee on Cancer (AJCC), Chicago, IL. The original source for this material is Edge SB, Byrd DR, Compton CC, et al. *AJCC Cancer Staging Manual.* 7th ed. New York, NY: Springer; 2010. Pages 87-89 TNM Definitions/Stage Grouping Thyroid.

Table 7.4

Risk Factors Used in Various Prognostic Schemes for Patients with Follicular Cell-Derived Thyroid Cancer

Risk Factors	Prognostic Schemes						
	EORTC	AGES	AMES	MACIS	OSU	MSKCC	NTCTCS
Age	√	√	√	√		√	√
Tumor size		√	√	√	√	√	√
Extrathyroidal extension	√	√	√	√	√	√	√
Distant metastasis	√	√	√	√	√	√	√
Gender	√		√				
Multicentricity					√		√
Lymph node metastasis					√	√	√
Histologic type	√	√	√	√		√	√
Histologic grade		√				√	
Completeness of resection					√		

EORTC, European Organization for Research on Treatment of Cancer; AGES, patient age, histologic grade of the tumor, tumor extent (extrathyroidal invasion or distant metastases), and size of the primary tumor; AMES, patient age, presence of distant metastases, extent, and size of the primary tumor; MACIS, metastasis, patient age, completeness of resection, local invasion, and tumor size; OSU, Ohio State University; MSKCC, Memorial Sloan–Kettering Cancer Center; NTCTCS, National Thyroid Cancer Treatment Cooperative Study.

Adapted with modifications from Dean DS, Hay ID. Prognostic indicators in differentiated thyroid carcinoma. *Cancer Control.* 2000;7:229–239.

REFERENCES

1. DeLellis RA, Lloyd RV, Heitz PU, et al, eds. *World Health Organization Classification of Tumours. Pathology and Genetics of Tumours of Endocrine Organs.* Lyon, France: IARC Press; 2004.
2. Volante M, Collini P, Nikiforov YE, et al. Poorly differentiated thyroid carcinoma: the Turin proposal for the use of uniform diagnostic criteria and an algorithmic diagnostic approach. *Am J Surg Pathol.* 2007;31:1256–1264.
3. Carney JA, Ryan J, Goellner JR. Hyalinizing trabecular adenoma of the thyroid gland. *Am J Surg Pathol.* 1987;11:583–591.
4. Cheung CC, Boerner SL, MacMillan CM, et al. Hyalinizing trabecular tumor of the thyroid: a variant of papillary carcinoma proved by molecular genetics. *Am J Surg Pathol.* 2000;24:1622–1626.
5. Papotti M, Volante M, Giuliano A, et al. RET/PTC activation in hyalinizing trabecular tumors of the thyroid. *Am J Surg Pathol.* 2000;24:1615–1621.
6. Williams ED. Guest editorial: two proposals regarding the terminology of thyroid tumors. *Int J Surg Pathol.* 2000;8:181–183.
7. American Cancer Society. *Cancer Facts & Figures 2011.* Atlanta, GA: American Cancer Society; 2011.
8. Ferlay J, Shin HR, Bray F, et al. Estimates of worldwide burden of cancer in 2008: GLOBOCAN 2008. *Int J Cancer.* 2010;127:2893–2917.
9. Howlader N, Noone AM, Krapcho M, et al. SEER cancer statistics review, 1975–2008. National Cancer Institute. SEER web site. http://seer.cancer.gov/csr/1975_2008/. Accessed July 12, 2011.
10. Ries LAG, Melbert D, Krapcho M, et al. SEER cancer statistics review, 1975–2004. National Cancer Institute. SEER web site. http://seer.cancer.gov/csr/1975_2004/. Accessed January 10, 2010.
11. Aschebrook-Kilfoy B, Ward MH, Sabra MM, et al. Thyroid cancer incidence patterns in the United States by histologic type, 1992–2006. *Thyroid.* 2011;21:125–134.
12. Hundahl SA, Fleming ID, Fremgen AM, et al. A National Cancer Data Base report on 53,856 cases of thyroid carcinoma treated in the U.S., 1985–1995 [see comments]. *Cancer.* 1998;83:2638–2648.
13. Burgess JR. Temporal trends for thyroid carcinoma in Australia: an increasing incidence of papillary thyroid carcinoma (1982–1997). *Thyroid.* 2002;12:141–149.
14. Davies L, Welch HG. Increasing incidence of thyroid cancer in the United States, 1973–2002. *JAMA.* 2006;295:2164–2167.

15. Leenhardt L, Grosclaude P, Cherie-Challine L. Increased incidence of thyroid carcinoma in France: a true epidemic or thyroid nodule management effects? Report from the French Thyroid Cancer Committee. *Thyroid.* 2004;14:1056–1060.

16. Albores-Saavedra J, Henson DE, Glazer E, et al. Changing patterns in the incidence and survival of thyroid cancer with follicular phenotype—papillary, follicular, and anaplastic: a morphological and epidemiological study. *Endocr Pathol.* 2007;18:1–7.

17. Colonna M, Guizard AV, Schvartz C, et al. A time trend analysis of papillary and follicular cancers as a function of tumour size: a study of data from six cancer registries in France (1983–2000). *Eur J Cancer.* 2007;43:891–900.

18. Hughes DT, Haymart MR, Miller BS, et al. The most commonly occurring papillary thyroid cancer in the United States is now a microcarcinoma in a patient older than 45 years. *Thyroid.* 2011;21:231–236.

19. Cramer JD, Fu P, Harth KC, et al. Analysis of the rising incidence of thyroid cancer using the Surveillance, Epidemiology and End Results national cancer data registry. *Surgery.* 2010;148:1147–1152; discussion 1152–1143.

20. Enewold L, Zhu K, Ron E, et al. Rising thyroid cancer incidence in the United States by demographic and tumor characteristics, 1980–2005. *Cancer Epidemiol Biomarkers Prev.* 2009;18:784–791.

21. Rojeski MT, Gharib H. Nodular thyroid disease. Evaluation and management. *N Engl J Med.* 1985;313:428–436.

22. Burgess JR, Tucker P. Incidence trends for papillary thyroid carcinoma and their correlation with thyroid surgery and thyroid fine-needle aspirate cytology. *Thyroid.* 2006;16:47–53.

23. Harach HR, Franssila KO, Wasenius VM. Occult papillary carcinoma of the thyroid. A "normal" finding in Finland. A systematic autopsy study. *Cancer.* 1985;56:531–538.

24. Suster S. Thyroid tumors with a follicular growth pattern: problems in differential diagnosis. *Arch Pathol Lab Med.* 2006;130:984–988.

25. Mathur A, Moses W, Rahbari R, et al. Higher rate of *BRAF* mutation in papillary thyroid cancer over time: a single-institution study. *Cancer.* 2011;117:4390–4395.

26. Sykorova V, Dvorakova S, Ryska A, et al. *BRAFV600E* mutation in the pathogenesis of a large series of papillary thyroid carcinoma in Czech Republic. *J Endocrinol Invest.* 2010;33:318–324.

27. Nose V. Familial thyroid cancer: a review. *Mod Pathol.* 2011;24(suppl 2):S19–S33.

28. Frich L, Glattre E, Akslen LA. Familial occurrence of nonmedullary thyroid cancer: a population-based study of 5673 first-degree relatives of thyroid cancer patients from Norway. *Cancer Epidemiol Biomarkers Prev.* 2001;10:113–117.

29. Hemminki K, Eng C, Chen B. Familial risks for nonmedullary thyroid cancer. *J Clin Endocrinol Metab.* 2005;90:5747–5753.

30. Plail RO, Bussey HJ, Glazer G, et al. Adenomatous polyposis: an association with carcinoma of the thyroid. *Br J Surg.* 1987;74:377–380.

31. Harach HR, Williams GT, Williams ED. Familial adenomatous polyposis associated thyroid carcinoma: a distinct type of follicular cell neoplasm. *Histopathology.* 1994;25:549–561.

32. Laury AR, Bongiovanni M, Tille JC, et al. Thyroid pathology in PTEN-hamartoma tumor syndrome: characteristic findings of a distinct entity. *Thyroid.* 2011;21:135–144.

33. Malchoff CD, Malchoff DM. Familial nonmedullary thyroid carcinoma. *Cancer Control.* 2006;13:106–110.

34. Burgess JR, Duffield A, Wilkinson SJ, et al. Two families with an autosomal dominant inheritance pattern for papillary carcinoma of the thyroid. *J Clin Endocrinol Metab.* 1997;82:345–348.

35. Charkes ND. On the prevalence of familial nonmedullary thyroid cancer. *Thyroid.* 1998;8:857–858.

36. Charkes ND. On the prevalence of familial nonmedullary thyroid cancer in multiply affected kindreds. *Thyroid.* 2006;16:181–186.

37. Cardis E, Kesminiene A, Ivanov V, et al. Risk of thyroid cancer after exposure to ^{131}I in childhood. *J Natl Cancer Inst.* 2005;97:724–732.

38. Ron E, Lubin JH, Shore RE, et al. Thyroid cancer after exposure to external radiation: a pooled analysis of seven studies. *Radiat Res.* 1995;141:259–277.

39. Schneider AB, Ron E, Lubin J, et al. Dose-response relationships for radiation-induced thyroid cancer and thyroid nodules: evidence for the prolonged effects of radiation on the thyroid. *J Clin Endocrinol Metab.* 1993;77:362–369.

40. Nikiforov YE. Radiation-induced thyroid cancer: what we have learned from Chernobyl. *Endocr Pathol.* 2006;17:307–317.

41. Adams MJ, Shore RE, Dozier A, et al. Thyroid cancer risk 40+ years after irradiation for an enlarged thymus: an update of the Hempelmann cohort. *Radiat Res.* 2010;174:753–762.

42. Nikiforov Y, Gnepp DR. Pediatric thyroid cancer after the Chernobyl disaster. Pathomorphologic study of 84 cases (1991–1992) from the Republic of Belarus. *Cancer.* 1994;74:748–766.

43. Ciampi R, Knauf JA, Kerler R, et al. Oncogenic *AKAP9-BRAF* fusion is a novel mechanism of MAPK pathway activation in thyroid cancer. *J Clin Invest.* 2005;115:94–101.

44. Nikiforov YE, Rowland JM, Bove KE, et al. Distinct pattern of ret oncogene rearrangements in morphological variants of radiation-induced and sporadic thyroid papillary carcinomas in children. *Cancer Res.* 1997;57:1690–1694.

45. Gandhi M, Evdokimova V, Nikiforov YE. Mechanisms of chromosomal rearrangements in solid tumors: the model of papillary thyroid carcinoma. *Mol Cell Endocrinol.* 2010;321:36–43.

46. D'Avanzo B, La Vecchia C, Franceschi S, et al. History of thyroid diseases and subsequent thyroid cancer risk. *Cancer Epidemiol Biomarkers Prev.* 1995;4:193–199.

47. Franceschi S, Preston-Martin S, Dal Maso L, et al. A pooled analysis of case-control studies of thyroid cancer. IV. Benign thyroid diseases. *Cancer Causes Control.* 1999;10:583–595.

48. Hundahl SA, Cady B, Cunningham MP, et al. Initial results from a prospective cohort study of 5583 cases of thyroid carcinoma treated in the United States during 1996. U.S. and German Thyroid Cancer Study Group. An American College of Surgeons Commission on Cancer Patient Care Evaluation study. *Cancer.* 2000;89:202–217.

49. Fagin JA. Minireview: branded from the start-distinct oncogenic initiating events may determine tumor fate in the thyroid. *Mol Endocrinol.* 2002;16:903–911.

50. Williams ED. Mechanisms and pathogenesis of thyroid cancer in animals and man. *Mutat Res.* 1995;333:123–129.

51. Boelaert K, Horacek J, Holder RL, et al. Serum thyrotropin concentration as a novel predictor of malignancy in thyroid nodules investigated by fine-needle aspiration. *J Clin Endocrinol Metab.* 2006;91:4295–4301.

52. Fiore E, Rago T, Provenzale MA, et al. Lower levels of TSH are associated with a lower risk of papillary thyroid cancer in patients with thyroid nodular disease: thyroid autonomy may play a protective role. *Endocr Relat Cancer.* 2009;16:1251–1260.

53. Haymart MR, Glinberg SL, Liu J, et al. Higher serum TSH in thyroid cancer patients occurs independent of age and correlates with extrathyroidal extension. *Clin Endocrinol (Oxf).* 2009;71:434–439.

54. Franco AT, Malaguarnera R, Refetoff S, et al. Thyrotropin receptor signaling dependence of *Braf*-induced thyroid tumor initiation in mice. *Proc Natl Acad Sci U S A.* 2011;108:1615–1620.

55. Walker RP, Paloyan E. The relationship between Hashimoto's thyroiditis, thyroid neoplasia, and primary hyperparathyroidism. *Otolaryngol Clin North Am.* 1990;23:291–302.

56. Mazzaferri EL. Thyroid cancer and Graves' disease. *J Clin Endocrinol Metab.* 1990;70:826–829.

57. Holm LE, Blomgren H, Lowhagen T. Cancer risks in patients with chronic lymphocytic thyroiditis. *N Engl J Med.* 1985;312:601–604.

58. Dobyns BM, Sheline GE, Workman JB, et al. Malignant and benign neoplasms of the thyroid in patients treated for hyperthyroidism: a report of the cooperative thyrotoxicosis therapy follow-up study. *J Clin Endocrinol Metab.* 1974;38:976–998.

59. Pettersson B, Coleman MP, Ron E, et al. Iodine supplementation in Sweden and regional trends in thyroid cancer incidence by histopathologic type. *Int J Cancer.* 1996;65:13–19.

60. Belfiore A, La Rosa GL, Padova G, et al. The frequency of cold thyroid nodules and thyroid malignancies in patients from an iodine-deficient area. *Cancer.* 1987;60:3096–3102.

61. Franceschi S, Boyle P, Maisonneuve P, et al. The epidemiology of thyroid carcinoma. *Crit Rev Oncog.* 1993;4:25–52.

62. Williams ED, Doniach I, Bjarnason O, et al. Thyroid cancer in an iodide rich area: a histopathological study. *Cancer.* 1977;39:215–222.

63. Harach HR, Escalante DA, Day ES. Thyroid cancer and thyroiditis in Salta, Argentina: a 40-yr study in relation to iodine prophylaxis. *Endocr Pathol.* 2002;13:175–181.

64. Negri E, Dal Maso L, Ron E, et al. A pooled analysis of case-control studies of thyroid cancer. II. Menstrual and reproductive factors. *Cancer Causes Control.* 1999;10:143–155.

65. Ron E, Curtis R, Hoffman DA, et al. Multiple primary breast and thyroid cancer. *Br J Cancer.* 1984;49:87–92.

66. Ron E, Kleinerman RA, Boice JD Jr, et al. A population-based case-control study of thyroid cancer. *J Natl Cancer Inst.* 1987;79:1–12.

67. Kolonel LN, Hankin JH, Wilkens LR, et al. An epidemiologic study of thyroid cancer in Hawaii. *Cancer Causes Control.* 1990;1:223–234.

68. Mijovic T, How J, Payne RJ. Obesity and thyroid cancer. *Front Biosci (Schol Ed).* 2011;3:555–564.

69. Renehan AG, Tyson M, Egger M, et al. Body-mass index and incidence of cancer: a systematic review and meta-analysis of prospective observational studies. *Lancet.* 2008;371:569–578.

70. Cooper DS, Doherty GM, Haugen BR, et al. Management guidelines for patients with thyroid nodules and differentiated thyroid cancer. *Thyroid.* 2006;16:109–142.

71. Sherman SI. Thyroid carcinoma. *Lancet.* 2003;361:501–511.

72. Gharib H, Papini E, Valcavi R, et al. American Association of Clinical Endocrinologists and Associazione Medici Endocrinologi medical guidelines for clinical practice for the diagnosis and management of thyroid nodules. *Endocr Pract.* 2006;12:63–102.

73. Jonklaas J, Sarlis NJ, Litofsky D, et al. Outcomes of patients with differentiated thyroid carcinoma following initial therapy. *Thyroid.* 2006;16:1229–1242.

74. Sawka AM, Prebtani AP, Thabane L, et al. A systematic review of the literature examining the diagnostic efficacy of measurement of fractionated plasma free metanephrines in the biochemical diagnosis of pheochromocytoma. *BMC Endocr Disord.* 2004;4:2.

75. Smallridge RC, Copland JA. Anaplastic thyroid carcinoma: pathogenesis and emerging therapies. *Clin Oncol (R Coll Radiol).* 2010;22:486–497.

76. Tuttle RM, Ball DW, Byrd D, et al. Medullary carcinoma. *J Natl Compr Canc Netw.* 2010;8:512–530.

77. Tuttle RM, Ball DW, Byrd D, et al. Thyroid carcinoma. *J Natl Compr Canc Netw.* 2010;8:1228–1274.

78. Sherman SI. Targeted therapies for thyroid tumors. *Mod Pathol.* 2011;24(suppl 2):S44–S52.

79. Edge SB, Byrd DR, Compton CC, et al. *AJCC Cancer Staging Manual.* 7th ed. New York, NY: Springer; 2010.

80. Kosary CL. Cancer of the thyroid. In: Lag R, Young JL, Keel GE, Eisner MP, Lin YD, Horner M-J, eds. *SEER Survival Monograph: Cancer Survival Among Adults: U.S. SEER Program, 1988–2001, Patient and Tumor Characteristics.* Bethesda, MD: National Cancer Institute; 2007:217–225.

81. Hay ID, Grant CS, Taylor WF, et al. Ipsilateral lobectomy versus bilateral lobar resection in papillary thyroid carcinoma: a retrospective analysis of surgical outcome using a novel prognostic scoring system. *Surgery.* 1987;102:1088–1095.

82. Sherman SI, Brierley JD, Sperling M, et al. Prospective multicenter study of thyroiscarcinoma treatment: initial analysis of staging and outcome. National Thyroid Cancer Treatment Cooperative Study Registry Group. *Cancer.* 1998;83:1012–1021.

83. Shaha AR, Loree TR, Shah JP. Prognostic factors and risk group analysis in follicular carcinoma of the thyroid. *Surgery.* 1995;118:1131–1136; discussion 1136–1138.

84. Hay ID, Bergstralh EJ, Goellner JR, et al. Predicting outcome in papillary thyroid carcinoma: development of a reliable prognostic scoring system in a cohort of 1779 patients surgically treated at one institution during 1940 through 1989. *Surgery.* 1993;114:1050–1057; discussion 1057–1058.

85. Mazzaferri EL. Long-term outcome of patients with differentiated thyroid carcinoma: effect of therapy. *Endocr Pract.* 2000;6:469–476.

86. Cady B, Rossi R. An expanded view of risk-group definition in differentiated thyroid carcinoma. *Surgery.* 1988;104:947–953.

87. Byar DP, Green SB, Dor P, et al. A prognostic index for thyroid carcinoma. A study of the E.O.R.T.C. Thyroid Cancer Cooperative Group. *Eur J Cancer.* 1979;15:1033–1041.

88. Tuttle RM, Leboeuf R, Martorella AJ. Papillary thyroid cancer: monitoring and therapy. *Endocrinol Metab Clin North Am.* 2007;36:753–778, vii.

89. Wartofsky L. Staging of thyroid cancer. In: Wartofsky L, Van Nostrand D, eds. *Thyroid Cancer: A Comprehensive Guide to Clinical Management.* 2nd ed. Totowa, NJ: Humana Press; 2006:87–95.

90. Dean DS, Hay ID. Prognostic indicators in differentiated thyroid carcinoma. *Cancer Control.* 2000;7:229–239.

Follicular Adenoma

 ## DEFINITION

Follicular adenoma is a benign, encapsulated, noninvasive tumor originating from thyroid follicular cells. When used without additional qualifiers, this term typically refers to a conventional type of follicular adenoma. The variants of follicular adenoma are designated using additional adjectives or other qualifiers. Oncocytic follicular adenoma is the most common variant of follicular adenoma.

 ## INCIDENCE AND EPIDEMIOLOGY

The true incidence of follicular adenomas is difficult to establish with high accuracy because they cannot be reliably discriminated from solitary hyperplasic nodules based on clinical parameters or fine needle aspiration (FNA) cytology. The incidence of adenomas in adults can be estimated at 3% to 5% based on autopsy series.[1–3] This estimate correlates well with the prevalence of thyroid nodules detected by palpation. Palpable thyroid nodules are found in 3% to 7% of adults living in iodine-sufficient areas, and three-fourths of those are solitary nodules on palpation and may represent adenomas.[4,5] Follicular adenomas more frequently affect females, with the female-to-male ratio ranging from 4:1 to 5:1. They are found on all age groups, although most patients present during the fifth and sixth decades of life.

 ## ETIOLOGIC FACTORS

Most follicular adenomas are sporadic, although some may arise as manifestations of known inherited syndromes. The risk factors implicated in the development of sporadic adenomas include radiation exposure and iodine deficiency. Exposure to X-ray or γ-radiation during childhood and adolescence increases the risk of follicular adenomas up to 15-fold.[6–8] The risk is radiation dose dependent and exists after a dose as small as 0.25 Gy. Most follicular adenomas develop 10 to 15 years after exposure, but elevated risk persists for at least 50 years. Follicular adenomas developing after radiation exposure are usually solitary and reveal conventional type histology, although oncocytic follicular adenomas may also be seen.[8]

Iodine deficiency is another risk factor that correlates with higher incidence of benign thyroid nodules including adenomas. Palpable thyroid nodules are two to three times more common in the areas of low iodine consumption as compared with iodine-sufficient areas, and a significant proportion of those are adenomas.[9,10] In support of this association, follicular adenomas can be induced in experimental animals by administration of low iodine diet or drugs that interfere with iodine uptake and metabolism in thyroid cells.[11,12] The exact mechanism of how iodine deficiency promotes adenoma formation is not clear, but it probably involves the increase in thyroid-stimulating hormone (TSH) levels that stimulate proliferation of thyroid cells.

A cholesterol-lowering agent, 3-hydroxymethylglutaryl coenzyme A (HMG CoA) 1 reductase inhibitor simvastatin, increases incidence of thyroid adenomas in female rats.[13] This is likely because of enhanced liver clearance of thyroid hormone, which is expected to cause elevation in TSH levels. It is unclear whether similar side effects occur in humans. To date, one case of thyroid follicular adenoma with oncocytic features has been reported in a patient treated with simvastatin.[14]

Follicular adenomas develop in patients affected by inherited diseases such as Cowden disease and Carney complex. Cowden disease (multiple hamartoma syndrome) is caused by germ line mutation of the phosphatase and tensin homolog (*PTEN*) tumor suppressor gene located on chromosome 10q23.[15–17] *PTEN* codes for a dual specificity phosphatase that functions as a negative regulator of the phosphatidylinositol 3-kinase (PI3K)/AKT signaling pathway responsible for cell survival and proliferation (illustrated in Fig. 10.5, Chapter 10). The inherited mutation, followed by inactivation of the gene on the second allele through a somatic event, results in the loss of PTEN function and chronic stimulation of AKT and its downstream targets. Follicular adenomas in the affected patients develop at young age and are almost always multiple and bilateral. They are typically follicular adenomas of conventional type, although oncocytic and clear cell adenomas and adenolipoma have also been reported in these patients.[18] Carney complex is another rare autosomal dominant disease caused by germ line mutations in the *PRKARIA* gene on chromosome 17q22-24 and in other still unknown genes.[19] *PRKARIA* encodes the regulatory 1-α subunit of the protein kinase A that mediates the cyclic AMP (cAMP) signaling. Patients affected by this disease frequently develop thyroid adenomas, which are often multiple and may show oncocytic features.[20]

 ## PATHOGENESIS AND MOLECULAR GENETICS

Clonality

Follicular adenomas are true neoplasms and therefore expected to have a monoclonal origin, that is, arise from a single cell. This is opposed to nonneoplastic lesions such as hyperplastic nodules, which have a polyclonal origin. Clonality of a lesion can be assessed in female tissue based on the randomness of inactivation of two X chromosomes. This can be achieved by several assays, including the PCR-based human androgen receptor gene (HUMARA) assay. The principles and limitations of clonality studies are discussed in more detail in Chapter 20. Most studies have confirmed that follicular adenomas diagnosed based on common morphologic criteria are monoclonal, which is consistent with their neoplastic nature.[21,22] Another way to establish clonal origin of a given tumor is through the detection of a mutation (such as *RAS* mutation) or a distinct cytogenetic abnormality (such as trisomy for chromosome 7). The presence of any of these molecular alterations detected in most cells within the lesion indicates its origin from a single cell, that is, its monoclonal origin.

Cytogenetic Abnormalities

Cytogenetically detectable chromosomal changes are found in 30% to 45% of follicular adenomas.[23,24] Most of those are numerical chromosome changes, typically gains, which involve one or several chromosomes. Chromosome 7 is most frequently affected with gains of one or more copies, followed by gains of chromosomes 12 and 5. These numerical chromosome changes can be visualized by G-band karyotyping, comparative genomic hybridization, or fluorescence in situ hybridization (FISH). By FISH, chromosome 7 gains are seen in ~15% of conventional follicular adenomas (typically trisomy 7) and in ~45% of oncocytic follicular adenomas (typically tetrasomy 7) (Fig. 8.1).[25]

The second most common cytogenetic alternation, found in approximately 10% of follicular adenomas, is a group of translocations involving chromosomal loci on 19q13 and 2p21, which are fused with various partners. These adenomas reveal no trisomy 7 or other numerical chromosomal changes and represent a cytogenetically distinct tumor group.[23,26] The gene participating in the fusion on 2p21 has been identified as *THADA*.[27] It is likely to be involved in the death receptor pathway, and its disruption by translocation may affect apoptosis.[28] A putative gene on 19q13 targeted by translocation has been identified as *ZNF331*.[29] The translocation apparently results in aberrant transcription of this gene, although how it promotes tumorigenesis remains clear.

DNA Ploidy

Change in DNA ploidy typically correlates with losses and gains of whole chromosomes. Overall, 20% to 30% of follicular adenomas have aneuploid cell populations.[30-32] Aneuploidy is more common in adenomas with high cellularity, particularly in those with a solid/trabecular growth pattern, where it can be found in >50% of tumors.[33,34] The frequency of aneuploidy tends to increase from hyperplastic nodules to follicular adenomas and then to follicular carcinomas, although a significant overlap between these groups exists.[30,31]

Loss of Heterozygosity

Loss of heterozygosity (LOH) results from deletions of small or large chromosomal regions and is an important genetic feature of neoplastic growth. Regions that are consistently deleted in tumors typically correspond to the location of tumor suppressor genes whose loss of function is required for tumor progression. Follicular adenomas have on average a 6% rate of LOH per chromosome arm, as compared with a 20% rate in follicular carcinomas.[35] The frequency of LOH tends to be higher in follicular adenomas of oncocytic type.[36] The regions most commonly deleted in follicular adenomas are on chromosomes 1q, 3q, 9p, 10q, 13q, and 18q.[35-37] LOH in those regions is found in 10% to 30% of adenomas. On 10q, the loss frequently affects the 10q22-24 region where the *PTEN* tumor suppression gene resides. Another potential target for deletion in this region is the *MINPP1* gene, which is located in proximity to *PTEN* and encodes a protein with similar functions.[38,39]

Somatic Mutations

RAS Mutations

Activating point mutations of the *RAS* genes are common in follicular adenomas. They may involve codons 12, 13, or 61 of the three *RAS* genes (*NRAS*, *KRAS*, and *HRAS*), although *NRAS* codon 61 and *HRAS* codon 61 mutations are by far the most prevalent. *RAS* mutations are found in approximately 30% of conventional type follicular adenomas.[40-42] The frequency may be higher in follicular adenomas with a microfollicular growth pattern.[40] One study has shown a significantly higher incidence of *RAS* mutations in adenomas from an area of iodine deficiency as compared with an iodine-rich region.[43] *RAS* mutations appear to be less frequent in oncocytic adenomas, although only few reported studies have examined this tumor type.[44,45] This is also supported by our experience.[46] In a series of 45 oncocytic and conventional type follicular adenomas, we observed *RAS* mutations in 7% of oncocytic adenomas as compared with 37% of conventional type adenomas.

RAS mutation results in chronic stimulation of various downstream signaling pathways, most notably the mitogen-activated protein kinase (MAPK) pathway and PI3K/AKT pathway, by the mutant RAS protein. This mutation is likely to be an initiating event in the development of follicular adenomas. This is supported by experiments on cultured human thyroid cells and by animal studies. RAS activation in cultured cells induces self-limited proliferation with formation of well-demarcated, differentiated cell colonies, recapitulating the growth of follicular adenomas.[47] Expression of mutant RAS in transgenic mice leads to the development of follicular adenomas and follicular carcinomas.[48,49]

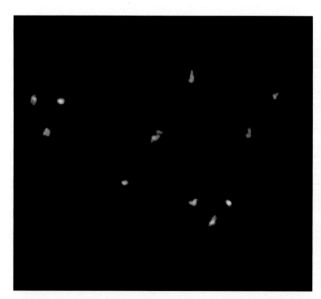 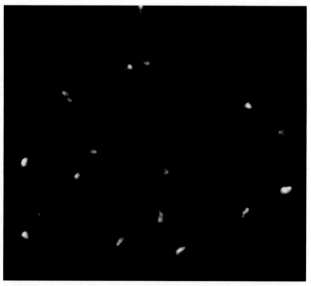

FIGURE 8.1. FISH with a chromosome 7 centromeric probe demonstrates three copies of chromosome 7 in a conventional follicular adenoma (left) and four copies in an oncocytic adenoma (right).

TSHR and *Gsα* Mutations

Somatic mutations in the TSH receptor (*TSHR*) and α subunit of the stimulatory G protein (*Gsα*) genes play a causal role in the development of hyperfunctioning (toxic) thyroid adenomas. These mutations lead to chronic stimulation of the cAMP signaling pathway, which is involved in the regulation of all major aspects of thyroid growth and function by TSH (Fig. 8.2). In hyperfunctioning adenomas, point mutations of the *TSHR* gene are found in 50% to 80% and of the *Gsα* genes in ~5% of cases.[50,51] Mutations cluster in the functionally important regions of both genes. In *TSHR*, they are primarily located in the transmembrane domain involved in interaction with the Gsα protein and in the region of the extracellular domain responsible for the receptor binding to TSH.[52] In the *Gsα* gene, mutations affect codons 201 and 227 and result in the inhibition of the intrinsic GTPase activity, so that the protein is permanently locked in the active form. These mutations invariably lead to the development of nodules with elevated thyroid function and increased iodine uptake. The causal role of these mutations in the development of hyperfunctioning thyroid nodules has been confirmed in transgenic mice carrying the mutant *Gsα*.[53] The animals develop thyroid nodules composed of cells with an elevated cAMP level and high uptake of radioiodine.

Other Mutations

Somatic mutations affecting the PI3K/PTEN/AKT pathway are rare in follicular adenomas. Mutations in the *PIK3CA* gene, coding for the subunit of PI3K, occur in ~5% of tumors.[54] No somatic

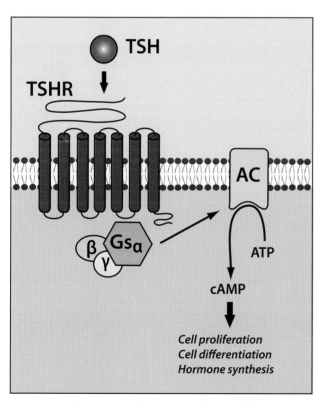

FIGURE 8.2. Schematic representation of the TSHR/Gsα/cAMP signaling pathway in thyroid cells. Physiologically, upon TSH binding, TSHR couples with the Gsα that leads to activation of adenylate cyclase, an enzyme that generates the secondary messenger cAMP. Elevated levels of cAMP in turn activate cAMP-dependent protein kinase A and other proteins, stimulating cell proliferation, iodine uptake and metabolism, thyroid hormone synthesis and release, and other aspects of thyroid physiology. Mutations in specific domains of the *TSHR* and *Gsα* genes result in permanent, TSH-independent activation of the cAMP pathway and development of hyperfunctioning thyroid adenomas.

mutations in the *PTEN* gene have been identified so far, despite the known role of *PTEN* germ line mutations in the development of thyroid adenomas in a setting of Cowden disease.

PAX8/PPARγ rearrangement, a feature of thyroid follicular carcinomas, is found in about 8% of tumors histologically diagnosed as follicular adenoma.[55–58] Many of these tumors are cellular and have thick capsule but fail to demonstrate invasion.[57] It remains to be determined whether the *PAX8/PPARγ* positive adenomas are actually follicular carcinomas in situ.

A single case of follicular adenoma carrying *BRAF* K601E mutation has been reported.[59]

Pathogenesis of Oncocytic Tumors

Oncocytic follicular adenomas are composed of cells with distinct cytoplasmic granularity because of accumulation of a large number of frequently abnormal mitochondria. The cause of the mitochondrial changes and their relationship to the neoplastic process are not fully understood. It remains unclear whether changes in the number and morphology of mitochondria are driven by specific mutations or whether they simply represent a secondary, compensatory change in the cell organelles.[60–62] Existing evidence supports each of the possibilities, and it is likely that the oncocytic cell appearance may develop through both pathways. In one pathway, tumors would be initiated and driven by the same oncogenes as nononcocytic follicular tumors, such as by mutant RAS, and would develop oncocytic features secondarily during the process of tumor progression. The increased replication of mitochondria in this setting may be a result of growth stimulation by cytokines and other mediators released from the inflammatory cells frequently seen in some tumors or a compensatory reaction to the functional deficiency of the existing abnormal mitochondria. These oncocytic tumors are expected to demonstrate either fully or partially developed oncocytic features and not to differ substantially in their biologic properties from nononcocytic tumors. In the other pathway, tumors would be driven by a specific somatic mutation that initiates tumorigenesis and also directly leads to the increased production of mitochondria. These tumors would have a uniform oncocytic appearance throughout and exhibit distinct biologic characteristics. It is likely that at least some oncocytic tumors develop after this pathway, although no specific mutations have been identified till date. Somatic mutations in mitochondrial DNA (mtDNA), including deletions and frameshift and missense point mutations, are frequently found in many oncocytic tumors.[63,64] These mutations predominantly affect the mitochondrial complex I genes and are predicted to disrupt gene function, although their role in tumor initiation remains unclear. This is because a high mutation rate is a general feature of mtDNA, as these mutations are also seen in non-neoplastic oncocytic cells and in nononcocytic tumors.[60,65]

CLINICAL PRESENTATION AND IMAGING

Thyroid adenomas typically present as a painless thyroid nodule incidentally discovered by palpation or during thyroid ultrasound performed for other reasons. Most adenomas are asymptomatic, although tumors of large size may cause difficulty in swallowing and other local symptoms. They grow very slowly, and some patients seek medical attention many years after discovering the nodule. Occasionally, bleeding into the tumor may occur and cause sudden pain, tenderness, and increase in nodule size. It may occur spontaneously or after vigorous neck palpation or FNA.

On palpation, adenomas are usually felt as a discrete mass that is not fixed to the neck and moves with the thyroid. Most patients are euthyroid. By radionuclide scan, adenomas typically appear as "cold" nodules because they concentrate radioiodine or other tracers less avidly than adjacent thyroid parenchyma (Fig. 8.3A). A small

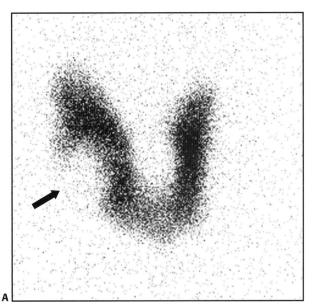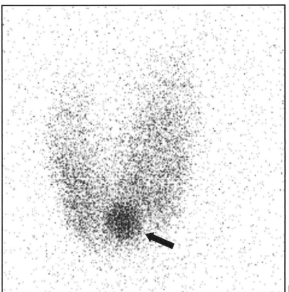

FIGURE 8.3. ¹²³I scans of two different thyroid lesions. A: A "cold" nodule is seen in the lateral aspect of the right lobe *(arrow)*. The lesion was diagnosed as a follicular adenoma after lobectomy. **B:** A small "hot" nodule is seen in the left side of isthmus *(arrow)*. This finding is consistent with a hyperfunctioning adenoma.

subset of adenomas are hyperfunctional and present with variably prominent symptoms of hyperthyroidism. Overt thyrotoxicosis, however, is rare, and many patients reveal subclinical hyperthyroidism manifested by the decreased serum TSH level and normal thyroid hormone levels. TSH suppression in these patients is a result of the negative feedback regulation of TSH secretion because of excess thyroid hormone production by the nodule. Hyperfunctioning adenomas appear "hot" on imaging in comparison with the adjacent thyroid tissue that is hypofunctional because of deprivation of TSH stimulation (Fig. 8.3B). On ultrasound examination, follicular adenoma is typically seen as a solid, homogeneous mass that may be hyperechoic, isoechoic, or hypoechoic as compared with the surrounding thyroid tissue (Fig. 8.4, top). The margins of the nodule are well defined and smooth. A peripheral hypoechoic halo that represents a fibrous capsule may be seen. Blood flow can be visualized by color Doppler ultrasound (Fig. 8.4 bottom). Low blood flow is more suggestive of a benign nodule, although no ultrasound features allow for a reliable diagnosis of adenoma.

Most adenomas that present as a solitary, "cold" nodule undergo FNA. Because FNA cytology cannot discriminate between follicular adenoma and follicular carcinoma, the patients are typically referred for surgery.

 GROSS FEATURES

Macroscopically, most follicular adenomas are solitary nodules that are clearly demarcated from the surrounding thyroid tissue by a well-formed fibrous capsule (Fig. 8.5A). Multiple adenomas are rare and should raise the possibility of an inherited disease. Adenomas usually have a round to ovoid shape. The size is highly variable and is typically between 1 and 3 cm. The color closely reflects the cellularity of tumors. Densely cellular, solid/trabecular adenomas have light, whitish to gray appearance, whereas colloid-rich adenomas are tan to brown in color. Oncocytic adenomas have characteristic mahogany brown color. Typical adenoma has rubbery consistency and a fleshy, homogeneous solid cut surface. Secondary changes may occur spontaneously or be precipitated by an FNA procedure and manifest as hemorrhage, infarction, cystic degeneration, fibrosis, or calcification (Fig. 8.5B). Oncocytic follicular adenomas are more prone to extensive hemorrhage and infarction.

Gross examination of surgically removed thyroid samples that contain an encapsulated solitary nodule requires careful inspection of the capsule in search for the areas of irregularity or overt

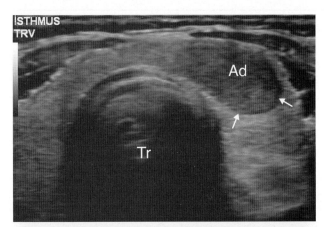

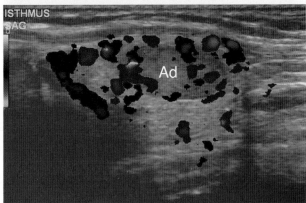

FIGURE 8.4. Ultrasonographic appearance of follicular adenoma. Top: Gray-scale transverse image shows a distinct ovoid mass (Ad) with homogeneous and hypoechoic appearance and relatively smooth margins *(arrows)*. Tr, trachea. **Bottom:** Longitudinal color Doppler image demonstrates rich vascularity within the nodule (Ad) and in adjacent thyroid parenchyma.

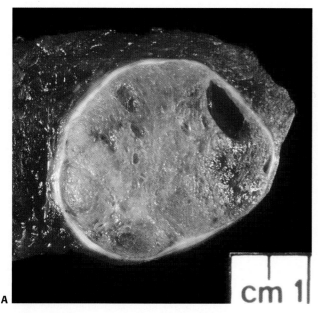
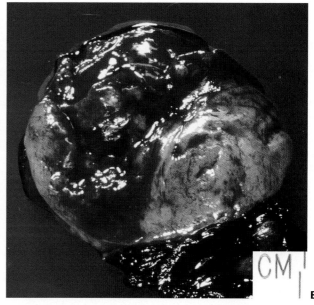

FIGURE 8.5. Gross appearance of follicular adenoma. A: This follicular adenoma of conventional type has a moderately thick capsule and light brown cut surface with focal cystic area, which is likely a consequence of previous FNA. **B:** Extensive hemorrhage in the oncocytic follicular adenoma induced by a recent FNA procedure.

invasion. Unless the nodule is very large, the entire peripheral zone of the nodule surrounding the capsule should be submitted for microscopic examination to rule out tumor invasion. The principles and details of gross examination are described in Chapter 19.

 MICROSCOPIC FEATURES

On microscopic examination, follicular adenoma appears as an encapsulated follicular lesion with architectural and cytologic features that are distinct from the surrounding thyroid parenchyma (Fig. 8.6). The capsule is complete and typically thin to moderately thick. The capsule is composed of parallel layers of collagen occasionally penetrated by smooth muscle-walled blood vessels (Fig. 8.7). Myxoid degeneration of collagen fibers and blood vessel walls within the capsule may be seen. Capsular calcification is sometimes found. Small aggregates of entrapped follicular cells may be seen within the capsule and should not be misinterpreted as evidence for invasion. A very thick capsule should raise the suspicion of carcinoma and prompt particularly

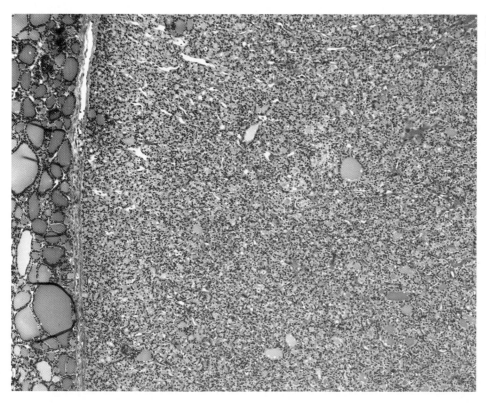

FIGURE 8.6. Low-power view of follicular adenoma. Note a distinct lesion with a homogeneous microfollicular appearance separated from normal thyroid tissue by a thin capsule.

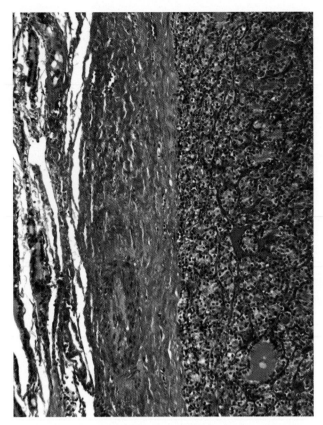

FIGURE 8.7. This follicular adenoma has a thick capsule that shows a blood vessel with myxoid changes in the wall.

thorough evaluation for invasion. However, in the absence of capsular or vascular invasion, the diagnosis of adenoma is rendered.

Follicular adenomas display various microscopic architectural patterns. Most commonly seen patterns are solid, trabecular, microfollicular, normofollicular, and macrofollicular (Fig. 8.8). The solid/trabecular pattern adenomas are sometimes designated as "embryonal" because they have an appearance of an early developmental stage of the thyroid. Those tumors are very cellular and depleted of colloid. Microfollicular adenomas are composed of small, round follicles and are referred to as "fetal" adenomas because of their resemblance to the thyroid tissue during the late fetal period of development. Small amounts of colloid are seen within the lumen of follicles. Normofollicular adenomas are composed of neoplastic follicles of size comparable with normal thyroid gland follicles. Macrofollicular adenomas have large follicles filled with colloid. Other growth pattern, such as nested/insular and papillary, may occasionally be found. One pattern usually predominates within an individual tumor nodule, although it is rarely pure and is typically seen in combination with other growth patterns. The patterns bare no diagnostic significance and do not have to be mentioned in the diagnostic line.

Inspissated colloid found in the lumen of some follicles may occasionally undergo calcification and show concentric laminations resembling psammoma bodies (Fig. 8.9). These pseudopsammoma bodies are more frequently seen in oncocytic adenomas and distinguished from true psammoma bodies based on their location within the lumen of follicles. In contrast, psammoma bodies in papillary carcinomas reside in the tumor stroma.

Adenomas are typically composed of uniform cells of cuboid or polygonal shape (Fig. 8.10A). The cells are tall in hyperfunctioning adenomas. The cytoplasm is moderately abundant, pale

eosinophilic to amphophilic. Cell borders are well defined. The nuclei are basally located and relatively evenly spaced along the basement membrane. They are typically small, round, uniform, hyperchromatic or normochromatic. The coarse or vesicular chromatin is rarely seen. The cells of conventional type adenomas have one or several inconspicuous, eccentrically located nucleoli. Some variation in the nuclear size, shape, and chromatin texture may be seen, with single cells showing very large, irregular, hyperchromatic nuclei (Fig. 8.10B). The most extreme manifestations of nuclear atypia are observed in follicular adenomas with bizarre nuclei, as discussed later in the chapter. Severe nuclear atypia affecting random cells is occasionally seen in follicular adenomas and other benign thyroid nodules and is not a feature of malignancy. Mitotic figures are rarely found except in the areas of recent aspiration and other regenerative changes. Finding several mitoses is rare in adenomas and requires careful evaluation for malignancy.

The stroma is typically scant. Some adenomas have abundant edematous or hyalinized stroma that is more pronounced in the central portion of the nodule (Fig. 8.11A). Thick fibrotic bands are rarely seen, and their presence raises suspicion for the follicular variant of papillary carcinoma. Adenomas are rich in delicate capillary vessels, which are not readily identifiable on routine hematoxylin and eosin (H&E) staining. Secondary changes include hemorrhage, edema, ischemic necrosis, cystic degeneration, fibrosis and hyalinization, calcification, and osseous or cartilaginous metaplasia (Fig. 8.11). Squamous metaplasia is rarely seen. The FNA-induced injury may mimic invasion or lead to other change that may be mistaken for malignancy. The term *worrisome histologic alterations following fine needle aspiration of the thyroid or WHAFFT* has been proposed for these changes,[66] which are described in more detail in Chapter 6.

Microscopic Variants

Oncocytic (Hürthle Cell) Adenoma

Oncocytic adenoma is a common microscopic variant of thyroid follicular adenomas. Approximately 10% to 15% of adenomas belong to this variant. These tumors are entirely or predominantly (at least 75%) composed of oncocytic cells. In all other aspects, that is, encapsulation, architectural patterns, and criteria for malignancy, they are not different from follicular adenomas of conventional type.

Oncocytes derive from thyroid follicular epithelial cells and are characterized by (1) abundant granular eosinophilic cytoplasm and (2) nuclei with prominent nucleoli (Fig. 8.12). The cytoplasmic granularity of oncocytic cells is because of the accumulation of large numbers of mitochondria, which frequently reveal abnormal morphology when studied by electron microscopy (see section on Ultrastructural Features). The cells have a polygonal shape. The nuclei are centrally located and have round shape with smooth contours and vesicular or dark chromatin. Some variability in the nuclear size, shape, and chromatin appearance is frequently seen in oncocytic adenomas. Occasionally, scattered single cells with large, highly irregular, hyperchromatic nuclei containing nuclear grooves or pseudoinclusions may be found.

Oncocytic adenomas are prone to spontaneous and FNA-induced secondary changes, and acute hemorrhage or infarction may involve a large area or the entire tumor (Fig. 8.13). The presence of ischemic necrosis should not be interpreted as evidence of malignancy.

As compared with thyroid nodules composed of nononcocytic follicular cells, a higher proportion of oncocytic nodules reveal capsular or vascular invasion on histologic examination and therefore are malignant.[60] It does not indicate, however, that oncocytic appearance by itself is a feature of malignancy. Conventional diagnostic criteria of malignancy in follicular tumors,

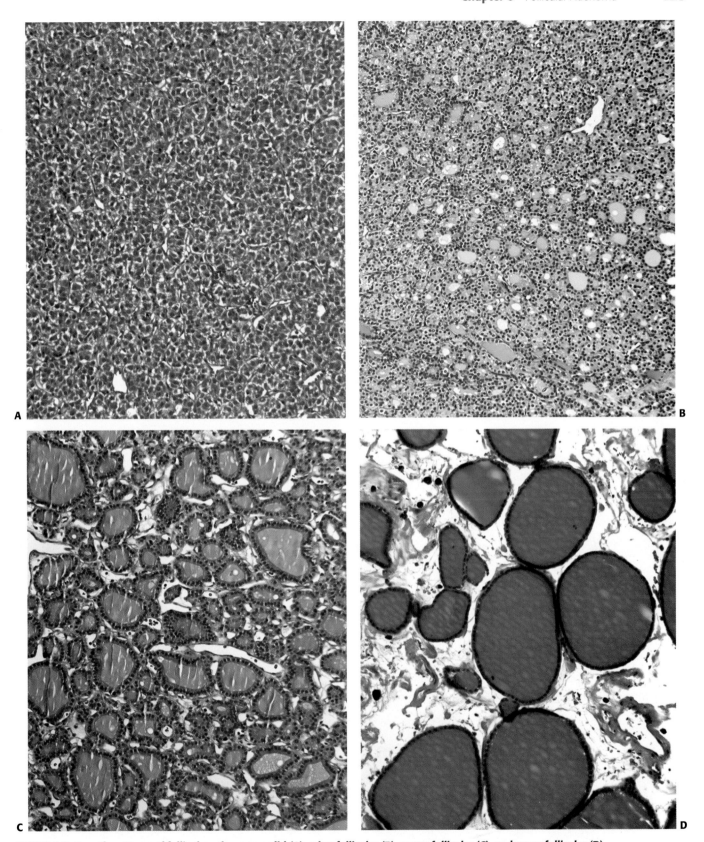

FIGURE 8.8. Growth patterns of follicular adenoma: solid (A), microfollicular (B), normofollicular (C), and macrofollicular (D).

FIGURE 8.9. Calcified colloid within the lumen of follicles that mimics psammoma bodies.

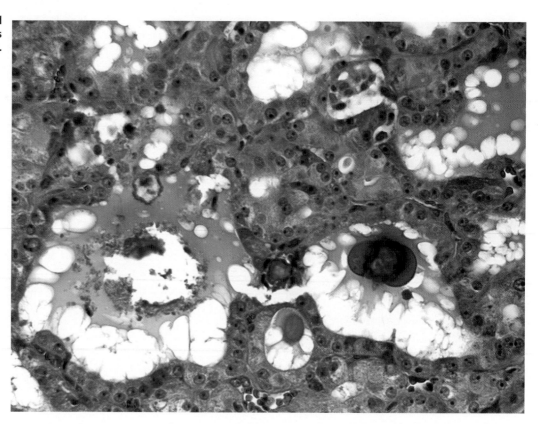

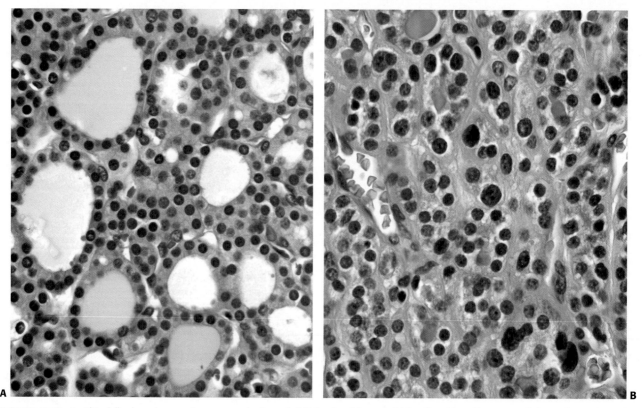

FIGURE 8.10. A: This follicular adenoma is composed of small follicles lined by cuboidal cells with uniform, round, hyperchromatic nuclei. **B:** Nuclei of this follicular adenoma cells are more irregular, and some are significantly larger and irregularly shaped. The chromatin is coarse, and nucleoli are more prominent.

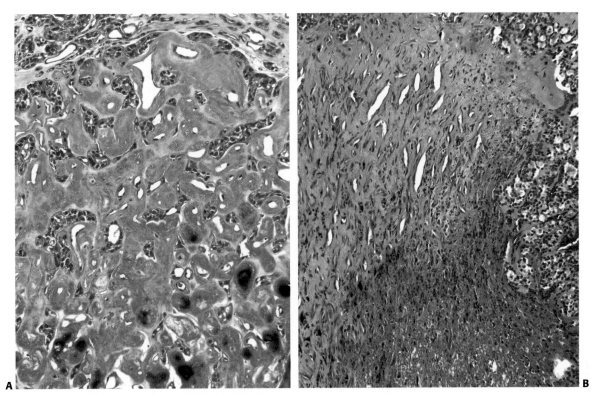

FIGURE 8.11. Secondary changes in follicular adenomas. A: Scattered calcifications embedded into abundant hyalinized stroma. **B:** FNA-induced necrosis with organization, fibrosis, vascular proliferation, and hemosiderin deposition.

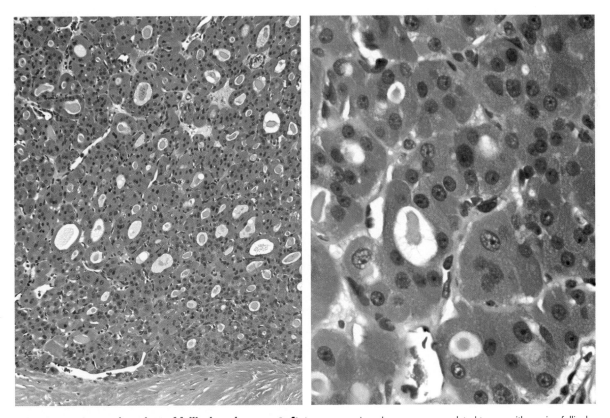

FIGURE 8.12. Oncocytic variant of follicular adenoma. Left: Low-power view shows an encapsulated tumor with a microfollicular growth pattern. **Right:** High-power view reveals oncocytic cells with large amount of finely granular, intense eosinophilic cytoplasm. The nuclei have prominent centrally located nucleoli. Some variation in the size and shape of nuclei is seen.

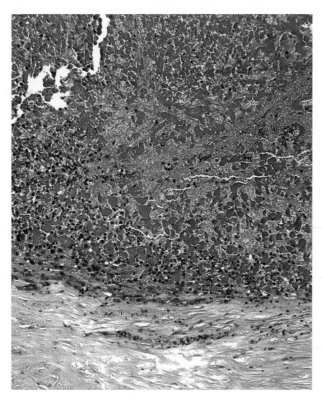

FIGURE 8.13. Confluent ischemic necrosis in the oncocytic adenoma.

that is, capsular and vascular invasion, reliably predict behavior of oncocytic tumors.

Oncocytic cells in the thyroid have been known by different names including Hürthle, Askanazy, and oxyphilic cells. The term *Hürthle cell*, although a misnomer, was frequently used in the past to designate these cells. Correspondingly, benign follicular tumors with this appearance were frequently called *Hürthle cell adenomas*. Currently, the term *oncocytic* is recommended to define these cells and tumors.[67] This is because of the general trend to depart from eponymous terms and because, in reality, Dr. Hürthle most likely described C cells instead of oncocytic follicular cells in his 1894 publication.[68] The term *oncocyte* comes from the Greek word *onkoustai*, to swell, and refers to the "swollen" appearance of the cytoplasm.

Hyperfunctioning (Toxic, Hot) Adenoma

Hyperfunctioning adenomas constitute approximately 1% of all follicular adenomas.[69] They are associated with variably prominent symptoms of hyperthyroidism caused by excessive thyroid hormone production by the tumor. The nodules are "hot" on radionuclide scans (Fig. 8.3B). As discussed earlier in the chapter, most of these tumors carry an activation mutation of the *TSHR* or *Gsα* genes, which leads to chronic upregulation of the cAMP signaling pathway that mimics constant TSH stimulation. As a result, the cells function autonomously, that is, in TSH-independent manner.

Microscopically, the tumors typically show normofollicular or microfollicular architecture (Fig. 8.14). The follicles are irregularly shaped and frequently show significant variation in size and shape. They are lined by tall, columnar epithelial cells. Delicate papillary projections into the lumen are often seen. The cells have abundant

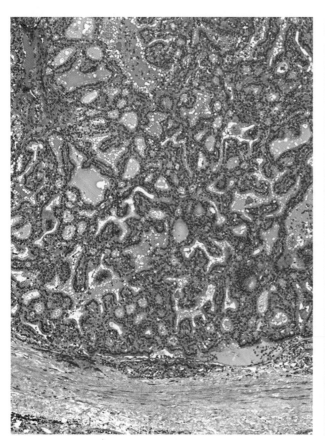

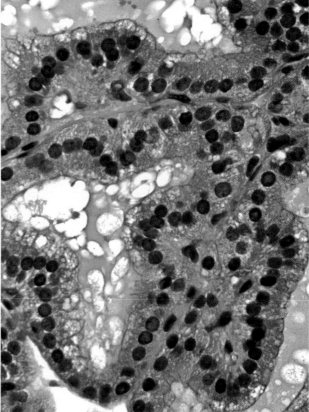

FIGURE 8.14. Hyperfunctioning adenoma. Left: Low-power view shows an encapsulated lesion composed of highly irregular follicles, many of which have delicate papillary infoldings. **Right:** High-power view reveals columnar cells with vacuolated cytoplasm and round, basally located nuclei. Vacuolation of cytoplasm is more pronounced in the apical portion of cells. Scalloping of colloid is also seen.

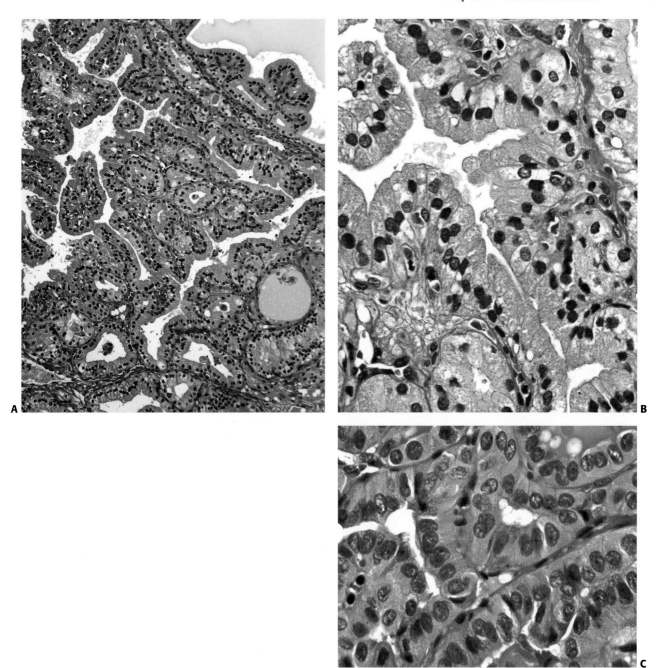

FIGURE 8.15. A and B: This hyperfunctioning adenoma was initially misdiagnosed as the tall cell variant of papillary thyroid carcinoma. Note that papillary structures have delicate cores that contain small follicles and lack fibrous stroma. The cells are tall but in contrast to the tall cell variant of papillary carcinoma (shown for comparison in **[C]**); they are basally located, small and round, with smooth contours and dark chromatin, and have no nuclear grooves or pseudoinclusions.

pale eosinophilic and frequently vacuolated cytoplasm and round, uniform, small to slightly enlarged, basally located nuclei. The colloid is bubbly, pale, watery, often with peripheral scalloping. Examination of thyroid parenchyma surrounding the adenoma typically shows evidence of suppressed TSH stimulation, that is, large follicles with dense colloid lined by flattened epithelium.

These microscopic features, particularly the tall shape of cells, micropapillary infoldings, and evidence of increased colloid resorption are characteristic of the hyperfunctional status, which should be confirmed by laboratory findings of hyperthyroidism or by radionuclide scan. The ultrastructural features of hyperfunctioning adenomas are consistent with the increased functional status of these cells.

Most importantly, the tall shape of cells and papillary growth pattern in hyperfunctioning adenomas should not be confused with the appearance of the tall cell variant of papillary carcinoma (Fig. 8.15). The latter contains papillae with dense fibrovascular cores lined by tall cells with large oval-shaped nuclei showing characteristic nuclear features of papillary carcinoma.

Follicular Adenoma with Papillary Hyperplasia

Rarely, follicular adenomas demonstrate a predominantly papillary architecture. These tumors are more common during the second and third decade of life. Some patients yield a history of exposure to ionizing radiation.[70] The tumor typically presents as

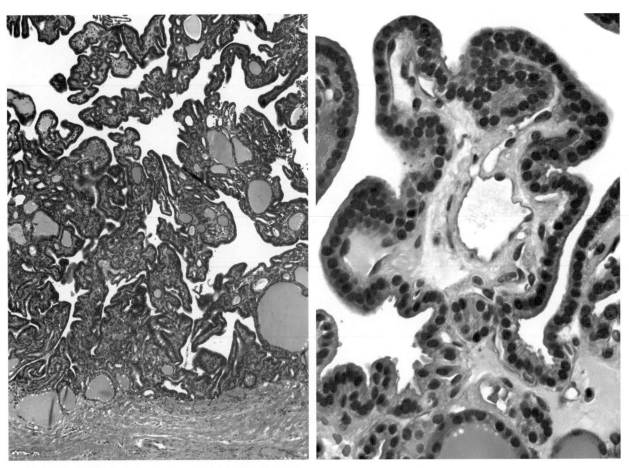

FIGURE 8.16. Follicular adenoma with papillary hyperplasia. Left: The tumor has a thick capsule and shows a predominantly papillary architecture. **Right:** The papillae have a loose, edematous stroma and are lined by a layer of cuboidal cells with round, uniform, basally located nuclei.

a solitary nodule that shows the following morphologic features: (1) moderately thick complete capsule, (2) predominantly papillary architecture, (3) partially cystic appearance, and (4) lack of diagnostic nuclear features of papillary carcinoma (Fig. 8.16). The papillae are delicate and typically nonbranching and have hypovascular edematous cores, which may contain follicles. Overall, the stroma is scant with poorly developed vasculature and no fibrosis. The cells lining the papillary structures have a cuboidal or columnar shape and basally located, uniform, round nuclei with dark chromatin. The cystic changes vary from moderate to extensive. In the most dramatic examples, only a narrow rim of epithelial tissue is identified lining the internal surface of the capsule. It is conceivable that these tumors may undergo progressive cystic degeneration to eventually transform to a cyst completely devoid of epithelial cells. Some tumors may be accompanied by clinical evidence of thyroid hyperfunction,[71] although this is rare in our experience. It is possible that the overproduction of thyroid hormone may be more pronounced at the early stages of tumor growth and declines with the progression of cystic changes.

Important differential diagnosis for this lesion is encapsulated papillary carcinoma. The distinction is based on the difference in the appearance of papillae, preserved cell polarity, and lack of characteristic nuclear features of papillary carcinoma and psammoma bodies. These adenomas have a benign course. Papillary carcinoma can arise in these lesions as it can develop in any benign thyroid nodule. If malignancy emerges, a sharp demarcation between the benign and malignant areas is seen within the nodule (Fig. 8.17).

The term *papillary adenoma* should not be used to designate these lesions. This term was utilized in the past for encapsulated papillary carcinomas, and it may be misinterpreted as a malignant diagnosis.

Adenolipoma (Lipoadenoma)

Adenolipoma is a rare type of follicular adenoma that reveals a mixture of mature fat and thyroid follicles.[72] These tumors have also been termed *lipoadenoma* and *thyrolipoma*. They are encapsulated and have a more yellow, greasy cut surface resembling the gross appearance of lipomas (Fig. 8.18). Highly variable proportions of adipose cells and follicular structures can be seen within the nodule. In one reported case, foci of extramedullary hematopoiesis could be seen within the fat.[73] The adjacent thyroid parenchyma may either have an unremarkable microscopic appearance or contain fat cells in the stroma.

The histogenesis of adenolipomas is not fully understood. They may represent either true mixed neoplasms consisting of different types of tumor cells or follicular adenomas with extensive fatty metaplasia. Single cases of adenolipoma have been reported in a setting of Cowden disease[18] and in a patient with a history of radiation exposure to the neck.[74] The presence of stromal fat within the adenoma bears no diagnostic significance because mature adipocytes can be seen in various thyroid lesions ranging from nonneoplastic conditions to papillary and follicular carcinomas.[74]

Follicular Adenoma with Signet-Ring Cells

This rare variant is characterized by cells with large intracytoplasmic vacuoles that displace and compress the nucleus to the side. In the H&E–stained sections, the vacuoles appear clear or pale eosinophilic with homogeneous or finely granular texture (Fig. 8.19). The vacuoles frequently reveal strong immunoreactivity for thyroglobulin and positive staining with periodic acid Schiff (PAS) after diastase digestion, whereas other mucin stains,

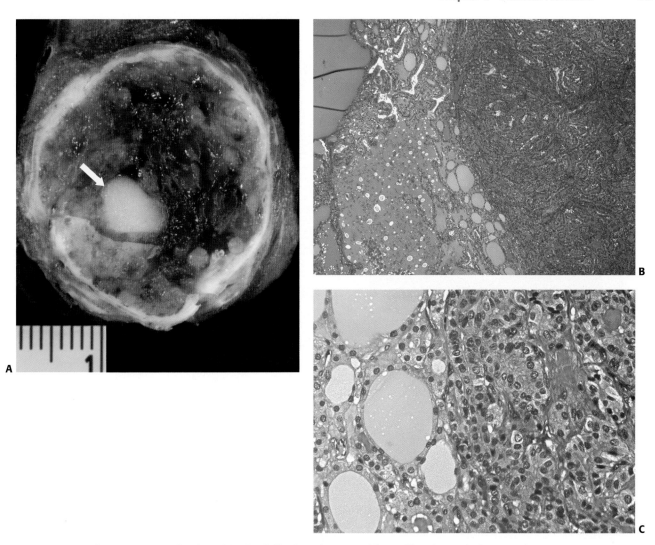

FIGURE 8.17. Papillary carcinoma developed in the follicular adenoma with papillary hyperplasia. A: In this case, gross examination revealed a 3.1-cm nodule that has a well-developed, complete fibrous capsule and shows a clearly demarcated, white-tan, 0.6-cm lesion located close to the center of the nodule *(arrow)*. **B and C:** Microscopic examination revealed that the 0.6-cm lesion (right side in B and C) was sharply demarcated from the rest of the nodule (left side in B and C) and composed of tightly packed papillary and follicular structured lined by epithelial cells with significantly enlarged nuclei showing characteristic nuclear features of papillary carcinoma.

such as mucicarmine and alcian blue at pH 2.5, are more often negative.[75–77] This pattern of staining of vacuoles is consistent with the presence of protein–polysaccharide complexes derived from partial degradation of thyroglobulin.[78] Ultrastructurally, the vacuoles represent intracytoplasmic lumens bordered by various numbers of microvilli.[75] Several tumors with such appearance have also been reported as mucin-producing adenomas.[79,80]

The presence of signet-ring cells in an adenoma is not a feature of malignancy and has no clinical implications. These adenomas may to be mistaken for metastatic carcinoma of signet-ring type, particularly from stomach or breast. Immunostaining for thyroglobulin and thyroid transcription factor 1 (TTF1) is helpful to resolve this issue.

Follicular Adenoma with Clear Cells

This uncommon variant is predominantly composed of cells with clear cytoplasm which is a result of the accumulation of glycogen, lipid, thyroglobulin, or distended mitochondria. The cytoplasm is abundant and watery clear or has a pale eosinophilic hue or fine granularity (Fig. 8.20). The nuclei are centrally placed and have smooth contours. The tumor may be composed entirely of clear cells or contain small clusters of cells with typical follicular cell cytoplasm or oncocytic cytoplasm. The cells retain thyroglobulin

immunoreactivity, but it is typically focal and weak. In some cases, they are PAS positive and diastase sensitive, which reflects their glycogen content. On the ultrastructural level, the cells contain multiple cytoplasmic vacuoles. In some cases, the vacuoles reveal the presence of residual cristae, suggesting that they represent massively dilated mitochondria.[69,81] This suggests that at least some clear-cell tumors may evolve from oncocytic adenomas as a result of progressive enlargement and conversion of mitochondria into vesicles.

Follicular adenomas with this unusual appearance should be distinguished from follicular, papillary, and medullary carcinomas with clear cells; metastatic renal cell carcinoma; and parathyroid tissue. Differentiation from follicular carcinoma follows the usual invasive criteria. Thyroglobulin and TTF1 immunoreactivity is helpful in distinguishing this tumor from parathyroid tissue or renal cell carcinoma. Papillary carcinoma is ruled out by the absence of characteristic nuclear features.

Follicular Adenoma with Lipid-Rich Cells

Rarely, follicular adenomas are composed of cells that have cytoplasm full of vacuoles containing lipid. Several reported cases of this peculiar variant of follicular adenoma were observed in

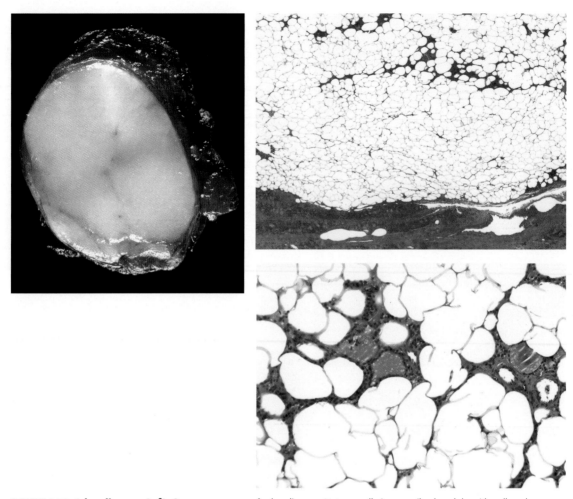

FIGURE 8.18. Adenolipoma. Left: Gross appearance of adenolipoma. Note a well-circumscribed nodule with yellow, homogeneous cut surface. **Right:** This tumor is composed predominantly of fat tissue with only few intermixed groups of thyroid follicles, which are better appreciated on the high-power examination **(bottom right)**.

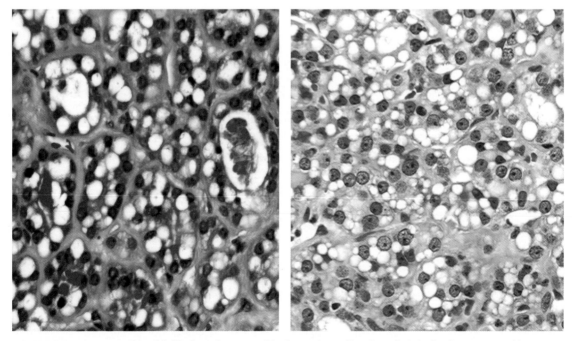

FIGURE 8.19. Two examples of follicular adenoma with signet-ring cells. The cells in both adenomas reveal large cytoplasmic vacuoles and peripherally displaced nuclei.

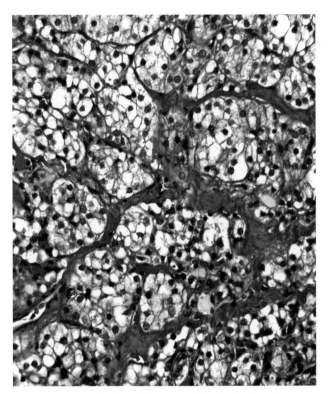

FIGURE 8.20. Follicular adenoma with clear cells. The tumor cells have sharply defined cell borders and clear cytoplasm. This tumor has a significant amount of hyalinized stroma.

middle-aged to older patients, mostly men, and ranged in size between 1.3 and 6 cm.[82–84] The tumor has a well-defined capsule and typically consists of microfollicles or solid sheets of cells with abundant vacuolated cytoplasm (Fig. 8.21). The vacuoles are smaller or larger in size, and have clear or finely granular appearance on H&E stain. The vacuoles contain lipid that can be confirmed by Sudan or other lipid stains and by electron microscopy. The accumulation of lipid in the adenoma cells is likely to be a result of the altered intracellular lipid metabolism rather than simple storage, as suggested by quantitative differences in triglyceride composition between cells of lipid-rich adenoma and subcutaneous fat.[84]

The follicular thyroid cell origin of these tumors can be confirmed by positive immunostaining for thyroglobulin and TTF1. These tumors are distinguished from adenomas with signet-ring cells based on the small size of vacuoles and rare displacement and indentation of the nucleus, although the vacuoles may coalesce and form large vesicles in some cells. In contrast to adenomas with clear cells, the cells of lipid-rich adenomas show multiple distinct intracytoplasmic vesicle. In adenolipomas, the fat is not intracytoplasmic but is rather present within mature adipose cells intermixed with thyroid follicles.

Follicular Adenoma with Bizarre Nuclei

Occasionally, otherwise typical follicular adenomas reveal scattered cells with highly enlarged, irregularly shaped, bizarre hyperchromatic nuclei (Fig. 8.22). There is significant variability in size and appearance between the atypical cells. Some may have nuclei with course chromatin and prominent nucleoli. These highly atypical cells are seen in single forms or in small clusters

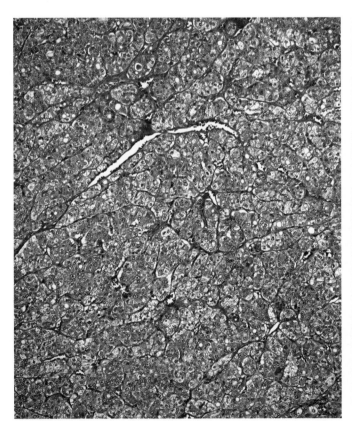
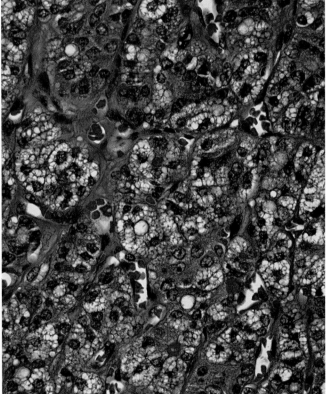

FIGURE 8.21. Follicular adenoma with lipid-rich cells. The tumor has a microfollicular and solid growth pattern and consists of cells with cytoplasm containing numerous small vesicles (left), which is better appreciated on high-power view (right). Images courtesy of Runjan Chetty, Oxford Radcliffe Hospitals NHS Trust and University of Oxford, UK.

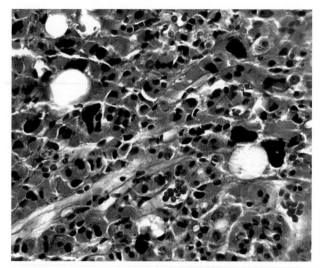

FIGURE 8.22. Follicular adenoma with bizarre nuclei. Scattered cells in the tumor have huge, highly irregular, dark nuclei.

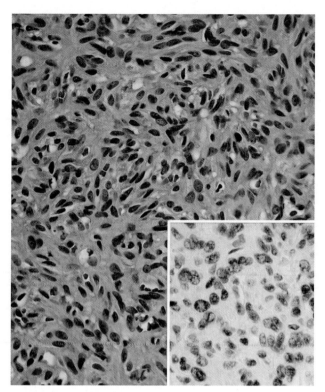

FIGURE 8.23. Follicular adenoma with spindle cells. Inset: Immunostaining for TTF1 confirms the thyroid origin of this tumor.

scattered in the background of the normal appearing follicular cells. These cells are never seen in mitosis, and proliferative activity of all cells comprising the lesion is low. The bizarre appearance of nuclei is likely because of cell degeneration that is seen in many endocrine tissues (so-called endocrine atypia), and it should not be regarded as a feature of malignancy. These cells are more commonly seen in oncocytic adenomas and in adenomas from patients with a history of treatment with radioactive iodine.[85] These cells may resemble the appearance of anaplastic thyroid carcinoma cells, where cells with large hyperchromatic nuclei are seen in sheets and in association with high mitotic activity and frequent tumor necrosis.

Atypical Follicular Adenoma

This term is occasionally used by some pathologists to designate follicular adenomas that display atypical features but reveal no definitive capsular or vascular invasion.[86,87] The atypical features that historically have been applied to place a tumor in this category include high cellularity, nuclear atypia, unusual cell appearance such as spindle shape, thick capsules with groups of adenoma cells entrapped within the capsule, increased mitotic activity, and spontaneous necrosis. As established more recently, these atypical features have no independent diagnostic or prognostic value, and tumors designated as atypical adenomas behave in a benign fashion as long as capsular and vascular invasion are not found.[86,88,89] The presence of unusual or worrisome features should trigger a vigorous search for invasion by examining the entire capsule, obtaining deeper levels of all suspicious areas, and possibly utilizing ancillary techniques. However, if no invasion is found, the tumor is expected to pursue a benign course and should be designated as a follicular adenoma. Some authors have proposed the term *hypercellular adenoma* for those tumors that one would designate as atypical based on high cellularity only.[69] The use of the term *atypical follicular adenoma* is generally discouraged.

Other Variants of Follicular Adenoma

Black adenomas of the thyroid have been reported in patients treated with minocycline.[90] The tumors have black discoloration on gross examination. The cells reveal abundant black pigment with appearance and staining qualities similar to cases of minocycline-associated diffuse black thyroid (Chapter 6). Thyroid

parenchyma surrounding these adenomas may show various degrees of pigment accumulation or may be completely devoid of it.

Single cases of follicular adenomas with extensive cartilagineous[91] and osseous[92] metaplasia have been reported. Rarely, tumors contain areas of spindle cell metaplasia or are composed predominantly of spindle cells (Fig. 8.23).[93,94] Those should be distinguished from anaplastic thyroid carcinoma and mesenchymal tumors. A case of follicular adenoma composed of spindle cells arranged in whorls that resemble meningioma appearance has been reported.[95] Immunoreactivity for thyroglobulin and TTF1 can establish the follicular cell origin of these cells.

IMMUNOHISTOCHEMISTRY

The diagnosis of adenoma is typically made based on microscopic evaluation alone. Some cases may benefit from additional diagnostic workup. The immunohistochemical profile of follicular adenoma cells is similar to that of normal thyroid cells. The cells are reactive for thyroglobulin, TTF1, PAX8, and low- and some intermediate-molecular weight cytokeratins. The thyroid follicular cell origin is best established using thyroglobulin, TTF1, and PAX8. Thyroglobulin is the most specific marker; the immunoreactivity is seen in the cytoplasm of cells and in the luminal colloid (Fig. 8.24B). The staining is diffuse and strong, although it may be slightly less intense than in the surrounding normal thyroid tissue. TTF1 exhibits strong nuclear staining in all tumors (Fig. 8.24C). However, TTF1 immunoreactivity is not specific for thyroid follicular cells and may also be found in thyroid C cells and medullary thyroid carcinomas, respiratory epithelium and lung tumors, and small cell carcinomas from different locations.[96,97] PAX8 immunostain is positive in adenomas, although it is not specific for thyroid follicular cells and may also be seen in thyroid C cells and medullary carcinomas as well as in renal, ovarian, and

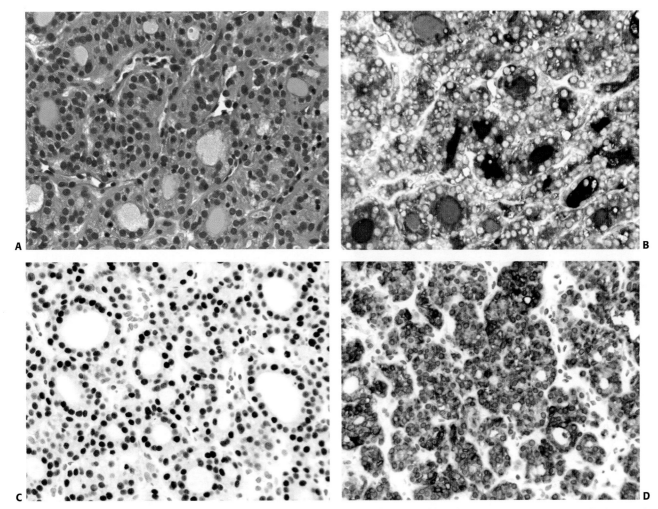

FIGURE 8.24. Immunohistochemical profile of follicular adenoma. This follicular adenoma with a predominantly microfollicular growth pattern (A) shows strong and diffuse immunoreactivity for thyroglobulin (B), TTF1 (C), and CK7 (D).

endometrial cancers but not in lung tumors.[98,99] Cytokeratins of low molecular weight (CAM 5.2) and pankeratin cocktails show strong reactivity, whereas stains for high molecular weight keratins are negative. Adenoma cells are CK7 positive and CK20 negative (Fig. 8.24D).[100] CK19 immunoreactivity is found in adenomas with variable frequency. Some authors have reported either a lack of or a weak staining in adenomas in contrast to positive staining in thyroid carcinomas, claiming the diagnostic usefulness of CK19.[101] Others have observed significant staining in many adenomas.[102,103] This has also been our experience, as we observed significant CK19 reactivity in about half of all follicular adenomas. Rich vascularity of adenomas can be confirmed by staining with CD34 or other endothelial markers. Important negative immunostains include calcitonin, CEA, and neuroendocrine markers.

Oncocytic adenomas show an overall similar pattern of immunoreactivity, although they frequently stain less intensely with thyroglobulin. Immunostaining with mitochondria-specific antibodies may be used to demonstrate the presence of abundant mitochondria in oncocytic cells,[104] although it is rarely used for diagnostic purposes. The immunohistochemical analysis of oncocytic cells has an important limitation that has to be taken into account to avoid false positive results. These cells frequently show nonspecific staining of the cytoplasm with various antibodies because of high endogenous biotin activity, which may be further enhanced by antigen-retrieval procedures.[105] It manifests as coarsely granular staining limited to the cytoplasm

(Fig. 8.25). The nonspecific immunoreactivity may be prevented, although not always completely, by endogenous biotin blocking procedures.

Follicular adenomas have Ki-67 proliferative index <5% and typically preserve Bcl-2 immunoreactivity.[102,106]

Immunoreactivity for galectin-3, HBME-1, and CITED1 is rarely seen in follicular adenomas and may be used to aid the differential diagnosis between follicular adenoma, follicular carcinoma, and follicular variant of papillary carcinoma. However, none of the stains are specific for malignancy, and they should be used in combination. In several large series, immunoreactivity have been observed for galectin-3 in 6% to 30% adenomas, for HBME-1 in 4% to 11%, and for CITED1 in 7% to 16%.[102,107,108] However, the positive staining for two or three markers has been seen in only 2% to 5% of adenomas. We use galectin-3, HBME-1, and CITED1 in combination as an ancillary test for diagnostically challenging follicular lesions and find it most useful in distinguishing follicular adenoma from the follicular variant of papillary carcinoma. Most importantly, these immunostains can be used diagnostically only after careful validation of each antibody in the particular laboratory and accumulation of significant experience in the interpretation of these stains. A detailed description of these immunostains is provided in Chapter 11.

Follicular adenomas rarely display strong and diffuse immunoreactivity for PPARγ. This pattern of immunoreactivity correlates well with the presence of *PAX8/PPARγ* rearrangement, which is the characteristic of thyroid follicular carcinoma.[57,109]

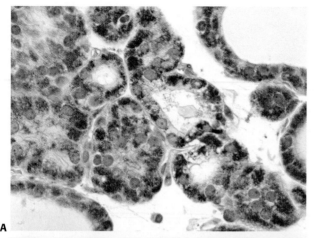

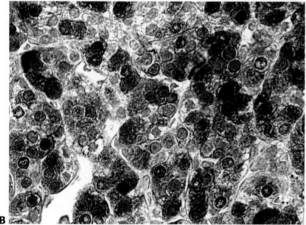

FIGURE 8.25. A: Nonspecific granular cytoplasmic *only* immunoreactivity for galectin-3 is seen in this oncocytic adenoma. **B:** For comparison, true positive staining for galectin-3 should involve nuclei and cytoplasm, as shown in this follicular carcinoma.

 MOLECULAR DIAGNOSTICS

PAX8/PPARγ rearrangement, a hallmark of follicular carcinomas, is detected in about 8% (range, 0% to 55%) of tumor diagnosed as follicular adenoma.[58] In our experience, most of the tumors positive for *PAX8/PPARγ* reveal vascular or capsular invasion, which may be identified only after submitting additional sections of the capsule and obtaining multiple levels of suspicious or randomly selected areas of the capsule. Diagnostic utility of *PAX8/PPARγ* in differentiation between follicular adenoma and follicular carcinoma is discussed more extensively in Chapter 10.

RAS mutations are not restricted to follicular adenomas and occur with significant frequency in follicular carcinomas and other thyroid tumors. The finding of mutant *RAS* indicates the presence of a neoplasm but cannot distinguish adenoma from carcinoma.

Biologically, follicular adenomas are true neoplasms and therefore should have a monoclonal cell population. This can be established by the clonality assays such as HUMARA or by detecting a clonal genetic alteration such as *RAS* mutation. The molecular techniques can unequivocally distinguish follicular adenomas from hyperplastic nodules in many cases because the latter are polyclonal lesions. Nevertheless, molecular assays are rarely used to address this differential diagnosis due to the lack of clinical importance in distinguishing these two types of benign lesions.

Follicular adenomas have an overall lower frequency of LOH than follicular carcinomas. Similarly, DNA aneuploidy is less common in follicular adenomas as compared with follicular carcinomas. However, a significant overlap between the tumors exists with respect to both the LOH frequency and DNA aneuploidy, which limits the use of these techniques as diagnostic separators.

 ULTRASTRUCTURAL FEATURES

The ultrastructural features of conventional follicular adenomas are similar to those of normal thyroid gland and hyperplastic nodules. The follicular cells rest on the continuous basal lamina that separates them from the adjacent capillaries. Reduplication of the basal lamina is occasionally seen.[110] The cells preserve polarity and have microvilli on the apical surface (Fig. 8.26). The nuclei are basally located and have round shape, finely distributed chromatin, and inconspicuous nucleoli. The usual cytoplasmic organelles are present, with well-developed granular endoplasmic reticulum, mitochondria, and Golgi complex. Small dense secretory vesicles and larger phagolysosomes containing colloid are found predominantly in the apical portion of the cell. Their number is highly variable between different adenomas and even between individual cells in one tumor and correlates with the functional status of the cell.

Oncocytic adenoma cells have the cytoplasm packed with innumerable mitochondria (Fig. 8.27). Many mitochondria are dilated and have irregular shape and diminished or almost entirely absent cristae. Some mitochondria contain electron-dense bodies or irregularly spaced cristae with the formation of filamentous bundles in the matrix.[111] Primary lysosomes, phagolysosomes, and secretory vesicles are identifiable in the apical location, whereas other organelles are difficult to find. Scanning electron microscopy identifies cells with smooth apical surface interspersed with cells containing abundant microvilli.[111] The ultramicroscopic features of oncocytes in adenomas are not different from those seen in carcinomas or in nonneoplastic oncocytic cells.

Clear cell adenomas show abundant cytoplasmic vacuoles that vary in size and typically have a smooth inner surface. The vacuoles may be of different origin. In some cases, they may develop from the Golgi complex or endocytotic vesicles.[112] Some vacuoles may reveal residual cristae, which suggests their mitochondrial derivation.[69,81]

Hyperfunctioning adenomas have a cytoplasm rich in organelles, particularly in rough endoplasmic reticulum, which reflects a high level of hormone production. The apical surface of cells shows a dense layer of long microvilli.[113]

 CYTOLOGIC FEATURES

The aspirated cytology specimens from microfollicular and solid/trabecular follicular adenomas are expected to be cellular with numerous microfollicular structures and generally contain very little colloid (Fig. 8.28). Microfollicles are composed of 6 to 12 follicular epithelial cells arranged in small spherical aggregates. A minute deposit of colloid may be seen in the center of the microfollicle. Normofollicular and macrofollicular adenomas yield more abundant colloid. The follicular epithelial cells are round to polygonal, show slight crowding, and lack the evenly spaced honeycomb pattern of benign follicular epithelial cells. The nuclei of most neoplastic follicular cells are round, slightly hyperchromatic with a homogeneous chromatin pattern and inconspicuous nucleoli. The nuclear membranes are smooth and without significant irregularities. Although some nuclear atypia with slight enlargement, pleomorphism, and occasional prominent nucleoli may be present, features associated with papillary carcinoma such as nuclear grooves and intranuclear pseudoinclusions are lacking.

The FNA procedure samples the substance of the nodule but not the capsule and therefore cannot document the presence or absence of capsular or vascular invasion. As a result, the typical FNA

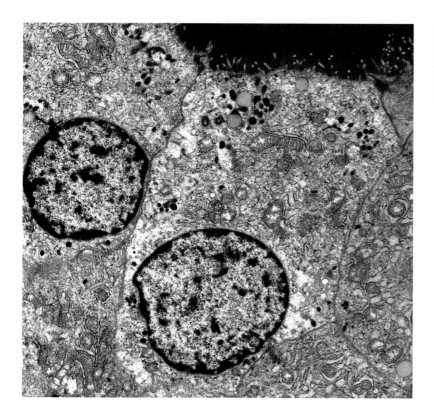

FIGURE 8.26. Ultramicroscopic appearance of follicular adenoma. The cells have a cuboidal shape, round basally located nuclei, apical microvilli protruding into the colloid-filled follicular lumen, and various cytoplasmic organelles. Electron-dense secretory vesicles and phagolysosomes are seen mostly in the apical portion of the cytoplasm.

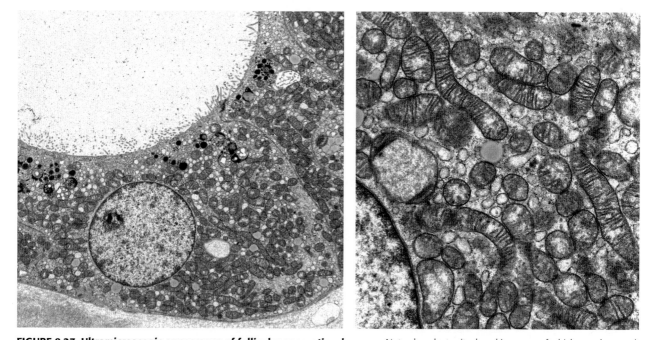

FIGURE 8.27. Ultramicroscopic appearance of follicular oncocytic adenoma. Note abundant mitochondria, some of which are elongated, are irregularly shaped, and show loss of cristae.

specimen of follicular adenoma with a microfollicular or solid/trabecular growth pattern yields the cytologic diagnosis of "follicular neoplasm" or "suspicious for follicular neoplasm" by the current Bethesda System for Reporting Thyroid Cytopathology (BSRTC).[114] This cytologic diagnosis entails the differential diagnosis of follicular adenoma, cellular hyperplastic nodule, follicular carcinoma, and follicular variant of papillary carcinoma. After surgery, approximately one-fourth of these lesions are found to be malignant,

and the rest represent either cellular hyperplastic nodules or follicular adenomas.[115,116] Follicular adenomas with a significant normofollicular or macrofollicular component typically produce a cytologic specimen with features of a benign colloid nodule.

Cytologic samples of oncocytic (Hürthle) cell adenomas contain large cells with a relatively low nuclear–cytoplasmic ratio and numerous fine granules in the cytoplasm (Fig. 8.29). The nuclei are typically round with smooth nuclear contours and

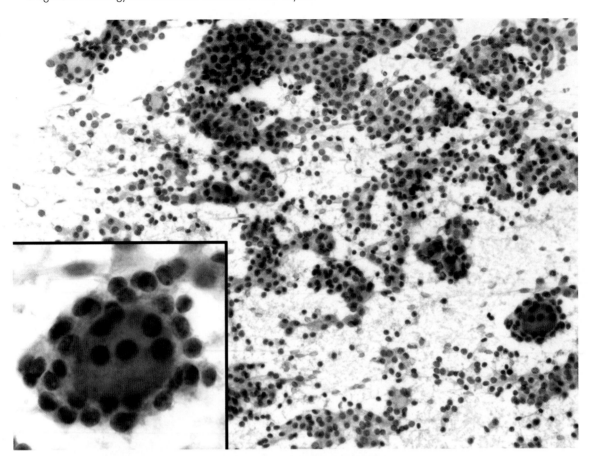

FIGURE 8.28. Cytologic appearance of conventional type follicular adenoma. Highly cellular smear shows numerous clusters of epithelial cells and occasional microfollicular structures. Microfollicles **(inset)** are composed of follicular epithelial cells in small spherical aggregates and contain a small amount of colloid in the center (Papanicolaou stain).

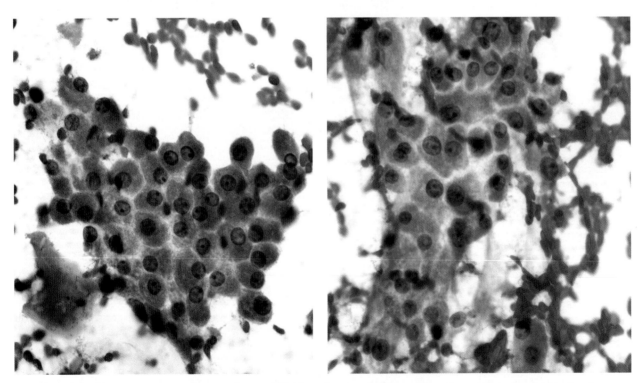

FIGURE 8.29. Cytologic appearance of oncocytic type follicular adenoma. Left: An aspirate shows polygonal cells with abundant cytoplasm containing copious cytoplasmic granules. The nuclei are round with even chromatin pattern and prominent nucleoli (Papanicolaou stain). **Right:** Another image from the same case shows mild nuclear pleomorphism (Papanicolaou stain).

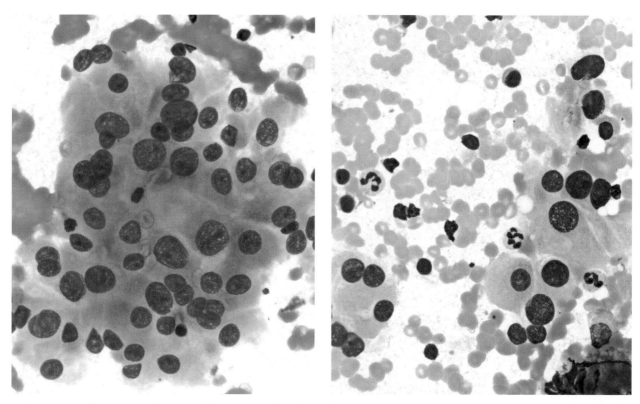

FIGURE 8.30. Left: An aspirate from a nodule in a case of lymphocytic thyroiditis may show oncocytic cell clusters that are similar to those of an oncocytic adenoma (Diff-Quik stain). **Right:** Other areas show occasional scattered lymphocytes suggesting the possibility of lymphocytic thyroiditis (Diff-Quik stain).

prominent nucleoli. Occasional cells may show nuclear membrane irregularities, groove formation, and intranuclear pseudoinclusions, although these are expected to be few in number in adenoma samples. Most FNA specimens from oncocytic (Hürthle) cell adenomas are cellular but do not show microfollicular pattern. These cytology specimens usually are reported as "follicular neoplasm, oncocytic (Hürthle cell) type" or "suspicious for follicular neoplasm, oncocytic (Hürthle cell) type," according to BSRTC. The differential diagnosis for this cytologic diagnosis includes cellular hyperplastic oncocytic (Hürthle) cell nodule (usually from lymphocytic/Hashimoto thyroiditis or goiter), hyperfunctioning follicular adenoma with or without papillary hyperplasia, oncocytic (Hürthle) cell carcinoma, and oncocytic (Hürthle) cell variant of papillary carcinoma. In cases of lymphocytic/Hashimoto thyroiditis, sampling of various areas may demonstrate the lymphocytic population typical for this entity, thus clarifying the nature of the lesion (Fig. 8.30). Cytology specimens from cellular hyperplastic oncocytic (Hürthle) cell nodules may show varying degrees of atypia. However, specimens with a uniform population of oncocytic (Hürthle) cells without atypia are mostly benign. If the oncocytic (Hürthle) cell population is sparse, the case may be diagnosed as "atypia of undetermined significance/follicular lesion of undetermined significance" because the distinction between an oncocytic (Hürthle) cell neoplasm and a hyperplastic process cannot be made. However, if there is a significant degree of atypia (especially features concerning for papillary carcinoma), the diagnosis of "suspicious for malignancy" may be considered.

Hyperfunctioning follicular adenoma with or without papillary hyperplasia may show monolayers of large cells with abundant cytoplasm, mimicking oncocytic (Hürthle) cells. Flame cells represented by marginal cytoplasmic vacuoles and red to pink cytoplasmic borders are hallmarks of the hyperplastic process. Papillary fragments may or may not be observed.

In cases showing significant nuclear atypia, clinical investigation regarding the possible history of radioactive iodine therapy should be made. Usually, the nuclei show significant enlargement, pleomorphism, and crowding but not the typical features of papillary thyroid carcinoma such as consistent nuclear groove and intranuclear pseudoinclusion formation. Also the radioactive iodine–induced atypia tends to be random. The atypical cells appear disproportionately enlarged and abnormal and stand out among other epithelial cells. In contrast, the "atypia" in low-grade neoplasms (adenomas and carcinomas) tends to affect the neoplastic cell uniformly. The nuclear changes are found throughout the lesional cell population. At the other end of the spectrum, anaplastic carcinoma typically shows numerous highly abnormal cells. Diagnostic dilemmas in cytology arise when there is a small focus of anaplasia in an otherwise well-differentiated neoplasm or when there is sparse sampling of the anaplastic carcinoma. Therefore, at times, changes induced by radiation atypia may be difficult to distinguish from malignancy in cytology samples.[85]

 DIFFERENTIAL DIAGNOSIS

The differential diagnosis of follicular adenoma frequently includes dominant hyperplastic nodule, follicular carcinoma, and encapsulated follicular variant of papillary carcinoma. The unusual variants of adenoma should be distinguished from encapsulated medullary carcinoma, metastatic carcinoma, and intrathyroidal parathyroid adenoma or hyperplasia.

The distinction between follicular adenoma and hyperplastic nodule is based on finding the histologic features that are more characteristic for each lesion (Table 8.1). In those cases where microscopic examination revealed a single well-encapsulated nodule with

Table 8.1	
Histopathologic and Molecular Features Helpful in Distinguishing Between Follicular Adenoma and Hyperplastic Nodule	

Follicular Adenoma	Hyperplastic Nodule
Histologic features	
Solitary nodule	One of several nodules
Complete capsule	No or partial capsule
Uniform, monotonous growth pattern within nodule	Variable growth patterns within nodule
High cellularity, microfollicular, or solid growth pattern	Abundant colloid
Microscopic appearance sharply different from adjacent thyroid	Microscopic appearance blends with adjacent thyroid
Compression of adjacent thyroid tissue	No compression of adjacent thyroid tissue
Molecular features	
Monoclonal lesion	Polyclonal lesion
Positive for clonal mutations (i.e., *RAS*)	Lack of genetic mutations
Presence of clonal cytogenetic alterations (i.e., trisomy 7)	Lack of clonal cytogenetic alterations

uniform microfollicular or solid growth pattern and compression of the adjacent normal-appearing thyroid gland, the diagnosis of an adenoma is straightforward. However, not infrequently, the nodule in question possesses some features of adenoma and other features more characteristic of hyperplastic nodules. In those instances, the distinction is difficult, if not impossible. The presence of a clonal cell population or *RAS* mutation is diagnostic of an adenoma.

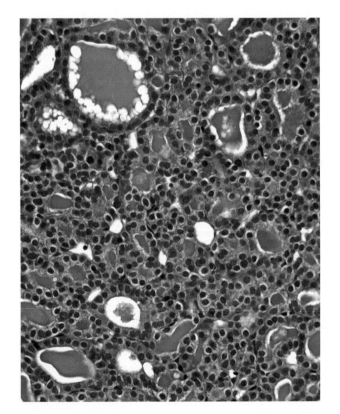

FIGURE 8.31. This intrathyroidal parathyroid adenoma mimics thyroid follicular adenoma. The tumor is composed exclusively of chief cells, contains numerous follicles filled with dense eosinophilic material resembling colloid, and lacks stromal fat, making it difficult to distinguish it from thyroid adenoma.

Follicular adenoma is distinguished from minimally invasive follicular carcinoma based on the absence of capsular or vascular invasion. The criteria for invasion are described in Chapter 10. The lack of immunoreactivity for galectin-3, HBME-1, CITED1, and PPARγ and absence of *PAX8/PPARγ* rearrangement support the diagnosis of an adenoma.

The lack of diagnostic nuclear features of papillary carcinoma allows separation of follicular adenoma from encapsulated follicular variant of papillary carcinoma. In difficult cases, immunostaining for galectin-3, HBME-1, and CITED1 may be of help as negative staining with all of the antibodies would be more consistent with an adenoma. The lack of *BRAF* and *RET/PTC* mutations is also more suggestive of an adenoma. The presence of *RAS* mutation is equally supportive of both conditions.

Medullary carcinoma should be ruled out when the tumor has a solid growth pattern with no colloid formation or reveals clear cells or spindle cells. Positive staining for thyroglobulin and lack of immunoreactivity for calcitonin, CEA, and chromogranin confirm the diagnosis. TTF1 is not helpful in this situation because it reveals positive staining in many medullary carcinomas.

Metastatic adenocarcinoma is an important differential diagnosis for adenomas that contain clear cells or signet-ring cells. Immunostaining for thyroglobulin establishes the thyroid cell origin. TTF1 may also be helpful, especially when lung adenocarcinoma is not a consideration.

Parathyroid adenoma or hyperplasia in the intrathyroidal location may be confused with thyroid follicular adenoma (Fig. 8.31). Immunostains for thyroglobulin, TTF1, and parathyroid hormone are helpful to establish the correct diagnosis.

 ## TREATMENT AND PROGNOSIS

Follicular adenomas cannot be reliably distinguished from carcinomas by imaging or FNA cytology, and therefore, most patients are referred for surgery.[5,117] A lobectomy is usually performed. Less frequently, patients are treated with levothyroxine to suppress TSH and are followed without surgery, particularly if the nodule decreases in size. Hyperfunctioning nodules are associated with a very low risk of malignancy and are typically managed conservatively; common modalities include administration of radioiodine, antithyroid drugs, and β-blockers.

Follicular adenomas are benign tumors and cured by surgical excision. Although some adenomas are likely to have potential to progress to follicular carcinomas, their removal at preinvasive stage is curative. Historically, concerns had existed that histologic criteria cannot reliably predict behavior of oncocytic follicular tumors and that all of them should be regarded as malignant.[118] However, it has been convincingly demonstrated over the last three decades that conventional histologic criteria, that is, capsular or vascular invasion, are entirely adequate in predicting the behavior of oncocytic follicular tumors.[119-121]

REFERENCES

1. Bisi H, Fernandes VS, de Camargo RY, et al. The prevalence of unsuspected thyroid pathology in 300 sequential autopsies, with special reference to the incidental carcinoma. *Cancer*. 1989;64:1888–1893.
2. Silverberg SG, Vidone RA. Adenoma and carcinoma of the thyroid. *Cancer*. 1966;19:1053–1062.
3. Avetisian IL, Petrova GV. Latent thyroid pathology in residents of Kiev, Ukraine. *J Environ Pathol Toxicol Oncol*. 1996;15:239–243.
4. Klonoff DC, Greenspan FS. The thyroid nodule. *Adv Intern Med*. 1982;27:101–126.
5. Cooper DS, Doherty GM, Haugen BR, et al. Management guidelines for patients with thyroid nodules and differentiated thyroid cancer. *Thyroid*. 2006;16:109–142.
6. Shore RE, Hildreth N, Dvoretsky P, et al. Benign thyroid adenomas among persons X-irradiated in infancy for enlarged thymus glands. *Radiat Res*. 1993;134:217–223.
7. Wong FL, Ron E, Gierlowski T, et al. Benign thyroid tumors: general risk factors and their effects on radiation risk estimation. *Am J Epidemiol*. 1996;144:728–733.
8. Acharya S, Sarafoglou K, LaQuaglia M, et al. Thyroid neoplasms after therapeutic radiation for malignancies during childhood or adolescence. *Cancer*. 2003;97:2397–2403.
9. Belfiore A, La Rosa GL, Padova G, et al. The frequency of cold thyroid nodules and thyroid malignancies in patients from an iodine-deficient area. *Cancer*. 1987;60:3096–3102.
10. Belfiore A, Sava L, Runello F, et al. Solitary autonomously functioning thyroid nodules and iodine deficiency. *J Clin Endocrinol Metab*. 1983;56:283–287.
11. Ohshima M, Ward JM. Dietary iodine deficiency as a tumor promoter and carcinogen in male F344/NCr rats. *Cancer Res*. 1986;46:877–883.
12. Thomas GA, Williams ED. Evidence for and possible mechanisms of nongenotoxic carcinogenesis in the rodent thyroid. *Mutat Res*. 1991;248:357–370.
13. Smith PF, Grossman SJ, Gerson RJ, et al. Studies on the mechanism of simvastatin-induced thyroid hypertrophy and follicular cell adenoma in the rat. *Toxicol Pathol*. 1991;19:197–205.
14. McCord EL, Goenka S. Development of thyroid follicular adenoma on simvastatin therapy. *Tenn Med*. 2000;93:210–212.
15. Eng C. Genetics of cowden syndrome: through the looking glass of oncology. *Int J Oncol*. 1998;12:701–710.
16. Nelen MR, van Staveren WC, Peeters EA, et al. Germline mutations in the *PTEN/MMAC1* gene in patients with cowden disease. *Hum Mol Genet*. 1997;6:1383–1387.
17. Hollander MC, Blumenthal GM, Dennis PA. *PTEN* loss in the continuum of common cancers, rare syndromes and mouse models. *Nat Rev Cancer*. 2011;11:289–301.
18. Harach HR, Soubeyran I, Brown A, et al. Thyroid pathologic findings in patients with cowden disease. *Ann Diagn Pathol*. 1999;3:331–340.
19. Kirschner LS, Carney JA, Pack SD, et al. Mutations of the gene encoding the protein kinase A type I-alpha regulatory subunit in patients with the carney complex. *Nat Genet*. 2000;26:89–92.
20. Stratakis CA, Courcoutsakis NA, Abati A, et al. Thyroid gland abnormalities in patients with the syndrome of spotty skin pigmentation, myxomas, endocrine overactivity, and schwannomas (carney complex). *J Clin Endocrinol Metab*. 1997;82:2037–2043.
21. Hicks DG, LiVolsi VA, Neidich JA, et al. Clonal analysis of solitary follicular nodules in the thyroid. *Am J Pathol*. 1990;137:553–562.
22. Namba H, Matsuo K, Fagin JA. Clonal composition of benign and malignant human thyroid tumors. *J Clin Invest*. 1990;86:120–125.
23. Belge G, Roque L, Soares J, et al. Cytogenetic investigations of 340 thyroid hyperplasias and adenomas revealing correlations between cytogenetic findings and histology. *Cancer Genet Cytogenet*. 1998;101:42–48.
24. Teyssier JR, Liautaud-Roger F, Ferre D, et al. Chromosomal changes in thyroid tumors. Relation with DNA content, karyotypic features, and clinical data. *Cancer Genet Cytogenet*. 1990;50:249–263.
25. Ciampi R, Zhu Z, Nikiforov YE. *BRAF* copy number gains in thyroid tumors detected by fluorescence in situ hybridization. *Endocr Pathol*. 2005;16:99–105.
26. Roque L, Gomes P, Correia C, et al. Thyroid nodular hyperplasia: chromosomal studies in 14 cases. *Cancer Genet Cytogenet*. 1993;69:31–34.
27. Rippe V, Drieschner N, Meiboom M, et al. Identification of a gene rearranged by 2p21 aberrations in thyroid adenomas. *Oncogene*. 2003;22:6111–6114.
28. Drieschner N, Kerschling S, Soller JT, et al. A domain of the thyroid adenoma associated gene (thada) conserved in vertebrates becomes destroyed by chromosomal rearrangements observed in thyroid adenomas. *Gene*. 2007;403:110–117.
29. Meiboom M, Murua Escobar H, Pentimalli F, et al. A 3.4-kbp transcript of *ZNF331* is solely expressed in follicular thyroid adenomas. *Cytogenet Genome Res*. 2003;101:113–117.
30. Grant CS, Hay ID, Ryan JJ, et al. Diagnostic and prognostic utility of flow cytometric DNA measurements in follicular thyroid tumors. *World J Surg*. 1990;14:283–289; discussion 289–290.
31. Czyz W, Joensuu H, Pylkkanen L, et al. P53 protein, pcna staining, and DNA content in follicular neoplasms of the thyroid gland. *J Pathol*. 1994;174:267–274.
32. Oyama T, Vickery AL Jr, Preffer FI, et al. A comparative study of flow cytometry and histopathologic findings in thyroid follicular carcinomas and adenomas. *Hum Pathol*. 1994;25:271–275.
33. Castro P, Eknaes M, Teixeira MR, et al. Adenomas and follicular carcinomas of the thyroid display two major patterns of chromosomal changes. *J Pathol*. 2005;206:305–311.
34. Castro P, Sansonetty F, Soares P, et al. Fetal adenomas and minimally invasive follicular carcinomas of the thyroid frequently display a triploid or near triploid DNA pattern. *Virchows Arch*. 2001;438:336–342.
35. Ward LS, Brenta G, Medvedovic M, et al. Studies of allelic loss in thyroid tumors reveal major differences in chromosomal instability between papillary and follicular carcinomas. *J Clin Endocrinol Metab*. 1998;83:525–530.
36. Segev DL, Saji M, Phillips GS, et al. Polymerase chain reaction-based microsatellite polymorphism analysis of follicular and Hürthle cell neoplasms of the thyroid. *J Clin Endocrinol Metab*. 1998;83:2036–2042.
37. Zedenius J, Wallin G, Svensson A, et al. Allelotyping of follicular thyroid tumors. *Hum Genet*. 1995;96:27–32.
38. Gimm O, Chi H, Dahia PL, et al. Somatic mutation and germline variants of *MINPP1*, a phosphatase gene located in proximity to *PTEN* on 10q23.3, in follicular thyroid carcinomas. *J Clin Endocrinol Metab*. 2001;86:1801–1805.
39. Yeh JJ, Marsh DJ, Zedenius J, et al. Fine-structure deletion mapping of 10q22-24 identifies regions of loss of heterozygosity and suggests that sporadic follicular thyroid adenomas and follicular thyroid carcinomas develop along distinct neoplastic pathways. *Genes Chromosomes Cancer*. 1999;26:322–328.
40. Lemoine NR, Mayall ES, Wyllie FS, et al. High frequency of ras oncogene activation in all stages of human thyroid tumorigenesis. *Oncogene*. 1989;4:159–164.
41. Namba H, Rubin SA, Fagin JA. Point mutations of ras oncogenes are an early event in thyroid tumorigenesis. *Mol Endocrinol*. 1990;4:1474–1479.
42. Esapa CT, Johnson SJ, Kendall-Taylor P, et al. Prevalence of *Ras* mutations in thyroid neoplasia. *Clin Endocrinol (Oxf)*. 1999;50:529–535.
43. Shi YF, Zou MJ, Schmidt H, et al. High rates of *ras* codon 61 mutation in thyroid tumors in an iodide-deficient area. *Cancer Res*. 1991;51:2690–2693.
44. Schark C, Fulton N, Jacoby RF, et al. N-ras 61 oncogene mutations in Hürthle cell tumors. *Surgery*. 1990;108:994–999; discussion 999–1000.
45. Tallini G, Hsueh A, Liu S, et al. Frequent chromosomal DNA unbalance in thyroid oncocytic (Hürthle cell) neoplasms detected by comparative genomic hybridization. *Lab Invest*. 1999;79:547–555.
46. Nikiforova MN, Lynch RA, Biddinger PW, et al. *RAS* point mutations and *PAX8-PPAR gamma* rearrangement in thyroid tumors: evidence for distinct molecular pathways in thyroid follicular carcinoma. *J Clin Endocrinol Metab*. 2003;88:2318–2326.
47. Bond JA, Wyllie FS, Rowson J, et al. In vitro reconstruction of tumour initiation in a human epithelium. *Oncogene*. 1994;9:281–290.
48. Santelli G, de Franciscis V, Portella G, et al. Production of transgenic mice expressing the *Ki-ras* oncogene under the control of a thyroglobulin promoter. *Cancer Res*. 1993;53:5523–5527.
49. Vitagliano D, Portella G, Troncone G, et al. Thyroid targeting of the *N-ras(Gln61Lys)* oncogene in transgenic mice results in follicular tumors that progress to poorly differentiated carcinomas. *Oncogene*. 2006;25:5467–5474.
50. Trulzsch B, Krohn K, Wonerow P, et al. Detection of thyroid-stimulating hormone receptor and *Gsalpha* mutations: in 75 toxic thyroid nodules by denaturing gradient gel electrophoresis. *J Mol Med*. 2001;78:684–691.
51. Parma J, Duprez L, Van Sande J, et al. Diversity and prevalence of somatic mutations in the thyrotropin receptor and Gs alpha genes as a cause of toxic thyroid adenomas. *J Clin Endocrinol Metab*. 1997;82:2695–2701.
52. Yen PM. Thyrotropin receptor mutations in thyroid diseases. *Rev Endocr Metab Disord*. 2000;1:123–129.
53. Michiels FM, Caillou B, Talbot M, et al. Oncogenic potential of guanine nucleotide stimulatory factor alpha subunit in thyroid glands of transgenic mice. *Proc Natl Acad Sci U S A*. 1994;91:10488–10492.
54. Hou P, Liu D, Shan Y, et al. Genetic alterations and their relationship in the phosphatidylinositol 3-kinase/Akt pathway in thyroid cancer. *Clin Cancer Res*. 2007;13:1161–1170.
55. Dwight T, Thoppe SR, Foukakis T, et al. Involvement of the *PAX8*/peroxisome proliferator-activated receptor gamma rearrangement in follicular thyroid tumors. *J Clin Endocrinol Metab*. 2003;88:4440–4445.
56. French CA, Alexander EK, Cibas ES, et al. Genetic and biological subgroups of low-stage follicular thyroid cancer. *Am J Pathol*. 2003;162:1053–1060.
57. Nikiforova MN, Biddinger PW, Caudill CM, et al. *PAX8-PPARgamma* rearrangement in thyroid tumors: RT-PCR and immunohistochemical analyses. *Am J Surg Pathol*. 2002;26:1016–1023.
58. Chia WK, Sharifah NA, Reena RM, et al. Fluorescence in situ hybridization analysis using *PAX8*- and *PPARG*-specific probes reveals the presence of *PAX8-PPARG* translocation and 3p25 aneusomy in follicular thyroid neoplasms. *Cancer Genet Cytogenet*. 2010;196:7–13.
59. Soares P, Trovisco V, Rocha AS, et al. *BRAF* mutations and RET/PTC rearrangements are alternative events in the etiopathogenesis of ptc. *Oncogene*. 2003;22:4578–4580.
60. Maximo V, Sobrinho-Simoes M. Hürthle cell tumours of the thyroid. A review with emphasis on mitochondrial abnormalities with clinical relevance. *Virchows Arch*. 2000;437:107–115.
61. Tallini G. Oncocytic tumours. *Virchows Arch*. 1998;433:5–12.
62. Katoh R, Harach HR, Williams ED. Solitary, multiple, and familial oxyphil tumours of the thyroid gland. *J Pathol*. 1998;186:292–299.
63. Gasparre G, Porcelli AM, Bonora E, et al. Disruptive mitochondrial DNA mutations in complex I subunits are markers of oncocytic phenotype in thyroid tumors. *Proc Natl Acad Sci U S A*. 2007;104:9001–9006.

64. Maximo V, Soares P, Lima J, et al. Mitochondrial DNA somatic mutations (point mutations and large deletions) and mitochondrial DNA variants in human thyroid pathology: a study with emphasis on Hürthle cell tumors. *Am J Pathol.* 2002;160:1857–1865.

65. Wallace DC. Diseases of the mitochondrial DNA. *Annu Rev Biochem.* 1992;61:1175–1212.

66. LiVolsi VA, Merino MJ. Worrisome histologic alterations following fine-needle aspiration of the thyroid (WHAFFT). *Pathol Annu.* 1994;29(pt 2):99–120.

67. DeLellis RA, Lloyd RV, Heitz PU, et al. *World Health Organization Classification of Tumours. Pathology and Genetics of Tumours of Endocrine Organs.* IARC Press, Lyon, France, 2004.

68. Hürthle K. Beiträge zur kenntniss des secretionsvorgangs in der schilddrüse. *Arch Gesammte Physiol.* 1894;56:1–44.

69. Rosai J, Carcangiu ML, DeLellis RA. *Tumors of the Thyroid Gland.* Washington, DC: Armed Forces Institute of Pathology; 1992.

70. Nikiforov YE, Heffess CS, Korzenko AV, et al. Characteristics of follicular tumors and nonneoplastic thyroid lesions in children and adolescents exposed to radiation as a result of the chernobyl disaster. *Cancer.* 1995;76:900–909.

71. Vickery AL Jr. Thyroid papillary carcinoma. Pathological and philosophical controversies. *Am J Surg Pathol.* 1983;7:797–807.

72. Hjorth L, Thomsen LB, Nielsen VT. Adenolipoma of the thyroid gland. *Histopathology.* 1986;10:91–96.

73. Schmid C, Beham A, Seewann HL. Extramedullary haematopoiesis in the thyroid gland. *Histopathology.* 1989;15:423–425.

74. Gnepp DR, Ogorzalek JM, Heffess CS. Fat-containing lesions of the thyroid gland. *Am J Surg Pathol.* 1989;13:605–612.

75. Schroder S, Bocker W. Signet-ring-cell thyroid tumors. Follicle cell tumors with arrest of folliculogenesis. *Am J Surg Pathol.* 1985;9:619–629.

76. el-Sahrigy D, Zhang XM, Elhosseiny A, et al. Signet-ring follicular adenoma of the thyroid diagnosed by fine needle aspiration. Report of a case with cytologic description. *Acta Cytol.* 2004;48:87–90.

77. Mendelsohn G. Signet-cell-simulating microfollicular adenoma of the thyroid. *Am J Surg Pathol.* 1984;8:705–708.

78. Gherardi G. Signet ring cell "mucinous" thyroid adenoma: a follicle cell tumour with abnormal accumulation of thyroglobulin and a peculiar histochemical profile. *Histopathology.* 1987;11:317–326.

79. Rigaud C, Peltier F, Bogomoletz WV. Mucin producing microfollicular adenoma of the thyroid. *J Clin Pathol.* 1985;38:277–280.

80. Brisigotti M, Lorenzini P, Alessi A, et al. Mucin-producing adenoma of the thyroid gland. *Tumori.* 1986;72:211–214.

81. Carcangiu ML, Sibley RK, Rosai J. Clear cell change in primary thyroid tumors. A study of 38 cases. *Am J Surg Pathol.* 1985;9:705–722.

82. Schroder S, Husselmann H, Bocker W. Lipid-rich cell adenoma of the thyroid gland. Report of a peculiar thyroid tumour. *Virchows Arch A Pathol Anat Histopathol.* 1984;404:105–108.

83. Chetty R. Thyroid follicular adenoma composed of lipid-rich cells. *Endocr Pathol.* 2011;22:31–34.

84. Toth K, Peter I, Kremmer T, et al. Lipid-rich cell thyroid adenoma: histopathology with comparative lipid analysis. *Virchows Arch A Pathol Anat Histopathol.* 1990;417:273–276.

85. Granter SR, Cibas ES. Cytologic findings in thyroid nodules after ^{131}I treatment of hyperthyroidism. *Am J Clin Pathol.* 1997;107:20–25.

86. Hazard JB, Kenyon R. Atypical adenoma of the thyroid. *AMA Arch Pathol.* 1954;58:554–563.

87. Lang W, Georgii A, Stauch G, et al. The differentiation of atypical adenomas and encapsulated follicular carcinomas in the thyroid gland. *Virchows Arch A Pathol Anat Histol.* 1980;385:125–141.

88. Fukunaga M, Shinozaki N, Endo Y, et al. Atypical adenoma of the thyroid. A clinicopathologic and flow cytometric DNA study in comparison with other follicular neoplasms. *Acta Pathol Jpn.* 1992;42:632–638.

89. Lang W, Choritz H, Hundeshagen H. Risk factors in follicular thyroid carcinomas. A retrospective follow-up study covering a 14-year period with emphasis on morphological findings. *Am J Surg Pathol.* 1986;10:246–255.

90. Koren R, Bernheim J, Schachter P, et al. Black thyroid adenoma. Clinical, histochemical, and ultrastructural features. *Appl Immunohistochem Mol Morphol.* 2000;8:80–84.

91. Visona A, Pea M, Bozzola L, et al. Follicular adenoma of the thyroid gland with extensive chondroid metaplasia. *Histopathology.* 1991;18:278–279.

92. Ardito G, Fadda G, Revelli L, et al. Follicular adenoma of the thyroid gland with extensive bone metaplasia. *J Exp Clin Cancer Res.* 2001;20:443–445.

93. Aker FV, Bas Y, Ozkara S, et al. Spindle cell metaplasia in follicular adenoma of the thyroid gland: case report and review of the literature. *Endocr J.* 2004;51:457–461.

94. Shikama Y, Mizukami H, Sakai T, et al. Spindle cell metaplasia arising in thyroid adenoma: characterization of its pathology and differential diagnosis. *J Endocrinol Invest.* 2006;29:168–171.

95. Magro G, Benkova K, Michal M. Meningioma-like tumor of the thyroid: a previously undescribed variant of follicular adenoma. *Virchows Arch.* 2005;446:677–679.

96. Katoh R, Miyagi E, Nakamura N, et al. Expression of thyroid transcription factor-1 (TTF-1) in human c cells and medullary thyroid carcinomas. *Hum Pathol.* 2000;31:386–393.

97. Lau SK, Luthringer DJ, Eisen RN. Thyroid transcription factor-1: a review. *Appl Immunohistochem Mol Morphol.* 2002;10:97–102.

98. Nonaka D, Tang Y, Chiriboga L, et al. Diagnostic utility of thyroid transcription factors Pax8 and TTF-2 (FoxE1) in thyroid epithelial neoplasms. *Mod Pathol.* 2008;21:192–200.

99. Tacha D, Zhou D, Cheng L. Expression of PAX8 in normal and neoplastic tissues: a comprehensive immunohistochemical study. *Appl Immunohistochem Mol Morphol.* 2011;19:293–299.

100. Bejarano PA, Nikiforov YE, Swenson ES, et al. Thyroid transcription factor-1, thyroglobulin, cytokeratin 7, and cytokeratin 20 in thyroid neoplasms. *Appl Immunohistochem Mol Morphol.* 2000;8:189–194.

101. Schelfhout LJ, Van Muijen GN, Fleuren GJ. Expression of keratin 19 distinguishes papillary thyroid carcinoma from follicular carcinomas and follicular thyroid adenoma. *Am J Clin Pathol.* 1989;92:654–658.

102. Nakamura N, Erickson LA, Jin L, et al. Immunohistochemical separation of follicular variant of papillary thyroid carcinoma from follicular adenoma. *Endocr Pathol.* 2006;17:213–223.

103. Sahoo S, Hoda SA, Rosai J, et al. Cytokeratin 19 immunoreactivity in the diagnosis of papillary thyroid carcinoma: a note of caution. *Am J Clin Pathol.* 2001;116:696–702.

104. Papotti M, Gugliotta P, Forte G, et al. Immunocytochemical identification of oxyphilic mitochondrion-rich cells. *Appl Immunohistochem Mol Morphol.* 1994;2:261–263.

105. Bussolati G, Gugliotta P, Volante M, et al. Retrieved endogenous biotin: a novel marker and a potential pitfall in diagnostic immunohistochemistry. *Histopathology.* 1997;31:400–407.

106. Hoos A, Stojadinovic A, Singh B, et al. Clinical significance of molecular expression profiles of Hürthle cell tumors of the thyroid gland analyzed via tissue microarrays. *Am J Pathol.* 2002;160:175–183.

107. Scognamiglio T, Hyjek E, Kao J, et al. Diagnostic usefulness of HBME1, galectin-3, CK19, and CITED1 and evaluation of their expression in encapsulated lesions with questionable features of papillary thyroid carcinoma. *Am J Clin Pathol.* 2006;126:700–708.

108. Saggiorato E, De Pompa R, Volante M, et al. Characterization of thyroid "follicular neoplasms" in fine-needle aspiration cytological specimens using a panel of immunohistochemical markers: a proposal for clinical application. *Endocr Relat Cancer.* 2005;12:305–317.

109. Kroll TG, Sarraf P, Pecciarini L, et al. PAX8-PPARgamma1 fusion oncogene in human thyroid carcinoma [corrected]. *Science.* 2000;289:1357–1360.

111. Nesland JM, Sobrinho-Simoes MA, Holm R, et al. Hürthle-cell lesions of the thyroid: a combined study using transmission electron microscopy, scanning electron microscopy, and immunocytochemistry. *Ultrastruct Pathol.* 1985;8:269–290.

112. Bocker W, Dralle H, Koch G, et al. Immunhistochemical and electron microscope analysis of adenomas of the thyroid gland. II. Adenomas with specific cytological differentiation. *Virchows Arch A Pathol Anat Histol.* 1978;380:205–220.

113. Panke TW, Croxson MS, Parker JW, et al. Triiodothyronine-secreting (toxic) adenoma of the thyroid gland: light and electron microscopic characteristics. *Cancer.* 1978;41:528–537.

114. Ali SZ, Cibas ES. *The Bethesda System for Reporting Thyroid Cytopathology: Definitions, Criteria, and Explanatory Notes.* Springer, New York, 2010.

115. Wang HH. Reporting thyroid fine-needle aspiration: literature review and a proposal. *Diagn Cytopathol.* 2006;34:67–76.

116. Yang GC, Liebeskind D, Messina AV. Should cytopathologists stop reporting follicular neoplasms on fine-needle aspiration of the thyroid? *Cancer.* 2003;99:69–74.

117. Gharib H, Papini E, Valcavi R, et al. American Association of Clinical Endocrinologists and Associazione Medici Endocrinologi medical guidelines for clinical practice for the diagnosis and management of thyroid nodules. *Endocr Pract.* 2006;12:63–102.

118. Thompson NW, Dunn EL, Batsakis JG, et al. Hürthle cell lesions of the thyroid gland. *Surg Gynecol Obstet.* 1974;139:555–560.

119. Carcangiu ML, Bianchi S, Savino D, et al. Follicular Hürthle cell tumors of the thyroid gland. *Cancer.* 1991;68:1944–1953.

120. Bronner MP, LiVolsi VA. Oxyphilic (Askanazy/Hürthle cell) tumors of the thyroid: microscopic features predict biologic behavior. *Surg Pathol.* 1988;1:137–150.

121. Grant CS. Operative and postoperative management of the patient with follicular and Hürthle cell carcinoma. Do they differ? *Surg Clin North Am.* 1995;75:395–403.

Hyalinizing Trabecular Tumor

DEFINITION

Hyalinizing trabecular tumor is a rare noninvasive follicular cell-derived thyroid neoplasm with a characteristic trabecular growth pattern and intratrabecular hyalinization. The malignant potential of this tumor is uncertain, but at most is very low. Synonyms include paraganglioma-like adenoma of the thyroid (PLAT), hyalinizing trabecular adenoma, hyalinizing trabecular neoplasm, and hyaline cell tumor of the thyroid with massive accumulation of cytoplasmic microfilaments.

HISTORICAL COMMENTS AND POINTS OF CONTROVERSY

The first detailed description of this tumor in the modern era was provided by Carney and colleagues,[1] who reported in 1987 a series of 11 tumors and called them *hyalinizing trabecular adenoma*. Prior to this publication, this tumor was apparently described and drawn by Rahel Zipkin in 1905 and by Pierre Masson in 1922 and reported in an abstract form by Ward and colleagues in 1982 (as recently reviewed by Carney[2]). All 11 tumors reported in 1987 were well circumscribed or encapsulated and revealed no invasion, no tumor recurrence, or metastases during a mean follow-up period of 10 years.[1] A year later, the same tumor was described as *paraganglioma-like adenoma of the thyroid* or PLAT by Bronner and colleagues[3] in a series of nine cases.

In 1991, a series of nine thyroid tumors with trabecular pattern and hyalinization was reported, and one of those cases had a lymph node metastasis at presentation.[4] Although in the latter case only an incisional biopsy of the tumor was available for review, the authors argued that tumors with this appearance may have malignant behavior and should be designated as hyalinizing trabecular tumors. Several subsequent studies have reported occasional cases with similar trabecular appearance and hyalinization but associated with blood vessel or tumor capsule invasion and distant metastases, as well as areas of classic papillary carcinoma merging with this tumor.[5–9] Together with the prominent nuclear features of papillary carcinoma typically seen in the tumor cells, these reports argued against the uniformly benign nature of hyalinizing trabecular adenoma. Although no well-documented cases of malignant behavior of tumors with no invasion at presentation have been published so far, many believe that this tumor is likely to represent a peculiar variant of papillary carcinoma.

The tumor relationship to papillary carcinoma was expected to be firmly proven by two simultaneously published reports demonstrating that hyalinizing trabecular tumors frequently harbor *RET/PTC* rearrangement,[10,11] which is a genetic feature of papillary carcinoma. However, these molecular findings did not provide full confirmation of the association and raised a controversy by themselves. In addition to some concerns about the uniformity of the criteria for tumor selection,[12] the problem was that these studies did not use a quantitative approach for *RET/PTC* detection and therefore failed to establish whether the rearrangement in these tumors was *clonal*, i.e., present in most tumor cells, or *nonclonal* and occurred only in

a small fraction of cells within the nodule. As nonclonal *RET/PTC* rearrangement is not specific for papillary carcinoma,[13,14] the results of these studies cannot be used to confirm that hyalinizing trabecular tumor is a variant of papillary carcinoma. As the controversy persists, the 2004 WHO classification places this tumor in a separate category and designates it as hyalinizing trabecular tumor.[15]

INCIDENCE AND EPIDEMIOLOGY

Hyalinizing trabecular tumor is a rare type of thyroid tumors. Its exact incidence is not known, although it would be unusual to encounter more than one in-house case of this tumor per year in an average size pathology laboratory. The age of patients at diagnosis ranges between 21 and 81 years, with approximately uniform distribution from the third until the seventh decade and a mean age of 46 to 50 years in the reported series with a substantial number of patients.[16–19] The tumor has a marked female predominance, with a female:male ratio of 5–6:1.

ETIOLOGY

The etiologic factors for hyalinizing trabecular tumor development are not well defined. In the original series of 11 cases, two patients (18%) had a history of radiation exposure.[1] However, in a larger series, a history of radiation was found in 5% of patients.[16] The tumor frequently arises in thyroid glands affected by chronic lymphocytic thyroiditis or multinodular goiter (Fig. 9.1) and may coexist with a typical follicular adenoma or papillary carcinoma, although whether these associations are coincidental or hyalinizing trabecular tumor shares common causal factors with these conditions remains unclear.

A case of hyalinizing trabecular tumor in a patient with Cowden disease[20] and a case of an invasive tumor with similar morphology in a patient with familial polyposis coli[7] have been reported. Adenomas with a growth pattern of hyalinizing trabecular tumor were described in individuals with familial oncocytic (oxyphilic) thyroid tumors linked to a locus on chromosome 19p13.2.[21] However, concrete evidence for the association between hyalinizing trabecular tumor and familial cancer syndromes is lacking.

PATHOGENESIS AND MOLECULAR GENETICS

DNA Ploidy

Most tumors have a diploid cell population. In one study, flow cytometric analysis of DNA ploidy revealed a diploid pattern in 5/6 (83%) tumors and evidence for aneuploidy in 1 (17%) tumor.[1]

Cytogenetic Abnormalities

In one reported case,[4] the tumor revealed a normal karyotype together with two clones, one with translocation t(2;3)(q21;p27) and another with the same translocation in addition to trisomy 7 and 12.

Somatic Mutations

RET/PTC

Two initial simultaneously published reports found *RET/PTC* rearrangement in a significant fraction of hyalinizing trabecular tumors.[10,11] In a series of 14 tumors reported by Papotti and colleagues,[11] 29% showed RET expression by immunohistochemistry and 21% revealed *RET/PTC1* rearrangement detected by RT-PCR. Cheung and colleagues[10] reported a series of eight tumors, including six hyalinizing trabecular adenomas and two hyalinizing trabecular carcinomas diagnosed as such based on the presence of invasion. They found RET expression by immunohistochemistry in six (75%) tumors and detected *RET/PTC1* rearrangement by RT-PCR in five of these cases. A subsequent report of a larger series of cases (28 cases) from the first group found *RET/PTC1* in 36% of cases and *RET/PTC3* in 11%.[22] A more recent study revealed no *RET/PTC* rearrangements in a series of 18 hyalinizing trabecular tumors studied by RT-PCR.[19]

Although the three positive studies suggested the association between this tumor and *RET/PTC*, the pathogenetic role of *RET/PTC* rearrangement remains unclear. This is because all these reports used (1) formalin-fixed and paraffin-embedded tissues to isolate tumor RNA, which is known to provide a suboptimal template for RNA-based studies (see Chapter 20), and (2) highly sensitive detection techniques, that is, 35 to 40 cycles of PCR amplification followed by hybridization with specific probes, which were performed in a qualitative rather than quantitative manner. As a result, these studies were not able to establish what portion of the tumor cells harbored *RET/PTC* rearrangement. The use of immunohistochemistry with a RET antibody developed in one of the author's laboratories and not cross-validated for specificity of staining[11] or the use of a commercially available RET antibody known for weak and irreproducible staining results[10] could not clarify this issue with confidence. *RET/PTC* are known to occur in a *clonal* fashion in papillary carcinoma and in a *nonclonal* fashion, that is, in only a few cells within the tumor mass, in many thyroid lesions.[13,14] The lack of understanding of the extent of *RET/PTC* occurrence in hyalinizing trabecular tumor cells does not allow to establish the link between this tumor and papillary carcinoma or to postulate the pathogenetic role of *RET/PTC* in the development of hyalinizing trabecular tumors. The conclusive resolution of these issues awaits additional studies that have to be performed using reliable quantitative techniques for the detection of *RET/PTC* (Chapter 20).

Other Mutations

The prevalence of *BRAF* and *RAS* point mutations in these tumors is very low. No *BRAF* mutation was found in six studies that analyzed 82 hyalinizing trabecular tumors.[17–19,22–24] One study, however, reported the presence of a *BRAF* V600E mutation in a hyalinizing trabecular tumor developed in black thyroid, although the report did not provide sufficient details of the detection technique and illustrated the tumor quite poorly.[25] By contrast, *BRAF* mutations are found with high prevalence in papillary carcinomas, including papillary carcinomas with a trabecular growth pattern.[24]

No *RAS* mutation was found in 31 tumors reported to date.[22,26] *RAS* mutations are common in follicular adenomas, follicular carcinomas, and the follicular variant of papillary carcinoma (30% to 50% incidence). As hyalinizing trabecular tumor is expected to be related to one of these tumor types, the lack of *RAS* mutations provides evidence for distinct molecular pathways involved in the development of hyalinizing trabecular tumor.

Dysregulation of miRNA

The expression levels of several miRNAs known to be consistently upregulated in papillary thyroid carcinomas were studied in a series of 18 hyalinizing trabecular tumors.[19] They included miR-146b, miR-181b, miR-21, miR-221, and miR-222. None of these miRNAs

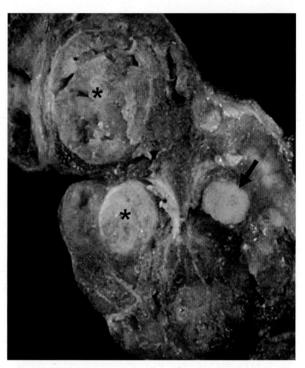

FIGURE 9.1. Gross appearance of hyalinizing trabecular tumor. Thyroid lobe showing two ill-defined hyperplastic nodules (*asterisk*) and a well-circumscribed but nonencapsulated 0.7 cm nodule of hyalinizing trabecular tumor with solid, homogeneous, yellow-tan cut surface (*arrow*).

were found to be upregulated in hyalinizing trabecular tumors, in contrast to papillary thyroid carcinoma samples assayed in the same study.[19] This provides further evidence suggesting that pathogenesis of hyalinizing trabecular tumor may be different from papillary thyroid carcinoma, at least from its most common variants.

CLINICAL PRESENTATION AND IMAGING

Hyalinizing trabecular tumor typically presents as a palpable thyroid nodule discovered during routine physical examination or incidentally by a patient. Small tumors may be found after surgery in a gland affected by multinodular goiter or removed because of a larger neoplastic or hyperplastic nodule. Patients are typically

Table 9.1

Microscopic Features of Hyalinizing Trabecular Tumor

Encapsulation:	Well circumscribed or encapsulated
Capsular/vascular invasion:	Absent
Architecture:	Trabecular, nested
Intratrabecular hyalinization:	Prominent*
Intertrabecular stroma:	Scant or more abundant, vascular
Cell arrangement:	Perpendicular to axis of trabecula
Cell shape:	Elongated, fusiform, polygonal
Cytoplasm:	Abundant, contains yellow bodies
Nuclei:	Oval or elongated with irregular contours, finely dispersed chromatin; common nuclear grooves and pseudoinclusions

*Can be highlighted by D-PAS stain.

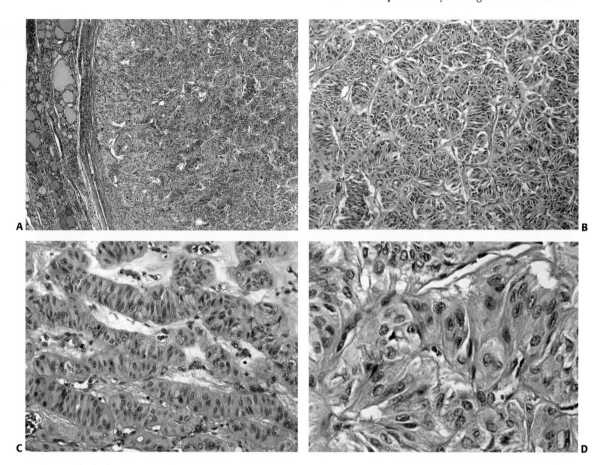

FIGURE 9.2. This hyalinizing trabecular tumor shows a thin capsule **(A)** and a trabecular architecture **(B)** with cells inserted perpendicular to the ace of a trabecula **(C)**. High-power view shows spindle, fusiform cells with oval shape nuclei containing multiple nuclear grooves **(D)**.

euthyroid. The nodule is usually "cold" on a radioactive scan. On ultrasound, the tumor is typically seen as a well-defined solid nodule of oval to round shape, either hypoechoic or with heterogeneous echogenicity, and with no microcalcifications.[18]

 ## GROSS FEATURES

The tumor is typically well circumscribed and may be encapsulated. The cut surface is solid or vaguely lobulated, yellow-tan or light-tan in color (Fig. 9.1). The size of the tumor varies from very small (0.3 to 0.5 cm) to large (5 to 7 cm) and is typically <3 cm.

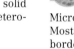 ## MICROSCOPIC FEATURES

Microscopic features of this tumor are summarized in Table 9.1.[27] Most tumors are well circumscribed with a smooth, pushing border but are not encapsulated (Fig. 9.2).[16] A fibrous capsule is seen in some tumors and can be thin or thick. No tumor capsule invasion or blood vessel invasion is noted.

The tumor typically shows a prominent trabecular pattern with straight or curvilinear bands of tumor cells two to four cells thick (Fig. 9.2). The cells and nuclei are frequently seen oriented perpendicular to the ace of a trabecula. In some tumors, a nested (alveolar and lobular) pattern is more pronounced (Fig. 9.3). The

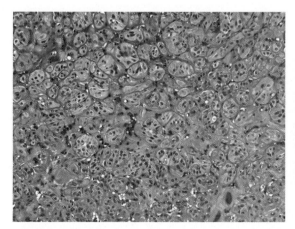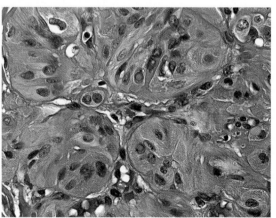

FIGURE 9.3. Hyalinizing trabecular tumor with a nested growth pattern. High-power view **(right)** shows polygonal cells with abundant cytoplasm and frequent intranuclear pseudoinclusions that are surrounded by a rim of nuclear membrane and stain densely eosinophilic, similar to the cytoplasm.

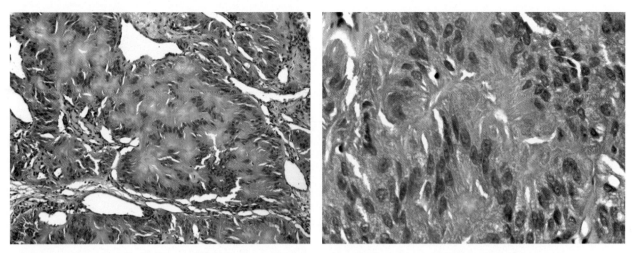

FIGURE 9.4. Depositions of a hyaline material in the center of cell nests with palisading of the surrounding cells nuclei.

intratrabecular stroma shows abundant homogeneous eosinophilic material of hyaline appearance (Fig. 9.4), which has yielded the tumor name. The hyalinization is more prominent at the peripheral zones of the trabeculae, although it may also be seen in the center of trabeculae and cell nests. This pattern of hyalinization should be distinguished from intertrabecular hyalinization, which is seen in various thyroid lesions and is a result of degenerative change. The hyaline material is highlighted by PAS stain and is diastase resistant. Small follicular spaces may be seen, and colloid formation is minimal or not found.

The cells are of medium to large size, elongated and may have polygonal, oval, spindled, or fusiform shapes (Figs. 9.2 to 9.5). The cytoplasm is abundant, eosinophilic or pale eosinophilic, amphophilic, or clear. It has a homogeneous, glassy or more granular texture. Distinct refractile yellow bodies are found in the cytoplasm, commonly in a perinuclear location (Fig. 9.5).[28]

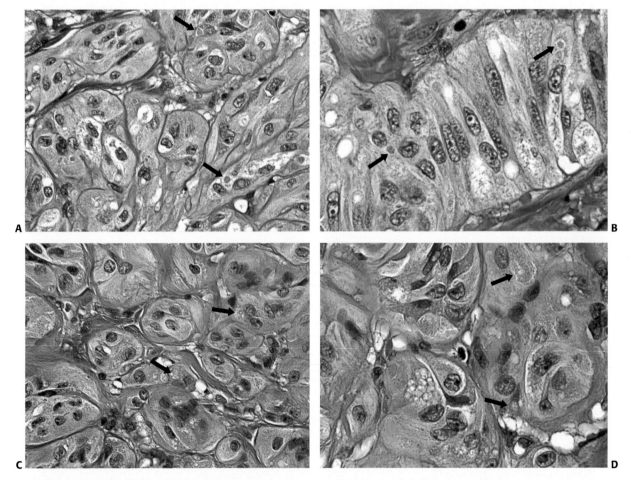

FIGURE 9.5. Yellow bodies in hyalinizing trabecular tumor. A, B: This tumor shows multiple homogeneous, smooth-contours bodies ranging in color from golden yellow to pink-yellow (*arrows*). Also note perinucleolar clearing in some cells **(B). C, D:** In this tumor, the bodies are pale yellow, crenated, and have granular and vesicular texture (*arrows*).

They are up to 5 μm in size, crenated or smooth-contoured, with homogeneous or granular texture. Their color is more often pale yellow, and may also be golden yellow, yellow-pink, or very pale. These bodies may be surrounded by a zone of cytoplasm clearing. They appear to be composed of glycosaminoglycans, proteoglycans, and lipids, and based on their ultrastructural characteristics are probably giant lysosomes.[28] Yellow bodies are found in most tumors; in one-third of cases, they are present in abundance and are easily identifiable in each tumor field, and in two-thirds of cases, they are less abundant and are found with difficulty.[28] These structures are characteristic of hyalinizing trabecular tumor but are not specific for it and are also found in other thyroid lesions such as follicular adenomas.[28]

The nuclei are round to oval, frequently elongated, and frequently have irregular contours (Fig. 9.5). The chromatin is finely dispersed. The nucleoli are of medium size, frequently with a zone of perinucleolar clearing. Intranuclear grooves and pseudoinclusion are common. These intranuclear formations are characteristically seen in papillary carcinoma nuclei and have a similar origin in both tumor types, that is, they reflect the irregularity of nuclear contours and are formed by invagination of the nuclear membrane with formation of a single deep fold (a groove) or a more round body filled with cytoplasmic material (a pseudoinclusion) (also see Chapter 11). Mitotic figures are rare, typically <1 per 10 high power fields.[19]

In addition to the accumulation of hyaline material within trabecular spaces or tumor nests, various amounts of stroma located between trabeculae or nests may be seen. The intertrabecular stroma is usually not prominent and contains capillary blood vessels surrounded by delicate fibrous bands. Some tumors may show more abundant perivascular fibrous or hyalinized stroma. Scattered calcifications are frequently seen, whereas stromal concentric lamination that meets the diagnostic criteria for psammoma bodies are less common and can be seen in about 20% of cases.[19]

The adjacent thyroid parenchyma frequently shows changes of chronic lymphocytic (Hashimoto) thyroiditis, hyperplastic nodules, or follicular adenomas with typical appearance. Concurrent papillary carcinoma is found in 5% of cases.[16]

CYTOCHEMISTRY AND IMMUNOHISTOCHEMISTRY

The hyaline material shows strong positivity for PAS and is diastase resistant. It is negative for amyloid by Congo red stain. By immunohistochemistry, it is reactive for type IV collagen and laminin.[29,30]

The tumor cells are strongly positive for thyroglobulin, thyroid transcription factor-1 (TTF1), and low molecular weight cytokeratins (Fig. 9.6A,B). The cells are uniformly negative for calcitonin and calcitonin-gene related peptide. They may show faint staining for neuron-specific enolase. Some authors reported immunoreactivity for chromogranin,[29] but in most studies this stain is negative. These tumors show an unusual pattern of immunoreactivity with the MIB-1 monoclonal antibody to Ki-67.[31] A membranous and peripheral cytoplasmic staining pattern (Fig. 9.6C) (as

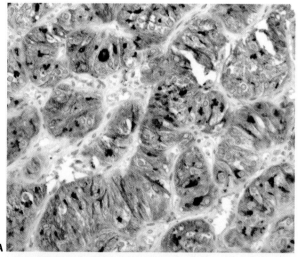

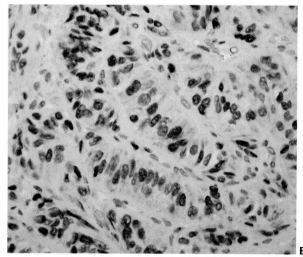

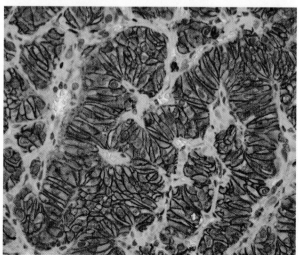

FIGURE 9.6. Immunohistochemical profile of hyalinizing trabecular tumor. Positive cytoplasmic and colloidal staining for thyroglobulin **(A)**, nuclear staining for TTF1 **(B)**, and membranous and peripheral cytoplasmic staining for MIB-1 **(C)**.

opposed to expected nuclear staining in other tissues) is seen only with MIB-1 antibody and not with other antibodies against Ki-67, and only when staining is performed at room temperature.[32] This staining pattern can also be seen in cytology aspirates from hyalinizing trabecular tumor.[33]

Reports on immunoreactivity for high molecular weight keratins and cytokeratin 19 are conflicting, with different studies reporting frequent,[34] occasional,[35] or consistently negative[30,36,37] staining with one or both of these antibodies. Galectin-3 reactivity has been reported in some but not all tumors.[38,39] HBME-1 staining is typically negative in hyalinizing trabecular tumors as opposed to positive staining in papillary carcinomas.[30,36]

MOLECULAR DIAGNOSTICS

As discussed above, it remains unclear whether *clonal RET/PTC* rearrangements are common in these tumors. Until this issue is resolved, *RET/PTC* status cannot be used as a diagnostic marker for hyalinizing trabecular tumor or to distinguish it from papillary carcinoma. The finding of a *BRAF* or *RAS* point mutation would offer evidence against hyalinizing trabecular tumor, as these mutations are rarely found in this tumor.[17-19,22-24]

ULTRASTRUCTURAL FEATURES

The ultrastructural examination reveals nests and cords of cells surrounded by a basal lamina and forming small lumens with protruding short microvilli (Fig. 9.7).[1] Lumpy accumulation of basement membrane material may be seen surrounding the tumor cell nests, and it corresponds to the deposits of hyaline material seen by light microscopy.[29,40] Fine cytoplasmic processes of tumor cells may be seen extending into the hyaline mass.[30] Usual organelles are present, including mitochondria, rough endoplasmic reticulum, lysosomes, and phagolysosomes. Some cells show bundles of intermediate filaments in the cytoplasm (Fig. 9.8A,B).[4,41] In addition, large membrane-bound structures, probably representing giant lysosomes, can be found.[28] They apparently correspond to yellow bodies seen by light microscopy. These structures contain vacuoles, granular material of different electron density, and regularly stacked membranes or "fingerprint" bodies as they were described by Rothenberg et al.[28] (Fig. 9.8C,D). The nuclei have irregular contours with multiple indentations and nicks and show intranuclear grooves and pseudoinclusions (Fig. 9.8B).

CYTOLOGIC FEATURES

The aspirated cytology specimens are typically moderately cellular to cellular and have a bloody background.[1,42,43] Cohesive clusters of cells with abundant cytoplasm are seen, frequently in association with dense homogeneous stromal material (Fig. 9.9). This hyaline material may be seen as irregularly shaped deposits located between cells or more round, centrally located aggregates with radially oriented surrounding cells. The nuclei have a round to elongated shape, with evenly dispersed chromatin and frequent nuclear pseudoinclusions and grooves. Cytoplasmic bodies, which correspond to yellow bodies of histologic sections, may be seen as green (Papanicolaou stain) or pink (Diff-Quik stain) color cytoplasmic structures.[44] Psammoma bodies and other calcifications may be found. The finding of the amorphous material resembling amyloid or dense colloid and cell nuclei with abundant grooves and pseudoinclusions makes it difficult to differentiate

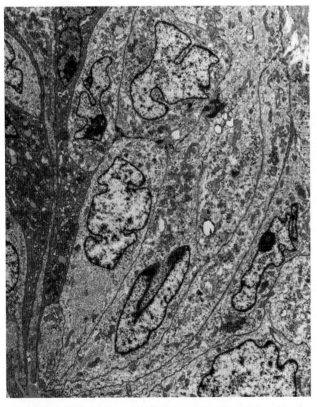
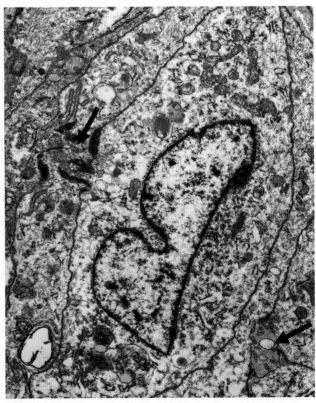

FIGURE 9.7. Ultramicroscopic features of hyalinizing trabecular tumor. *Left:* A nest of elongated, fusiform cells with irregularly shaped nuclei. ***Right:*** Small lumens are formed between cells with associated tight junctions *(arrows)*. Short microvolli protruding into the lumens are seen. (Images courtesy of Dr. J Aidan Carney, Mayo Clinic, Rochester, MN.)

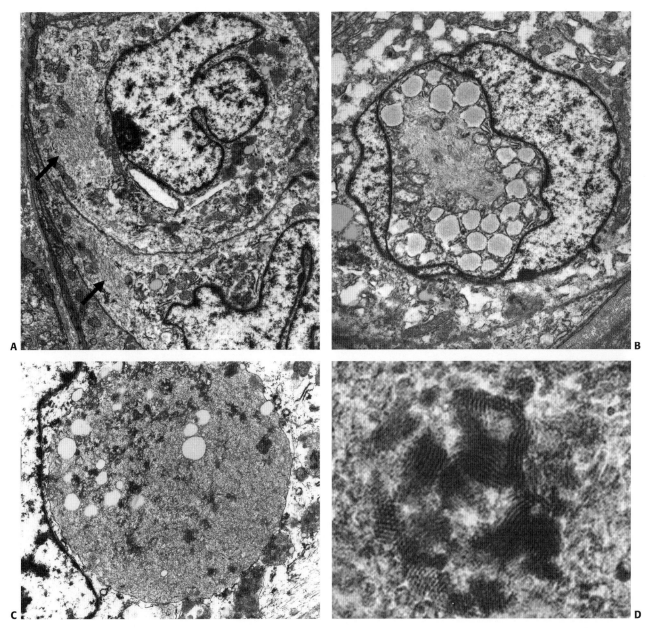

FIGURE 9.8. Ultramicroscopic features of hyalinizing trabecular tumor. A: Accumulation of cytoplasmic microfilaments (*arrows*). **B:** A nucleus with large intranuclear pseudoinclusion that is rimmed by nuclear membrane and contains cytoplasmic organelles and microfilaments. **C:** A perinuclear, membrane-bound structure probably representing a giant lysosome, which corresponds to a yellow body seen on light microscopy. It contains vacuoles and material of various electron densities, as well as substructures composed of regularly stacked membranes and forming "fingerprint bodies," which are shown on the higher magnification image from a different field in panel **D**. (Images courtesy of Dr. J Aidan Carney, Mayo Clinic, Rochester, MN.)

this tumor cytologically from papillary carcinoma and medullary carcinoma.[18,45]

 DIFFERENTIAL DIAGNOSIS

The differential diagnosis of hyalinizing trabecular tumor includes papillary carcinoma, follicular adenoma, medullary carcinoma, and paraganglioma. Papillary carcinoma has to be excluded because of the overlapping nuclear features. However, extensive stromal hyalinization, particularly intratrabecular hyalinization, is rare in papillary carcinomas, even in those with trabecular and nested architecture. The presence of a papillary growth pattern, significant amount of colloid, more than occasional stromal psammoma bodies (as opposed to calcified intraluminal colloid), or invasive growth in a setting of a tumor with abundant nuclear grooves and pseudoinclusions favors the diagnosis of a papillary carcinoma. A membranous and cytoplasmic pattern of immunoreactivity with MIB-1 antibody and lack of HBME-1 and galectin-3 staining would favor hyalinizing trabecular tumor. Molecular detection of *BRAF* mutation is virtually diagnostic of papillary carcinoma, and finding of *RAS* mutations argues strongly against the diagnosis of hyalinizing trabecular tumor.

Separation from follicular adenoma is based on the distinct pattern of hyalinization, oval and spindle cell and nuclei, and common nuclear grooves and pseudoinclusions. Medullary

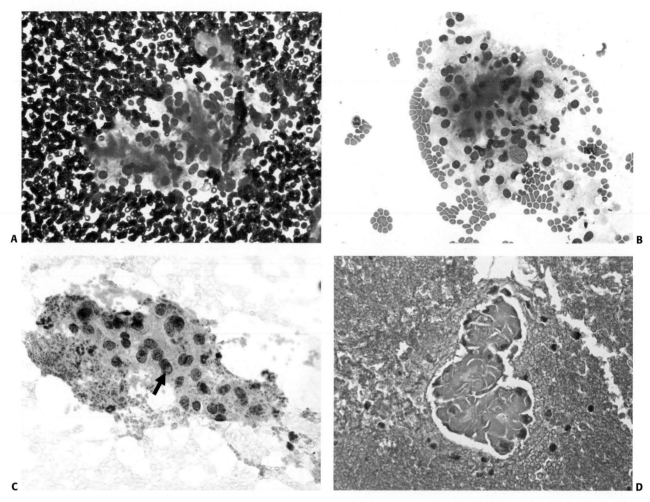

FIGURE 9.9. Cytologic features of hyalinizing trabecular tumor. A: Two clusters of neoplastic cells show irregular aggregates of dense pink hyaline material. **B:** A round-shape deposit of hyaline material in the center of a cell cluster. (**A, B:** Diff-Quik stain). **C:** A cluster of cells with round to oval nuclei, evenly dispersed chromatin, and nuclear pseudoinclusion *(arrow)* (Papanicolaou stain). **D:** Cell block section showing an aggregate of polygonal cells associated with hyaline material (Hematoxylin and Eosin stain).

thyroid carcinoma is an invasive tumor that produces amyloid and demonstrates calcitonin and CEA immunoreactivity, and is negative for thyroglobulin.

Primary thyroid paraganglioma is an exceedingly rare tumor that is difficult to separate on the basis of histology. However, immunohistochemistry provides sufficient help, as hyalinizing trabecular tumor is positive for thyroglobulin and cytokeratin and typically negative for synaptophysin or chromogranin and S-100, and the pattern of staining is reversed in paraganglioma.

 TREATMENT AND PROGNOSIS

The malignant potential of hyalinizing trabecular tumor is extremely low. In a series of 112 patients, 83 of whom were followed for >5 years and 46 for >10 years, no tumor recurrence or metastases was observed in 111 patients, whereas one patient developed pulmonary metastases.[16] The latter patient had a 3-cm tumor with grossly identifiable capsular invasion and microscopically detectable capsular and vascular invasion at presentation. Therefore, one can conclude that noninvasive hyalinizing trabecular tumors have extremely low risk of recurrence or metastasis when completely excised. Therefore, surgical excision of the tumor is expected to be curative, even if only a lobectomy was performed. In fact, in the above discussed analysis of 112

patients, half of them underwent simple lobectomy.[16] Therefore, the prognosis is excellent.

REFERENCES

1. Carney JA, Ryan J, Goellner JR. Hyalinizing trabecular adenoma of the thyroid gland. *Am J Surg Pathol.* 1987;11:583–591.
2. Carney JA. Hyalinizing trabecular tumors of the thyroid gland: quadruply described but not by the discoverer. *Am J Surg Pathol.* 2008;32:622–634.
3. Bronner MP, LiVolsi VA, Jennings TA. Plat: paraganglioma-like adenomas of the thyroid. *Surg Pathol.* 1988;1:383–389.
4. Sambade C, Franssila K, Cameselle-Teijeiro J, et al. Hyalinizing trabecular adenoma: a misnomer for a peculiar tumor of the thyroid gland. *Endocr Pathol.* 1991;2:83–91.
5. Gonzalez-Campora R, Fuentes-Vaamonde E, Hevia-Vazquez A, et al. Hyalinizing trabecular carcinoma of the thyroid gland: report of two cases of follicular cell thyroid carcinoma with hyalinizing trabecular pattern. *Ultrastruct Pathol.* 1998;22:39–46.
6. McCluggage WG, Sloan JM. Hyalinizing trabecular carcinoma of thyroid gland. *Histopathology.* 1996;28:357–362.
7. Molberg K, Albores-Saavedra J. Hyalinizing trabecular carcinoma of the thyroid gland. *Hum Pathol.* 1994;25:192–197.
8. Rosai J, Carcangiu ML, DeLellis RA. *Tumors of the Thyroid.* Washington, DC: AFIP; 1992.
9. Gowrishankar S, Pai SA, Carney JA. Hyalinizing trabecular carcinoma of the thyroid gland. *Histopathology.* 2008;52:529–531.
10. Cheung CC, Boerner SL, MacMillan CM, et al. Hyalinizing trabecular tumor of the thyroid: a variant of papillary carcinoma proved by molecular genetics. *Am J Surg Pathol.* 2000;24:1622–1626.

11. Papotti M, Volante M, Giuliano A, et al. Ret/ptc activation in hyalinizing trabecular tumors of the thyroid. *Am J Surg Pathol.* 2000;24:1615–1621.
12. Lloyd RV. Hyalinizing trabecular tumors of the thyroid: a variant of papillary carcinoma? *Adv Anat Pathol.* 2002;9:7–11.
13. Nikiforov YE. Molecular diagnostics of thyroid tumors. *Arch Pathol Lab Med.* 2011;135:569–577.
14. Zhu Z, Ciampi R, Nikiforova MN, et al. Prevalence of ret/ptc rearrangements in thyroid papillary carcinomas: effects of the detection methods and genetic heterogeneity. *J Clin Endocrinol Metab.* 2006;91:3603–3610.
15. DeLellis RA, Lloyd RV, Heitz PU, et al. *World Health Organization Classification of Tumours: Pathology and Genetics of Tumours of Endocrine Organs.* Lyon, France: IARC Press; 2004
16. Carney JA, Hirokawa M, Lloyd RV, et al. Hyalinizing trabecular tumors of the thyroid gland are almost all benign. *Am J Surg Pathol.* 2008;32:1877–1889.
17. Kim T, Oh YL, Kim KM, et al. Diagnostic dilemmas of hyalinizing trabecular tumours on fine needle aspiration cytology: a study of seven cases with BRAF mutation analysis. *Cytopathology.* 2011; 22:407–413.
18. Lee S, Han BK, Ko EY, et al. The ultrasonography features of hyalinizing trabecular tumor of the thyroid are more consistent with its benign behavior than cytology or frozen section readings. *Thyroid.* 2011;21:253–259.
19. Sheu SY, Vogel E, Worm K, et al. Hyalinizing trabecular tumour of the thyroid-differential expression of distinct mirnas compared with papillary thyroid carcinoma. *Histopathology.* 2010;56:632–640.
20. Harach HR, Soubeyran I, Brown A, et al. Thyroid pathologic findings in patients with Cowden disease. *Ann Diagn Pathol.* 1999;3:331–340.
21. Harach HR, Lesueur F, Amati P, et al. Histology of familial thyroid tumours linked to a gene mapping to chromosome 19p13.2. *J Pathol.* 1999;189:387–393.
22. Salvatore G, Chiappetta G, Nikiforov YE, et al. Molecular profile of hyalinizing trabecular tumours of the thyroid: high prevalence of ret/ptc rearrangements and absence of b-raf and n-ras point mutations. *Eur J Cancer.* 2005;41:816–821.
23. Nakamura N, Carney JA, Jin L, et al. Rassf1a and nore1a methylation and brafv600e mutations in thyroid tumors. *Lab Invest.* 2005;85:1065–1075.
24. Baloch ZW, Puttaswamy K, Brose M, et al. Lack of braf mutations in hyalinizing trabecular neoplasm. *Cytojournal.* 2006;3:17.
25. Kang SW, Hong SW, Yeon PJ, et al. A case of black thyroid associated with hyalinizing trabecular tumor. *Endocr J.* 2008;55:1109–1112.
26. Capella G, Matias-Guiu X, Ampudia X, et al. Ras oncogene mutations in thyroid tumors: polymerase chain reaction-restriction-fragment-length polymorphism analysis from paraffin-embedded tissues. *Diagn Mol Pathol.* 1996;5:45–52.
27. Nose V, Volante M, Papotti M. Hyalinizing trabecular tumor of the thyroid: an update. *Endocr Pathol.* 2008;19:1–8.
28. Rothenberg HJ, Goellner JR, Carney JA. Hyalinizing trabecular adenoma of the thyroid gland: recognition and characterization of its cytoplasmic yellow body. *Am J Surg Pathol.* 1999;23:118–125.
29. Katoh R, Jasani B, Williams ED. Hyalinizing trabecular adenoma of the thyroid. A report of three cases with immunohistochemical and ultrastructural studies. *Histopathology.* 1989;15:211–224.
30. Ohtsuki Y, Kimura M, Murao S, et al. Immunohistochemical and electron microscopy studies of a case of hyalinizing trabecular tumor of the thyroid gland, with special consideration of the hyalinizing mass associated with it. *Med Mol Morphol.* 2009;42:189–194.
31. Hirokawa M, Carney JA. Cell membrane and cytoplasmic staining for mib-1 in hyalinizing trabecular adenoma of the thyroid gland. *Am J Surg Pathol.* 2000;24:575–578.
32. Leonardo E, Volante M, Barbareschi M, et al. Cell membrane reactivity of mib-1 antibody to ki67 in human tumors: fact or artifact? *Appl Immunohistochem Mol Morphol.* 2007;15:220–223.
33. Casey MB, Sebo TJ, Carney JA. Hyalinizing trabecular adenoma of the thyroid gland identification through mib-1 staining of fine-needle aspiration biopsy smears. *Am J Clin Pathol.* 2004;122:506–510.
34. Fonseca E, Nesland JM, Sobrinho-Simoes M. Expression of stratified epithelial-type cytokeratins in hyalinizing trabecular adenomas supports their relationship with papillary carcinomas of the thyroid. *Histopathology.* 1997;31:330–335.
35. Papotti M, Riella P, Montemurro F, et al. Immunophenotypic heterogeneity of hyalinizing trabecular tumours of the thyroid. *Histopathology.* 1997;31:525–533.
36. Galgano MT, Mills SE, Stelow EB. Hyalinizing trabecular adenoma of the thyroid revisited: a histologic and immunohistochemical study of thyroid lesions with prominent trabecular architecture and sclerosis. *Am J Surg Pathol.* 2006;30:1269–1273.
37. Hirokawa M, Carney JA, Ohtsuki Y. Hyalinizing trabecular adenoma and papillary carcinoma of the thyroid gland express different cytokeratin patterns. *Am J Surg Pathol.* 2000;24:877–881.
38. Gaffney RL, Carney JA, Sebo TJ, et al. Galectin-3 expression in hyalinizing trabecular tumors of the thyroid gland. *Am J Surg Pathol.* 2003;27:494–498.
39. Caraci P, Fulcheri A, Ondolo C, et al. Hyalinizing trabecular tumor of the thyroid: a case report. *Head Neck Pathol.* 2011;5:423–427.
40. Katoh R, Kakudo K, Kawaoi A. Accumulated basement membrane material in hyalinizing trabecular tumors of the thyroid. *Mod Pathol.* 1999;12:1057–1061.
41. Katoh R, Muramatsu A, Kawaoi A, et al. Alteration of the basement membrane in human thyroid diseases: an immunohistochemical study of type iv collagen, laminin and heparan sulphate proteoglycan. *Virchows Arch A Pathol Anat Histopathol.* 1993;423:417–424.
42. LiVolsi VA, Gupta PK. Thyroid fine-needle aspiration: intranuclear inclusions, nuclear grooves and psammoma bodies—paraganglioma-like adenoma of the thyroid. *Diagn Cytopathol.* 1992;8:82–83; discussion 83–84.
43. Kuma S, Hirokawa M, Miyauchi A, et al. Cytologic features of hyalinizing trabecular adenoma of the thyroid. *Acta Cytol.* 2003;47:399–404.
44. Casey MB, Sebo TJ, Carney JA. Hyalinizing trabecular adenoma of the thyroid gland: cytologic features in 29 cases. *Am J Surg Pathol.* 2004;28:859–867.
45. Bishop JA, Ali SZ. Hyalinizing trabecular adenoma of the thyroid gland. *Diagn Cytopathol.* 2011;39:306–310.

CHAPTER 10

Yuri E. Nikiforov and N. Paul Ohori

Follicular Carcinoma

DEFINITION

Follicular carcinoma is a malignant well-differentiated tumor of thyroid follicular cells that lacks the diagnostic nuclear features of papillary carcinoma. When used without additional qualifiers, this term typically refers to the conventional type of follicular carcinoma. Oncocytic (Hürthle cell) follicular carcinoma represents the main histopathologic variant of follicular carcinoma.

INCIDENCE AND EPIDEMIOLOGY

Follicular carcinoma is the second most common type of thyroid cancer after papillary carcinoma. The data collected over the past 20 to 30 years indicate that follicular carcinoma, when combining both the conventional type and oncocytic variant, accounts for approximately 15% of all thyroid cancer cases.[1] In recent years, this number has decreased to 10% and even lower.[1,2] Several reasons are likely to be responsible for this trend. First, the incidence of thyroid papillary cancer has been on a rise in many countries around the world; it has practically tripled in the United States over the past 30 years, making the frequency of follicular carcinoma proportionally smaller.[1] Second, as described in the next section, a higher incidence of follicular carcinoma is associated with dietary iodine deficiency. Severe iodine deficiency has been largely eliminated or diminished by widespread iodization of salt and other food supplies. Third, in the late 1980s to early 1990s, diagnostic histopathologic criteria for the follicular variant of papillary carcinoma became better recognized. As a result, many follicular-pattern carcinomas that would be previously diagnosed as follicular carcinomas are now classified as papillary carcinoma.[2,3]

The absolute incidence of follicular carcinoma has not changed significantly during the last several decades.[1,4,5] On the basis of the Surveillance, Epidemiology and End Results (SEER) database, the annual incidence in the United States during the time interval between 1973 and 2008 remained at 0.8 to 1.1 per 100,000 persons per year.[1]

Most follicular carcinomas are tumors of conventional type, and 25% to 30% are of oncocytic type.[1,6,7] Females are more commonly affected than males, with a gender ratio of approximately 2.5:1 for conventional and oncocytic types of follicular carcinomas based on the SEER database.[1] Some studies have found a slightly lower female predominance among oncocytic carcinomas (1.7:1).[7,8] These tumors are rare in children. Their incidence increases with age, reaching a peak during the fifth decade of life for conventional follicular carcinomas (Fig.10.1). For oncocytic tumors, the incidence continues to climb beyond the fifth decade of life. In fact, more than half of oncocytic follicular carcinomas are diagnosed in patients older than 60 years.[8]

ETIOLOGIC FACTORS

Etiologic factors implicated in the development of this tumor are summarized in Table 10.1. Most follicular carcinomas show no familial occurrence and occur as sporadic tumors. Two environmental factors implicated in the etiology of this disease are iodine deficiency and exposure to ionizing radiation. Residing in areas of low-dietary iodine intake is associated with an up to 2- to 3-fold increase in risk when compared with areas of sufficient iodine consumption.[9–11] Active iodine supplementation in the regions of severe iodine deficiency has resulted in a significant decrease of follicular carcinoma incidence, which provides additional

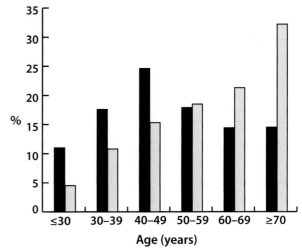

FIGURE 10.1. Age distribution of patients with conventional type follicular carcinoma *(black bars)* and oncocytic follicular carcinoma *(gray bars).* Based on the data reported by Hundahl SA, Cady B, Cunningham MP, et al. Initial results from a prospective cohort study of 5583 cases of thyroid carcinoma treated in the United States during 1996. U.S. and German Thyroid Cancer Study Group. An American College of Surgeons Commission on Cancer Patient Care Evaluation study. *Cancer.* 2000;89:202–217.

Table 10.1
Etiologic Factors for Thyroid Follicular Carcinomas

- Iodine deficiency
- Radiation exposure
- Preexisting benign thyroid disease
  - Solitary nodule
  - Goiter
- Familial syndromes
  - PHTS (including Cowden syndrome)
  - Werner syndrome
  - Carney complex

PHTS: PTEN hamartoma tumor syndrome.

evidence for this etiologic factor.[12,13] Low-iodine diet is associated with the increased thyroid-stimulating hormone (TSH) stimulation and development of thyroid hyperplasia in a form of endemic goiter, both of which are likely to be involved in promoting follicular carcinogenesis. A low-iodine diet administered to laboratory animals produces thyroid hyperplasia and nodular disease, followed by carcinoma development in some animals, simulating the disease progression in humans.[14,15]

Exposure to ionizing radiation is associated with predisposition to follicular carcinoma, although the risk is not as high as it is for papillary carcinoma. Cumulative analysis of several irradiated cohorts has demonstrated the relative risk of 5.2 for radiation-induced follicular carcinoma, about half the risk for papillary cancer.[16] In the United States, a history of radiation exposure is found in approximately 4% of follicular carcinoma patients.[8]

Preexisting benign thyroid disease is a well-established risk factor for follicular carcinoma and is identified in approximately 15% of patients.[8] Benign thyroid nodules/adenomas confer a higher risk as compared with nontoxic goiter (relative risk 60 to 70 vs. 7 to 8).[17,18] The risk is highest during the first 2 years after diagnosis of a benign thyroid disease, and it persists for >10 years. Preexisting benign thyroid disease may affect the incidence of carcinomas in several ways. Follicular adenoma may serve as a direct precursor lesion for follicular carcinoma. This has been directly demonstrated in mice lacking the *PTEN* gene function,[19] and further evidence for the follicular adenoma to follicular carcinoma progression is discussed later in the chapter. Goiter may predispose to follicular carcinoma by increasing the rate of cell proliferation owing to prolonged TSH stimulation, which enhances the chance for mutations in dividing cells.[20] This is supported by more common occurrence of follicular carcinomas than papillary carcinomas in patients with dyshormonogenetic goiter.[21,22] This condition is caused by an inherited defect in thyroid hormone production that leads to highly elevated TSH levels and marked thyroid hyperplasia. In addition, experimental animals with chronically increased TSH levels caused by antithyroid drugs develop thyroid hyperplasia, adenomas, and carcinomas, and cancer formation is enhanced by additional treatment with a mutagen.[23,24] Chronic TSH stimulation apparently provides a "fertile ground" for mutagenesis to occur, but it is likely not a mutagen by itself and relies on other genotoxic events, such as radiation or chemicals, to produce a mutation that would initiate the carcinogenesis.[20]

The role of hormonal and reproductive factors is not fully understood, despite a significant female predominance among patients with follicular carcinomas. A pooled analysis of 14 case–control studies revealed an increased relative risk of follicular carcinoma in women with artificially induced menopause and in those who miscarried during their first pregnancy, although no specific association with estrogens was found.[25] More recently, it has been shown experimentally that circulating estrogens were directly responsible for the increased proliferation rate of thyroid cells in mice that developed thyroid follicular carcinomas as a result of loss of function of the *PTEN* gene.[19] These data provide strong evidence for the role of estrogens in thyroid follicular carcinogenesis in a setting of *PTEN* loss, although it remains unclear whether this influence remains in human thyroid cells and when *PTEN* function is preserved.

Familial forms of follicular carcinoma are rare. Some are found in patients with PHTS, which encompasses Cowden syndrome, Bannayan–Riley–Ruvalcaba syndrome, and other rare syndromes caused by a germ line mutation of the *PTEN* gene located on chromosome 10q23.31. Cowden syndrome is characterized by multiple mucocutaneous hamartomas and a predisposition to malignant tumors, mostly of breast and thyroid. Thyroid lesions are seen in two-thirds of the affected patients, with 10% to 20% developing follicular carcinomas.[26–28] Thyroid glands from patients affected by this syndrome have characteristic microscopic appearance discussed later in the chapter. Follicular carcinoma may also arise as a manifestation of Werner syndrome. This

rare autosomal recessive disease is caused by germ line mutations in the *WRN* gene on chromosome 8p11-12. It is characterized by premature aging and a higher rate of various malignant tumors. On the basis of a large cohort of Japanese patients affected by this disease, thyroid cancer occurs in approximately 3% of these patients and is typically a follicular carcinoma.[29] Thyroid tumors in patients with Werner syndrome manifest at a younger age when compared with the general population and have a lower female to male ratio. Follicular carcinoma may be a rare manifestation of the Carney complex, an autosomal dominant disorder caused by germ line mutations in *PRKARIA* and other genes and characterized by spotty skin pigmentations, myxomatosis, and other endocrine and nonendocrine tumors.[30,31] Isolated familial follicular carcinomas, that is, tumors that are not a part of the known cancer syndromes, are very uncommon. Only few families with isolated conventional or oncocytic follicular carcinoma have been reported.[32] In the United States, a family history of thyroid carcinoma (follicular or papillary) is found in 3.7% of patients diagnosed with conventional follicular carcinoma and in 2% of those diagnosed with oncocytic carcinoma.[8]

PATHOGENESIS AND MOLECULAR GENETICS

Cytogenetic Abnormalities

Clonal chromosomal changes are detected by conventional cytogenetics in approximately 60% of follicular carcinomas.[33] They manifest either as chromosome copy number change or as structural chromosomal abnormalities, such as translocations. Numerical chromosomal changes involve loss and/or gain of whole chromosomes or chromosome arms. Most common are gains of chromosome 7 and losses of chromosomes 8, 11, 17, and 18.[33–37] Losses of chromosome arms most frequently affect 3p, 11q, and 13q. Recurrent chromosomal translocations are also found, and those tumors rarely show numerical chromosome changes. A t(2;3) (q13;p25) translocation is known to produce the *PAX8/PPARγ* fusion.[38,39] Single cases of tumors with other translocations involving 3p25, such as t(3;7)(p25;q34) and t(1;3)(p13;p25), have been described.[38,40] More recently, a tumor with t(3;7)(p25;q34) was found to have another type of *PPARγ* fusion, *CREB3L2/PPARγ*[41] Follicular carcinomas with t(7;18)(p15;q24) and t(6;7)(q16;p15) have been reported, suggesting the presence of an important gene on 7p15.[33,34]

Using comparative genomic hybridization, chromosomal alterations are detected in 60% to 90% of follicular carcinomas.[37,42,43] Gains on 1q, 5p, 7p/7q, 12p/12q, and 16p and losses on 3p, 2p, and 8q are most common. Loss of the entire chromosome 22 or 22q appears to be more frequent in widely invasive tumors.[42,44] Oncocytic carcinomas more often show losses on 9q.[43,45] By fluorescent in situ hybridization (FISH), gains of chromosome 7 are seen in about half of conventional and oncocytic follicular carcinomas.[46,47] FISH can also be used for the detection of *PAX8/PPARγ* rearrangement (Fig. 10.2).[39]

DNA Ploidy

An aneuploid cell population is found in 50% to 60% of follicular carcinomas and typically correlates with multiple numerical chromosomal changes that are seen cytogenetically.[48–50] Some, but not all, studies have reported a general tendency of an increased aneuploidy rate from follicular adenomas to follicular carcinomas and from minimally invasive to widely invasive follicular carcinomas.[49–51]

Loss of Heterozygosity

Loss of heterozygosity (LOH) results from a deletion of discrete, small or large chromosomal regions. During tumorigenesis, LOH frequently affects the regions where important tumor suppressor

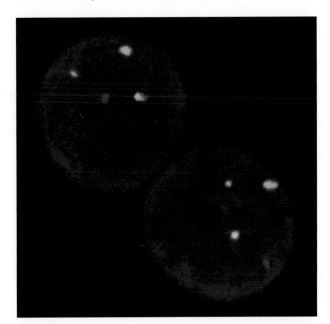

FIGURE 10.2. Detection of *PAX8/PPARγ* rearrangement in follicular carcinoma cells by FISH. Note that each cell contains one intact *PAX8* (red) and one intact *PPARγ* (green) signals, as well as two fused signal pairs corresponding to the rearrangement between the two gene probes.

genes reside. A high rate of LOH is a characteristic feature of follicular carcinomas and of the follicular tumorigenesis in general. A meta-analysis of the data reported in the literature demonstrates a 20% average rate of LOH per chromosome arm in follicular carcinoma, 6% in follicular adenoma, and only 2.5% in papillary carcinoma (Fig. 10.3).[52] The different levels of chromosome regions loss signify a fundamental difference in the pathogenesis between follicular and papillary thyroid carcinomas.

The reported data on LOH in specific chromosomal regions show high variability between individual studies owing to the difference in the locations of microsatellite markers used for each study. Regions on 2p, 3p, 10q, 11p, and 17p were found to be deleted in several studies.[36,53-56] Several of these regions harbor known tumor suppressor genes such as *VHL* on 3p25-26, *TP53* on 17p13, and *PTEN* on 10q23. Although results vary, investigators have found a higher rate of LOH in oncocytic carcinomas when compared with conventional follicular carcinomas.[53,54] LOH may more often affect the regions that are imprinted (i.e., have parent-specific expression of genes) as compared with nonimprinted regions.[57]

Somatic Mutations

The prevalence of somatic mutations found in follicular carcinoma is summarized in Table 10.2.

RAS Mutations

RAS is the most common mutation known to occur in follicular carcinomas. It is found in almost half of conventional follicular carcinomas and with lower prevalence in oncocytic carcinomas.[58-61] Point mutations involve codons 12, 13, and 61 of the three human *RAS* genes (*HRAS*, *KRAS*, and *NRAS*). The most frequently affected hot spots are *NRAS* codon 61 and *HRAS* codon 61.[60,62] These mutations stabilize the protein in its active guanosine triphosphate (GTP)-bound form, leading to constant stimulation of the downstream signaling pathways, particularly the mitogen-activated protein kinase (MAPK) and phosphatidylinositol-3-kinase (PI3K)/AKT cascades (Fig. 10.4).

RAS mutation is likely to serve as an early and initiating event in thyroid follicular carcinogenesis. However, it may not be sufficient

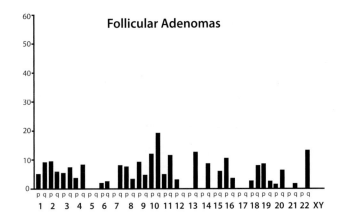

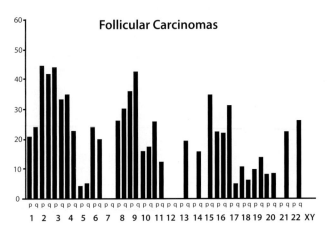

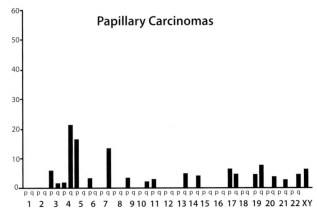

FIGURE 10.3. Rate of LOH per chromosome arm in various types of thyroid tumors. Note a sharp difference in the extent and frequency of LOH between papillary carcinoma and follicular tumors. Reproduced with permission from Ward LS, Brenta G, Medvedovic M, et al. Studies of allelic loss in thyroid tumors reveal major differences in chromosomal instability between papillary and follicular carcinomas. *J Clin Endocrinol Metab.* 1998;83:525–530. Copyright, *The Endocrine Society.*

by itself for full malignant transformation. This is supported by occurrence of this mutation not only in carcinomas but also in follicular adenomas. In experiments on cultured cells, the mutant RAS initiates self-limited cell proliferation and promotes chromosome instability, which may predispose the cells for acquiring additional mutations and a more malignant phenotype.[63,64] Expression of mutant RAS in transgenic mice leads mostly to the development of hyperplastic nodules and follicular adenomas, whereas additional loss of PTEN results in the rapid development of follicular carcinomas.[65-67]

Table 10.2

Prevalence of Somatic Mutations in Thyroid Follicular Carcinomas

Mutation Type	Conventional Type Follicular Carcinoma	Oncocytic Type Follicular Carcinoma
RAS point mutations (%)	40–50	10–15
*PAX8/PPAR*γ rearrangement (%)	30–40	0–5
PIK3CA point mutations (%)	5–10	NR
PTEN point mutations, small deletions (%)	5–10	NR
GRIM-19 point mutations (%)	0	~10

NR, not reported.

*PAX8/PPAR*γ Rearrangement and Other *PPAR*γ Fusions

*PAX8/PPAR*γ rearrangement is the second most common genetic alteration in follicular carcinoma. It is found in approximately 35% (range, 0% to 78%) of conventional follicular carcinomas and <5% of oncocytic carcinomas.[68] This rearrangement can also be seen in a small proportion (1% to 5%) of the follicular variant papillary carcinomas and in some (~8%) of follicular adenomas.[60,68–72] It is a result of the cytogenetically detectable translocation t(2;3)(q13;p25), which leads to the fusion between the *PAX8* gene on 2q13 and the *PPAR*γ gene on 3p25 (Fig. 10.2).[39] *PAX8/PPAR*γ-positive tumors tend to present in patients at a younger age and be smaller, and more often show a solid growth pattern and vascular invasion as compared with follicular carcinomas negative for this rearrangement.[60,69] Tumors with *PAX8/PPAR*γ almost never show

RAS mutations, suggesting that follicular carcinomas develop through two distinct molecular pathways, associated with either *PAX8/PPAR*γ or *RAS* mutation.[60]

The *PAX8/PPAR*γ fusion results in strong overexpression of the *PPAR*γ gene. However, the mechanisms of cell transformation induced by this rearrangement are not fully understood. Several proposed possibilities, some of which contradict each other, include inhibition of normal PPARγ function by the chimeric PAX8/PPARγ protein through a dominant negative effect, activation of normal PPARγ targets because of the overexpression of the chimeric protein that contains all functional domains of wild-type PPARγ, deregulation of PAX8 function, and activation of a set of genes unrelated to both wild-type PPARγ and wild-type PAX8 pathways.[39,73,74] Some studies that utilized experimental models have observed, in addition to the oncogenic properties, a paradoxical, tumor suppressor effect of this chimeric protein in the form of inhibition of angiogenesis.[75,76]

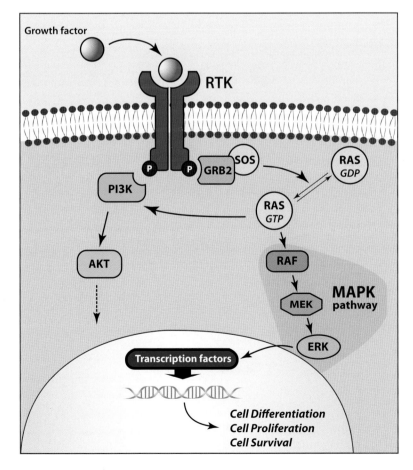

FIGURE 10.4. Molecular pathways activated by mutant RAS in thyroid cells. RAS proteins function as a molecular switch propagating signals from cell membrane receptor tyrosine kinases (RTK) to multiple cytoplasmic targets. On activation, RAS shifts from its inactive, guanosine diphosphate (GDP) bound form to the active, GTP-bound form and phosphorylates downstream cytoplasmic targets before returning to the inactive, RAS–GDP form. Point mutations stabilize the protein in its active form, leading to constitutive stimulation of the RAF–MEK–ERK pathway, also known as MAPK pathway, and PI3K/AKT pathway.

In addition to follicular carcinomas, *PAX8/PPARγ* is found in about 8% of follicular adenomas.[68] Although some interpret these data as evidence that the signaling from PAX8/PPARγ is insufficient for the development of malignancy, it is more likely that follicular adenomas positive for this rearrangement are in fact preinvasive or in situ follicular carcinomas, or tumors where invasion was overlooked or not sampled during examination. In support of this possibility, most of *PAX8/PPARγ*-positive follicular adenomas are highly cellular tumors that show a microfollicular or solid/trabecular growth pattern, have a thick capsule, and express immunohistochemical markers of malignancy such as galectin-3 and/or HBME-1.[60,71,77]

In addition to *PAX8/PPARγ*, the *PPARγ* gene can be fused to other partners. Another fusion partner is *CREB3L2*; however, this type of *PPARγ* fusion is rare and has been reported in 1 out of 42 (2.4%) follicular carcinomas in one series.[41]

PI3K/PTEN/AKT Pathway Mutations

The PI3K/PTEN/AKT signaling pathway plays an important role in the regulation of cell survival, proliferation, and migration.[78] In thyroid cancer, the activation of this pathway may be more important for the development and progression of follicular carcinomas than papillary carcinomas.[79]

In follicular carcinomas, this pathway can be chronically stimulated by activating mutation in the *RAS* or *PIK3CA* gene or by inactivating mutation in the *PTEN* gene (Fig. 10.5). The activation of this pathway induces thyroid cell proliferation and other effects, which particularly rely on the activation of the downstream mammalian target of rapamycin (mTOR) protein.[80]

The *PIK3CA* gene, which codes for a catalytic subunit (p110) of PI3K, is mutated in 6% to 13% of follicular carcinomas.[81–83] The mutations are typically located in exon 20 and exon 9 of the *PIK3CA* gene that code for the kinase domain and helical domain, respectively. In addition, *PIK3CA* gene copy number gains are found in up to 25% of follicular carcinomas.[84] However, whether the gain of several gene copies is functionally sufficient for the activation of this pathway remains unclear.

Somatic mutations of the *PTEN* tumor suppressor gene are identified in 6% to 12% of follicular carcinomas.[82,83,85] They are point mutations or small frameshift deletions that most frequently affect exons 5 and 7 of the gene. These alterations lead to a loss of function of the PTEN protein, which results in the activation of AKT, mTOR, and other downstream targets. It appears that mutations of *RAS*, *PTEN*, and *PIK3CA* are rarely found in combination in the same tumor.[82] This suggests that one of these mutations may be sufficient for the activation of the PI3K/PTEN/AKT pathway. However, the experimental studies have demonstrated that, although mice with thyroid-specific expression of mutant RAS at physiologic levels and mice with loss of PTEN do not develop follicular carcinomas, the double-mutant mice quickly develop invasive and metastatic follicular carcinomas.[67] The mice carrying both *RAS* and *PTEN* mutations show strong activation of both PI3K and MAPK signaling pathways, which was probably responsible for the accelerated follicular carcinogenesis.

Mitochondria-Related Mutations in Oncocytic Carcinomas

Oncocytic follicular carcinomas are composed of cells with distinct cytoplasmic granularity because of the accumulation of frequently abnormal mitochondria. The cause of the mitochondrial changes and their relationship to the neoplastic process are not fully understood. It is likely that they may represent either a primary change induced by a tumor initiation mutation or a secondary, phenotypic change.[2,86–88]

Mutations of the *GRIM-19* gene have been recently identified in oncocytic thyroid tumors.[89] This gene encodes a protein that regulates cell death, promotes apoptosis, and affects mitochondrial metabolism, serving as an essential component of complex I of the mitochondrial respiratory chain.[90] In one study, somatic missense mutations in *GRIM-19* were found in 1 out of 11 of oncocytic follicular carcinomas and in 2 out of 10 of oncocytic variants of

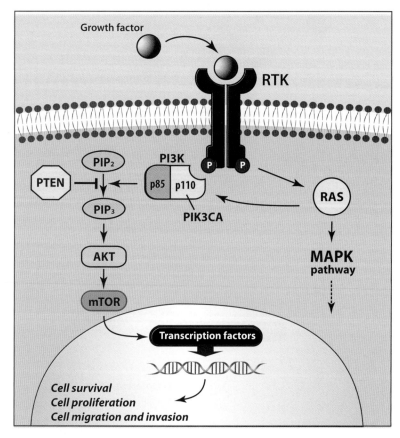

FIGURE 10.5. PI3K/PTEN/AKT signaling pathway and location of mutations in thyroid follicular carcinoma. This pathway transmits signals from cell membrane growth factor receptors (RTK), which activate PI3K directly or through RAS. AKT is activated downstream of PI3K and regulates multiple genes that oppose apoptosis and promote cell survival, proliferation, and migration/invasion. PTEN negatively regulates PI3K signaling and prevents AKT activation. PI3K consists of two subunits, one of which, p110, is coded by the *PIK3CA* gene. In thyroid follicular carcinomas, this pathway can be activated by gain-of-function mutations of *RAS* and *PIK3CA* and loss-of-function mutations of *PTEN*. PIP2, phosphatidylinositol-3,4-diphosphate; PIP3, phosphatidylinositol-3,4,5-triphosphate.

papillary carcinoma.[89] These mutations may disrupt the function of this antiapoptotic tumor suppressor gene and promote tumorigenesis. However, the prevalence of *GRIM-19* mutations in oncocytic follicular carcinomas and their role in carcinogenesis have yet to be fully established.

Mutations in mitochondrial DNA (mtDNA) are found with a high frequency in oncocytic carcinomas.[91,92] These mutations, which include deletions and frameshift and missense point mutations, predominantly affect the mitochondrial complex I genes and are predicted to disrupt the gene function. Whether they play the causative role in tumor initiation remains unclear because mtDNA generally has a high mutation rate and these mutations also occur in nonneoplastic oncocytic cells and in nononcocytic tumors.

Alterations in Gene Expression Profiles

High-density cDNA microarrays were used in several studies to identify alterations in gene expression profiles in follicular carcinomas. These studies have identified a large number of genes in which expression was dysregulated in follicular carcinomas as compared with normal thyroid tissue and with follicular adenomas.[73,93–96] Many of these genes are involved in the regulation of cellular growth and proliferation, programmed cell death, thyroid differentiation, development, and cell migration. However, there is little overlap between specific genes found to be differentially upregulated or downregulated in different studies, which makes it difficult to define the role of alteration in the expression of specific genes and follicular carcinogenesis.

PATHOGENETIC RELATIONSHIP BETWEEN FOLLICULAR ADENOMA AND FOLLICULAR CARCINOMA

The relationship between follicular adenoma and follicular carcinoma is not fully understood. Several lines of evidence suggest that these tumors are related biologic entities and point toward the existence of the adenoma to carcinoma progression.

- The two tumor types have similar histopathologic appearance in all aspects except for the presence of invasion.
- Follicular carcinomas are rarely very small. Only 3% to 8% of follicular carcinomas are ≤1 cm as opposed to 27% to 45% of papillary carcinomas.[1,4,8] This suggests that many follicular carcinomas may develop from preexisting lesions rather than arise de novo.

- Follicular carcinomas typically present at a patient age 8 to 10 years older than adenomas and are larger in size than adenomas, implying a progression over time.[26,88,97,98]
- Experimental mice carrying mutations in the *RAS*, *PTEN*, and *PRKARIA* genes develop first follicular adenomas and then develop follicular carcinomas at an older age or after additional goitrogen stimulation.[19,65,66,99,100] Similarly, dietary iodine deficiency in experimental animals leads first to follicular adenoma and after longer intervals to follicular carcinoma.[15]
- Both tumor types share similar molecular and cytogenetic alterations. Mutations of *RAS* are common, and mutations of *PTEN* and *PIK3CA* occur in both tumor types but with higher frequency in carcinomas. Chromosomal gains and losses are frequent and show similar patterns, with polysomy 7 being the most common cytogenetic change in adenomas and carcinomas. Considerable similarity in the comparative genomic hybridization (CGH) profiles also exists.[37,43] Both tumor types reveal substantial rates and similar profiles of LOH, but the overall frequency of chromosome arm loss is significantly higher in carcinomas,[52] supporting the progression.

Other data suggest that progression from adenoma to carcinoma is not a paradigm of follicular carcinogenesis.

- Balanced translocations involving chromosomal loci on 19q13 or 2p21 are common in adenomas but are exceptionally rare in carcinomas, suggesting that adenomas harboring these translocations have low potential for progression to carcinomas. Similarly, hyperfunctioning ("toxic") thyroid adenomas caused by mutations in the *TSHR* and *Gsα* genes (see Chapter 8) exceedingly rarely progress to follicular carcinoma.
- *PAX8/PPARγ* rearrangement occurs in a significant portion of follicular carcinomas but is rarely found in adenomas, suggesting that tumors with this genetic alteration develop without a preexisting stage of adenoma.

These findings provide evidence, although indirect, for the existence of three different pathways in thyroid follicular tumorigenesis (Fig. 10.6).

CLINICAL PRESENTATION AND IMAGING

Follicular carcinomas typically present as a slowly enlarging, painless, solitary thyroid nodule. Patients are usually asymptomatic, although dysphagia, hoarseness, and/or stridor may

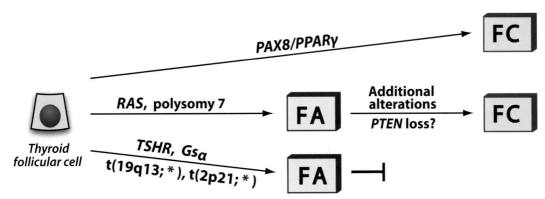

FIGURE 10.6. Putative pathways in the development of follicular tumors and progression from follicular adenoma to follicular carcinoma. Some carcinomas are likely to arise from preexisting adenomas that carry *RAS* mutation or numerical chromosomal alterations, most frequent of which is chromosome 7 polysomy. Additional alterations are likely required for malignant transformation, possibly loss of function of PTEN. Other carcinomas, such as those harboring *PAX8/PPARγ* rearrangement, may develop directly, bypassing the adenoma stage. Finally, some adenomas, such as those with translocations involving 19q13 and 2p21 and hyperfunctioning adenomas with *TSHR* and *Gsα* mutations, lack the propensity to progress to carcinomas. *These translocations involve fusions to several different partners. FC, follicular carcinoma; FA, follicular adenoma.

sometimes accompany the mass. In rare cases, the presenting symptoms are caused by distant metastases, such as bone pain or pathologic bone fracture. On physical examination, the nodule typically moves with swallowing. Nodules that are fixed to surrounding tissues raise strong suspicion for invasive malignancy. Thyroid function tests are normal. Radionuclide scans typically reveal a "cold" nodule because follicular carcinomas concentrate radioiodine or other tracers less avidly than adjacent thyroid parenchyma. Although single cases of "hot," hyperfunctioning follicular carcinomas of both conventional and oncocytic type have been described,[101-103] they are exceedingly rare. On ultrasound examination, tumors usually appear as a solid hypoechoic nodule with a peripheral halo, the latter representing the fibrous capsule (Fig. 10.7). The outlines of the nodule are well defined and smooth, unless the tumor is widely invasive. Ultrasound features do not reliably differentiate follicular carcinomas from adenomas. However, the presence of irregular, poorly defined margins, a thick irregular capsule, and chaotic intranodular blood flow on color Doppler imaging is more suggestive of carcinoma. A routine chest x-ray that includes the neck may reveal tracheal deviation and pulmonary metastases. CT and MRI can be used when invasion is suspected to better evaluate the extension of tumor into the adjacent neck structures. Fine needle aspiration (FNA) is routinely performed on solitary thyroid nodules. Because FNA cytology typically reveals a cellular aspirate suggestive of a follicular tumor, the patients are referred for surgery.

 ## GROSS FEATURES

On gross examination, follicular carcinomas typically appear as an encapsulated nodule of oval or round shape (Fig. 10.8A). Most are 2 to 4 cm in size, although they can be larger. The cut surface is solid and fleshy, and in fresh, nonfixed samples, the tumor is frequently seen bulging from the confines of the capsule. The color of the nodule is gray-white in conventional type carcinomas and brown-tan or mahogany-brown in oncocytic carcinomas. A thick fibrotic capsule frequently surrounds the tumor. A very thick capsule is more suggestive of malignancy. Invasion of the capsule is rarely found on gross examination, although it can be identified in some cases (Fig. 10.8A). Widely invasive tumors have widespread invasion through the capsule, and in some cases, no residual capsule is recognized (Fig. 10.9). Foci of hemorrhage, infarction, and other secondary changes, either spontaneous or FNA induced, may be seen.

Macroscopic evaluation of an encapsulated solitary nodule requires careful inspection of the capsule to identify areas of invasion. Unless the nodule is very large, the entire pericapsular zone should to be submitted for microscopic examination. If this is not possible, at least 10 sections from the capsule should be processed because the chance of detecting invasion progressively increases when 1 to 10 blocks are examined.[104] The details of gross examination are described in Chapter 19.

Most follicular carcinomas present as a solitary nodule in the background of normal appearing thyroid parenchyma, although macroscopic changes suggestive of lymphocytic thyroiditis or nodular hyperplasia may also be seen in the adjacent thyroid tissue. The presence of multiple well-defined solid thyroid nodules, particularly in a young patient, should raise the possibility of an inherited disease, such as PHTS, as discussed later in the chapter.

 ## MICROSCOPIC FEATURES

Follicular carcinomas typically have a well-formed and complete capsule, which is thick (0.1 to 0.3 cm) or at least moderately thick (0.1 cm) (Fig. 10.10).[105,106] The capsule consists of parallel layers of collagen fibers and frequently contains medium caliber blood vessels; the

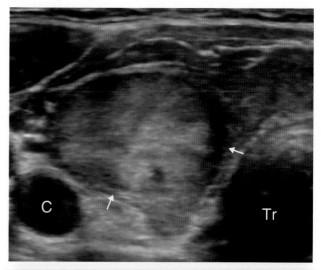

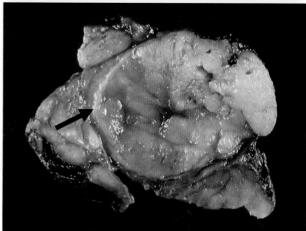

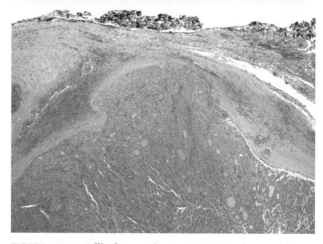

FIGURE 10.7. Follicular carcinoma. Top: An ultrasound image shows a large ovoid nodule with variable echogenicity, slightly irregular outlines, and hypoechoic, focally irregular halo *(arrows)*. Tr, trachea; C, carotid artery. **Middle:** Gross photograph showing an encapsulated nodule *(arrow)* with no obvious invasion. Whitish appearance of the adjacent thyroid tissue is because of marked chronic lymphocytic thyroiditis. **Bottom:** Microscopic image demonstrating capsular invasion, which is diagnostic for follicular carcinoma.

latter may show an edematous and irregularly thick smooth muscle wall. In rare cases, carcinomas have a thin or incomplete capsule.

Architectural patterns of follicular carcinomas are similar to those seen in follicular adenomas, although the proportion of more

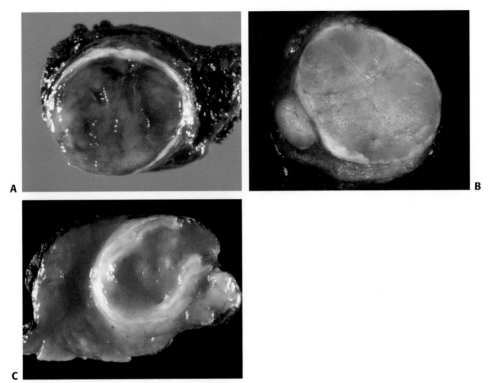

FIGURE 10.8. Gross appearance of follicular carcinoma. A: This follicular carcinoma of conventional type shows a moderately thick capsule and solid cut surface with foci of hemorrhage. The gross appearance is indistinguishable from that of follicular adenoma. **B:** This follicular carcinoma of conventional type shows a well-defined moderately thick capsule with a focus of tumor located outside of the capsule. **C:** This follicular carcinoma of oncocytic type shows characteristic mahogany-brown cut surface and a very thick capsule with a clearly identifiable focus of tumor invasion through the capsule.

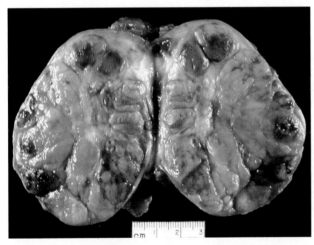

FIGURE 10.9. Widely invasive follicular carcinoma of oncocytic type. The tumor replaces the entire lobe of the thyroid and shows multifocal hemorrhage and necrosis.

cellular growth patterns is higher in carcinomas. A microfollicular or solid/trabecular growth pattern is found in approximately 80% of cases and normofollicular or macrofollicular pattern with high colloid content in approximately 20%.[104] A nested or insular architecture may also be seen. Although the growth pattern has no diagnostic value per se, it should alert a pathologist to search more extensively for invasion, especially if the lesion is very cellular. Likewise, the architectural patterns do not correlate with the frequency of metastases or cancer-related death.[107,108] Tumors with solid, trabecular, and insular growth patterns should be distinguished from poorly differentiated thyroid carcinoma, which has a significantly more aggressive behavior.

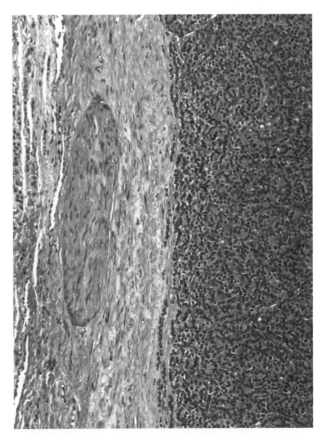

FIGURE 10.10. Low-power view of follicular adenoma. Note a thick fibrous capsule containing a medium-sized artery.

The cells are typically cuboidal (Fig. 10.11). The cytoplasm is moderately abundant, light eosinophilic to amphophilic. The nuclei are usually small to medium and round, with smooth contours and dark or more vesicular chromatin. Small nucleoli are frequently seen in conventional type carcinomas but are much more prominent in oncocytic follicular carcinoma. Some tumors have more irregular nuclei and coarse chromatin. The irregular nuclear contours raise suspicion for papillary carcinoma, but other nuclear features of papillary carcinoma are lacking (Fig. 10.12A). Rarely, random cells with very large, hyperchromatic, and highly irregular nuclei may be found (Fig. 10.12B). This exuberant nuclear atypia of single cells does not increase the likelihood of malignancy in thyroid tumors, as it is also seen in follicular adenomas and hyperplastic nodules.

Mitotic figures may be found, typically 1 to 2 per 10 high-power fields (Fig. 10.11B). Higher mitotic activity may mark the

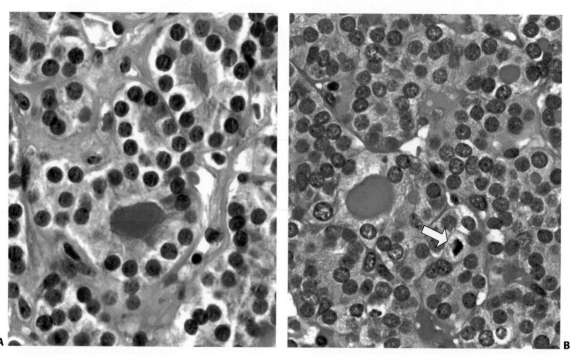

FIGURE 10.11. High-power views of two follicular carcinomas. A: This tumor shows cells with uniform, dark nuclei with smooth contours. **B:** Cells of this tumor have more atypical, enlarged nuclei with coarse chromatin and significant variability in nuclear size and shape. A mitotic figure is seen *(arrow)*.

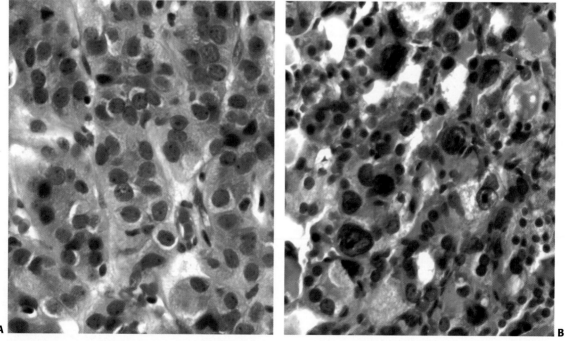

FIGURE 10.12. Appearance of nuclei in follicular carcinoma cells. A: Nuclei of this follicular carcinoma have substantial irregularity of contours, although overall the nuclear features are insufficient to classify this tumor as papillary carcinoma. **B:** Cells with highly atypical hyperchromatic nuclei are seen in this follicular carcinoma. The presence of scattered bizarre cells does not constitute evidence for malignancy.

areas of recent aspiration of other secondary changes. Atypical mitoses are rare. Well-differentiated follicular carcinomas do not show tumor necrosis unless seen in association with spontaneous or FNA-induced secondary changes. When present, it suggests the emergence of poorly differentiated thyroid carcinoma.[109]

The stroma is scant and may show some hyalinization and edema. Cystic changes may be present as a consequence of previous FNA procedure, although spontaneous cystic transformation is uncommon. Intratumoral areas of dense fibrosis are rarely found in follicular carcinomas and are more characteristic of the follicular variant of papillary carcinoma.

The growth pattern, thickness of the capsule, or cytologic features do not distinguish between follicular adenoma and follicular carcinoma. The only diagnostic criteria for carcinoma are capsular invasion and vascular invasion, and either one is sufficient for malignancy.

Vascular Invasion

Vascular invasion is defined as direct tumor extension into the blood vessel lumen or a tumor aggregate present within the vessel lumen (Fig. 10.13). Diagnostic criteria for invasion

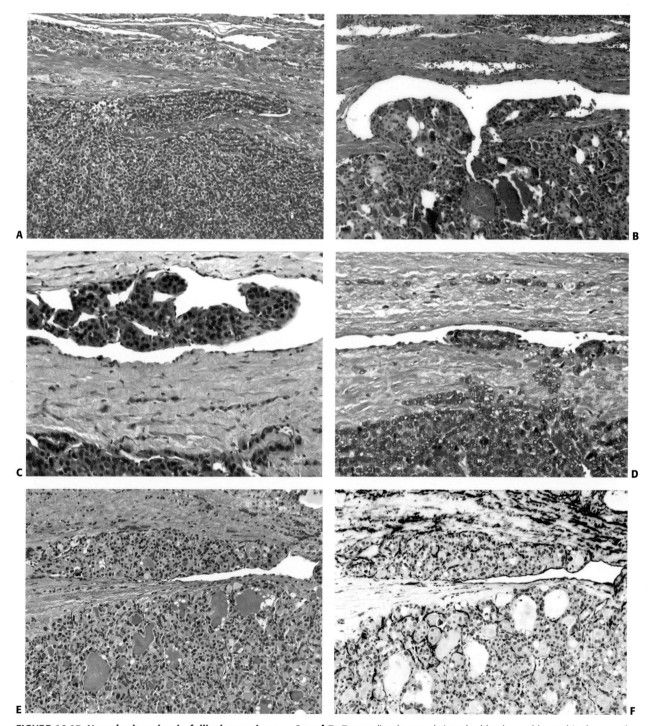

FIGURE 10.13. Vascular invasion in follicular carcinoma. A and B: Tumor directly extends into the blood vessel located in the capsule. **C–E:** Aggregates of tumor cells are seen within the vessel lumen attached to the wall and covered by endothelium. **F:** CD34 immunostain highlights the endothelial lining of the blood vessel and endothelium covering the tumor aggregate.

Table 10.3

Diagnostic Criteria for Vascular Invasion and Potential Mimickers

Criteria for Vascular Invasion	Potential Mimickers of Vascular Invasion
Invaded blood vessel is located in the capsule or immediately outside it	Invaded blood vessel within the tumor nodule parenchyma
Invaded vessel has a clearly identifiable wall lined by endothelium	Tumor cells entrapped within the capsule with artifactual crack in the capsule or retraction artifact
Invading tumor forms a polypoid mass projecting into the lumen	Tumor aggregate located outside of the vessel wall slightly bulging into the vessel lumen
Intravascular plug is a true epithelial cell aggregate	Reactive endothelial cell proliferation, intravascular organizing thrombus
Tumor aggregate is attached to the vessel wall and/or covered by an endothelial layer	Free floating tumor aggregates within the vessel lumen

are summarized in Table 10.3. The affected vessel must be located within the capsule or immediately outside the capsule but not within the tumor nodule itself. The vessel should have a clearly identifiable wall with endothelial lining. If tumor extends directly into the vessel lumen, it should form a polypoid mass protruding into the lumen, not just slightly bulge into the lumen (Figs. 10.13B vs. 10.14B). The cell aggregates within the lumen should be histologically identical to the tumor cells and be composed of epithelial cells, not of reactive endothelial cells (Fig. 10.14F). Finally, the intravascular tumor aggregate should be attached to the wall of the blood vessel and covered by a layer of endothelial cells (Fig. 10.13). The presence of thrombus adjacent to the tumor aggregate provides confirmation of vascular invasion but is not required for it. Finding both, attachment to the wall and endothelial covering of the intravascular tumor aggregate, provides undisputable evidence for vascular invasion. However, several authors accept the presence of only one of these two criteria as sufficient evidence for invasion.[110] The following rationale is offered: (1) finding an endothelialized but not-attached tumor aggregate may reflect the sampling of a floating tail of the tumor aggregate whose attachment site is not in the section plain and (2) a freshly formed tumor thrombus may be caught at a stage when it has not developed an endothelial covering yet.[111] Although these scenarios are possible, they should not expected to be seen often; in most cases, both of the criteria should be met. Irregularly shaped tumor aggregates that are floating in the vessel lumen and not covered by an endothelial layer should not be mistaken for vascular invasion (Fig. 10.14E). They typically represent an artifactual displacement of tumor cells during surgical and postsurgical handing or gross sectioning of the sample.[112]

Immunostains for endothelial markers may help to establish whether the tumor is covered by endothelial cells and the space is indeed a blood vessel (Figs. 10.13 and 10.14).

Capsular Invasion

Capsular invasion manifests as penetration of the full thickness of the capsule by the tumor cells (Fig. 10.15A,B). In more advanced cases, the tumor extends beyond the capsule into thyroid parenchyma, frequently in a mushroom-like or a hook-like manner (Fig. 10.15C,D). Direct contact of tumor cells with normal thyroid parenchyma is rarely seen because of the formation of one or several secondary fibrotic layers at the advancing, invasive border of the tumor. When sectioned

not in the plane of tumor penetration through the capsule, the tumor extension may present as a satellite nodule adjacent to the capsule (Fig. 10.15E). Connection to the main mass through a defect in the capsule is usually found in deeper sections (Fig. 10.15F). In tumors with extensive, widespread invasion, the original capsule may be largely destroyed by the tumor and not recognizable.

The following findings should *not* be considered as capsular invasion:

- Tumor projection into the capsule but not through the entire thickness of the capsule (Fig. 10.16A). Encapsulated tumors with partial capsular invasion *only* do not show recurrence or metastases[104,113] and, in our opinion, should be diagnosed as a follicular adenoma. This more stringent requirement for capsular invasion, that is, through-and-through penetration of the capsule, is accepted by many authors.[110,111,114–117] Nevertheless, others consider the partial invasion of the capsule sufficient to qualify for capsular invasion.[118]
- Small groups of tumor cells confined within the capsule (Fig. 10.16B). These cells are simply entrapped within the capsule during formation of new collagen layers and do not represent invasion by the neoplastic cells.
- A nodule located beyond the tumor capsule and not connected to the main tumor mass (Fig. 10.16C). If a thorough search reveals no connection to the main tumor through a defect in the capsule (as illustrated on Fig. 10.15E,F), this nodule likely represents a separate lesion rather than an extension from the main tumor. Differences in the growth pattern, cellularity, and cellular morphology between the two nodules help with the distinction.
- A folding of the capsule at the very edge of the section (Fig. 10.16D). This artifact, which typically has a "V" shape, is created by higher pressure within the tumor limited by the capsule and is found when sections of the tumor nodule were taken perpendicularly to the surface of the initial bisection.
- Capsular pseudoinvasion induced by a FNA procedure (Fig. 10.16E). The needle penetration site may show capsular distortion, reactive endothelial cell proliferation, and sometimes direct protrusion of tumor cells through the defect in the capsule. It is distinguished from true invasion by the linear shape of the capsular defect and presence of other changes induced by an aspirating needle. The spectrum of "worrisome histologic alterations following fine needle aspiration of the thyroid" or "WHAFFT"[119] is described in more detail in Chapter 6.

Chapter 10   Follicular Carcinoma   **163**

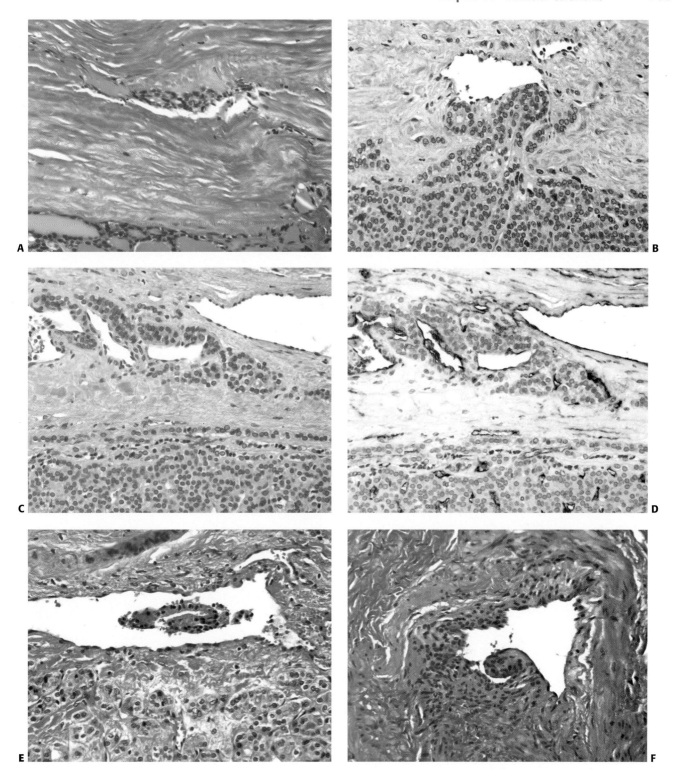

FIGURE 10.14. Findings that mimic vascular invasion. A: Tumor cells entrapped within the capsule and located adjacent to a crack that is not covered by endothelium and therefore does not represent a blood vessel. **B:** Tumor cells located outside of a blood vessel slightly protruding into a lumen but not forming a plug or polypoid mass in the lumen. **C:** Tumor cells intermingle with blood vessels in the capsule with no invasion into the vessel lumen. **D:** CD34 immunostaining of the area shown in **(C)** confirms the lack of invasion into the vessel lumen. **E:** An irregularly shaped tumor aggregate not attached to the wall and not covered by endothelium. **F:** Reactive proliferation of endothelial cells with polypoid projection into the lumen.

TUMOR INVASIVENESS

Finding a single focus of capsular or vascular invasion is diagnostic of follicular carcinoma. The extent of invasion is also important because it is used to further categorize these tumors to predict their behavior. Traditionally, follicular carcinomas have been subdivided into minimally invasive (encapsulated) and widely invasive.[117] In this classification scheme, minimally invasive carcinomas are fully encapsulated tumors with microscopically identifiable foci of capsular or vascular invasion, whereas widely invasive carcinomas are tumors with extensive, frequently extrathyroidal, invasion. Other and more recent classification schemes employ three or more categories.[60,120–122] They have been proposed to

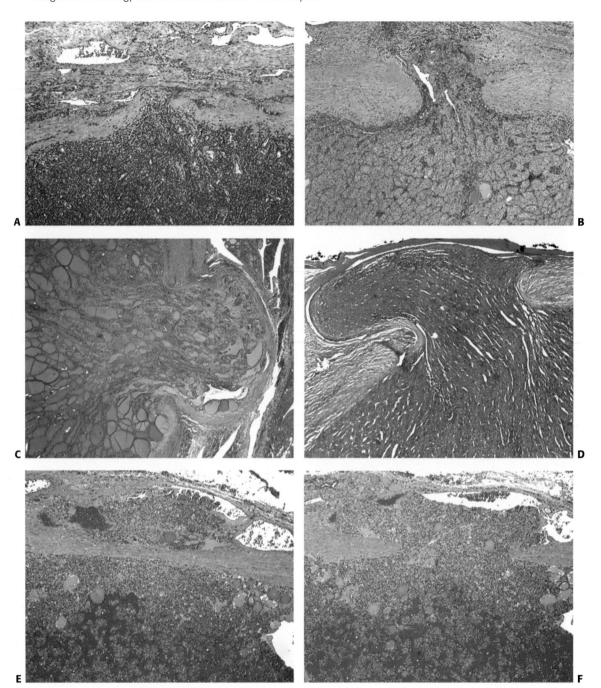

FIGURE 10.15. Capsular invasion in follicular carcinoma. A and B: Tumor penetrates through the full thickness of the capsule, with no extension into thyroid parenchyma. **C and D:** More pronounced capsular invasion with either mushroom-like **(C)** or hook-like **(D)** tumor extension into pericapsular thyroid parenchyma. **E:** A nodule with similar microscopic appearance is located outside of the main tumor capsule. Although highly suspicious for invasion, it does not fully qualify for it because a point of penetration through the capsule is not present. Connection between the two nodules through the capsular defect is found in the deeper sections **(F)**, fulfilling the criterion for invasion.

(1) incorporate more recent findings suggesting that angioinvasive carcinomas behave more aggressively and (2) accommodate those tumors that are difficult to fit into the two main categories. Analysis of the literature, specifically excluding series that included follicular variant of papillary carcinoma, leads to the following conclusions:

1. The traditional two-tier classification scheme, that is, minimally invasive and widely invasive follicular carcinomas, highlights a dramatic difference in outcome between the two groups: the average recurrence rate is 18% and mortality rate is 14% for minimally invasive tumors as compared

with a 56% recurrence rate and 50% mortality rate for widely invasive carcinomas (based on the meta-analysis of the literature by D'Avanzo et al.).[122]

2. Among minimally invasive carcinomas, tumors with capsular invasion *only* appear to have a slightly better outcome as compared with those with vascular invasion, particularly during the first 5 to 10 years.[122–124] The disease-free survival appears to be significantly different, at least on short follow-up.[125] The overall survival may not be too different, such as 89% versus 86% or 100% versus 98%, respectively.[122,126] One study has reported a dramatic difference in tumor-associated

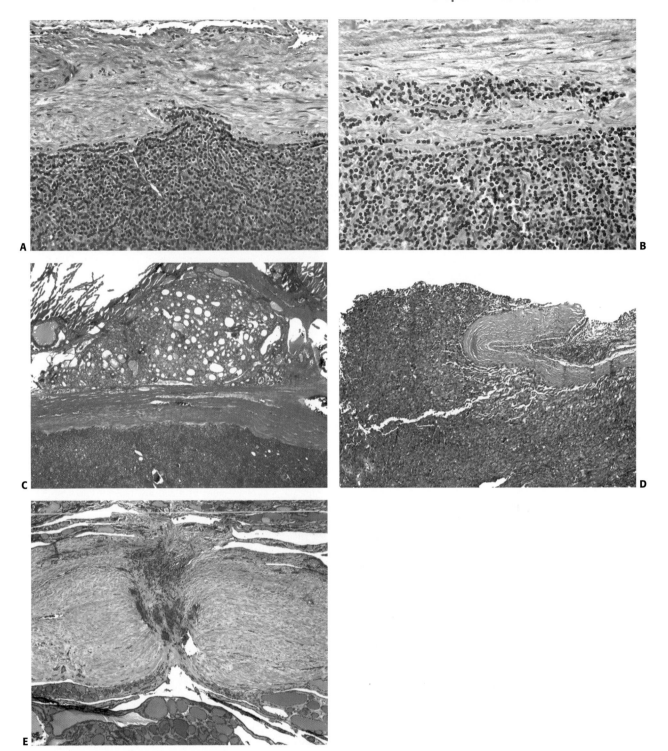

FIGURE 10.16. Findings that mimic capsular invasion. A: Tumor extension into the capsule but not through the full thickness of the capsule. **B:** Groups of cells entrapped within the capsule. **C:** A nodule located outside of the capsule and not connected to the main tumor through a defect in the capsule. This nodule has a different microscopic appearance, providing additional evidence that it does not represent a satellite nodule formed by invasion from the main tumor mass. **D:** An artifactual V-shaped folding of the capsule at the edge of a section. **E:** A post-FNA change in the capsule with vascular proliferation and inflammatory infiltration that resembles capsular invasion.

mortality between carcinomas with capsular invasion *only* and vascular invasion (0% vs. 34%), although it is not entirely clear whether this study was limited to minimally invasive carcinomas or also included widely invasive tumors.[127]

3. The extent of vascular invasion appears to affect survival.[128] In several studies, vascular invasion of four or more blood vessels corresponded to a major increase in the rate of tumor recurrence and/or tumor-related mortality.[107,129,130]

4. Some evidence also suggests that more extensive capsular invasion, such as extension into thyroid parenchyma, correlates with a higher metastatic rate and mortality.[108,131]

On the basis of the reported data summarized above and our own experience, we subdivide follicular carcinomas into four categories: (1) encapsulated follicular carcinoma with microscopic capsular invasion (true minimally invasive carcinoma),

Table 10.4

Histologic Types of Follicular Carcinoma Based on the Extent of Invasion

Tumor Type	Current WHO Category	Diagnostic Criteria	Estimated Cumulative Mortality Rate (%)
Follicular carcinoma, encapsulated with microscopic capsular invasion	Minimally invasive	–Encapsulated tumor –Capsular invasion detected microscopically –No vascular invasion	0–5
Follicular carcinoma, encapsulated with gross capsular invasion	NC[a]	–Encapsulated tumor –Capsular invasion grossly identifiable –No vascular invasion	5–15
Follicular carcinoma, encapsulated with angioinvasion	Minimally invasive	–Encapsulated tumor –Vascular invasion –Capsular invasion is or is not present	5–30[b]
Follicular carcinoma, widely invasive	Widely invasive	–Loss of encapsulation –Extensive invasion, frequently extrathyroidal	50

[a]Not readily classifiable based on the current WHO classification.[110]
[b]Higher rate within this range correlates with larger number (≥4) of blood vessels involved.

(2) encapsulated follicular carcinoma with gross capsular invasion, (3) encapsulated follicular carcinoma with angioinvasion, and (4) widely invasive follicular carcinoma (Table 10.4).

Encapsulated Follicular Carcinoma with Microscopic Capsular Invasion

These are encapsulated tumors that are indistinguishable from follicular adenomas based on clinical presentation, imaging, and gross pathologic evaluation. The diagnosis is established on microscopic examination by finding one or several foci of transcapsular invasion with no significant tumor extension into adjacent thyroid parenchyma. No vascular invasion is present. These tumors have a very low chance of metastases, recurrence, or tumor-associated mortality, with the probability of these developments in <5% of cases.

Encapsulated Follicular Carcinoma with Gross Capsular Invasion

These tumors are overall encapsulated and reveal grossly identifiable but still limited capsular invasion. The capsular invasion is found macroscopically as a disruption of the capsule with tumor extension into thyroid parenchyma or as a satellite nodule connected to the main tumor capsule (Fig. 10.8B,C). There is no vascular invasion. These tumors are expected to have a low but slightly higher rate of metastases, recurrence, and tumor-related mortality. Tumors that belong to this intermediate group have been also designated as *overtly invasive follicular carcinomas*.[60]

Encapsulated Follicular Carcinoma with Angioinvasion

These are encapsulated lesions that reveal vascular invasion that involves one or several blood vessels. Capsular invasion may be present or absent. These tumors are associated with a more substantial probability of metastases, recurrence, or death from disease. The latter can be estimated at 5% to 30% based on the literature data summarized above. Within this range, the rate of adverse events is expected to be progressively higher with increasing number of blood vessels involved, particularly when four or more foci of vascular invasion are identified. Tumors that belong to this group have been designated by others as

angioinvasive grossly encapsulated follicular carcinomas[118] and *moderately invasive follicular carcinomas*.[122]

Widely Invasive Follicular Carcinoma

These tumors are not encapsulated and show widespread extension into thyroid parenchyma and frequently into extrathyroidal soft tissues. The tumors appear malignant on radiographic imaging studies and gross examination. They show multiple fronts of invasion and the remainder of the capsule may or may not be identified. Multiple foci of vascular invasion are typically present. The main differential diagnosis is poorly differentiated thyroid carcinoma. The rate of recurrence and metastases in these patients is approximately 55%, and mortality rate is approximately 50%. Owing to increased physician and patient awareness, superior radiographic techniques, and advances in surgical management, this type of follicular carcinoma is seldom diagnosed in modern clinical practice.

 ## SPREAD AND METASTASES

Follicular carcinoma grows as a solitary nodule expanding by progressive broad-based invasion into thyroid parenchyma, perithyroidal soft tissues, trachea, and neck blood vessels (Fig. 10.17A). A pushing, relatively smooth invasive border is common. The tumor does not disseminate throughout the thyroid gland and usually does not recur in the opposite lobe after lobectomy. If local recurrence occurs after surgery, it typically involves the thyroid bed or perithyroidal soft tissues (Fig. 10.17B). Follicular carcinomas characteristically disseminate hematogenously to distant sites. Distant metastases are found at presentation in approximately 10% of patients, and as many patients develop them during follow-up.[122,123,132] The most frequent sites of tumor spread are bones (Fig. 10.17C) and lungs, whereas brain/spinal cord, liver, kidney, skin, and other organs are involved less commonly.[122,128,133]

The frequency of lymph node metastases has been reported in the range of 3% to 20% for conventional tumor types and 0% to 56% for oncocytic types.[134] However, it is likely that most of the tumors reported in older series as metastatic to lymph nodes are actually follicular variant of papillary carcinoma. Using current diagnostic criteria (i.e., tumors showing nuclear features of papillary carcinoma are papillary carcinomas irrespective of the growth pattern), the lymph node metastases from *conventional type* follicular carcinomas are exceedingly rare and probably do not occur

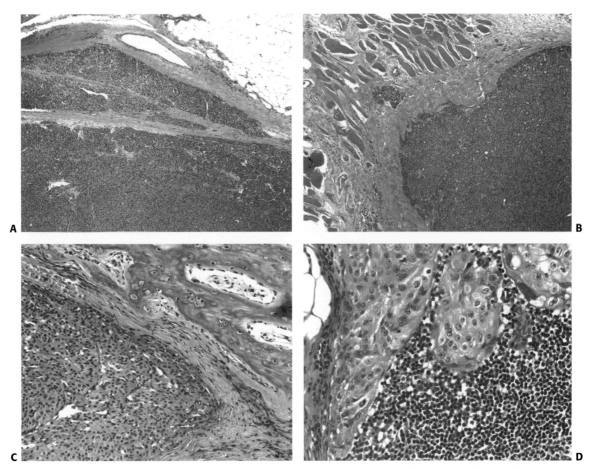

FIGURE 10.17. Spread of follicular carcinoma. A: Tumor invasion into perithyroidal adipose tissue with a pushing border and formation of new fibrotic layers at the invasive edge. **B:** Local recurrence of the follicular carcinoma in soft tissues of the neck. **C:** Oncocytic follicular carcinoma metastatic to the rib. **D:** Lymph node metastasis from oncocytic follicular carcinoma.

at all, other than by direct tumor extension into the lymph node. In *oncocytic type* follicular carcinomas, lymph node metastases do occur even when stringent diagnostic criteria are applied (Fig. 10.17D). However, they are found in only 5% to 10% of tumors and typically in those cases that also show locally advanced disease or distant metastases.[7,135] For practical purposes, it can be assumed that thyroid carcinoma metastatic to the cervical lymph nodes is a papillary carcinoma, unless the tumor is oncocytic or shows wide local invasion and direct extension into the lymph node.

 MICROSCOPIC VARIANTS

Oncocytic (Hürthle Cell) Follicular Carcinoma

Oncocytic follicular carcinoma is a common tumor variant that comprises 25% to 30% of all follicular carcinomas.[1,7,8] These tumors are composed of follicular cells that have abundant granular eosinophilic cytoplasm because of the accumulation of innumerable mitochondria. The mitochondria frequently reveal abnormal morphology on ultrastructural examination, as discussed later in the chapter.

In order to be classified as the oncocytic variant of follicular carcinoma, the tumor should be composed of at least 75% by oncocytic cells and should not reveal diagnostic nuclear features of papillary carcinoma (Fig. 10.18). The cells are large and have polygonal shape with well-defined cell borders. The cytoplasm is abundant, finely granular, deeply eosinophilic, and opacified or "smooth." The nuclei

are small or medium sized and round and have vesicular chromatin and prominent nucleoli. Slight variability in the nuclear size and shape is common. Some tumors demonstrate substantial nuclear pleomorphism (Fig. 10.19A). Scattered cells with nuclear grooves and intranuclear cytoplasmic inclusions may be found, although they are not expected to be present in more than single numbers.

Various growth patterns can be seen, most commonly microfollicular and solid. Oncocytic carcinomas are rarely colloid rich, and colloid is frequently amphophilic. Laminated calcification of the colloid, mimicking psammoma bodies, can be seen (Fig. 10.19B), but not true psammoma bodies that are seen within the fibrous stroma of papillary carcinoma. Oncocytic tumors have fragile parenchyma and frequently reveal foci of hemorrhage, infarction, and other secondary changes.

The diagnosis of malignancy requires the identification of capsular or vascular invasion. The criteria for invasion are identical to those described for conventional type follicular carcinomas, as are tumor categories based on degree of invasion. Using the diagnostic criteria for malignancy, a higher proportion of solitary encapsulated oncocytic nodules reveal invasion and are diagnosed as carcinoma as compared with solitary encapsulated nodules composed of nononcocytic follicular cells.[86] The proportion of carcinoma in oncocytic nodules varies (5% to >50%) but on average is close to 20%.[136,137]

The debate continues about whether oncocytic carcinoma is a variant of follicular carcinoma or represents a distinct type of thyroid cancer. In favor of the first possibility is the fact that oncocytic tumors resemble conventional follicular carcinoma in all major histopathologic aspects such as encapsulation, growth pattern, and

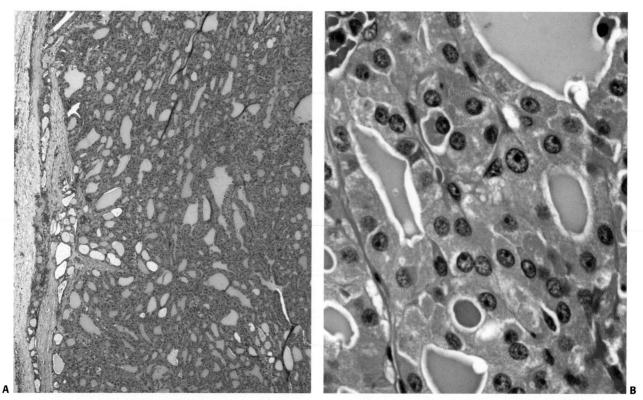

FIGURE 10.18. Oncocytic variant of follicular carcinoma. A: Low-power view showing a predominantly microfollicular growth pattern of the tumor. **B:** High-power view demonstrates cells with abundant finely granular cytoplasm and round to oval nuclei with prominent nucleoli.

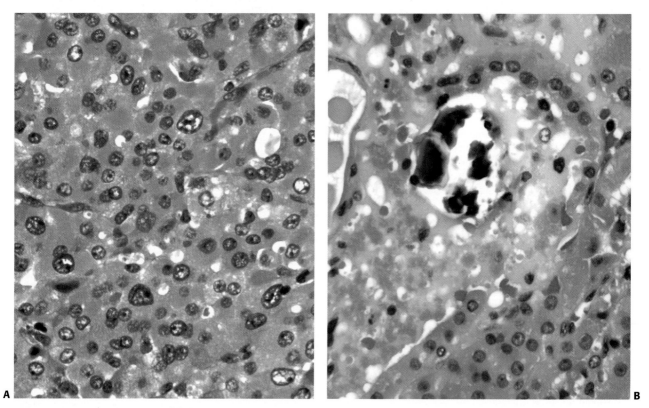

FIGURE 10.19. Oncocytic variant of follicular carcinoma. A: This oncocytic carcinoma shows significant variability in nuclear size and shape. Scattered cells have highly irregular nuclei, and some of them reveal nuclear grooves. These findings, present in single cells, are not sufficient for the diagnosis of papillary carcinoma. **B:** Laminated calcification of the colloid debris mimics psammoma bodies.

invasiveness and differ only in the characteristics of the cytoplasm. In favor of the second possibility is the fact that these tumors have some differences in biologic behavior, including the ability to metastasize to lymph nodes, and a possibly higher rate of recurrence and tumor-related mortality. Future genetic investigations may resolve this controversy. At present, they are considered a variant of follicular carcinoma, a concept promulgated by the 2004 WHO Classification of Endocrine Tumours.[110] The term *Hürthle cell*, although widely used in the past, is now discouraged and replaced by the preferred and recommended term *oncocytic*.[110]

Clear Cell Variant of Follicular Carcinoma

This rare variant designates carcinomas that are predominantly (>75%) composed of cells with clear cytoplasm (Fig. 10.20). This quality of cytoplasm can reflect the accumulation of glycogen, lipid, thyroglobulin, other vesicles, or distended mitochondria.[138–140] In the routine hematoxylin and eosin (H&E)-stained sections, the cytoplasm is watery clear or has fine, pale eosinophilic granularity. The nuclei are small, dark, and centrally placed. They have smooth or slightly irregular contours. The tumor may be composed entirely of clear cells or contain small areas of cells with nonclear cytoplasm. The cells retain thyroglobulin immunoreactivity, which is usually focal and more pronounced in the colloid and in the cytoplasm of nonclear cells. In some cases, the cytoplasm is PAS positive and diastase sensitive, which reflects the accumulation of glycogen.

Clear cell follicular carcinomas frequently present with extrathyroidal extension and reveal distant metastases, although the number of reported cases is too small to establish whether these tumors as a group have more aggressive behavior. In one series of eight clear cell follicular carcinomas, half of the patients died from disease and more than three-fourth developed distant metastases during the mean follow-up of 7 years, although this outcome was not significantly different from that of nonclear cell follicular carcinomas analyzed in the same study.[141]

Follicular carcinomas composed of clear cells should be distinguished from metastatic carcinoma, particularly from the kidney, and from clear cell medullary carcinoma. Immunohistochemical studies can resolve this issue.

Mucinous Variant of Follicular Carcinoma

Rarely, follicular carcinomas reveal large stromal pools of mucinous material surrounding the follicular structures.[142,143] This material may also be seen in the lumens of thyroid follicles. It stains positive with Alcian blue (pH 2.5), PAS after diastase digestion, and mucicarmine. It remains unclear whether this material represents true mucin secreted by thyroid epithelial cells or originates from breakdown of thyroglobulin. As various carbohydrates constitute 2% to 4% of the molecular weight of thyroglobulin, these components and products of their degradation are likely to stain positively for mucin.[142,143] Electron microscopy demonstrates abundant clear vesicles or vacuoles within the epithelial cells, but it cannot discriminate between true mucin production and thyroglobulin products-containing vesicles.[144]

The criteria for malignancy in the mucin-rich tumors are the same as in other follicular carcinomas. The prognosis appears to be similar to conventional type follicular carcinoma.[144,145] The differential diagnosis of mucin-rich follicular carcinoma typically includes metastatic carcinoma and mucinous variant of medullary thyroid carcinoma. It can be facilitated by using immunohistochemistry. Primary mucinous carcinoma of the thyroid may also be considered in the differential diagnosis (Chapter 15).

Follicular Carcinoma with Signet-Ring Cells

This rare variant is characterized by cells with large intracytoplasmic vacuoles that displace and compress the nucleus to the side (Fig. 10.21). In H&E-stained sections, the vacuoles have a finely granular texture. The material within vacuoles typically shows immunoreactivity for thyroglobulin and positive staining for PAS after diastase digestion, whereas other mucin stains, such as mucicarmine and Alcian blue, are negative.[146] By electron microscopy, the cells contain large cytoplasmic vacuoles bordered by various numbers of microvilli.[146]

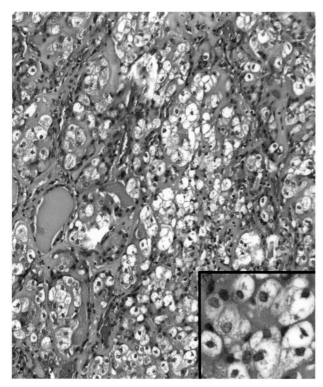

FIGURE 10.20. Clear cells variant of follicular carcinoma.

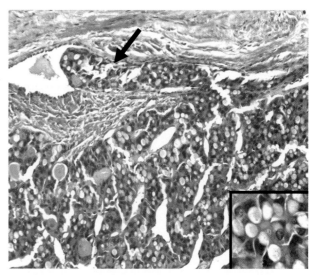

FIGURE 10.21. Follicular carcinoma with signet-ring cells. The tumor invades a blood vessel within the capsule (arrow).

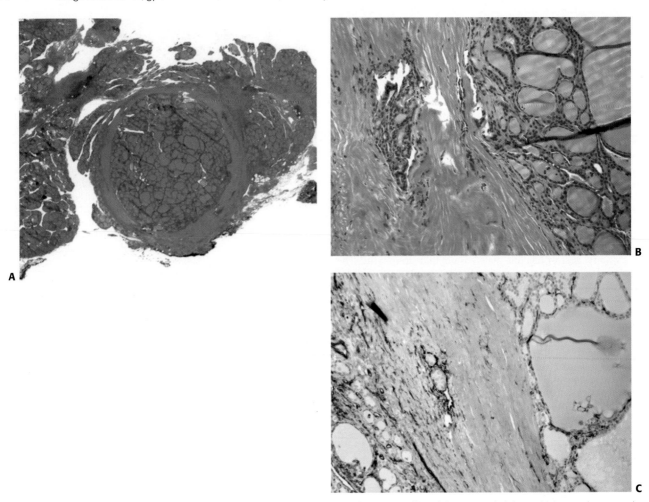

FIGURE 10.22. A 0.4-cm follicular microcarcinoma. A: Low-power scan shows a small nodule surrounded by a thick complete capsule. **B:** Focus of vascular invasion. **C:** CD31 immunostain confirming the endothelialized tumor aggregate present within the lumen of a blood vessel.

The presence of signet-ring cells is not a feature of malignancy by itself because these cells can also be seen in follicular adenomas and hyperplastic nodules. The diagnosis of cancer rests on the identification of invasion. Signet-ring carcinoma may be mistaken for metastatic carcinoma from stomach or breast, which can be ruled out by demonstrating immunoreactivity for thyroglobulin and/or thyroid transcription factor 1 (TTF1).

Follicular Microcarcinoma

This term is occasionally used for accidentally found follicular carcinomas that are 1 cm or less in size.[147] These tumors are rare. On the basis of the data reported in large registry-type databases, 3% to 8% of follicular carcinomas were ≤1 cm as opposed to 27% to 45% of papillary carcinomas.[1,4,8] However, the true incidence of follicular carcinomas of such size is likely to be even lower than 3-8%, as careful histopathologic review of cases submitted to one cancer registry resulted in reclassification of most of these tumors as a benign adenoma or follicular variant of papillary carcinoma or changing the tumor size to above 1 cm.[147] In a reported series of four verified follicular microcarcinomas, all tumors occurred in females of the age ranging from 33 to 75 years and were found after surgery performed for euthyroid goiter or Graves disease.[147] The size of tumors was between 0.5 and 0.7 cm. The smallest follicular carcinoma observed in our practice was a 0.4-cm tumor diagnosed in a 45-year-old woman. Despite small size, the tumor showed several foci of vascular invasion (Fig. 10.22). The biologic behavior of these tumors is not well defined and is likely to depend on the degree of invasiveness similar to the follicular carcinomas of larger size.

Follicular Carcinoma in Patients with the PHTS

Follicular carcinoma is a well-known manifestation of the PTEN hamartoma tumor syndrome (PHTS), which includes Cowden syndrome, Bannayan–Riley–Ruvalcaba syndrome, Proteus syndrome, and Proteus-like syndrome, all of which are associated with a germ line mutation of the *PTEN* gene.[28,148,149] In addition to the increased risk of thyroid cancer, typically of follicular carcinoma, the affected individuals are also at a high risk for malignant tumors of breast and endometrium.

Most of the patients who undergo thyroidectomy are females ratio, 2-3:1 and typically present at young age, although age at diagnosis varies; it ranged 9 to 76 years (mean age, 33.7 years) in a series of 20 patients affected by the PHTS.[28] The gross and microscopic appearance of thyroid glands in these patients is very characteristic[28,149] and should allow to suspect this syndrome even when family history is not known. On gross examination, the gland shows multiple well-defined, frequently encapsulated solid yellow-tan thyroid nodules (Fig. 10.23A). The nodules vary greatly in size and number, with >100 discrete nodules reported in one gland.[26,28,149,150] Microscopically, the nodules are well delineated, with no, partial or full encapsulation and variable growth

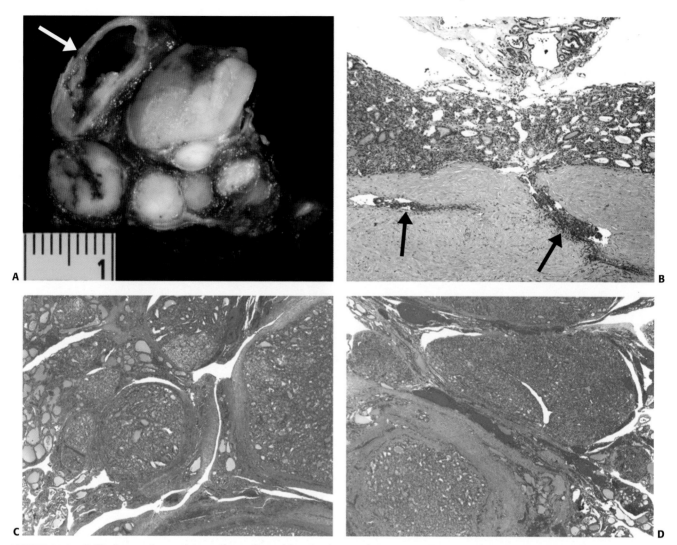

FIGURE 10.23. Follicular carcinoma in a patient affected by Cowden syndrome. A: Multiple well-defined solid thyroid nodules are seen macroscopically. A nodule subsequently diagnosed as follicular carcinoma *(arrow)* has a thick capsule and cystic changes resulted from the previously performed FNA procedure. **B:** Several foci of vascular invasion *(arrows)* were identified in the capsule of the follicular carcinoma. **C and D:** Low-power view of two areas showing multiple well-defined partially or completely encapsulate nodules. Changes of focal chronic lymphocytic thyroiditis are also noted (**D,** right lower corner).

patterns (Fig. 10.23C,D). They typically have microscopic features of conventional type follicular adenoma or cellular hyperplastic nodule. Occasionally, oncocytic and clear cell nodules and adenolipomas can be seen.[26,150] In addition, chronic lymphocytic thyroiditis, C-cell hyperplasia, and papillary microcarcinomas may be seen in the background thyroid.[26,28] Follicular carcinomas are diagnosed based on the presence of vascular and/or capsular invasion. Finding of a follicular carcinoma in such a setting should raise suspicion for this familial syndrome and trigger genetic counseling.

Other Variants of Follicular Carcinoma

Rarely, follicular carcinomas may contain focal areas or be entirely composed of spindle cells (Fig. 10.24A). Mature fat tissue may also be found in some carcinomas (Fig. 10.24B).[151] These findings are of no particular diagnostic or prognostic significance.

Single cases of hyperfunctioning ("hot," "toxic") follicular carcinoma have been described. These tumors appear as "hot" nodules on radioisotope scanning and may produce clinical symptoms of hyperthyroidism. Most of the reported cases carry mutations in the *TSHR* gene, which causes chronic stimulation of the cyclic AMP signaling pathway.[152,153] Distant metastases may preserve the

autonomous production of thyroid hormone. The histopathologic features of hyperfunctioning follicular carcinomas are not well defined.

Mixed medullary and follicular carcinomas of the thyroid are discussed in Chapter 14.

 ## IMMUNOHISTOCHEMISTRY

Immunostains can aid the diagnosis of follicular carcinomas in two ways: (1) by establishing the thyroid follicular cell origin of distant metastases or primary thyroid tumors with unusual appearance and (2) by assisting the diagnosis of malignancy.

The first application typically utilizes immunostains for thyroglobulin and TTF1. Thyroglobulin is produced only by thyroid follicular cells and is the most specific marker. The reactivity is seen in the luminal colloid and cell cytoplasm (Fig. 10.25B). The staining is diffuse and overall strong, although its intensity in most follicular carcinomas is slightly weaker than in the surrounding thyroid tissue. TTF1, a nuclear transcription factor, shows diffuse and strong nuclear reactivity (Fig. 10.25C). The nuclear pattern and high intensity of staining makes it a robust and reliable diagnostic marker, although TTF1 is not specific for thyroid follicular cells and

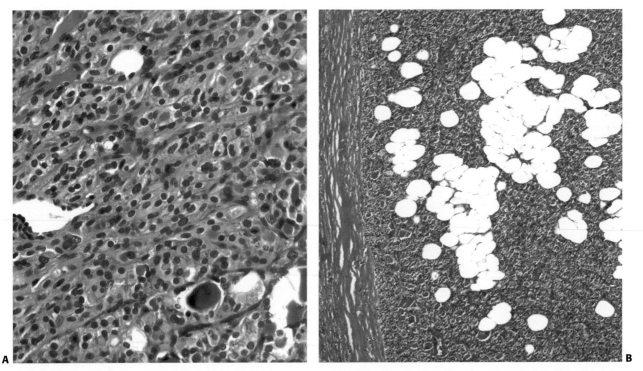

FIGURE 10.24. A: This follicular carcinoma contains areas of spindle cells (*top*) merging with the areas of more typical cuboidal cells (*bottom right*). **B:** Islands of adipose tissue are seen in this follicular carcinoma.

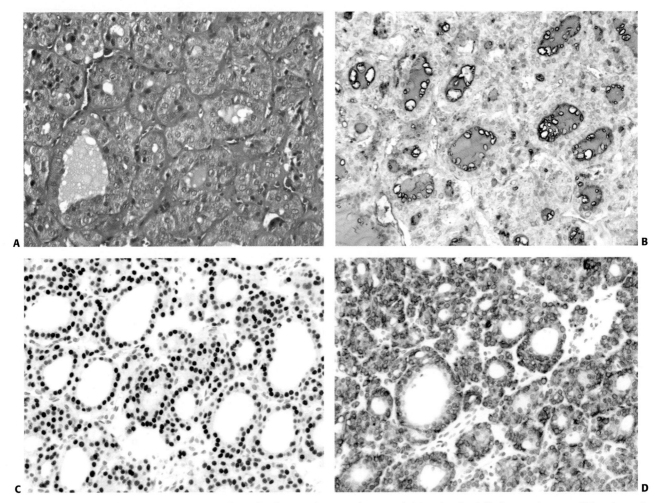

FIGURE 10.25. Follicular carcinoma metastatic to the femur. The tumor has a predominantly microfollicular growth pattern **(A)** and reveals strong and diffuse immunoreactivity for thyroglobulin **(B)**, TTF1 **(C)**, and CK7 **(D)**.

also highlights lung tumors, small-cell carcinomas from different locations, diencephalic lesions, and some medullary thyroid carcinomas.[154,155] Two other thyroid transcription factors, PAX8 and TTF2, may also be used to establish follicular cell origin. A recent study found diffuse nuclear reactivity for both markers in follicular carcinoma but not in lung carcinoma.[156] The specificity of these antibodies needs further validation. The pattern of reactivity for cytokeratins in follicular carcinomas is similar to normal thyroid cells. The cells are positive for CK7 (Fig. 10.25D), CAM 5.2, and AE1/AE3, whereas they are negative for CK20.[157,158] Immunoreactivity for AE1/AE3 and thyroglobulin is preserved in many necrotic thyroid nodules and can be used to confirm the thyroid origin of tumors with massive necrosis.[159] Important negative markers are calcitonin, CEA, and neuroendocrine markers (chromogranin, synaptophysin, CD56, NSE).

Oncocytic carcinomas show a similar pattern of immunoreactivity, although they typically demonstrate a lower intensity of thyroglobulin staining. Mitochondria-specific antibodies may be used to demonstrate the presence of abundant mitochondria.[160] It is important to note that oncocytic cells are prone to nonspecific staining of the cytoplasm with various antibodies because of high endogenous biotin activity.[161] It manifests as coarsely granular cytoplasmic staining that should not be confused with true positive staining (for illustration, see Chapter 8, Fig. 8.25A). The nonspecific immunoreactivity may be prevented in many, but not all cases, by endogenous biotin blocking procedures.

Several immunostains have been explored to assist the diagnosis of malignancy in follicular thyroid lesions. When vascular invasion is suspected, endothelial markers such as CD34 and CD31 are helpful to confirm the tumor location within the lumen of a blood vessel and to visualize the endothelial lining of the tumor plug (Fig. 10.13F).

PPARγ immunostain can be used as a marker of *PAX8/PPARγ*, exploiting the fact that this rearrangement results in dramatic overexpression of the PPARγ protein.[39,70] Most importantly, only strong and diffuse immunoreactivity correlates with the presence of the rearrangement (Fig. 10.26A). Moderate and weak intensity of staining, as well as focal strong reactivity of epithelial cells in areas of intense inflammation in Hashimoto thyroiditis, should be discounted (Fig. 8.24B,C).[70] The finding of strong PPARγ immunoreactivity requires confirmation of the presence of the *PAX8/PPARγ* rearrangement by a different technique (see next section) and should prompt thorough search for invasion.

Galectin-3, HBME-1, and CITED1 stains can also be used to assist in the diagnosis of malignancy. In several large series, follicular carcinomas were positive for galectin-3 in 50% to 90%, for HBME-1 in 40% to 90%, and for CITED1 in 15% to 50% of cases.[162-166] More than half of tumors showed reactivity for two or three markers. These stains are not specific for malignancy because 10% to 30% of follicular adenomas also revealed positivity for any one of these markers. However, reactivity for two or three markers was observed in these series in only 2% to 5% of adenomas.[162-166] In our experience, these stains may serve as a helpful adjunct to the workup of diagnostically challenging cases but have to be applied and interpreted as a panel and after appropriate validation in each laboratory. Most follicular carcinomas show patchy staining with these antibodies, and the intensity of staining is usually not as strong and diffuse as it is seen in papillary carcinomas (Fig. 10.27).

Many other immunohistochemical markers have been explored for use in the diagnosis of follicular carcinoma, including thyroperoxidase (TPO), cytokeratin 19, fibronectin-1, S100A4, cyclin D1, and p27.[167] Although many of them show statistically

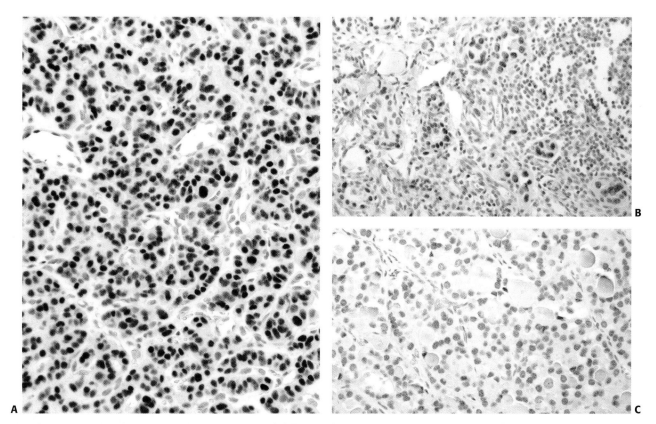

FIGURE 10.26. PPARγ immunostaining. A: Strong and diffuse nuclear immunoreactivity for PPARγ in the follicular carcinoma carrying *PAX8/PPARγ* rearrangement. Focal strong reactivity seen in the areas of dense lymphocytic infiltration in Hashimoto thyroiditis **(B)** and weak diffuse staining of the follicular tumor **(C)** does not correlate with the presence of *PAX8/PPARγ* rearrangement. Of note, PPARγ immunostain may be challenging to set up because not all currently available antibodies give a reliable result and the staining is difficult to optimize using an automated slide stainer.

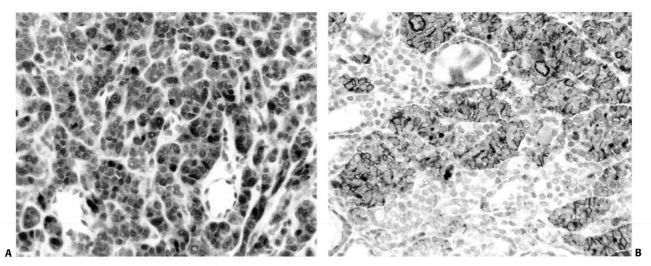

FIGURE 10.27. A: Moderate intensity of galectin-3 immunoreactivity in the nuclei and cytoplasm of the follicular carcinoma cells. **B:** Membranous staining for HBME 1 is seen in ~50% of the follicular carcinoma cells.

significant difference in expression levels between follicular carcinomas and follicular adenomas, their diagnostic usefulness has not been clearly demonstrated.

The proliferative index detected by Ki-67 (MIB-1) immunostaining is typically <5% in minimally invasive carcinomas, 5% to 10% in widely invasive tumors, and 10% to 20% in metastatic follicular carcinomas.[98,162,168] Most follicular carcinomas reveal no TP53 staining and preserve Bcl-2 and E-cadherin immunoreactivity, although Bcl-2 and E-cadherin expression are frequently decreased in widely invasive follicular carcinomas.[168,169]

 MOLECULAR DIAGNOSTICS

PAX8/PPARγ rearrangement occurs in approximately 35% of conventional follicular carcinomas and can be detected in thyroid resection specimens and FNA samples. The presence of *PAX8/PPARγ* can be suspected based on the positive PPARγ immunostaining or finding t(2;3)(q13;p25) translocation by karyotyping and can be confirmed by RT-PCR or FISH. In follicular carcinomas positive for *PAX8/PPARγ*, transcripts of various size

are found, which are formed by alternative splicing of the *PAX8* part of the fusion (Fig. 10.28A).[39] As a result, amplification of tumor RNA by conventional RT-PCR is expected to yield various size products (Fig. 8.26B). The finding of *PAX8/PPARγ* provides strong evidence for malignancy, despite the fact that this rearrangement can also be seen in approximately 8% of adenomas. In fact, in our experience, a significant proportion of tumors that originally had been diagnosed as follicular adenomas and later found to harbor *PAX8/PPARγ* revealed vascular or capsular invasion in deeper levels or in additional sections (Fig. 10.29). Therefore, finding the rearrangement in tumor cells should justify examining the entire tumor capsule irrespective of tumor size and obtaining multiple levels of all suspicious areas in search of capsular or vascular invasion. Those rearrangement-positive tumors that did not reveal invasion after thorough and complete examination should be designated as follicular adenomas. It is most likely that biologically they represent preinvasive or in situ follicular carcinomas.

Detection of *RAS* mutation has a limited diagnostic value in thyroid resection specimens and plays a bigger role in thyroid FNA samples. The limitation of its usefulness is attributed to the

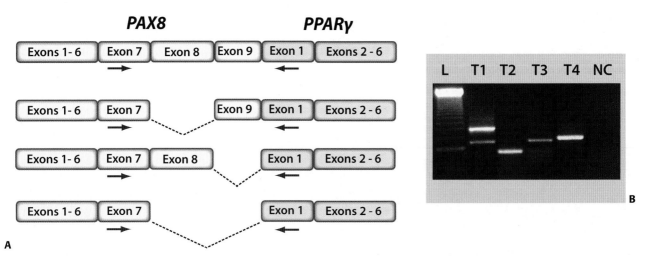

FIGURE 10.28. PAX8/PPARγ rearrangement. A: Schematic representation of various transcripts of *PAX8/PPARγ* formed by alternative splicing of *PAX8* mRNA. All transcripts can be amplified with primers located in exon 7 of *PAX8* and exon 1 of *PPARγ (arrows)* but are expected to yield amplification products of various size. **B:** Agarose gel electrophoresis of PCR products from four follicular carcinomas (T1 to T4) showing different size bands. L, 123-bp ladder; NC, negative control.

fact that *RAS* mutations are not specific for malignancy. They are found not only in 40% to 50% of conventional follicular carcinomas and approximately 40% of follicular variant of papillary carcinoma but also in approximately 30% of follicular adenomas. Despite lacking specificity for malignancy, *RAS* mutations mark carcinomas that are difficult to diagnose by FNA cytology. Testing for *RAS* mutations improves the diagnostic accuracy of FNA cytology.[166,170–172] In one study, *RAS* mutations found in several thyroid samples with negative or suboptimal cytology led to surgical treatment and subsequent detection of carcinoma.[173] In addition, because *RAS* mutation is likely to predispose to progression from follicular adenoma to carcinoma and to further tumor dedifferentiation, it may be justifiable to surgically remove *RAS*-positive adenomas to prevent their progression. More detailed information on the role of *RAS* and other mutations in the diagnosis of follicular carcinoma and other types of cancer in thyroid FNA samples is provided in Chapter 21.

Follicular carcinomas have overall a higher frequency of LOH and DNA aneuploidy than follicular adenomas. However, a significant overlap exists with respect to both alteration types, particularly between follicular adenomas and minimally invasive follicular carcinomas. This limits the diagnostic utility of these markers. However, higher frequency of LOH and loss of specific chromosomal loci appear to correlate with more aggressive behavior and can be exploited for prognostic purposes, as discussed later in the chapter.

ULTRASTRUCTURAL FEATURES

The ultrastructural features of conventional follicular carcinomas resemble those of follicular adenomas and normal thyroid tissue (Fig. 10.30A,B). The follicular cells generally preserve polarity, although it is less apparent than in normal thyroid cells. The cells rest on the continuous basal lamina and are linked together by tight junctions and desmosomes. Microvilli and occasional cilia are seen on the apical surface. The number and size of microvilli tend to vary between individual cells, and they are unevenly distributed on the apical surface of each cell.[174] The nuclei have a regular shape, finely dispersed chromatin, and typically inconspicuous nucleoli. The cytoplasm contains usual organelles, including well-developed granular endoplasmic reticulum, mitochondria, and Golgi complex. Small dense exocytotic vesicles and larger phagolysosomal bodies containing colloid may be seen.

Oncocytic carcinomas have more abundant cytoplasm that is packed with mitochondria (Fig. 10.30C,D). Many mitochondria show abnormalities in size, shape, and contents. They are frequently elongated and dilated and have diminished or

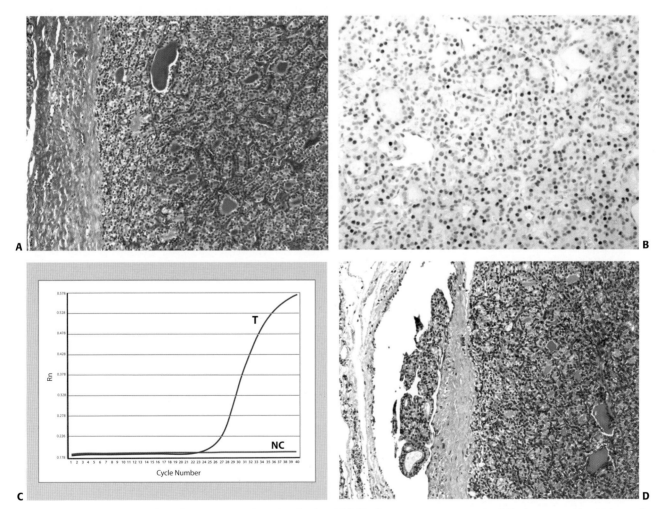

FIGURE 10.29. Diagnostic utility of *PAX8/PPARγ* detection in thyroid follicular tumors. A 2.0-cm microfollicular tumor with a thick capsule **(A)** had no invasion at the time of initial examination and was diagnosed as follicular adenoma. After discovery of *PAX8/PPARγ* the tumor was reexamined and found positive for PAX8 by immunohistochemistry **(B)** and for *PAX8/PPARγ* by real-time RT-PCR **(C)**. All tumor blocks were retrieved and serially sectioned, and deeper sections from one of the blocks revealed vascular invasion **(D)**, so that the diagnosis was changed to follicular carcinoma.

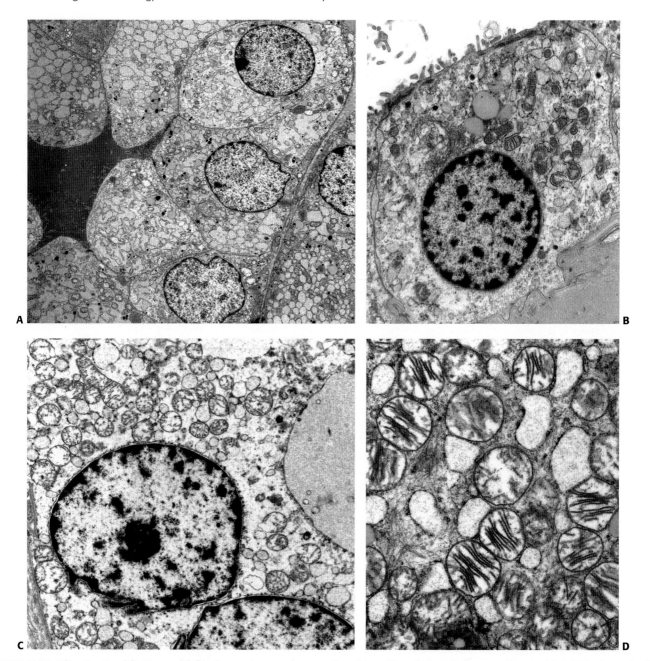

FIGURE 10.30. Ultrastructural features of follicular carcinoma of conventional type (A and B) and of oncocytic type (C and D). A: A microfollicular structure lined by cells with basally located round nuclei with no or slight irregularity of nuclear contours. **B:** A cuboidal cell rests on the basal lamina and shows microvilli on the apical surface. Various cytoplasmic organelles, including dilated endoplasmic reticulum, mitochondria, and lysosomes are seen. A few dense secretory vesicles are identifiable. **C:** Numerous mitochondria in the cytoplasm of the oncocytic follicular carcinoma. The apical surface lacks microvilli. Many mitochondria are abnormal, with irregularly spaced or absent cristae and bundles of cristae in the matrix **(D).**

almost entirely disappeared cristae. Some mitochondria reveal irregularly spaced cristae, filamentous bundles of cristae, and electron-dense bodies in the matrix.[175] Sparse dense vesicles and phagolysosomes are identifiable in the apical location, whereas other organelles are present in low numbers. Many oncocytic cells have a decreased number of apical microvilli. Scanning electron microscopy typically reveals a mixture of cells with a smooth surface interspersed with cells containing more abundant microvilli.[175] The ultramicroscopic features of oncocytic cells in oncocytic carcinomas are not different from those seen in oncocytic adenomas or nonneoplastic oncocytic cells.

Clear cell carcinomas show abundant cytoplasmic vacuoles of variable size. The vacuoles may be of different origins. Some

contain glycogen or lipids.[176] Others may develop from the Golgi complex or endocytotic vesicles[177] or reveal residual cristae suggesting their mitochondrial derivation.[117,138] In some clear cell tumors, the cytoplasm is packed with dilated cisternae of rough endoplasmic reticulum.[178]

 # CYTOLOGIC FEATURES

Cytologic sampling of follicular carcinoma typically yields a moderate to highly cellular specimen (Fig. 10.31A). Most of the tumors are well differentiated and represent minimally invasive follicular carcinoma. Many of the neoplastic epithelial cells are arranged in

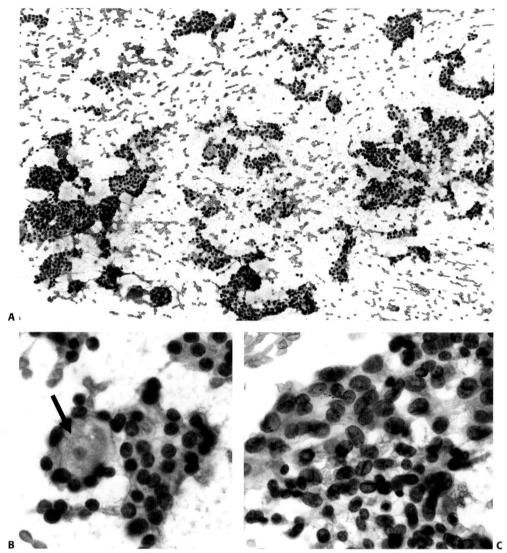

A

B

C

FIGURE 10.31. Cytologic features of conventional type follicular carcinoma. A: The cytology smear from follicular carcinoma shows multiple clusters of cells and small amount of colloid. **B:** At higher magnification, epithelial cells have bland nuclear features and form sheets and microfollicles containing colloid in the center *(arrow)*. This cytologic appearance is characteristic of well-differentiated carcinoma as well as microfollicular follicular adenoma. **C:** FNA smear from widely invasive follicular carcinoma reveals significant variability in nuclear size and shape. Some nuclei show irregular outlines; however, the nuclear contours of most cells are smooth. (Papanicolaou stain).

microfollicular structures, which are small spherical aggregates of 6 to 15 cells (Fig. 10.31B). The individual cells are cuboidal, although the cytoplasmic borders may be indistinct. The nuclei are round with minimal enlargement and the nuclear contours are smooth and regular. The chromatin pattern is even, and nucleoli are inconspicuous. The amount of colloid is usually small. In some clusters, a minute droplet of colloid may be seen in the center of the microfollicle. Widely invasive follicular carcinoma frequently shows architectural disorganization and additional nuclear abnormalities, such as nuclear enlargement, cellular and nuclear overlapping, pleomorphism, nuclear membrane irregularities, clumping of chromatin, and prominent nucleoli (Fig. 10.31C). These cytologic features are not specific for follicular carcinoma and may be encountered in benign and other malignant follicular-patterned thyroid lesions, including cellular hyperplastic nodule, follicular adenoma, and follicular variant of papillary carcinoma.[121] In practice, the cytologic diagnosis of "follicular neoplasm" or "suspicious for follicular neoplasm" (FN/SFN) by the current Bethesda System for Reporting Thyroid Cytopathology is given to these cases.[179,180] However, the microfollicular pattern is not specific for follicular carcinoma, and only 5% or fewer cases diagnosed as FN/SFN are found to be follicular carcinoma after resection.[181,182]

On occasion, aspirates of follicular carcinoma with normofollicular or macrofollicular areas produce smears with relatively abundant colloid. Such cases may produce smears showing a mixed pattern of follicular cells with flat sheets of follicular cells (from macrofollicular areas) and microfollicular structures (from more densely cellular areas) and often are diagnosed as "atypia/follicular lesion of undetermined significance" (AUS/FLUS) according to the Bethesda System. Cases in which the macrofollicular areas predominate are potential pitfalls resulting in false negative diagnoses. Aspirates from widely invasive follicular carcinoma typically show greater degrees of cytologic atypia. However, there are no specific cytologic features that allow for a prospective diagnosis of follicular carcinoma by cytologic sampling. These cases of widely invasive follicular carcinoma often are diagnosed as AUS/FLUS (if the cellularity is low), FN/SFN, or suspicious for malignancy (in cases of pronounced nuclear atypia). If cell block material is available, immunohistochemical stains for PPARγ, galectin-3, HBME1, and/or CITED1 may be utilized. Positive immunoreactivity by any of these markers increases the probability of malignancy. However, these markers are not specific for follicular carcinoma and the results should be interpreted in the appropriate context (see section above on Immunohistochemistry).

The oncocytic variant of follicular carcinoma also shows features overlapping with oncocytic follicular adenoma. Cytology smears reveal large round to oval cells with a relatively low nuclear:cytoplasmic ratio and numerous fine granules in the cytoplasm (Fig. 10.32). The nuclei are typically round and centrally or eccentrically located. The nuclear contours are smooth in most but

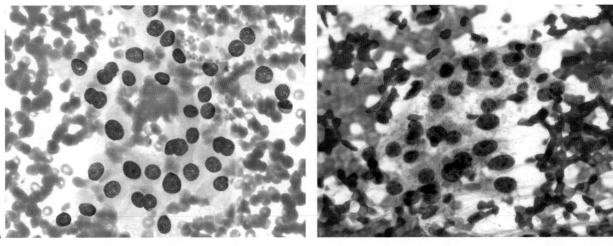

FIGURE 10.32. Cytologic features of oncocytic type follicular carcinoma. The sample was reported as "oncocytic lesion" and found to be an oncocytic follicular carcinoma after surgery (**A:** Diff-Quik stain; **B:** Papanicolaou stain).

irregular in some neoplastic cells. Bi- or multinucleation may be seen in occasional cells. The chromatin pattern is typically finely granular, and the nucleoli are prominent. In cytologic samples, these cases are diagnosed as "follicular neoplasm, Hürthle cell type" or "suspicious for follicular neoplasm, Hürthle cell type" (FNHCT/SFNHCT) according to the Bethesda System. Approximately a quarter of the cytologic diagnoses of "FNHCT/SFNHCT" result in oncocytic follicular carcinoma.[183,184] The outcome for the remainder includes oncocytic adenoma, nodular hyperplasia with oncocytic cells, hyperplastic nodule in lymphocytic (Hashimoto) thyroiditis, papillary carcinoma, and medullary carcinoma. For the cytopathologist, the presence of oncocytic (Hürthle) cells may present a challenge in making the appropriate diagnosis. A case that is highly cellular and exclusively composed of these cells is typically reported as FNHCT/SFNHCT. However, if the clinical scenario suggests the possibility of lymphocytic thyroiditis or multinodular goiter, the category of AUS/FLUS may be suitable. In addition, some cases may be hypocellular, but the predominant cell population may be oncocytes (Hürthle cells). In such cases, the distinction of benign processes (lymphocytic thyroiditis or multinodular goiter) from neoplastic processes is impossible, and the AUS/FLUS category may be used. However, if there are relatively few Hürthle cells in the background of abundant colloid and flat sheets of bland follicular cells (and no other concerning features), a benign diagnosis would be appropriate. Individual oncocytic cells are notorious for demonstrating worrisome nuclear changes under reactive situations. Nuclear membrane irregularities, grooves, and pseudoinclusion formation have been reported in cases of lymphocytic thyroiditis; however, these findings tend to be sparse. Therefore, the diagnosis of papillary carcinoma should be reserved for cases in which the background changes are appropriate and diagnostic nuclear changes are found reproducibly in multiple areas.

 # DIFFERENTIAL DIAGNOSIS

The differential diagnosis of follicular carcinoma includes follicular adenoma, cellular hyperplastic nodule, follicular variant of papillary carcinoma, poorly differentiated carcinoma, medullary carcinoma, and metastatic tumors.

The distinction between follicular carcinoma and follicular adenoma or hyperplastic nodule is based solely on the detection of capsular or vascular invasion. Other findings, such as very thick capsule, highly cellular tumors, and presence of mitoses, indicate a higher probability of malignancy and should serve as indicators for a more thorough examination of the lesion. However, none

of these features are diagnostic for malignancy in the absence of invasion. The diagnosis of carcinoma is supported by strong and diffuse immunoreactivity for PPARγ and by the presence of *PAX8/PPARγ* rearrangement, as well as by positive staining for galectin-3, HBME1, or CITED1, particularly when more than one of these markers are positive and the staining is diffuse and strong. The presence of *RAS* mutation strongly supports the neoplastic rather than hyperplastic nature of the lesion but cannot differentiate between follicular carcinoma and adenoma.

The distinction between follicular carcinoma and follicular variant of papillary carcinoma rests primarily on the finding of several diagnostic nuclear features of papillary carcinoma. Simple clearing of chromatin in random nuclei is not sufficient, and more widespread nuclear changes are needed for the diagnosis of papillary carcinoma. Thick fibrotic bands dissecting the nodule and elongated, slender follicles are more suggestive of papillary carcinoma. True psammoma bodies, if found in this setting, are virtually diagnostic of papillary carcinoma. The finding of *PAX8/PPARγ* rearrangement supports the diagnosis of follicular carcinoma, whereas *BRAF* and *RET/PTC* mutations are consistent with papillary carcinoma. Positive immunostaining for galectin-3, HBME1, and CITED1 helps support a malignant diagnosis but does not allow separation between the two cancer types.

Oncocytic follicular carcinoma is distinguished from oncocytic follicular variant of papillary carcinoma based on the lack of characteristic nuclear features of papillary carcinoma. Oncocytic follicular carcinomas not infrequently show concentric laminated calcifications of the luminal colloid, which should not be confused with true psammoma bodies.

Widely invasive follicular carcinomas with solid, trabecular, and insular growth patterns should be separated from poorly differentiated carcinomas. The separation is based on the lack of tumor necrosis or mitotic activity ≥3 per 10 high-power fields, both of which serve as diagnostic features of poorly differentiated thyroid carcinoma in this setting.[109]

Medullary carcinoma may enter the differential diagnosis, particularly when the tumor has a solid or trabecular growth pattern, reveals clear cells, and shows no colloid formation. Moreover, some medullary carcinomas may reveal a pseudofollicular growth or have oncocytic cytoplasm, mimicking the classic microfollicular appearance of follicular carcinoma and its main variant. The possibility of medullary carcinoma should be suspected when finding spindle-shaped cells, speckled ("salt and pepper") nuclear chromatin, and stromal deposits of amorphous material that represent amyloid. Once this possibility is considered, the distinction is straightforward and relies on the complementary pattern of immunoreactivity with the follicular cell marker thyroglobulin and the C-cell markers calcitonin, CEA, and chromogranin. TTF1 cannot be used for this distinction.

A metastatic carcinoma should be excluded if the tumor contains clear or signet-ring cells, shows mucin production, or lacks colloid. Immunoreactivity for thyroglobulin establishes the thyroid cell origin. However, positive staining of entrapped thyroid follicles should not be misinterpreted as evidence for the thyroid cell origin of the tumor mass.[138] More recently introduced markers, PAX8 and TTF2, may also be helpful.[156] TTF1 is a valuable marker when lung cancer and small-cell carcinomas from other locations are not a possibility. Distinction from parathyroid tumor may utilize staining for parathyroid hormone and chromogranin.

 ## TREATMENT AND PROGNOSIS

The treatment of follicular carcinomas is surgery. Because the diagnosis is rarely established preoperatively, the initial surgical approach is lobectomy. If invasion is identified in intraoperative frozen sections from a lobectomy specimen, the surgery may be expanded to total or near-total thyroidectomy. However, most minimally invasive follicular carcinomas are diagnosed only during microscopic evaluation of routine sections. The necessity of second surgery to remove the remaining lobe is debatable. Many studies find that total thyroidectomy has an overall positive effect on outcome, particularly in patients with tumors >1 to 1.5 cm and in high-risk groups,[185,186] whereas other studies report no effect of the extended surgery on survival.[97,187,188] Most of the current consensus guidelines recommend total thyroidectomy for patients with follicular carcinomas.[189,190] The main rationale for completion thyroidectomy is to allow subsequent radioiodine therapy and monitoring of tumor recurrence by measuring serum thyroglobulin. Most patients with follicular carcinoma undergo postoperative therapy with ^{131}I, which improves the outcome.[97,185,187] External beam radiation therapy is reserved for tumors that cannot be completely excised.[97,187]

On follow-up, tumor recurrence at local site or distant metastases occurs in 15% to 30% of cases.[122,185] Most of these complications happen within the first 5 years after initial surgery, although some may manifest one or two decades later.[108] Early recurrence of follicular carcinoma appears to predict a worse outcome.[191]

The 10-year survival in US patients for tumors diagnosed in the 1980s to 1990s was 83% to 85% for conventional follicular carcinoma and 73% to 76% for oncocytic follicular carcinoma,[7,192] and the survival continues to improve. Factors consistently found to negatively affect survival are older age (older than 50), larger tumor size (>4 cm), distant metastases at presentation, and extrathyroidal extension.[7,132,185,193-195] Those factors are used in most staging and prognostic scoring systems for well-differentiated thyroid cancer, including TNM staging (see Chapter 7, Table 7.3).[196] These systems offer an overall good prediction of prognosis, although patients in the low-stage/low-risk category still die of disease.[186,197]

Additional factors that correlate with mortality and/or recurrence include degree of invasiveness, that is, minimally invasive versus widely invasive carcinomas,[107,122,132] marked vascular invasion (≥4 vessels),[107,128,130] and oncocytic appearance.[193] The difference in survival between conventional and oncocytic carcinomas found in some studies may be because of older age of patients and decrease in iodine uptake by oncocytic tumors. Indeed, approximately 75% of metastases from conventional follicular carcinomas concentrate radioiodine as compared with 10% to 40% of oncocytic carcinoma metastases.[134]

Several potentially promising molecular and immunohistochemical markers have been offered for tumor prognostication, although most of them need further validation before widespread clinical use. It has been suggested that an increased rate of LOH, and particularly loss of the *VHL* gene locus on 3p25-26, has significant correlation with recurrent disease and death from tumor.[198,199]

In oncocytic tumors, a greater number of chromosomal gains appear to correlate with tumor recurrence.[43] The presence of *RAS* mutation in follicular carcinomas has been correlated with tumor dedifferentiation, distant metastases, and shorter survival.[200-202] Some studies have found that reduced expression of Bcl-2 and E-cadherin and high Ki-67 proliferative index are associated with distant metastases and/or tumor-related mortality.[98,168,169]

REFERENCES

1. Howlader N, Noone AM, Krapcho M, et al. SEER cancer statistics review, 1975–2008. National Cancer Institute. SEER web site. http://seer.cancer.gov/csr/1975_2008/. Accessed on July 10, 2011.
2. Sobrinho-Simoes M, Eloy C, Magalhaes J, et al. Follicular thyroid carcinoma. *Mod Pathol.* 2011;24(suppl 2):S10–S18.
3. LiVolsi VA, Asa SL. The demise of follicular carcinoma of the thyroid gland. *Thyroid.* 1994;4:233–236.
4. Colonna M, Guizard AV, Schvartz C, et al. A time trend analysis of papillary and follicular cancers as a function of tumour size: a study of data from six cancer registries in France (1983–2000). *Eur J Cancer.* 2007;43:891–900.
5. Albores-Saavedra J, Henson DE, Glazer E, et al. Changing patterns in the incidence and survival of thyroid cancer with follicular phenotype—papillary, follicular, and anaplastic: a morphological and epidemiological study. *Endocr Pathol.* 2007;18:1–7.
6. Hundahl SA. Perspective: National Cancer Institute summary report about estimated exposures and thyroid doses received from iodine 131 in fallout after Nevada atmospheric nuclear bomb tests. *CA Cancer J Clin.* 1998;48:285–298.
7. Haigh PI, Urbach DR. The treatment and prognosis of Hürthle cell follicular thyroid carcinoma compared with its non-Hürthle cell counterpart. *Surgery.* 2005;138:1152–1157; discussion 1157–1158.
8. Hundahl SA, Cady B, Cunningham MP, et al. Initial results from a prospective cohort study of 5583 cases of thyroid carcinoma treated in the United States during 1996. U.S. and German Thyroid Cancer Study Group. An American College of Surgeons Commission on Cancer Patient Care Evaluation study. *Cancer.* 2000;89:202–217.
9. Cuello C, Correa P, Eisenberg H. Geographic pathology of thyroid carcinoma. *Cancer.* 1969;23:230–239.
10. Pettersson B, Coleman MP, Ron E, et al. Iodine supplementation in Sweden and regional trends in thyroid cancer incidence by histopathologic type. *Int J Cancer.* 1996;65:13–19.
11. Belfiore A, La Rosa GL, Padova G, et al. The frequency of cold thyroid nodules and thyroid malignancies in patients from an iodine-deficient area. *Cancer.* 1987;60:3096–3102.
12. Franceschi S, Boyle P, Maisonneuve P, et al. The epidemiology of thyroid carcinoma. *Crit Rev Oncog.* 1993;4:25–52.
13. Harach HR, Escalante DA, Day ES. Thyroid cancer and thyroiditis in Salta, Argentina: a 40-yr study in relation to iodine prophylaxis. *Endocr Pathol.* 2002;13:175–181.
14. Schaller RT Jr, Stevenson JK. Development of carcinoma of the thyroid in iodine-deficient mice. *Cancer.* 1966;19:1063–1080.
15. Ward JM, Ohshima M. The role of iodine in carcinogenesis. *Adv Exp Med Biol.* 1986;206:529–542.
16. Shore RE. Issues and epidemiological evidence regarding radiation-induced thyroid cancer. *Radiat Res.* 1992;131:98–111.
17. D'Avanzo B, La Vecchia C, Franceschi S, et al. History of thyroid diseases and subsequent thyroid cancer risk. *Cancer Epidemiol Biomarkers Prev.* 1995;4:193–199.
18. Franceschi S, Preston-Martin S, Dal Maso L, et al. A pooled analysis of case-control studies of thyroid cancer. IV. Benign thyroid diseases. *Cancer Causes Control.* 1999;10:583–595.
19. Antico-Arciuch VG, Dima M, Liao XH, et al. Cross-talk between PI3K and estrogen in the mouse thyroid predisposes to the development of follicular carcinomas with a higher incidence in females. *Oncogene.* 2010;29:5678–5686.
20. Williams ED. Mechanisms and pathogenesis of thyroid cancer in animals and man. *Mutat Res.* 1995;333:123–129.
21. Cooper DS, Axelrod L, DeGroot LJ, et al. Congenital goiter and the development of metastatic follicular carcinoma with evidence for a leak of nonhormonal iodide: clinical, pathological, kinetic, and biochemical studies and a review of the literature. *J Clin Endocrinol Metab.* 1981;52:294–306.
22. Medeiros-Neto G, Gil-Da-Costa MJ, Santos CL, et al. Metastatic thyroid carcinoma arising from congenital goiter due to mutation in the thyroperoxidase gene. *J Clin Endocrinol Metab.* 1998;83:4162–4166.
23. Mitsumori K, Onodera H, Takahashi M, et al. Effect of thyroid stimulating hormone on the development and progression of rat thyroid follicular cell tumors. *Cancer Lett.* 1995;92:193–202.
24. Thomas GA, Williams ED. Evidence for and possible mechanisms of non-genotoxic carcinogenesis in the rodent thyroid. *Mutat Res.* 1991;248:357–370.
25. Negri E, Dal Maso L, Ron E, et al. A pooled analysis of case-control studies of thyroid cancer. II. Menstrual and reproductive factors. *Cancer Causes Control.* 1999;10:143–155.
26. Harach HR, Soubeyran I, Brown A, et al. Thyroid pathologic findings in patients with Cowden disease. *Ann Diagn Pathol.* 1999;3:331–340.
27. Starink TM, van der Veen JP, Arwert F, et al. The Cowden syndrome: a clinical and genetic study in 21 patients. *Clin Genet.* 1986;29:222–233.
28. Laury AR, Bongiovanni M, Tille JC, et al. Thyroid pathology in PTEN-hamartoma tumor syndrome: characteristic findings of a distinct entity. *Thyroid.* 2011;21:135–144.

29. Ishikawa Y, Sugano H, Matsumoto T, et al. Unusual features of thyroid carcinomas in Japanese patients with Werner syndrome and possible genotype-phenotype relations to cell type and race. *Cancer.* 1999;85:1345–1352.
30. Nwokoro NA, Korytkowski MT, Rose S, et al. Spectrum of malignancy and premalignancy in Carney syndrome. *Am J Med Genet.* 1997;73:369–377.
31. Stratakis CA, Courcoutsakis NA, Abati A, et al. Thyroid gland abnormalities in patients with the syndrome of spotty skin pigmentation, myxomas, endocrine overactivity, and schwannomas (Carney complex). *J Clin Endocrinol Metab.* 1997;82:2037–2043.
32. Rubén Harach H. Familial nonmedullary thyroid neoplasia. *Endocr Pathol.* 2001;12:97–112.
33. Roque L, Clode A, Belge G, et al. Follicular thyroid carcinoma: chromosome analysis of 19 cases. *Genes Chromosomes Cancer.* 1998;21:250–255.
34. Teyssier JR, Liautaud-Roger F, Ferre D, et al. Chromosomal changes in thyroid tumors. Relation with DNA content, karyotypic features, and clinical data. *Cancer Genet Cytogenet.* 1990;50:249–263.
35. Roque L, Serpa A, Clode A, et al. Significance of trisomy 7 and 12 in thyroid lesions with follicular differentiation: a cytogenetic and in situ hybridization study. *Lab Invest.* 1999;79:369–378.
36. Herrmann MA, Hay ID, Bartelt DH Jr, et al. Cytogenetic and molecular genetic studies of follicular and papillary thyroid cancers. *J Clin Invest.* 1991;88:1596–1604.
37. Roque L, Rodrigues R, Pinto A, et al. Chromosome imbalances in thyroid follicular neoplasms: a comparison between follicular adenomas and carcinomas. *Genes Chromosomes Cancer.* 2003;36:292–302.
38. Jenkins RB, Hay ID, Herath JF, et al. Frequent occurrence of cytogenetic abnormalities in sporadic nonmedullary thyroid carcinoma. *Cancer.* 1990;66:1213–1220.
39. Kroll TG, Sarraf P, Pecciarini L, et al. *PAX8-PPARgamma1* fusion oncogene in human thyroid carcinoma [corrected]. *Science.* 2000;289:1357–1360.
40. Lui WO, Kytola S, Anfalk L, et al. Balanced translocation (3;7)(p25;q34): another mechanism of tumorigenesis in follicular thyroid carcinoma? *Cancer Genet Cytogenet.* 2000;119:109–112.
41. Lui WO, Zeng L, Rehrmann V, et al. *CREB3L2-PPARgamma* fusion mutation identifies a thyroid signaling pathway regulated by intramembrane proteolysis. *Cancer Res.* 2008;68:7156–7164.
42. Hemmer S, Wasenius VM, Knuutila S, et al. DNA copy number changes in thyroid carcinoma. *Am J Pathol.* 1999;154:1539–1547.
43. Wada N, Duh QY, Miura D, et al. Chromosomal aberrations by comparative genomic hybridization in Hürthle cell thyroid carcinomas are associated with tumor recurrence. *J Clin Endocrinol Metab.* 2002;87:4595–4601.
44. Hemmer S, Wasenius VM, Knuutila S, et al. Comparison of benign and malignant follicular thyroid tumours by comparative genomic hybridization. *Br J Cancer.* 1998;78:1012–1017.
45. Frisk T, Kytola S, Wallin G, et al. Low frequency of numerical chromosomal aberrations in follicular thyroid tumors detected by comparative genomic hybridization. *Genes Chromosomes Cancer.* 1999;25:349–353.
46. Ciampi R, Zhu Z, Nikiforov YE. *BRAF* copy number gains in thyroid tumors detected by fluorescence in situ hybridization. *Endocr Pathol.* 2005;16:99–105.
47. Erickson LA, Jalal SM, Goellner JR, et al. Analysis of Hurthle cell neoplasms of the thyroid by interphase fluorescence in situ hybridization. *Am J Surg Pathol.* 2001;25:911–917.
48. Joensuu H, Klemi P, Eerola E, et al. Influence of cellular DNA content on survival in differentiated thyroid cancer. *Cancer.* 1986;58:2462–2467.
49. Grant CS, Hay ID, Ryan JJ, et al. Diagnostic and prognostic utility of flow cytometric DNA measurements in follicular thyroid tumors. *World J Surg.* 1990;14:283–289; discussion 289–290.
50. Oyama T, Vickery AL Jr, Preffer FI, et al. A comparative study of flow cytometry and histopathologic findings in thyroid follicular carcinomas and adenomas. *Hum Pathol.* 1994;25:271–275.
51. Salmon I, Gasperin P, Remmelink M, et al. Ploidy level and proliferative activity measurements in a series of 407 thyroid tumors or other pathologic conditions. *Hum Pathol.* 1993;24:912–920.
52. Ward LS, Brenta G, Medvedovic M, et al. Studies of allelic loss in thyroid tumors reveal major differences in chromosomal instability between papillary and follicular carcinomas. *J Clin Endocrinol Metab.* 1998;83:525–530.
53. Tung WS, Shevlin DW, Kaleem Z, et al. Allelotype of follicular thyroid carcinomas reveals genetic instability consistent with frequent nondisjunctional chromosomal loss. *Genes Chromosomes Cancer.* 1997;19:43–51.
54. Segev DL, Saji M, Phillips GS, et al. Polymerase chain reaction-based microsatellite polymorphism analysis of follicular and Hürthle cell neoplasms of the thyroid. *J Clin Endocrinol Metab.* 1998;83:2036–2042.
55. Kitamura Y, Shimizu K, Ito K, et al. Allelotyping of follicular thyroid carcinoma: frequent allelic losses in chromosome arms 7q, 11p, and 22q. *J Clin Endocrinol Metab.* 2001;86:4268–4272.
56. Grebe SK, McIver B, Hay ID, et al. Frequent loss of heterozygosity on chromosomes 3p and 17p without *VHL* or *p53* mutations suggests involvement of unidentified tumor suppressor genes in follicular thyroid carcinoma. *J Clin Endocrinol Metab.* 1997;82:3684–3691.
57. Sarquis MS, Weber F, Shen L, et al. High frequency of loss of heterozygosity in imprinted, compared with nonimprinted, genomic regions in follicular thyroid carcinomas and atypical adenomas. *J Clin Endocrinol Metab.* 2006;91:262–269.
58. Schark C, Fulton N, Jacoby RF, et al. *N-ras 61* oncogene mutations in Hürthle cell tumors. *Surgery.* 1990;108:994–999; discussion 999–1000.
59. Esapa CT, Johnson SJ, Kendall-Taylor P, et al. Prevalence of *Ras* mutations in thyroid neoplasia. *Clin Endocrinol (Oxf).* 1999;50:529–535.
60. Nikiforova MN, Lynch RA, Biddinger PW, et al. *RAS* point mutations and *PAX8-PPAR gamma* rearrangement in thyroid tumors: evidence for distinct molecular pathways in thyroid follicular carcinoma. *J Clin Endocrinol Metab.* 2003;88:2318–2326.
61. Lemoine NR, Mayall ES, Wyllie FS, et al. Activated *ras* oncogenes in human thyroid cancers. *Cancer Res.* 1988;48:4459–4463.
62. Vasko V, Ferrand M, Di Cristofaro J, et al. Specific pattern of RAS oncogene mutations in follicular thyroid tumors. *J Clin Endocrinol Metab.* 2003;88:2745–2752.
63. Fagin JA. Minireview: branded from the start-distinct oncogenic initiating events may determine tumor fate in the thyroid. *Mol Endocrinol.* 2002;16:903–911.
64. Saavedra HI, Knauf JA, Shirokawa JM, et al. The *RAS* oncogene induces genomic instability in thyroid PCCL3 cells via the MAPK pathway. *Oncogene.* 2000;19:3948–3954.
65. Santelli G, de Franciscis V, Portella G, et al. Production of transgenic mice expressing the *Ki-ras* oncogene under the control of a thyroglobulin promoter. *Cancer Res.* 1993;53:5523–5527.
66. Vitagliano D, Portella G, Troncone G, et al. Thyroid targeting of the *N-ras(Gln61Lys)* oncogene in transgenic mice results in follicular tumors that progress to poorly differentiated carcinomas. *Oncogene.* 2006;25: 5467–5474.
67. Miller KA, Yeager N, Baker K, et al. Oncogenic *Kras* requires simultaneous PI3K signaling to induce ERK activation and transform thyroid epithelial cells in vivo. *Cancer Res.* 2009;69:3689–3694.
68. Chia WK, Sharifah NA, Reena RM, et al. Fluorescence in situ hybridization analysis using PAX8- and PPARG-specific probes reveals the presence of PAX8-PPARG translocation and 3p25 aneusomy in follicular thyroid neoplasms. *Cancer Genet Cytogenet.* 2010;196:7–13.
69. French CA, Alexander EK, Cibas ES, et al. Genetic and biological subgroups of low-stage follicular thyroid cancer. *Am J Pathol.* 2003;162:1053–1060.
70. Nikiforova MN, Biddinger PW, Caudill CM, et al. *PAX8-PPARgamma* rearrangement in thyroid tumors: RT-PCR and immunohistochemical analyses. *Am J Surg Pathol.* 2002;26:1016–1023.
71. Dwight T, Thoppe SR, Foukakis T, et al. Involvement of the *PAX8*/peroxisome proliferator-activated receptor gamma rearrangement in follicular thyroid tumors. *J Clin Endocrinol Metab.* 2003;88:4440–4445.
72. Marques AR, Espadinha C, Catarino AL, et al. Expression of *PAX8-PPAR gamma 1* rearrangements in both follicular thyroid carcinomas and adenomas. *J Clin Endocrinol Metab.* 2002;87:3947–3952.
73. Giordano TJ, Au AY, Kuick R, et al. Delineation, functional validation, and bioinformatic evaluation of gene expression in thyroid follicular carcinomas with the PAX8-PPARG translocation. *Clin Cancer Res.* 2006;12:1983–1993.
74. Reddi HV, McIver B, Grebe SK, et al. The paired *box-8*/peroxisome proliferator-activated receptor-gamma oncogene in thyroid tumorigenesis. *Endocrinology.* 2007;148:932–935.
75. Reddi HV, Madde P, Marlow LA, et al. Expression of the PAX8/PPARgamma fusion protein is associated with decreased neovascularization in vivo: impact on tumorigenesis and disease prognosis. *Genes Cancer.* 2010;1:480–492.
76. Reddi HV, Madde P, Milosevic D, et al. The putative PAX8/PPARgamma fusion oncoprotein exhibits partial tumor suppressor activity through up-regulation of micro-RNA-122 and dominant-negative PPARgamma activity. *Genes Cancer.* 2011;2:46–55.
77. Cheung L, Messina M, Gill A, et al. Detection of the *PAX8-PPAR gamma* fusion oncogene in both follicular thyroid carcinomas and adenomas. *J Clin Endocrinol Metab.* 2003;88:354–357.
78. Cully M, You H, Levine AJ, et al. Beyond *PTEN* mutations: the PI3K pathway as an integrator of multiple inputs during tumorigenesis. *Nat Rev Cancer.* 2006;6:184–192.
79. Shinohara M, Chung YJ, Saji M, et al. AKT in thyroid tumorigenesis and progression. *Endocrinology.* 2007;148:942–947.
80. Yeager N, Brewer C, Cai KQ, et al. Mammalian target of rapamycin is the key effector of phosphatidylinositol-3-OH-initiated proliferative signals in the thyroid follicular epithelium. *Cancer Res.* 2008;68:444–449.
81. Sobrinho-Simoes M, Maximo V, Castro IV, et al. Hürthle (oncocytic) cell tumors of thyroid: etiopathogenesis, diagnosis and clinical significance. *Int J Surg Pathol.* 2005;13:29–35.
82. Hou P, Liu D, Shan Y, et al. Genetic alterations and their relationship in the phosphatidylinositol 3-kinase/Akt pathway in thyroid cancer. *Clin Cancer Res.* 2007;13:1161–1170.
83. Wang Y, Hou P, Yu H, et al. High prevalence and mutual exclusivity of genetic alterations in the phosphatidylinositol-3-kinase/akt pathway in thyroid tumors. *J Clin Endocrinol Metab.* 2007;92:2387–2390.
84. Wu G, Mambo E, Guo Z, et al. Uncommon mutation, but common amplifications, of the *PIK3CA* gene in thyroid tumors. *J Clin Endocrinol Metab.* 2005;90:4688–4693.
85. Halachmi N, Halachmi S, Evron E, et al. Somatic mutations of the *PTEN* tumor suppressor gene in sporadic follicular thyroid tumors. *Genes Chromosomes Cancer.* 1998;23:239–243.
86. Maximo V, Sobrinho-Simoes M. Hürthle cell tumours of the thyroid. A review with emphasis on mitochondrial abnormalities with clinical relevance. *Virchows Arch.* 2000;437:107–115.
87. Tallini G. Oncocytic tumours. *Virchows Arch.* 1998;433:5–12.
88. Katoh R, Harach HR, Williams ED. Solitary, multiple, and familial oxyphil tumours of the thyroid gland. *J Pathol.* 1998;186:292–299.
89. Maximo V, Botelho T, Capela J, et al. Somatic and germline mutation in GRIM-19, a dual function gene involved in mitochondrial metabolism and cell death, is linked to mitochondrion-rich (Hurthle cell) tumours of the thyroid. *Br J Cancer.* 2005;92:1892–1898.
90. Angell JE, Lindner DJ, Shapiro PS, et al. Identification of GRIM-19, a novel cell death-regulatory gene induced by the interferon-beta and retinoic acid combination, using a genetic approach. *J Biol Chem.* 2000;275:33416–33426.
91. Gasparre G, Porcelli AM, Bonora E, et al. Disruptive mitochondrial DNA mutations in complex I subunits are markers of oncocytic phenotype in thyroid tumors. *Proc Natl Acad Sci U S A.* 2007;104:9001–9006.
92. Maximo V, Soares P, Lima J, et al. Mitochondrial DNA somatic mutations (point mutations and large deletions) and mitochondrial DNA variants in

human thyroid pathology: a study with emphasis on Hürthle cell tumors. *Am J Pathol.* 2002;160:1857–1865.
93. Aldred MA, Huang Y, Liyanarachchi S, et al. Papillary and follicular thyroid carcinomas show distinctly different microarray expression profiles and can be distinguished by a minimum of five genes. *J Clin Oncol.* 2004;22:3531–3539.
94. Barden CB, Shister KW, Zhu B, et al. Classification of follicular thyroid tumors by molecular signature: results of gene profiling. *Clin Cancer Res.* 2003;9:1792–1800.
95. Williams MD, Zhang L, Elliott DD, et al. Differential gene expression profiling of aggressive and nonaggressive follicular carcinomas. *Hum Pathol.* 2011;42:1213–1220.
96. Zhao J, Leonard C, Gemsenjager E, et al. Differentiation of human follicular thyroid adenomas from carcinomas by gene expression profiling. *Oncol Rep.* 2008;19:329–337.
97. Lopez-Penabad L, Chiu AC, Hoff AO, et al. Prognostic factors in patients with Hürthle cell neoplasms of the thyroid. *Cancer.* 2003;97:1186–1194.
98. Erickson LA, Jin L, Goellner JR, et al. Pathologic features, proliferative activity, and cyclin D1 expression in Hurthle cell neoplasms of the thyroid. *Mod Pathol.* 2000;13:186–192.
99. Yeager N, Klein-Szanto A, Kimura S, et al. *PTEN* loss in the mouse thyroid causes goiter and follicular adenomas: insights into thyroid function and Cowden disease pathogenesis. *Cancer Res.* 2007;67:959–966.
100. Kirschner LS, Carney JA, Pack SD, et al. Mutations of the gene encoding the protein kinase A type I-alpha regulatory subunit in patients with the Carney complex. *Nat Genet.* 2000;26:89–92.
101. Niepomniszcze H, Suarez H, Pitoia F, et al. Follicular carcinoma presenting as autonomous functioning thyroid nodule and containing an activating mutation of the TSH receptor *(T620I)* and a mutation of the *Ki-RAS (G12C)* genes. *Thyroid.* 2006;16:497–503.
102. Giovanella L, Fasolini F, Suriano S, et al. Hyperfunctioning solid/trabecular follicular carcinoma of the thyroid gland. *J Oncol.* 2010;2010:pii:635984.
103. Yalla NM, Reynolds LR. Hürthle cell thyroid carcinoma presenting as a “hot” nodule. *Endocr Pract.* 2011;17:e68–e72.
104. Lang W, Georgii A, Stauch G, et al. The differentiation of atypical adenomas and encapsulated follicular carcinomas in the thyroid gland. *Virchows Arch A Pathol Anat Histol.* 1980;385:125–141.
105. Evans HL. Follicular neoplasms of the thyroid. A study of 44 cases followed for a minimum of 10 years, with emphasis on differential diagnosis. *Cancer.* 1984;54:535–540.
106. Yamashina M. Follicular neoplasms of the thyroid. Total circumferential evaluation of the fibrous capsule. *Am J Surg Pathol.* 1992;16:392–400.
107. Lang W, Choritz H, Hundeshagen H. Risk factors in follicular thyroid carcinomas. A retrospective follow-up study covering a 14-year period with emphasis on morphological findings. *Am J Surg Pathol.* 1986;10:246–255.
108. Kahn NF, Perzin KH. Follicular carcinoma of the thyroid: an evaluation of the histologic criteria used for diagnosis. *Pathol Annu.* 1983;18(pt 1):221–253.
109. Volante M, Collini P, Nikiforov YE, et al. Poorly differentiated thyroid carcinoma: the Turin proposal for the use of uniform diagnostic criteria and an algorithmic diagnostic approach. *Am J Surg Pathol.* 2007;31:1256–1264.
110. DeLellis RA, Lloyd RV, Heitz PU, et al, eds. *World Health Organization Classification of Tumours. Pathology and Genetics of Tumours of Endocrine Organs.* Lyon, France: IARC Press; 2004.
111. Franssila KO, Ackerman LV, Brown CL, et al. Follicular carcinoma. *Semin Diagn Pathol.* 1985;2:101–122.
112. Mete O, Asa SL. Pathological definition and clinical significance of vascular invasion in thyroid carcinomas of follicular epithelial derivation. *Mod Pathol.* 2011; 24:1545-1552.
113. Jorda M, Gonzalez-Campora R, Mora J, et al. Prognostic factors in follicular carcinoma of the thyroid. *Arch Pathol Lab Med.* 1993;117:631–635.
114. Suster S. Thyroid tumors with a follicular growth pattern: problems in differential diagnosis. *Arch Pathol Lab Med.* 2006;130:984–988.
115. Franc B, de la Salmoniere P, Lange F, et al. Interobserver and intraobserver reproducibility in the histopathology of follicular thyroid carcinoma. *Hum Pathol.* 2003;34:1092–1100.
116. Schmid KW, Farid NR. How to define follicular thyroid carcinoma? *Virchows Arch.* 2006;448:385–393.
117. Rosai J, Carcangiu ML, DeLellis RA. *Tumors of the Thyroid Gland.* 3rd ed. Washington, DC: Armed Forces Institute of Pathology; 1992.
118. LiVolsi VA, Baloch ZW. Follicular neoplasms of the thyroid: view, biases, and experiences. *Adv Anat Pathol.* 2004;11:279–287.
119. LiVolsi VA, Merino MJ. Worrisome histologic alterations following fine-needle aspiration of the thyroid (WHAFFT). *Pathol Annu.* 1994;29(pt 2):99–120.
120. Rosai J. Handling of thyroid follicular patterned lesions. *Endocr Pathol.* 2005;16:279–283.
121. Baloch ZW, Livolsi VA. Follicular-patterned lesions of the thyroid: the bane of the pathologist. *Am J Clin Pathol.* 2002;117:143–150.
122. D’Avanzo A, Treseler P, Ituarte PH, et al. Follicular thyroid carcinoma: histology and prognosis. *Cancer.* 2004;100:1123–1129.
123. Segal K, Arad A, Lubin E, et al. Follicular carcinoma of the thyroid. *Head Neck.* 1994;16:533–538.
124. Mai KT, Khanna P, Yazdi HM, et al. Differentiated thyroid carcinomas with vascular invasion: a comparative study of follicular, Hürthle cell and papillary thyroid carcinoma. *Pathology.* 2002;34:239–244.
125. O’Neill CJ, Vaughan L, Learoyd DL, et al. Management of follicular thyroid carcinoma should be individualised based on degree of capsular and vascular invasion. *Eur J Surg Oncol.* 2011;37:181–185.
126. Gemsenjager E, Heitz PU, Seifert B, et al. Differentiated thyroid carcinoma. Follow-up of 264 patients from one institution for up to 25 years. *Swiss Med Wkly.* 2001;131:157–163.
127. van Heerden JA, Hay ID, Goellner JR, et al. Follicular thyroid carcinoma with capsular invasion alone: a nonthreatening malignancy. *Surgery.* 1992;112:1130–1136; discussion 1136–1138.
128. Brennan MD, Bergstralh EJ, van Heerden JA, et al. Follicular thyroid cancer treated at the Mayo Clinic, 1946 through 1970: initial manifestations, pathologic findings, therapy, and outcome. *Mayo Clin Proc.* 1991;66:11–22.
129. Ghossein RA, Hiltzik DH, Carlson DL, et al. Prognostic factors of recurrence in encapsulated Hurthle cell carcinoma of the thyroid gland: a clinicopathologic study of 50 cases. *Cancer.* 2006;106:1669–1676.
130. Collini P, Sampietro G, Pilotti S. Extensive vascular invasion is a marker of risk of relapse in encapsulated non-Hürthle cell follicular carcinoma of the thyroid gland: a clinicopathological study of 18 consecutive cases from a single institution with a 11-year median follow-up. *Histopathology.* 2004;44:35–39.
131. Sanders LE, Silverman M. Follicular and Hürthle cell carcinoma: predicting outcome and directing therapy. *Surgery.* 1998;124:967–974.
132. Lo CY, Chan WF, Lam KY, et al. Follicular thyroid carcinoma: the role of histology and staging systems in predicting survival. *Ann Surg.* 2005;242:708–715.
133. Machens A, Holzhausen HJ, Dralle H. The prognostic value of primary tumor size in papillary and follicular thyroid carcinoma. *Cancer.* 2005;103:2269–2273.
134. Phitayakorn R, McHenry CR. Follicular and Hürthle cell carcinoma of the thyroid gland. *Surg Oncol Clin N Am.* 2006;15:603–623, ix–x.
135. Grant CS. Operative and postoperative management of the patient with follicular and Hürthle cell carcinoma. Do they differ? *Surg Clin North Am.* 1995;75:395–403.
136. Gosain AK, Clark OH. Hürthle cell neoplasms. Malignant potential. *Arch Surg.* 1984;119:515–519.
137. Gundry SR, Burney RE, Thompson NW, et al. Total thyroidectomy for Hürthle cell neoplasm of the thyroid. *Arch Surg.* 1983;118:529–532.
138. Carcangiu ML, Sibley RK, Rosai J. Clear cell change in primary thyroid tumors. A study of 38 cases. *Am J Surg Pathol.* 1985;9:705–722.
139. Civantos F, Albores-Saavedra J, Nadji M, et al. Clear cell variant of thyroid carcinoma. *Am J Surg Pathol.* 1984;8:187–192.
140. Ropp BG, Solomides C, Palazzo J, et al. Follicular carcinoma of the thyroid with extensive clear-cell differentiation: a potential diagnostic pitfall. *Diagn Cytopathol.* 2000;22:398–399.
141. Schroder S, Bocker W. Clear-cell carcinomas of thyroid gland: a clinicopathological study of 13 cases. *Histopathology.* 1986;10:75–89.
142. Cretney A, Mow C. Mucinous variant of follicular carcinoma of the thyroid gland. *Pathology.* 2006;38:184–186.
143. Diaz-Perez R, Quiroz H, Nishiyama RH. Primary mucinous adenocarcinoma of thyroid gland. *Cancer.* 1976;38:1323–1325.
144. Rigaud C, Bogomoletz WV. “Mucin secreting” and “mucinous” primary thyroid carcinomas: pitfalls in mucin histochemistry applied to thyroid tumours. *J Clin Pathol.* 1987;40:890–895.
145. Deligdisch L, Subhani Z, Gordon RE. Primary mucinous carcinoma of the thyroid gland: report of a case and ultrastructural study. *Cancer.* 1980;45:2564–2567.
146. Schroder S, Bocker W. Signet-ring-cell thyroid tumors. Follicle cell tumors with arrest of folliculogenesis. *Am J Surg Pathol.* 1985;9:619–629.
147. Clerici T, Kolb W, Beutner U, et al. Diagnosis and treatment of small follicular thyroid carcinomas. *Br J Surg.* 2010;97:839–844.
148. Hollander MC, Blumenthal GM, Dennis PA. *PTEN* loss in the continuum of common cancers, rare syndromes and mouse models. *Nat Rev Cancer.* 2011;11:289–301.
149. Nose V. Familial thyroid cancer: a review. *Mod Pathol.* 2011;24(suppl 2):S19–S33.
150. Hemmings CT. Thyroid pathology in four patients with Cowden’s disease. *Pathology.* 2003;35:311–314.
151. Gnepp DR, Ogorzalek JM, Heffess CS. Fat-containing lesions of the thyroid gland. *Am J Surg Pathol.* 1989;13:605–612.
152. Fuhrer D, Tannapfel A, Sabri O, et al. Two somatic TSH receptor mutations in a patient with toxic metastasising follicular thyroid carcinoma and non-functional lung metastases. *Endocr Relat Cancer.* 2003;10:591–600.
153. Russo D, Wong MG, Costante G, et al. A Val 677 activating mutation of the thyrotropin receptor in a Hürthle cell thyroid carcinoma associated with thyrotoxicosis. *Thyroid.* 1999;9:13–17.
154. Katoh R, Miyagi E, Nakamura N, et al. Expression of thyroid transcription factor-1 (TTF-1) in human C cells and medullary thyroid carcinomas. *Hum Pathol.* 2000;31:386–393.
155. Lau SK, Luthringer DJ, Eisen RN. Thyroid transcription factor-1: a review. *Appl Immunohistochem Mol Morphol.* 2002;10:97–102.
156. Nonaka D, Tang Y, Chiriboga L, et al. Diagnostic utility of thyroid transcription factors Pax8 and TTF-2 (FoxE1) in thyroid epithelial neoplasms. *Mod Pathol.* 2008;21:192–200.
157. Bejarano PA, Nikiforov YE, Swenson ES, et al. Thyroid transcription factor-1, thyroglobulin, cytokeratin 7, and cytokeratin 20 in thyroid neoplasms. *Appl Immunohistochem Mol Morphol.* 2000;8:189–194.
158. Wilson NW, Pambakian H, Richardson TC, et al. Epithelial markers in thyroid carcinoma: an immunoperoxidase study. *Histopathology.* 1986;10:815–829.
159. Judkins AR, Roberts SA, Livolsi VA. Utility of immunohistochemistry in the evaluation of necrotic thyroid tumors. *Hum Pathol.* 1999;30:1373–1376.
160. Papotti M, Gugliotta P, Forte G, et al. Immunocytochemical identification of oxyphilic mitochondrion-rich cells. *Appl Immunohistochem Mol Morphol.* 1994;2:261–263.
161. Bussolati G, Gugliotta P, Volante M, et al. Retrieved endogenous biotin: a novel marker and a potential pitfall in diagnostic immunohistochemistry. *Histopathology.* 1997;31:400–407.
162. Nakamura N, Erickson LA, Jin L, et al. Immunohistochemical separation of follicular variant of papillary thyroid carcinoma from follicular adenoma. *Endocr Pathol.* 2006;17:213–223.
163. Scognamiglio T, Hyjek E, Kao J, et al. Diagnostic usefulness of HBME1, galectin-3, CK19, and CITED1 and evaluation of their expression in encapsulated lesions with questionable features of papillary thyroid carcinoma. *Am J Clin Pathol.* 2006;126:700–708.
164. Saggiorato E, De Pompa R, Volante M, et al. Characterization of thyroid “follicular neoplasms” in fine-needle aspiration cytological specimens using a

panel of immunohistochemical markers: a proposal for clinical application. *Endocr Relat Cancer*. 2005;12:305–317.

165. Prasad ML, Pellegata NS, Huang Y, et al. Galectin-3, fibronectin-1, CITED-1, HBME1 and cytokeratin-19 immunohistochemistry is useful for the differential diagnosis of thyroid tumors. *Mod Pathol*. 2005;18:48–57.

166. Barut F, Onak Kandemir N, Bektas S, et al. Universal markers of thyroid malignancies: galectin-3, HBME-1, and cytokeratin-19. *Endocr Pathol*. 2010;21:80–89.

167. Asa SL. The role of immunohistochemical markers in the diagnosis of follicular-patterned lesions of the thyroid. *Endocr Pathol*. 2005;16:295–309.

168. Hoos A, Stojadinovic A, Singh B, et al. Clinical significance of molecular expression profiles of Hürthle cell tumors of the thyroid gland analyzed via tissue microarrays. *Am J Pathol*. 2002;160:175–183.

169. Brecelj E, Frkovic Grazio S, Auersperg M, et al. Prognostic value of E-cadherin expression in thyroid follicular carcinoma. *Eur J Surg Oncol*. 2005;31:544–548.

170. Nikiforov YE, Steward DL, Robinson-Smith TM, et al. Molecular testing for mutations in improving the fine-needle aspiration diagnosis of thyroid nodules. *J Clin Endocrinol Metab*. 2009;94:2092–2098.

171. Cantara S, Capezzone M, Marchisotta S, et al. Impact of proto-oncogene mutation detection in cytological specimens from thyroid nodules improves the diagnostic accuracy of cytology. *J Clin Endocrinol Metab*. 2010;95:1365–1369.

172. Ohori NP, Nikiforova MN, Schoedel KE, et al. Contribution of molecular testing to thyroid fine-needle aspiration cytology of "follicular lesion of undetermined significance/atypia of undetermined significance." *Cancer Cytopathol*. 2010;118:17–23.

173. Nikiforova MN, Zhaowen Z, Robinson-Smith T, et al. Molecular testing of thyroid FNA samples: feasibility and significance for preoperative diagnosis of thyroid tumors (abstract). *Modern Pathology*. 2004;17(suppl 1):77A.

174. Johannessen JV, Sobrinho-Simoes M. Follicular carcinoma of the human thyroid gland: an ultrastructural study with emphasis on scanning electron microscopy. *Diagn Histopathol*. 1982;5:113–127.

175. Nesland JM, Sobrinho-Simoes MA, Holm R, et al. Hürthle-cell lesions of the thyroid: a combined study using transmission electron microscopy, scanning electron microscopy, and immunocytochemistry. *Ultrastruct Pathol*. 1985;8:269–290.

176. Valenta LJ, Michel-Bechet M. Electron microscopy of clear cell thyroid carcinoma. *Arch Pathol Lab Med*. 1977;101:140–144.

177. Bocker W, Dralle H, Koch G, et al. Immunohistochemical and electron microscope analysis of adenomas of the thyroid gland. II. Adenomas with specific cytological differentiation. *Virchows Arch A Pathol Anat Histol*. 1978;380:205–220.

178. Ishimaru Y, Fukuda S, Kurano R, et al. Follicular thyroid carcinoma with clear cell change showing unusual ultrastructural features. *Am J Surg Pathol*. 1988;12:240–246.

179. Baloch ZW, LiVolsi VA, Asa SL, et al. Diagnostic terminology and morphologic criteria for cytologic diagnosis of thyroid lesions: a synopsis of the National Cancer Institute Thyroid Fine-Needle Aspiration State of the Science Conference. *Diagn Cytopathol*. 2008;36:425–437.

180. Ali SZ, Cibas ES. *The Bethesda System for Reporting Thyroid Cytopathology*. New York, NY: Springer; 2010.

181. Deveci MS, Deveci G, LiVolsi VA, et al. Fine-needle aspiration of follicular lesions of the thyroid. Diagnosis and follow-up. *Cytojournal*. 2006;3:9.

182. Yang J, Schnadig V, Logrono R, et al. Fine-needle aspiration of thyroid nodules: a study of 4703 patients with histologic and clinical correlations. *Cancer*. 2007;111:306–315.

183. Giorgadze T, Rossi ED, Fadda G, et al. Does the fine-needle aspiration diagnosis of "Hürthle-cell neoplasm/follicular neoplasm with oncocytic features" denote increased risk of malignancy? *Diagn Cytopathol*. 2004;31:307–312.

184. Pu RT, Yang J, Wasserman PG, et al. Does Hurthle cell lesion/neoplasm predict malignancy more than follicular lesion/neoplasm on thyroid fine-needle aspiration? *Diagn Cytopathol*. 2006;34:330–334.

185. Mazzaferri EL, Jhiang SM. Long-term impact of initial surgical and medical therapy on papillary and follicular thyroid cancer. *Am J Med*. 1994; 97:418–428.

186. Wu HS, Young MT, Ituarte PH, et al. Death from thyroid cancer of follicular cell origin. *J Am Coll Surg*. 2000;191:600–606.

187. Taylor T, Specker B, Robbins J, et al. Outcome after treatment of high-risk papillary and non-Hürthle-cell follicular thyroid carcinoma. *Ann Intern Med*. 1998;129:622–627.

188. Thompson LD, Wieneke JA, Paal E, et al. A clinicopathologic study of minimally invasive follicular carcinoma of the thyroid gland with a review of the English literature. *Cancer*. 2001;91:505–524.

189. Cooper DS, Doherty GM, Haugen BR, et al. Management guidelines for patients with thyroid nodules and differentiated thyroid cancer. *Thyroid*. 2006;16:109–142.

190. Sherman SI. Thyroid carcinoma. *Lancet*. 2003;361:501–511.

191. Lin JD, Hsueh C, Chao TC. Early recurrence of papillary and follicular thyroid carcinoma predicts a worse outcome. *Thyroid*. 2009;19:1053–1059.

192. Hundahl SA, Fleming ID, Fremgen AM, et al. A National Cancer Data Base report on 53,856 cases of thyroid carcinoma treated in the U.S., 1985–1995 [see comments]. *Cancer*. 1998;83:2638–2648.

193. Shaha AR, Loree TR, Shah JP. Prognostic factors and risk group analysis in follicular carcinoma of the thyroid. *Surgery*. 1995;118:1131–1136; discussion 1136–1138.

194. Simpson WJ, McKinney SE, Carruthers JS, et al. Papillary and follicular thyroid cancer. Prognostic factors in 1,578 patients. *Am J Med*. 1987;83:479–488.

195. Sugino K, Ito K, Nagahama M, et al. Prognosis and prognostic factors for distant metastases and tumor mortality in follicular thyroid carcinoma. *Thyroid*. 2011;21:751–757.

196. Zeiger MA, Dackiw AP. Follicular thyroid lesions, elements that affect both diagnosis and prognosis. *J Surg Oncol*. 2005;89:108–113.

197. Dean DS, Hay ID. Prognostic indicators in differentiated thyroid carcinoma. *Cancer Control*. 2000;7:229–239.

198. Hunt JL, Yim JH, Tometsko M, et al. Loss of heterozygosity of the *VHL* gene identifies malignancy and predicts death in follicular thyroid tumors. *Surgery*. 2003;134:1043–1047; discussion 1047–1048.

199. Hunt JL, Yim JH, Carty SE. Fractional allelic loss of tumor suppressor genes identifies malignancy and predicts clinical outcome in follicular thyroid tumors. *Thyroid*. 2006;16:643–649.

200. Basolo F, Pisaturo F, Pollina LE, et al. *N-ras* mutation in poorly differentiated thyroid carcinomas: correlation with bone metastases and inverse correlation to thyroglobulin expression. *Thyroid*. 2000;10:19–23.

201. Garcia-Rostan G, Zhao H, Camp RL, et al. *Ras* mutations are associated with aggressive tumor phenotypes and poor prognosis in thyroid cancer. *J Clin Oncol*. 2003;21:3226–3235.

202. Karga H, Lee JK, Vickery AL Jr, et al. *Ras* oncogene mutations in benign and malignant thyroid neoplasms. *J Clin Endocrinol Metab*. 1991;73:832–836.

Papillary Carcinoma

DEFINITION

Papillary carcinoma is a well-differentiated malignant tumor of thyroid follicular cells that shows a set of characteristic nuclear features. Although a papillary growth pattern is frequently seen, it is not required for the diagnosis.

INCIDENCE AND EPIDEMIOLOGY

Papillary carcinoma is the most common type of thyroid cancer. Its incidence in absolute numbers and in proportion to other types of thyroid cancer has been steadily increasing in the United States and many other countries around the world.[1-4] In the United States, based on the Surveillance, Epidemiology and End Results (SEER) data, the annual incidence of papillary carcinoma has more than tripled during the last 35 years, as it was 2.7 per 100,000 persons in 1973 and 11.2 per 100,000 in 2008.[5] Whereas in 1973 papillary carcinoma accounted for 74% of all thyroid cancer cases in the United States, its proportion increased to 86% in 2004 to 2008.[5] Papillary cancer more frequently affects women, with the female:male ratio of about 3:1 in the United States and many other countries.[5,6] The increase in incidence affects both genders but is more pronounced in females (Fig. 11.1).

Several factors may be responsible for the increase. First would be a widespread use of ultrasonography, which can detect thyroid nodules down to 0.2 cm in size and guide a fine needle aspiration (FNA) procedure to sample these small lesions. This leads to the detection of occult papillary carcinomas of <1 cm in size, which are common in the general population based on autopsy series.[7,8] Indeed, papillary carcinomas of 1 cm or smaller in size are responsible for over 50% of the observed increase in incidence (Fig. 11.2, left).[2,5,9,10] However, another half of the increase is still attributed to the tumors >1 cm in size. Overall, currently about 40% of newly diagnosed cases are 1 cm or less in size. Second, the increase may be due to the better recognition of the follicular variant of papillary carcinoma and changes in the histopathologic criteria for its diagnosis. As a result, tumors with partially developed nuclear features of papillary carcinoma are more likely to be interpreted as malignant today than 15 to 20 years ago.[11-13] This may not, however, provide a full explanation for the increase because the increase in incidence has affected both classic papillary carcinoma and the follicular variant (Fig. 11.2, right).

Overall, it is unlikely that the detection of small, clinically irrelevant cancers due to better imaging and change in the diagnostic criteria are solely responsible for the entire increase in thyroid cancer incidence. In fact, recent studies, although limited and restricted to specific types of papillary carcinoma, suggest that the proportion of tumors carrying a *BRAF* mutation, a marker of more aggressive cancer, has been constant or even increasing during the last decades.[14,15] Therefore, other factors may contribute to the rapidly growing incidence of papillary carcinoma, such as more common exposure to radiation and/or a more iodine-rich diet, as discussed later in this section.

Worldwide, the incidence of papillary carcinoma has significant geographic variability, which largely follows the variation in the cumulative rates of thyroid cancer observed in different countries (see Chapter 7, Fig. 7.2). The incidence also varies among different ethnic groups. In the United States, the average incidence in whites between 1973 to 2003 was 11.5 per 100,000 per year in females and 4.8 in males, which was higher than in blacks, where the incidence was 8.1 in females and 3.7 in males.[9] The incidence was observed to be higher among Israeli Jews than among Israeli Arabs.[16]

Although uncommon in early childhood, papillary carcinoma accounts for the most thyroid cancers in this age group.[17] The incidence increases sharply during adolescence and early adulthood. Surprisingly, the age of patients who develop papillary carcinoma has been continuously increasing over the last three decades (Fig. 11.3). Based on the SEER data, the mean age of patients was 37.8 years in 1975, 41.6 years in 1985, 43.7 years in 1995, and 46.8 years in 2005.[5]

ETIOLOGIC FACTORS

Although familial occurrence of follicular carcinomas has gained more recognition in the recent years, most tumors are sporadic, nonfamilial cases.

Ionizing Radiation

Exposure to ionizing radiation is a major known risk factor for papillary carcinoma (Table 11.1). Both external X-ray and γ-radiation as well as internal exposure to radioiodine during childhood lead to an increased cancer risk. This includes external beam radiation therapy for malignant and benign conditions as well as accidental exposure to radioiodine or γ-radiation as a result of nuclear weapon explosion or nuclear reactor accidents. Widespread use

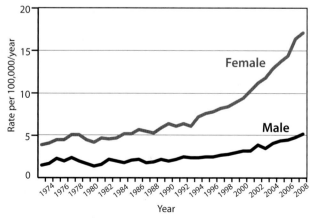

FIGURE 11.1. Incidence of papillary carcinoma in the United States in 1973–2008. Based on the SEER data.[5]

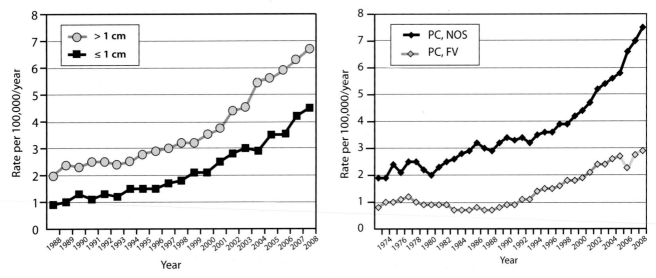

FIGURE 11.2. (Left) Incidence of papillary carcinomas 1 cm or less and >1 cm in 1988–2008 based on the SEER data.[5] **(Right)** Incidence of papillary carcinoma, not otherwise specified (PC, NOS) and the follicular variant (PC, FV) in 1973–2008 based on the SEER data.[5]

of external beam radiation therapy for benign conditions of the head and neck, common in the United States and several other countries in the 1930s to 1940s, resulted in a significant increase of thyroid cancer incidence in individuals exposed during childhood.[18,19] However, the use of radiation for treatment of benign conditions was abandoned in the 1950s. As a result, the impact of radiation as an etiologic agent has been gradually decreasing. For example, a history of radiation exposure was documented in 12% of patients with thyroid cancer diagnosed in 1978 to 1980 as compared with 5% of patients diagnosed in 1996.[20,21] However, radiation therapy for malignant tumors, such as Hodgkin disease, remains a source of radiation-induced papillary carcinoma. The Chernobyl nuclear power accident in 1986 has lead to the development of papillary carcinomas in >5,000 individuals exposed to radioiodines during childhood and adolescence.[22–24] The increase in cancer risk due to diagnostic X-ray procedures, occupational radiation exposure, and high dose ^{131}I therapy for hyperthyroidism has not been found.[21,25]

The risk of radiation-induced cancer has a linear correlation with dose received by the thyroid in the dose range of 0.2 to 2 Gy,

and it reaches a plateau at higher doses.[18,26,27] The risk has strong inverse correlation with age at exposure and is highest in children exposed during infancy. The excess relative risk of cancer after childhood exposure ranges widely in different studies and depends on the source of radiation, age at exposure, and length of follow-up, but most frequently is in the range of 5 to 9 per 1 Gy of radiation.[18,26–31] The risk of exposure during the adulthood is significantly lower and may not be detectable at all.[31]

The shortest time interval between exposure and cancer development is 4 years, and the risk remains elevated for 50 years and longer.[32–34] Papillary carcinomas is by far the most common type of radiation-induced thyroid cancer, and many of them reveal a solid or mixed solid-follicular growth pattern.[24,35,36] Molecular mechanisms of radiation-associated papillary carcinogenesis involve primarily chromosomal rearrangements, such as *RET/PTC*, whereas point mutations in *BRAF, RAS,* and other genes are rare in these tumors.[37,38]

Iodine-rich Diet

High iodine consumption represents another potential risk factor. The incidence of papillary carcinoma appears to be higher in regions with high dietary iodine intake, such as Iceland, Japan, and the Pacific islands.[39,40] In addition, the ratio of papillary carcinoma to follicular carcinoma is significantly higher in the areas of high iodine intake as compared with the areas of moderate and low intake.[41] In areas of severe iodine deficiency, widespread iodine supplementation coincided with the reduction in the prevalence of follicular and anaplastic carcinoma and a proportional increase in papillary carcinoma.[42–44] It remains unclear, however, whether the increase was caused by an iodine-rich diet or it reflected the reduction in other thyroid tumor types and a general increase in the incidence of papillary cancer observed in many countries.

A recent study of thyroid cancer in several regions of China with very high iodine content in drinking water and regions with normal iodine content has shown a significantly higher ratio of papillary cancer to non-papillary cancer in the former regions (7 to 8:1 vs. 3 to 4:1).[45] Moreover, the study has also identified a significantly higher prevalence of *BRAF* V600E mutation in papillary carcinoma from regions with high iodine content (69% vs. 53%), suggesting that correlation between this mutation and iodine-rich diet may serve as a biologic mechanism behind the increasing incidence of papillary carcinoma.

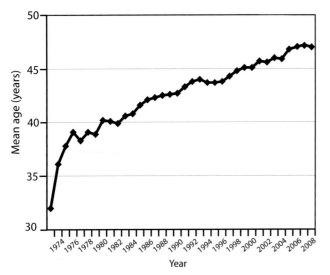

FIGURE 11.3. Mean age of patients with papillary carcinomas in the United States in 1974–2008. Based on the SEER data.[5]

Table 11.1

Radiation Exposure and Thyroid Papillary Carcinoma

Radiation type: External (X-ray, γ) radiation and internal exposure to ^{131}I impose increased cancer risk

Dose dependence: Risk is dose dependent and close to linear in 0.2–2 Gy dose range

Age dependence: Risk has strong inverse correlation with age at exposure; highest risk is in youngest children

Shortest time interval between exposure and cancer development: 4 years

Persistence of elevated risk: 50 years and longer after exposure

Histologic features: Many radiation-induced papillary cancers have solid or mixed solid-follicular architecture

Typical genetic alterations: Chromosomal rearrangements, particularly *RET/PTC*; point mutations *(BRAF, RAS)* are rare

Other Environmental Factors

A recent study of thyroid cancer in Sicily has identified a significantly higher incidence of papillary cancer, but not follicular or medullary cancer, in the volcanic region with high concentration of boron, iron, vanadium, manganese, and other chemicals in drinking water as compared with the neighboring regions with normal concentration of these elements.[46] Moreover, this region had a significantly higher incidence of *BRAF* mutations in papillary carcinomas (52% vs. 33% in other regions of Sicily).[46] This finding raises the possibility that mutagenesis leading to *BRAF* point mutation may be related to the excessive exposure to specific chemical compounds found in the volcanic areas. In support of this possibility, Hawaiian islands and Iceland belong to the regions of the world with the highest incidence of thyroid cancer, and they host multiple volcanoes, many of which are active.[6] However, no data linking papillary cancer and *BRAF* mutation to exposure to specific chemical compounds are available yet.

Preexisting Benign Thyroid Disease and Thyroid-Stimulating Hormone levels

A history of benign thyroid disease is a well-documented risk factor for papillary carcinoma. Preexisting solitary thyroid nodules and/or adenomas increase the carcinoma risk by 27 to 29 folds and multiple hyperplastic nodules (multinodular goiter) by 6 to 9 folds.[47,48] The mechanisms underlying the association between benign thyroid disease and papillary cancer are not fully understood. Mutations in the *RAS* genes are common in follicular adenomas and may predispose to malignant transformation.[49] Another possibility is an increased cell proliferation rate in adenomas and hyperplastic nodules, which may promote carcinogenesis by increasing the chances for mutation to occur in dividing cells[50] or by cooperating with an oncogenic event in tumor progression, particularly in patients with higher levels of thyroid-stimulating hormone (TSH). Three epidemiologic studies have found the association between higher serum TSH levels and risk of thyroid cancer, particularly of papillary carcinoma, in patients with thyroid nodules.[51–53] The risk of cancer was found to increase incrementally with higher levels of TSH, even within the normal range. Recently, strong experimental evidence has been offered indicating that expression of mutant *BRAF* at physiologic levels requires simultaneous TSH stimulation in order to transform thyroid cells and initiate papillary carcinoma development in transgenic mice.[54]

The association between papillary carcinoma and two other benign thyroid diseases, Graves disease and chronic lymphocytic (Hashimoto) thyroiditis, remains controversial. Several studies have reported a higher than expected frequency of papillary carcinoma in surgically removed thyroid glands of patients with Graves disease and Hashimoto thyroiditis.[55,56] However, epidemiologic case-control and large retrospective cohort studies failed to establish the association between these conditions and increased cancer risk.[57–60] Recent retrospective[61] and prospective[62] studies confirmed the lack of an increased risk of cancer in patients with Hashimoto thyroiditis. Moreover, although some reports have suggested that *RET/PTC* rearrangement, a molecular event characteristic for papillary carcinoma, can be found in most thyroid glands affected by Hashimoto thyroiditis,[63,64] the presence of this molecular alteration has not been confirmed in the recent studies.[65,66] As a result, to date there is no undisputable evidence for the causal association between Hashimoto thyroiditis and papillary carcinoma.[67]

In the United States, a personal history of Graves disease, thyroiditis, and goiter is reported in 2%, 8%, and 14%, respectively, of patients with papillary carcinoma.[20]

Hormonal and Reproductive Factors

The role of hormones and reproductive factors in papillary carcinoma development is suggested by the higher cancer incidence in women of reproductive age. However, no definitive association between estrogens or other specific hormonal factors or interventions and cancer development has been unraveled yet. A pooled analysis of 14 case-control studies demonstrated that the risk of papillary carcinoma is slightly increased in those with miscarriage of the first pregnancy (odds ratio of 1:7 as compared with nulligravidae) and in those with artificial menopause (odds ratio 1:7 as compared with premenopausal).[68] Some studies have found a slight increase in thyroid cancer risk in association with the number of pregnancies, late age at first birth, and use of estrogen-containing preparations including oral contraceptives, although other studies have not confirmed those associations.[39] Obesity has been linked to thyroid cancer in several, but not all, studies, with no specific reference to papillary carcinoma.[21,69–71]

Hereditary Factors

The risk of developing papillary carcinoma is 5- to 9-fold higher among first-degree relatives of patients with thyroid cancer than in the general population.[21,72,73] About 5% of papillary carcinomas are familial; the familial cancers occur in two settings: (1) as a component of known hereditary multi-cancer syndromes and (2) as tumors occurring in families with isolated thyroid cancer and little or no risk of other tumors.

In the first group, the best recognized association is between papillary carcinoma and familial adenomatous polyposis (FAP). FAP is an autosomal dominant disease caused by a germline mutation of the *APC* gene located on 5q21 and characterized by numerous colonic adenomatous polyps, colon cancer, and various extracolonic tumors and nonneoplastic lesions. Approximately 1% to 2% of the affected patients develop thyroid tumors, chiefly papillary carcinomas, and the incidence may be higher when thyroid glands are examined by ultrasonography.[74,75] Papillary carcinomas in this setting frequently manifest during the third decade of life and affect predominantly females (female:male ratio 8:1).[73,76] In fact, women under the age of 35 with FAP have 100- to 160-fold higher risk of thyroid carcinoma than unaffected individuals.[76,77] The FAP-associated papillary carcinomas are more frequently multifocal and exhibit distinct histologic features characteristic of the cribriform-morular variant, as described later in the chapter.

A higher incidence of papillary carcinoma is seen in patients with Carney complex[78] and possibly in those with Werner syndrome,[79] although both are rare diseases and the overall number of reported cases of papillary carcinoma in these patients is low.

Another subset of familial papillary carcinomas encompasses those cases which are not associated with known hereditary multi-cancer syndromes. The inherited nature of these papillary carcinomas can be established with certainty when three or more first-degree relatives develop thyroid cancer, whereas those with two affected family members have an equal chance of having either inherited or sporadic tumors.[80,81] Familial papillary carcinomas are likely to show autosomal dominant inheritance with incomplete penetrance, the latter increasing with age.[82,83] Familial cancers show more common multifocality and coexistence of multiple benign thyroid nodules, but typically do not differ from sporadic cancers with regard to female predominance and age at diagnosis.[73,84] Several susceptibility loci have been mapped, although specific genes have not been identified yet. A locus on 19p13.2 has been linked to familial papillary carcinoma with and without oncocytic (oxyphilic) change,[85,86] a locus on 1q21 to papillary carcinoma associated with papillary renal neoplasms,[87] and a locus on 2q21 to familial papillary carcinoma associated with multinodular goiter.[83,88]

PATHOGENESIS AND MOLECULAR GENETICS

Clonality and Multifocality

Most papillary carcinomas have a monoclonal origin, which means that they originate from a single cell.[89] Clonality assays, such as the human androgen receptor assay assay (see Chapter 20), have also revealed that multiple distinct foci of papillary carcinoma found within the thyroid gland are often (50%) of different clonal origin and therefore represent independent primary tumors rather than intraglandular spread from a single tumor.[90] Additional confirmation of the independent clonal origin of several tumor nodules within one gland comes from the studies showing that different tumor nodules frequently have distinct genetic alterations, such as different types of *RET/PTC* rearrangement, or vary in the presence of *BRAF* mutation.[91-93]

DNA Ploidy

Aneuploidy, which reflects losses or gains of whole chromosomes or large chromosomal regions, is not a common feature of papillary carcinomas. These tumors typically show normal DNA content, and aneuploidy is found in <10% of papillary carcinomas, which is significantly lower than in follicular carcinomas and even follicular adenomas.[94,95] The follicular variant of papillary carcinoma may have a slightly higher frequency of aneuploidy.[96]

Cytogenetic Abnormalities

Cytogenetic abnormalities are relatively infrequent in papillary carcinomas and are found by conventional karyotyping in 20% to 40% of all tumors.[97,98] Approximately half of those are numerical changes, which typically involve one or several chromosomes, the most common of which are loss of chromosome Y or 22, and gain of chromosome 7. Trisomy 17 as a sole abnormality is more commonly seen in encapsulated follicular variant of papillary carcinoma.[99] Some tumors reveal structural abnormalities, the most frequent of which is inversion inv(10)(q11.2;q21),[100] which leads to *RET/PTC1* rearrangement. Other translocations or inversions involving 10q11.2, the region where the *RET* gene resides, correspond to less frequent types of *RET/PTC* rearrangements that are discussed below. Single cases of translocation involving breakpoints at 1p32-36, 1q22, 3p25-26, and 7q32-36, among others, have been reported.[98,101,102]

Using comparative genomic hybridization (CGH), chromosomal imbalances are detected in about 40% of papillary carcinomas, and their frequency may be higher in aggressive tumors and in the tall cell variant.[103-105] The most common losses detected by CGH are at 22q and 9q (particularly 9q21.3-32) and gains are at 17q, 1q, and 9q33-qter. Wreesmann and colleagues[96] have found that the pattern of chromosomal imbalances detected by CGH in follicular variant of papillary carcinoma was closer to that of follicular carcinoma and adenoma than to the pattern seen in classic papillary carcinoma.

Loss of Heterozygosity

Loss of heterozygosity (LOH) results from a deletion of discrete chromosomal regions and frequently correlates with the loss of important tumor suppressor genes residing in these areas. Papillary carcinomas are characterized by a quite stable genotype and low overall rate of LOH. For example, a meta-analysis of the data reported in the literature demonstrates only a 2.5% average rate of LOH per chromosome arm in papillary carcinomas in contrast to a 20% rate in follicular carcinomas (for illustration see Chapter 10, Fig. 10.03).[106] The foci on 3p, 4q, and 10q are among the more frequently deleted.[106,107] The frequency of LOH may be higher in the follicular, oncocytic, and tall cell variants as compared with classic papillary carcinoma.[108]

Somatic Mutations

The pathogenesis of papillary carcinoma involves the perturbation of multiple signaling pathways, the most essential of which is the mitogen-activated protein kinase (MAPK) pathway that regulates cell growth, differentiation, and survival (Fig. 11.4).[109] Activation of this pathway in thyroid cells results from point mutation of the *BRAF* and *RAS* genes or chromosomal rearrangement involving the *RET* and *NTRK1* genes. These mutational events rarely overlap in the same tumor, and one of these alterations is found in >70% of papillary carcinomas.[110-112] Despite the common ability to activate the MAPK pathway, each of these mutations is likely to have additional and unique effects on cell transformation, as they are associated with distinct phenotypical and biologic properties of papillary carcinoma (Table 11.2).[113]

BRAF

Mutations of the *BRAF* gene represent the most common genetic alteration in papillary carcinomas as they are found in 40% to 45% of these tumors. The spectrum of mutations affecting this gene includes point mutations, small in-frame deletions or insertions, and chromosomal rearrangement. The most common mutation in papillary carcinoma is a point mutation that involves a thymine to adenine substitution at nucleotide position 1799,

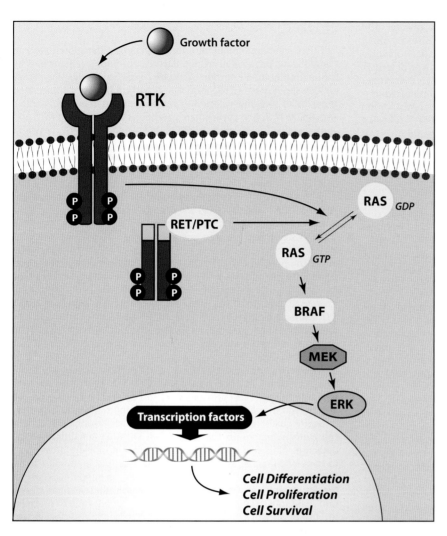

FIGURE 11.4. Schematic representation of the MAPK signaling pathway. Physiologically, binding of growth factors to a receptor tyrosine kinase (RTK), such RET and NTRK1, results in receptor dimerization and activation via autophosphorylation of tyrosine residues in the intracellular domain. The activated receptor through a series of adaptor proteins leads to activation of RAS, located at the inner surface of the plasma membrane, by substitution of GDP with GTP. The active, GTP-bound form of RAS binds to and recruits RAF proteins, mainly BRAF in thyroid follicular cells, to the plasma membrane. Activated BRAF phosphorylates and activates MEK and ERK. Once activated, ERK phosphorylates cytoplasmic proteins and translocates into the nucleus, where it regulates transcription of the genes involved in cell differentiation, proliferation, and survival. Activation of this pathway in papillary carcinoma occurs as a result of point mutation or chromosomal rearrangement affecting the *RET*, *RAS*, and *BRAF* genes.

Table 11.2

MAPK-activating Mutations in Papillary Carcinomas and Their Clinical and Phenotypical Associations

Mutation Type	Average Prevalence (%)	Common Associations
BRAF point mutation	40–45	Older age at presentation Classic papillary carcinoma, tall cell variant Extrathyroidal extension Higher tumor stage at presentation Higher rate of tumor recurrence Propensity for dedifferentiation
RET/PTC rearrangement	10–20	Younger age at presentation Classic papillary carcinoma, diffuse sclerosing variant History of radiation exposure Lymph node metastasis Lower tumor stage at presentation
RAS point mutation	10–20	Follicular variant of papillary carcinoma Tumor encapsulation More frequent vascular invasion Lack of lymph node metastasis Possibly more frequent distant metastasis
TRK rearrangement	<5	Not well defined

resulting in a valine-to-glutamate replacement at residue 600 (V600E).[110,114] *BRAF* V600E comprises 98% to 99% of all *BRAF* mutations found in thyroid cancer. Other alterations involve K601E point mutation and small in-frame insertions or deletions surrounding codon 600,[115–119] as well as *AKAP9/BRAF* rearrangement.[37] The rearrangement is a paracentric inversion of chromosome 7q leading to the fusion between the portion of *BRAF* gene encoding the protein kinase domain to the *AKAP9* gene.[37] All point mutations and the rearrangement lead to the activation of BRAF kinase and chronic stimulation of the MAPK pathway.

The causal role of *BRAF* mutation in tumor initiation has been confirmed in transgenic mice with thyroid-specific expression of V600E.[54,120] These animals frequently developed papillary carcinomas with microscopic features similar to tumors found in humans, although when expressed at physiologic levels in thyroid cells, the mutant BRAF apparently requires TSH stimulation to initiate papillary carcinoma development.[54]

BRAF V600E mutation is typically found in classic papillary carcinomas and in the tall cell variant and is rare in the follicular variant.[113,121,122] Tumors harboring *BRAF* K601E mutation usually have the follicular variant of papillary carcinoma histology.[115,119]

As discussed in more detail later in the chapter, the presence of *BRAF* V600E mutation correlates with aggressive tumor characteristics such as extrathyroidal extension, tumor recurrence, and distant metastases.[123] The association between this mutation and older patient age has also been seen in many studies.[123] *BRAF* association with more invasive tumor characteristics is likely due to the upregulation of expression of vascular endothelial growth factor (VEGF), matrix metalloproteinases, and other tumor cancer-promoting targets by mutant BRAF.[124,125] The mutation may predispose to tumor dedifferentiation, as it is found in papillary carcinomas that undergo anaplastic transformation.[121,126] These properties of mutant *BRAF* are confirmed in transgenic animals, which develop papillary carcinomas with frequent wide invasion into perithyroidal tissues and progression to poorly differentiated carcinoma.[120] A process of dedifferentiation of *BRAF*-mutated cancers coincides with profound deregulation of the expression of genes involved in cell adhesion and intracellular junction, providing evidence for epithelial-mesenchymal transition.[127,128]

RET/PTC

RET/PTC rearrangement is another genetic alteration found in a significant proportion of papillary carcinomas. It is formed by fusion among the 3' portion of the *RET* gene, coding for the receptor tyrosine kinase (RTK), and the 5' portion of various unrelated genes. The two most common rearrangement types, *RET/PTC1* and *RET/PTC3*, are paracentric inversions because both *RET* and its respective fusion partner, *H4* or *NCOA4 (ELE1; RFG)*, reside in the long arm of chromosome 10.[129–132] *RET/PTC2* and nine more recently identified types of *RET/PTC* are all interchromosomal translocations (Table 11.3). Most of these rare *RET/PTC* types have been found in papillary carcinomas from patients with a history of exposure to ionizing radiation,[133–139] with the exception of the *ELKS/RET* and *HOOK3/RET* fusions that have been identified in tumors from patients with no radiation exposure history.[140,141]

RET is not expressed in normal thyroid follicular cells in contrast to thyroid C cells. As a consequence of *RET/PTC* rearrangement, the portion of *RET* coding for the tyrosine kinase domain is fused in frame with an active promoter of the fusion partner gene. As a result, the truncated RET receptor becomes constitutively expressed and activated, stimulating the MAPK signaling. *RET/PTC* transforms thyroid cells in culture[142] and leads to the development of papillary carcinomas in transgenic mice, which has been shown in animals with thyroid-specific expression of *RET/PTC1* and *RET/PTC3*.[143–145]

The prevalence and specificity of *RET/PTC* rearrangement varies dramatically in the reported series.[146–148] In part, this is due to true difference in the prevalence of this alteration in specific age groups and in individuals exposed to ionizing radiation. However, in many cases, this is due to heterogeneous distribution of this rearrangement within the tumor and variable sensitivity of the detection. This rearrangement can be present in a significant proportion of tumor cells and detected by multiple methods (*clonal RET/PTC*) or can occur in a small fraction or single cells within the lesion and can be detectable only using ultrasensitive detection techniques (*nonclonal RET/PTC*).[149,150] Clonal *RET/PTC* occurs in 10% to 20% of papillary thyroid carcinomas and is specific for this tumor type,[150,151] whereas nonclonal rearrangements have been reported with a significantly higher prevalence in papillary

Table 11.3

Types of *RET/PTC* Rearrangement in Papillary Carcinoma

N	*RET/PTC* Type	Partner Gene Fused with RET	Cytogenetic Alteration	Frequency among *RET/PTC* types
1	*RET/PTC1*[129]	H4 (CCDC6, D10S170)	inv(10)(q11.2;q21)	65%
2	*RET/PTC2*[133]	PRKAR1A	t(10;17)(q11.2;q23)	3%
3	*RET/PTC3*[130,131] (*RET/PTC4*)[132]**	NCOA4 (RFG, ELE1)	inv(10)(q11.2;q10)	30%*
4	*RET/PTC5*[134]	GOLGA5 (RFG5)	t(10;14)(q11.2;q32)	Rare
5	*RET/PTC6*[135]	HTIF1 (TRIM24)	t(7;10)(q32;q11.2)	Rare
6	*RET/PTC7*[135]	TIF1G (RFG7, TRIM33)	t(1;10)(p13;q11.2)	Rare
7	*ELKS/RET*[140]	ELKS (RAB6IP2)	t(10;12)(q11.2;p13.3)	Rare
8	*RET/PTC8*[137]	KTN1	t(10;14)(q11.2;q22.1)	Rare
9	*RET/PTC9*[136]	RFG9	t(10;18)(q11.2;q21)	Rare
10	*PCM1/RET*[138]	PCM1	t(8;10)(p21;q11.2)	Rare
11	*RFP/RET*[139]	RFP (TRIM27)	t(6;10)(p21;q11.2)	Rare
12	*HOOK3/RET*[141]	HOOK3	t(8;10)(p11.21;q11.2)	Rare

**RET/PTC4* type has the same fusion partner genes as *RET/PTC3*, but a different location of a breakpoint in the *RET* gene.

carcinomas and also in various other thyroid tumors and benign lesions.[146]

Clonal *RET/PTC* is more common in papillary carcinomas from children and young adults and in patients with a history of radiation exposure. This includes individuals subjected to either accidental (mostly radioiodine) irradiation or therapeutic (mostly external beam) irradiation, as 50% to 80% of those papillary carcinomas harbor *RET/PTC*.[152,153] *RET/PTC* can be induced by ionizing radiation in cultured human thyroid cells and in human thyroid tissue grafted into mice.[154,155] The rearrangement may be a direct result of misrejoining of DNA breaks induced by radiation; this may be facilitated by close spatial positioning of chromosomal regions involved in *RET/PTC* generation, which can be seen by fluorescence in-situ hybridization (FISH) in normal human thyroid cells (Fig. 11.5).[156,157]

In most series of radiation-induced and sporadic tumors, *RET/PTC1* is more common. The notable expression is a population of papillary carcinomas that developed in children shortly (4 to 10 years) after radiation exposure at Chernobyl. Among those, *RET/PTC3* was the most prevalent rearrangement type.[152,158]

RET/PTC-positive papillary carcinomas typically present at younger age and have classic papillary histology, a high rate of lymph node metastases, but low stage at presentation. These findings are particularly characteristic of tumors harboring *RET/PTC1*.[113] Among papillary carcinomas associated with radiation exposure, *RET/PTC1* is associated with classic papillary carcinoma, whereas *RET/PTC3* type is associated with the solid variant.[38] *RET/PTC*-positive tumors lack the predisposition for progression to poorly differentiated and anaplastic carcinomas.[159]

The pathogenetic role of nonclonal *RET/PTC* rearrangement, i.e. *RET/PTC* detected at a very low level or in single cells within the thyroid nodule or in a gland affected by Hashimoto thyroiditis, is not clear.[147,149] A claim that frequent detection of *RET/PTC* using highly sensitive techniques in glands affected by Hashimoto thyroiditis provides evidence for multiple occult papillary carcinomas that are not detectable histologically[63,64] cannot be accepted at this time.[67]

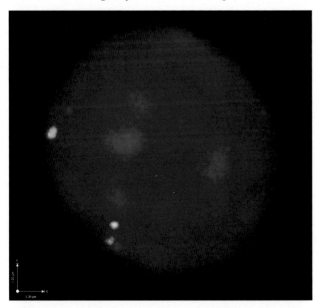

FIGURE 11.5. Nuclear architecture predisposes to the generation of *RET/PTC* rearrangements in thyroid cells. Nucleus of normal human thyroid follicular cell hybridized with probes for the *RET* (green color), *H4* (red), and *NCOA4* (orange) genes showing close proximity of *RET* and *NCOA4* (fusion partners in *RET/PTC3*) on one copy of chromosome 10 *(upper left)* and proximity of *RET* and *H4* (fusion partners in *RET/PTC1*) on another copy of chromosome 10 *(bottom)*.

RAS

Point mutations involving *RAS* genes are found in about 10% of papillary carcinomas and affect almost exclusively the follicular variant of this tumor.[160,161] The mutations are located at several specific sites (codons 12, 13, and 61) of the *NRAS*, *HRAS*, and *KRAS* genes.[162–164] The mutation stabilizes the protein in its active, GTP-bound conformation, resulting in chronic stimulation of several signaling pathways, most importantly the MAPK and phosphatidylinositol-3-kinase (PI3K/AKT) pathways. In addition to strong correlation with the follicular variant histology, this mutation is also associated with more frequent tumor encapsulation, less prominent nuclear features of papillary carcinoma, and a lower rate of lymph node metastases.[113,160] Some studies have reported an association between *RAS* mutation and a higher frequency of distant metastases.[165]

TRK

Rearrangement of the *NTRK1* gene, named TRK rearrangement, is the least frequent type of mutation capable of activating the MAPK pathway. *NTRK1* is located on chromosome 1q22 and encodes a cell membrane receptor with tyrosine kinase activity.[166,167] Similar to the *RET* gene, *NTRK1* is not expressed in normal thyroid follicular cells. The rearrangement juxtaposes the portion of *NTRK1* coding for the intracellular tyrosine kinase domain to the 5' terminal sequence of one of three genes that are highly expressed in thyroid follicular cells.[167] Two of them, the *TPM3* gene[168,169] and the *TPR* gene,[170,171] are also located on chromosome 1q, and therefore, these fusions are intrachromosomal inversions. The third fusion partner, the *TFG* gene, resides on chromosome 3, and this fusion is a result of the t(1;3) translocation.[172] All fusion types lead to the expression and activation of the tyrosine kinase domain of *NTRK1*. The fusion is tumorogenic for thyroid follicular cells, as *TPR/NTRK1* drives the development of papillary carcinomas in transgenic mice.[173]

TRK rearrangements occur in <5% of papillary carcinomas,[174,175] although in some regions of the world the reported frequency is in the range of 10% to 15%.[167,176,177] All three fusion types are found with approximately similar incidence, and several tumors with *NTRK1* fused to still unknown genes have been reported.[176,177] Approximately 5% of radiation-induced papillary carcinomas carry this rearrangement, most commonly the *NTRK1/TPM3* type.[178]

PAX8/PPARγ

This rearrangement is a prototypic alteration found in follicular thyroid carcinoma. However, the published data[179] and our own experience indicate that this rearrangement can be found in a small proportion (1% to 5%) of the follicular variant papillary carcinoma. Single reports of a much higher prevalence of this rearrangement in the follicular variant of papillary carcinoma also exist,[180] although the difference likely reflects the stringency of diagnostic criteria used to define the follicular variant of papillary carcinoma.

PI3K/PTEN/AKT Pathway Mutations

The PI3K/PTEN/AKT signaling pathway may be activated as a result of *RAS* mutation as well as mutation of the *PIK3CA* and *PTEN* genes (see Chapter 10, Fig. 10.5 for illustration). These mutations are common in anaplastic (undifferentiated) carcinoma and occur with lower prevalence in follicular carcinoma. However, *PIK3CA* and *PTEN* mutations are rare in papillary carcinomas, found in only 2% to 5% of tumors.[181–183]

Mutations in the Oncocytic Variant of Papillary Carcinoma

The oncocytic variant of papillary carcinoma reveals the characteristic nuclear features of papillary carcinoma along with cytoplasmic granularity due to accumulation of numerous and frequently abnormal mitochondria. The cause of the mitochondrial change and its relationship to the neoplastic process are not fully understood. It is likely that it may represent either a primary process induced by a distinct tumor initiation mutation or a secondary, probably compensatory change.[184-186]

Mutations of the *GRIM-19* (*NDUFA13*) gene, which encodes a protein that regulates cell death as well as mitochondrial metabolism, occur in oncocytic thyroid tumors. In one study of 10 oncocytic papillary carcinomas, two tumors revealed somatic missense mutations and one a germline mutation of *GRIM-19*.[187] The mutations may disrupt the function of this anti-apoptotic tumor suppressor gene and promote tumorigenesis. However, the prevalence of *GRIM-19* mutations in oncocytic thyroid tumors and their role in carcinogenesis remains to be fully characterized.

In some studies, a high prevalence of *RET/PTC* rearrangements has been found in oncocytic variant papillary carcinomas using highly sensitive detection techniques.[188-190] The significance of these findings is not clear because these ultrasensitive methods also led to the detection of nonclonal *RET/PTC* in many oncocytic follicular adenomas and carcinomas.

Alterations in Gene Expression Profiles

Using high-density cDNA microarrays, widespread alterations in gene expression can be detected in papillary carcinomas. Although the pathogenetic role of these changes awaits further analysis, several important observations have been made already. It has been found that gene expression profiles of papillary carcinoma (including follicular variant) are different from those of follicular carcinomas and other thyroid tumor types,[191-193] supporting the current classification scheme that is based primarily on histopathologic criteria. Furthermore, distinct sets of differently expressed genes have been found in classic papillary carcinoma and in the follicular variant, and possibly in some other variants (such as tall cell variant), pointing toward the pathogenetic and biologic

differences between these microscopic tumor variants (Fig. 11.6, left).[192,194] It appears that variation in gene expression profiles between papillary carcinomas carrying *BRAF, RAS, RET/PTC,* and *TRK* mutations can be detected, providing molecular basis for distinct phenotypical and biologic features associated with each mutation type (Fig. 11.6, right).[194,195]

Gene expression array studies have also confirmed the overexpression of several genes previously known to be upregulated in papillary carcinoma, such as *MET, LGALS3* (galectin-3), and *KRT19* (cytokeratin 19). Other characteristic findings included general downregulation of genes responsible for specialized thyroid function such as thyroid hormone synthesis, upregulation of many genes involved in cell adhesion, motility, and cell–cell interaction, and disregulation of the expression of genes coding for cytokines and other proteins involved in inflammation and immune response.[191,193,194] Dysregulation of expression of genes involved in cell adhesion and intracellular junction, consistent with epithelial-mesenchymal transition, is particularly prominent during invasion and dedifferentiation of *BRAF*-mutated cancers.[127,128]

Alterations in miRNA Expression

MicroRNAs (miRNAs) are small endogenous RNA molecules that do not code for proteins but act as negative regulators of the expression of protein-coding genes.[196,197] The miRNAs regulate the expression of well-known oncogenes and tumor suppressor genes. Upregulation and downregulation of specific miRNAs are common in cancer cells and may be involved in carcinogenesis. miRNA expression profiles of papillary carcinoma are different from those of follicular carcinoma and other thyroid tumors.[198] Within the papillary carcinoma group, the patterns of miRNA expression correlate with specific somatic mutations found in these tumors.[198] Several specific miRNAs, such as miR-221, miR-222, miR-187, miR-181b, and miR-146b, are consistently found to be strongly upregulated in papillary carcinomas, suggesting that they may play a pathogenetic role in the development of these tumors (Fig. 11.7).[198-200] Possible target genes affected by these miRNAs are the regulators of the cell cycle *p27(Kip1)* gene and the thyroid hormone receptor gene.[201,202] Other miRNAs upregulated in papillary carcinoma at lower levels are miR-155, miR-181b, miR-187, miR- 21, miR-31.[199,203,204]

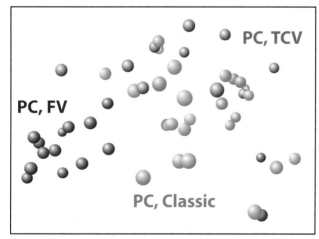
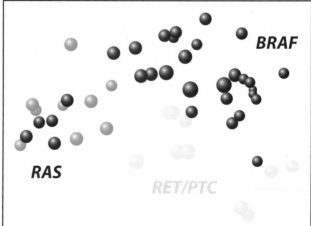

FIGURE 11.6. Correlation between gene expression profiles and histologic variants and mutations in papillary carcinoma. *(Left)* Principal component analysis based on the expression data for over 22,000 genes shows distinct clusters formed by cases of classic papillary carcinoma (orange spheres), follicular variant (purple), and tall cell variant (grey). *(Right)* Similar analysis with reference to mutational status demonstrates clusters of tumors carrying *BRAF* mutation (red), *RET/PTC* rearrangement (yellow), and *RAS* mutation (blue). Green spheres represent papillary carcinomas with no mutation. (Based on the data reported by Giordano TJ, Kuick R, Thomas DG, et al. Molecular classification of papillary thyroid carcinoma: distinct *BRAF, RAS,* and *RET/PTC* mutation-specific gene expression profiles discovered by DNA microarray analysis. *Oncogene.* 2005;24:6646–6656.)

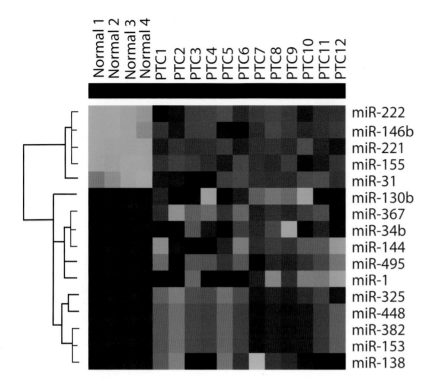

FIGURE 11.7. miRNAs dysregulation in papillary thyroid carcinoma. Cluster dendrogram demonstrates several upregulated (red) and downregulated (green) miR-NAs in papillary carcinomas (PTC) as compared with normal thyroid cells. (Based on data reported by Nikiforova MN, Tseng GC, Steward D, et al. MicroRNA expression profiling of thyroid tumors: biological significance and diagnostic utility. *J Clin Endocrinol Metab.* 2008;93:1600–1608 and Yip L, Kelly L, Shuai Y, et al. MicroRNA signature distinguishes the degree of aggressiveness of papillary thyroid carcinoma. *Ann Surg Oncol.* 2011;18:2035–2041.)

Differences in miRNA expression were also observed between papillary carcinomas with aggressive features as compared with nonaggressive tumors. Several miRNAs have been found to be significantly upregulated (miR-146b, miR-221, and miR-222) or downregulated (miR-34b and miR-130b) in aggressive tumors.[205,206] The *MET* gene is a potential target for two downregulated miRNAs (miR-34b and miR-1), and significantly higher level of *MET* expression was observed in aggressive papillary carcinomas,[205] suggesting that this may represent a mechanism of tumor progression.

CLINICAL FEATURES AND IMAGING

Patients typically present with a painless thyroid nodule. Other local symptoms, such as dysphagia, hoarseness, and stridor, are found in about 20% of patients and are indicative of vocal cord paralysis or tracheal compression.[20] Enlarged cervical lymph nodes may sometimes provide the first evidence of disease. Overall, neck lymphadenopathy is found at presentation in 27% of patients.[20] In some cases, patients are totally asymptomatic, and the nodule in the thyroid is identified incidentally using ultrasound or other imaging studies performed for other reasons. Thyroid function tests are typically normal.

Thyroid radioisotope scan typically reveals a "cold" nodule, although this diagnostic modality has fallen out of favor. Hyperfunctioning papillary carcinoma that appears as a "hot" nodule on thyroid scan have been described, but they are exceedingly rare.[207] On ultrasound, papillary carcinoma typically appears as a hypoechoic or isoechoic solid nodule with ill-defined margins (Fig. 11.8). Cystic change may be present, although rarely extensive. Finding punctate microcalcifications (that correspond to psammoma bodies) and high central blood flow within the nodule on color Doppler are more commonly seen in papillary carcinoma although none of the ultrasonographic features are entirely diagnostic of malignancy.[208,209] Tumor harboring *BRAF* mutations appear to have a more elongated shape and less frequently show microcalcifications.[210] Cervical

lymph nodes may reveal internal nodularity, cystic change, and microcalcification on ultrasound, all of which are suspicious for papillary carcinoma.

Other imaging modalities, such as CT, MRI, and [^{18}F]fluorodeoxyglucose (FDG)-positron emission tomography/computed tomography (PET/CT), can be used to evaluate substernal masses and to assess the extent of extrathyroidal disease. Distant metastases at diagnosis are rare and occur in 2% to 5% of patients.[211,212]

FNA is performed on almost all solitary thyroid nodules. Cytologic evaluation of the FNA material typically establishes or at least raises the possibility of the diagnosis of papillary carcinoma, resulting in a referral for surgery.

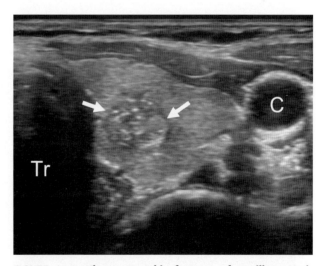

FIGURE 11.8. Ultrasonographic features of papillary carcinoma. Transverse grey scale image of the left thyroid lobe shows an irregularly-shaped isoechoic nodule *(arrows)* with ill-defined borders and several punctuate hyperechoic foci of microcalcifications, which correspond to psammoma bodies found on microscopic examination. Tr, trachea; C, carotid artery.

GROSS FEATURES

On gross examination, papillary carcinoma typically appears as a discrete but ill-defined nodule with irregular borders (Fig. 11.9 A,B). A capsule is typically absent. Some tumors, particularly the follicular variant of papillary carcinoma, may be well demarcated or encapsulated (Fig. 11.9 C). Tumor size varies widely but most frequently is in the range of 1 to 3 cm.[20] The cut surface is tan-brown or grey-white, irregular, firm and solid or more friable with small or larger cystic spaces. Papillary structures may be evident or suspected based on a granular or shaggy texture of the cut surface. Irregularly-shaped whitish areas of fibrosis are frequently seen. Foci of hemorrhage and necrosis can be found in tumors following a recent FNA procedure, whereas spontaneous necrosis and hemorrhage are rare. Calcifications may be occasionally seen. Focal cystic change is identifiable in many tumors, and some tumors may show extensive cystic change, presenting as an ill-defined multicystic lesion. Tumor multifocality is fairly common. In rare instances, diffuse changes are noticed in the thyroid with no discrete tumor mass; this presentation is common for the diffuse sclerosing variant of papillary carcinoma.

Because papillary carcinoma is frequently associated with areas of fibrosis, all whitish, fibrotic-appearing foci found during gross examination should to be sampled for microscopic evaluation.

Perithyroidal lymph nodes may be received with a thyroidectomy specimen. Metastatic disease frequently manifests as an enlarged firm lymph node that may also contain cystic areas filled with brownish, hemorrhagic fluid (Fig. 11.9 D).

 MICROSCOPIC FEATURES

On microscopic examination, papillary carcinoma typically shows infiltrative growth with an irregular, invasive border (Fig. 11.10). In some cases, the tumor may show a pushing border, although true encapsulation is rare with the exception of the follicular variant of papillary carcinoma. Characteristic microscopic features of papillary carcinoma include growth pattern, nuclear features, psammoma bodies, and tumor fibrosis, but only the nuclear features are *required* for the diagnosis (Table 11.4).

Architectural Patterns

The most characteristic growth pattern is papillary, although it is rarely pure and typically admixed with a variable proportion of neoplastic follicles. In approximately two-thirds of tumors, a papillary growth predominates, whereas another one-third have a predominantly follicular (including macrofollicular) architecture.[213] Other growth patterns include solid and trabecular, which are seen in about 20% of cases but rarely predominate.[213]

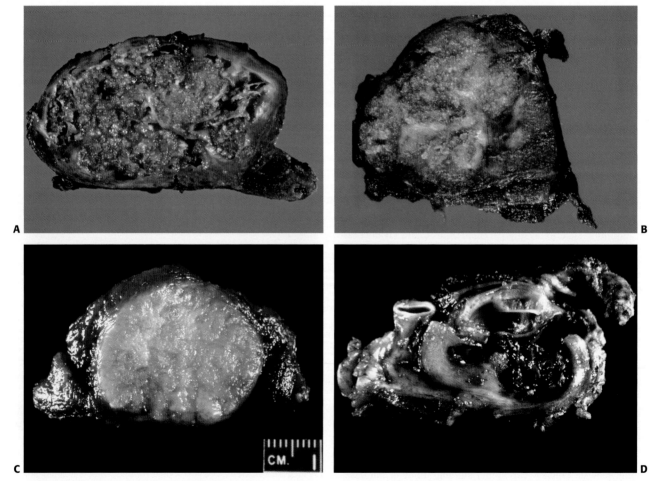

FIGURE 11.9. Gross appearance of papillary carcinoma. A, B: Two examples of classic papillary carcinoma. **C:** Follicular variant of papillary carcinoma. The tumor is well demarcated and has smooth borders but shows no capsule. **D:** Metastastatic papillary carcinoma to a lymph node with marked cystic change.

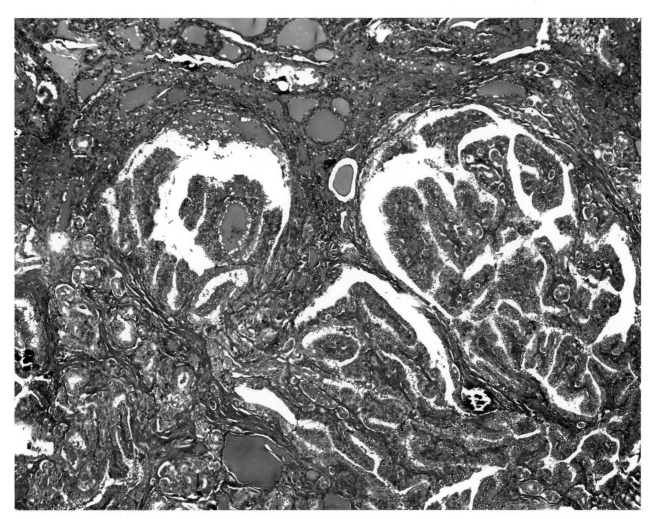

FIGURE 11.10. Low-power view of papillary carcinoma. Note an infiltrative border and a predominantly papillary architecture with occasional neoplastic follicles and scattered calcifications.

Papillae are finger-like projections composed of delicate strands of fibrovascular stroma that are covered by epithelial cells. The papillae are usually irregular, complex, arborizing, ramifying, and branching, with well-developed cores formed by cellular fibrous tissue and capillary blood vessels (Fig. 11.11). In some tumors, the stalks contain loose myxoid edematous stroma or virtually acellular hyalinized material. Occasionally, dense lymphoid infiltration can be seen in the tumor stroma extending into papillae stalks. The papillae are typically covered by a single layer of epithelial cells. Although some polarity of nuclei with location closer to the basement membrane may be seen, many cells show haphazard (up and down) position of nuclei within the cell. Cellular overlapping and multilayering may be seen as a true phenomenon or more commonly due to tangential sectioning of papillae tips.

Papillary growth is a valuable diagnostic feature. Nevertheless, it is important to remember that *not all papillary carcinomas have a papillary growth pattern and not all papillary-patterned thyroid lesions are papillary carcinomas.* An example of the former is the follicular variant of papillary carcinoma (discussed later in the chapter) and of the latter is papillary hyperplasia in goiter (see Chapter 5) and follicular adenoma with papillary hyperplasia (see Chapter 8). The hyperplastic papillae have a simple, typically nonbranching (nonforking) architecture, delicate hypocellular stalks, and uniform basally located nuclear of epithelial cells that lack the characteristic nuclear features of papillary carcinoma.

Tumor Cells

The cells typically have a cuboidal or low columnar shape and rest on the basal membrane that borders papillary stalks and neoplastic follicles. The cells are larger than adjacent nonneoplastic thyrocytes and usually have abundant, pale, eosinophilic cytoplasm.

Table 11.4

Main Microscopic Features of Papillary Carcinoma

I. **Architecture**
  Papillary growth pattern
II. **Nuclear features**
  1. Nuclear enlargement
  2. Nuclear crowding and overlapping
  3. Chromatin clearing
  4. Irregularity of nuclear contours
  5. Nuclear pseudoinclusions
  6. Nuclear grooves
III. **Psammoma bodies**
IV. **Tumor fibrosis**

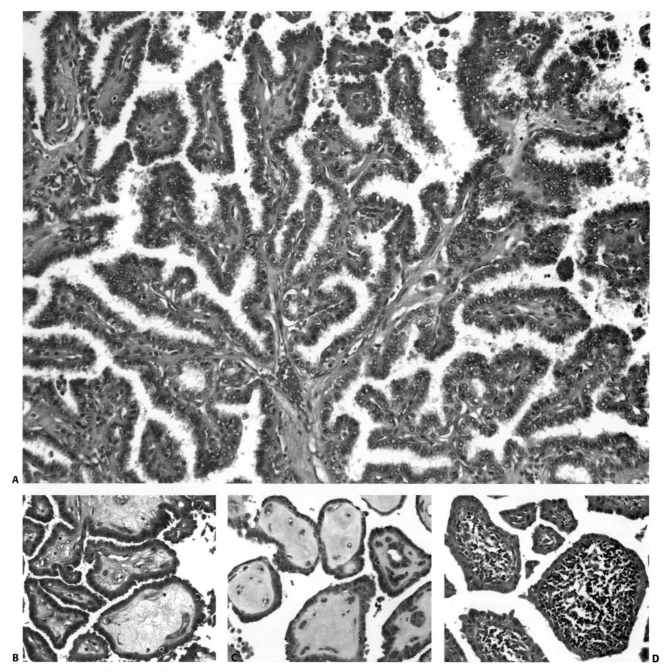

FIGURE 11.11. Papillae of papillary carcinoma. A: Typical tumor papillae with well-developed fibrovascular cores and complex branching. Some papillae may have stalks composed of loose myxoid stroma **(B)** or acellular hyalinized stroma **(C)** or contain dense lymphoid infiltration in the stalks **(D).**

The nuclei exhibit characteristic microscopic changes that serve as a core requirement for the diagnosis of papillary carcinoma. The following main diagnostic nuclear features are recognized:

1. Nuclear enlargement

The nuclei of papillary carcinoma cells are typically 2 to 3 times larger than those of nonneoplastic thyroid cells, as the nuclear area increases from 30 to 50 μm^2 to 97 to 110 μm^2.[214,215] The difference in nuclear size is best appreciated when the tumor cells are compared side by side with the adjacent nonneoplastic cells (Fig. 11.12 A). A sharp distinction between the tumor cells containing large nuclei and the nonneoplastic cells with smaller nuclei is required to fulfill this criterion, as opposed to a gradual change in the nuclear size focally seen in benign reactive conditions such as Hashimoto thyroiditis.

2. Nuclear overlapping and crowding

Overlapping of nuclei in cells lining the neoplastic papillae or follicles is common. It reflects the larger size of the haphazardly arranged nuclei within the cell volume (Fig. 11.12 B). Tangentially sectioned tips of the papillae appear as "crowds" or "lakes" of overlapping nuclei, which is also described as the "egg-basket" appearance.[216]

3. Chromatin clearing

Dispersion of nuclear chromatin with its margination along the nuclear membrane appears microscopically as optically clear nuclei with thickened nuclear membrane (Fig. 11.12). This finding, also known as empty, pale, clear, water-clear, ground-glass or "Orphan Annie Eye" nuclei,[217,218] had been considered for a long time as the most characteristic nuclear feature of papillary carcinoma. This nuclear

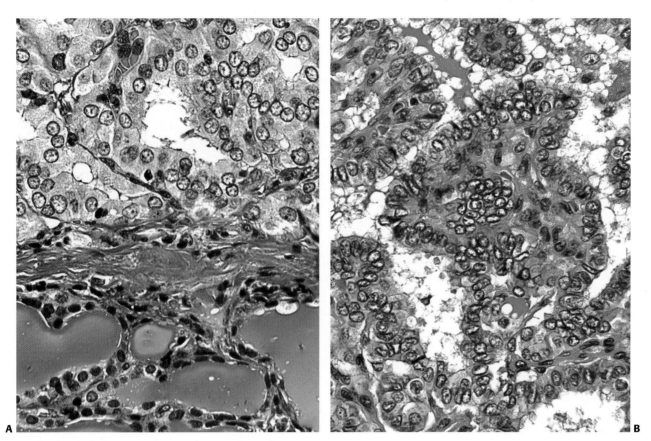

FIGURE 11.12. Nuclear features of papillary carcinoma. A: Enlarged size of tumor nuclei *(top)* is easier to appreciate when compared with adjacent normal thyroid tissue *(bottom).* **B:** Nuclear overlapping and crowding with "lakes" of overlapping nuclei. Many nuclei have finely dispersed chromatin and empty appearance with prominent nuclear membrane due to chromatin margination.

appearance requires a tissue fixation step, as it is not seen in frozen sections or FNA smears.[217] Formalin fixation most consistently yields nuclear clearing, which is also seen after fixation in Bouin fluid, Zenker fluid, or B5.[216] However, other fixatives such as SafeFix and HistoChoice tend not to show this nuclear appearance (Lester D. R. Thompson, unpublished data). Although changes in the distribution of chromatin and ribonucleoproteins have been seen in these tumors by electron microscopy,[219,220] the exact mechanism of nuclear clearing is not well understood.

4. Irregularity of nuclear contours

In contrast to the round, smooth-contoured nuclei of normal thyroid cells or follicular lesions, the nuclei of papillary carcinomas cells have (1) elongated, oval shape, (2) asymmetric, irregular configuration with angulated, crescent-moon, and triangular shapes, and (3) highly irregular, jagged nuclear membrane with indentations, "rat bites," and folds of various sizes and directions (Fig. 11.13 A). This light microscopic appearance reflects a marked irregularity of the nuclear contours that is seen ultramicroscopically (Fig. 11.13 B), as discussed later in the chapter. Importantly, the assessment of this feature should be performed in sections from tissue blocks that were not previously frozen during intraoperative consultation, as freezing introduces a prominent artifactual irregularity of the nuclear membrane.

5. Nuclear grooves

This is a direct consequence of marked irregularity of the nuclear contours, which manifests as a discrete, longitudinal fold typically situated along to the long axis of the nucleus.[221] The fold may be linear and regular (a "coffee bean" appearance)

or curved and irregular (a "piece of popcorn" appearance) (Fig. 11.14 A). By electron microscopy, it represents a deep invagination of the nuclear membrane (Fig. 11.14 B). This is a common finding and in most tumors, and one or more grooved nuclei are typically found in every high-power field.

6. Nuclear pseudoinclusions

This is another result of nuclear membrane irregularity, as an intranuclear cytoplasmic pseudoinclusion is formed by invagination of the nuclear membrane that drags a portion of the cytoplasm into the nuclear volume. The pseudoinclusion appears as a round or more irregular area within the nucleus that has staining qualities of the cytoplasm and is sharply demarcated by a thick nuclear membrane (Fig. 11.15).[222,223] Nuclear pseudoinclusions are the least common feature seen in papillary carcinoma, identified in only about 50% of cases.[113,221]

The pseudoinclusions may be mimicked by punched out defects in the staining of nuclei, which is common in frozen sections (Fig. 11.16A). The pseudoinclusion-like nuclear bubbles or vacuoles may also be seen in routinely processed sections that are poorly fixed (Fig. 11.16 B).[224,225] These artifactual formations typically have empty appearance or pale staining, are structureless, and lack a rim of the nuclear membrane. The bubbles may contain a nucleolus within its space, which rules out the possibility of a true cytoplasmic pseudoinclusion. In addition, these artifactual patches are frequently seen in numerous nuclei in a field, a finding that should immediately raise a question about their authenticity. This is because true intranuclear cytoplasmic pseudoinclusions are rarely seen in abundance and typically found in no more than 1 to 2 cells per high power field.[226]

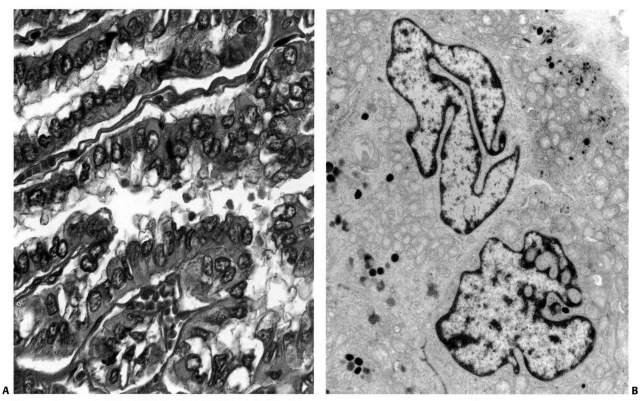

FIGURE 11.13. Marked irregularity of the nuclear contours. This important feature of papillary carcinoma can be seen on light microscopy **(A)** and electron microscopy **(B).**

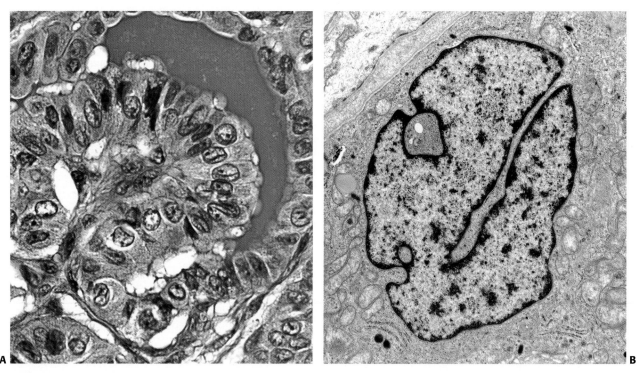

FIGURE 11.14. Nuclear grooves. These structures are often seen in papillary carcinoma cells on light microscopy **(A).** They are formed by linear invagination of the nuclear membrane that travels deep into the nuclear volume, which is best appreciated on electron microscopy **(B).**

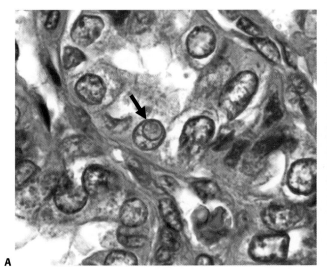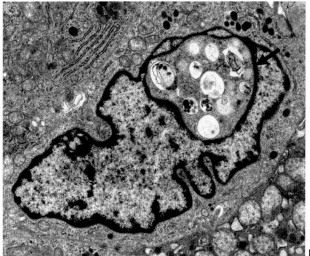

FIGURE 11.15. Nuclear pseudoinclusions. A: Light microscopy image showing a cell in the center of the field that contains an eosinophilic intranuclear body *(arrow)*, which is demarcated by a rim of nuclear membrane and stained more like the cytoplasm than the remainder of the nucleus. **B:** Ultramicroscopic image of a cell containing a nuclear pseudoinclusion *(arrow)*, which is surrounded by a nuclear membrane and contains phagolysosomes and other cytoplasmic organelles.

Frequency and Specificity of the Nuclear Features

In many papillary carcinomas, all or almost all of the nuclear features are readily identifiable, and this is diagnostic of papillary carcinoma irrespective of the growth pattern and other findings. However, some tumors exhibit most, but not all, of these features, or they are found focally within the nodule. There is no consensus on how many nuclear features are sufficient for the diagnosis and how widespread they should be.[227] In our experience, most papillary carcinomas reveal at least four of these nuclear features, and they are identifiable in many areas of the tumor.[113] We particularly rely on finding enlarged nuclei with nuclear contour irregularity. In our opinion, these two features are the most common and specific diagnostic features, particularly when they are present in a lesion sharply demarcated from the benign parenchyma. However, none of these features are pathognomonic for papillary carcinoma and a single feature may be seen, particularly focally, in many benign lesions.[217,224,228,229] This is particularly true for the grooved nuclei, which can be found in scattered cells of various benign and malignant lesions of the thyroid. True nuclear

pseudoinclusions have a relatively high specificity, but they are the least common feature and not found in a significant proportion of papillary carcinomas. Thyroid lesions composed of cells showing several, but not all, nuclear features are most challenging diagnostically, especially when they are encapsulated and lack papillary architecture, which is typically seen in the encapsulated follicular variant of papillary carcinoma.

Psammoma Bodies

Psammoma (from Greek "salt-like") bodies are distinctive calcifications that are found in 40% to 50% of papillary carcinomas.[113,213] In order to qualify as a psammoma body, the calcification must have the following characteristics:

(1) have a round or spherical shape,
(2) show concentric layers of calcium deposition, and
(3) be located in association with tumor cells, in the tumor stroma, or in a lymphatic channel, but not within the lumen of a follicle (Fig. 11.17).

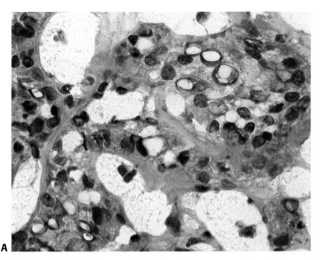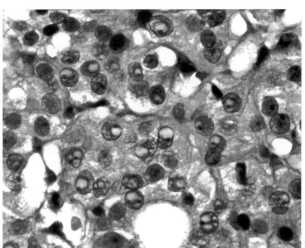

FIGURE 11.16. Structures mimicking nuclear pseudoinclusions. A: An intraoperative frozen section showing numerous nuclei with sharped-edged, punched-out empty spaces. **B:** A routine formalin fixed section showing multiple nuclei with bubbles that are pale stained and lack the texture of the adjacent cytoplasm. Many of the bubbles contain nucleoli.

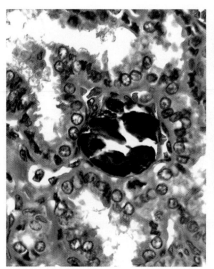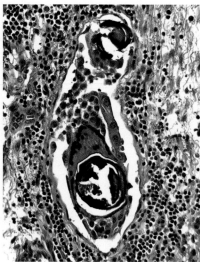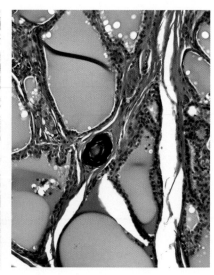

FIGURE 11.17. Psammoma bodies. True psammoma bodies are located either in a stalk of the papillae *(left)* or in association with tumor cells and multinucleated giant cells within a lymphatic channel *(middle)*, or in isolation within thyroid stroma *(right)*.

The intrafollicular calcifications can be seen in follicular adenomas and carcinomas, particularly of oncocytic type, and represent inspissated and calcified colloid. True psammoma bodies are believed to be formed by successive layering of calcium centered on a single or a small group of necrotic tumor cells, which serves as a nidus for calcium deposition.[216,230] Cell necrosis may develop at the tip of the papillae as a result of vascular thrombosis of a vessel within the stalk or in the intralymphatic tumor aggregate.[230] Psammoma bodies may be found in isolation, that is, with no tumor cells in the vicinity, and this is believed to represent a "tombstone," marking the site of prior viable tumor cells (Fig. 11.17, right).[231] However, the precise mechanism of psammoma body formation is not fully understood. The possible role of the immune response is suggested by the frequent presence of multinucleated giant cells intimately associated with psammoma bodies (Fig. 11.17, middle). Furthermore, macrophages in the vicinity of psammoma bodies overexpress a bone matrix protein osteopontin that participates in mineralization of bones and in ectopic calcification.[232] Psammoma bodies are particularly abundant in the diffuse sclerosing variant of papillary carcinoma and in tumors that carry *RET/PTC* rearrangement.[113] They are least common in the follicular variant and in tumors with *RAS* point mutations.

Psammoma bodies are not entirely specific for papillary carcinoma and have been reported in some benign lesions, such as nodular goiter with papillary hyperplasia.[233] However, true psammoma bodies are exceedingly rare in lesions other than papillary carcinomas, and their finding in the lesion with at least moderately expressed nuclear features of papillary carcinoma is virtually diagnostic of this tumor. Finding isolated psammoma bodies in the lymphatic channels, lymph nodes, or in the stroma of otherwise normal thyroid tissue provides strong evidence for papillary carcinoma present either in the adjacent thyroid tissue or in the contralateral lobe of the thyroid. In one study of 29 cases of isolated psammoma bodies found either in thyroid parenchyma (27 cases) or in perithyroidal lymph nodes (2 cases), 27 (93%) cases revealed either papillary (25 cases) or oncocytic (2 cases) carcinoma.[234] Two cases revealed no malignant tumor, but both of these patients underwent only lobectomy and the removed single lobe was not entirely submitted for microscopic examination. Of interest, most papillary carcinomas found in this study were incidental tumors <1 cm in size, and 44% of cases had psammoma bodies found in the opposite lobe from the carcinoma (intraglandular spread).

Tumor Fibrosis

In addition to the fibrous stroma of papillary stalks, discrete areas of fibrosis are frequently seen in papillary carcinomas. Discrete or interconnected fibrous bands traversing the tumor nodule in different directions or located at the periphery and forming a pseudocapsule may be found, as well as large, irregularly shaped, sometime stellate fibrous areas (Fig. 11.18). The fibrosis is typically paucicellular (sclerotic type) and less frequently cellular (desmoplastic type).[229] Considerable fibrosis is found in 50% to 90% of all tumors.[113,213,235] This type of densely eosinophilic fibrosis is not specific for papillary carcinoma, although it is far more characteristic of these tumors than of other thyroid follicular neoplasms. It serves as a particularly helpful diagnostic hint in two specific situations: (1) at the time of gross examination, when all small whitish, fibrotic-appearing areas should be sampled for microscopic evaluation as they often mark the areas of papillary carcinoma and (2) in the encapsulated follicular-pattern nodules, the presence of significant fibrosis not associated with degeneration or post-FNA injury provides support for the diagnosis of follicular variant of papillary carcinoma rather than follicular adenoma.

Other Microscopic Features

Colloid within neoplastic follicles frequently has a more intense, darkly eosinophilic tincture as compared with colloid in the adjacent nonneoplastic follicles (Fig. 11.19 A).[236] Multinucleated giant cells and foamy macrophages can be seen in the lumen of neoplastic follicles and between papillae (Fig. 11.19 B).

Squamous metaplasia is seen in about 20% of papillary carcinomas[213,237] and is more common in the diffuse sclerosing variant and tumors with classic papillary growth. In most cases, it appears as discrete concentric whorls of cells with keratinization and/or intercellular bridges (Fig. 11.19 C). Staining for thyroglobulin in these foci is often negative.[224]

Some degree of cystic change is common (Fig. 11.19 D), but it is usually not extensive. Approximately 10% of tumors reveal marked cystic transformation.[213]

Mitotic figures are uncommon. Typically, <1 to 2 mitoses per 10 high power fields (400× magnification: 40× objective combined with 10× eyepiece) are identified.[238,239] Atypical mitoses are exceedingly rare. If high mitotic activity is found, it should raise the possibility of poorly differentiated thyroid carcinoma.

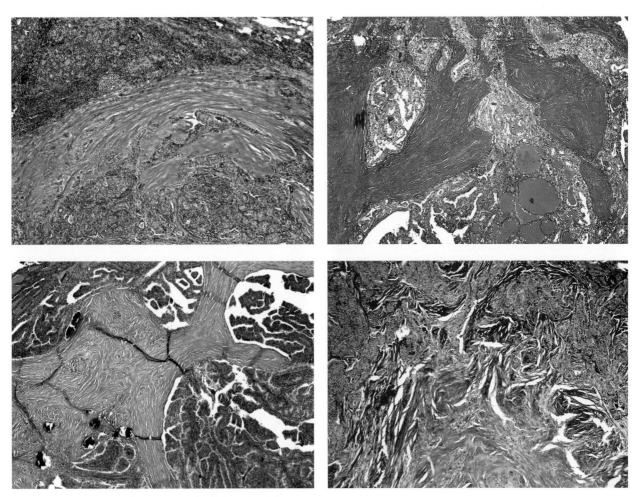

FIGURE 11.18. Various appearances of fibrosis in papillary carcinoma.

Significant lymphocytic infiltration is found within the tumor stroma or in thyroid tissue surrounding the tumor in 25% to 40% of cases.[113,213,237] Prominent stromal infiltration is a characteristic feature of the Warthin-like variant as described later in the chapter. Infiltration in the adjacent thyroid tissue may be either reactive (peritumor thyroiditis, see Chapter 4) or a part of chronic lymphocytic (Hashimoto) thyroiditis. As peritumoral lymphocytic infiltration is common in papillary carcinoma, this finding should not lead to the diagnosis of chronic lymphocytic (Hashimoto) thyroiditis, unless the same changes are found in thyroid tissue remote from the tumor, preferably in the opposite lobe.

 ## SPREAD AND METASTASES

Multicentricity versus Intraglandular Spread

Papillary carcinoma presents as a multifocal disease in 22% to 35% of cases,[213,240] which may represent either multiple independent primary tumors or intraglandular dissemination from a single primary tumor. As discussed earlier, clonality studies have shown that many discrete tumor foci in multifocal disease are of independent clonal origin.[90–93] In addition to the true multicentricity, the intraglandular dissemination of the tumor via lymphatic channels is very common, and multiple small or larger satellite foci are found in the vicinity or even more remotely from the main tumor mass in 27% to 78% of cases.[241,242] The distinction between independent primary tumors and intraglandular spread on one tumor is not always possible. In our experience, true independent primary tumors (judged based on the presence of different mutations) are more commonly:

(1) located in different thyroid lobes, (2) have distinct histologic appearance and/or belong to different variants of papillary carcinoma, (3) show partial or complete encapsulation, and (4) show no smaller satellite tumor foci surrounding the main tumor nodule.

Lymphatic and Blood Vessel Invasion

Papillary carcinoma is frequently seen invading *lymphatic* vessels in the thyroid parenchyma. In contrast, invasion of *blood* vessel located within the thyroid or in adjacent soft tissues is seen in less than 10% of cases.[213,243–245] Vascular invasion is more common in the follicular variant of papillary carcinoma than in other variants.[160,245] In order to qualify for vascular invasion, the tumor aggregates should be seen attached to the vessel wall and covered by a layer of endothelial cells (see detail description and illustration of vascular invasion in Chapter 10). The presence of vascular invasion is an unfavorable prognostic factor, as it correlated with higher risk of distant metastases[243–245] and tumor-related mortality.[243]

Extrathyroidal Extension

Papillary carcinomas typically have an infiltrative border and may extend beyond the confines of the gland by direct invasion. Extrathyroidal extension is defined as tumor penetration through the thyroid gland capsule into adjacent tissues. It is an important parameter used in the AJCC TNM-based staging system (Table 7.3.).[246] For tumor staging, extrathyroidal extension is subdivided into *minimal*, which is tumor invasion into immediate perithyroidal soft tissues or sternothyroid muscle (corresponds to T3) (Fig. 11.20 A) and *extensive*, which is tumor invasion into

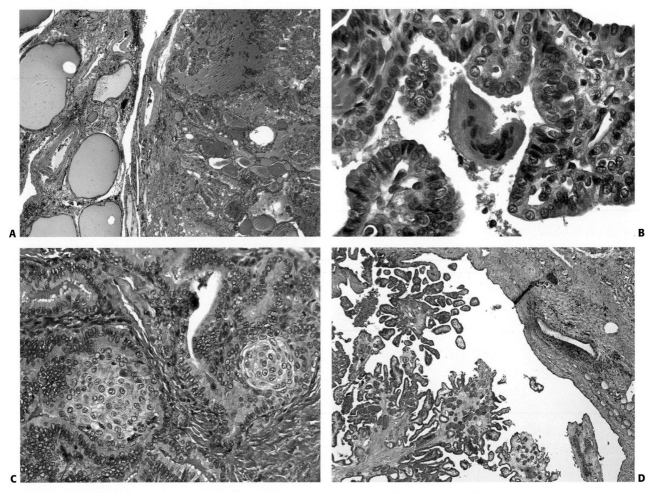

FIGURE 11.19. Additional changes seen in papillary carcinoma. A: Darker eosinophilic colloid in papillary carcinoma *(right)* as compared with adjacent thyroid *(left)*. **B:** Multinucleated giant cell in a space between papillae. **C:** Two foci of squamous metaplasia. **D:** Cystic change in papillary carcinoma.

subcutaneous soft tissues, larynx, trachea, esophagus, or recurrent laryngeal nerve (corresponds to T4) (Fig. 11.20 B). Extrathyroidal extension is found in 20% to 25% of tumors[213,240] and is more common in *BRAF*-positive papillary carcinomas and less common in the follicular variant.[113] As discussed later in the chapter, extrathyroidal extension is an important prognostic factor, although some more recent studies suggest that only extensive extrathyroidal invasion correlates with prognosis.[247,248]

Local and Distant Metastases

Spread to the cervical lymph nodes is a common feature of thyroid papillary carcinoma, whereas hematogenous tumor spread to

distant sites is rare. At the time of initial diagnosis, regional lymph node metastases are found in 30% to 50% and distant metastases in 2% to 5% of tumors.[211,212,249] The most common pattern of tumor growth in the metastatic deposits in lymph nodes is papillary, even if the primary tumor has a predominantly follicular architecture (Fig. 11.21 A). Cystic changes in lymph node metastases are common, and they are prominent in about 25% of cases (Fig. 11.21 B).[250] Tumor extension beyond the capsule of a lymph node can be seen in rare cases, and this is an unfavorable prognostic factor (Fig. 11.21 C).[251]

Distant metastases most frequently involve lungs (70%) (Fig. 11.21 D), followed by bones (20%) and other rare sites such as soft tissues of the mediastinum and brain.[252–254]

FIGURE 11.20. Extrathyroidal extension. A: Minimal extrathyroidal extension into adjacent soft tissue (TNM, T3). **B:** Extensive extrathyroidal extension involving tracheal cartilage (TNM, T4a).

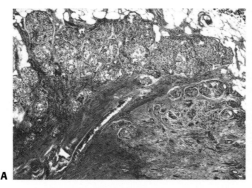

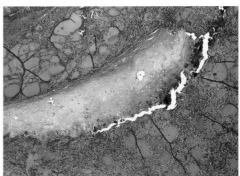

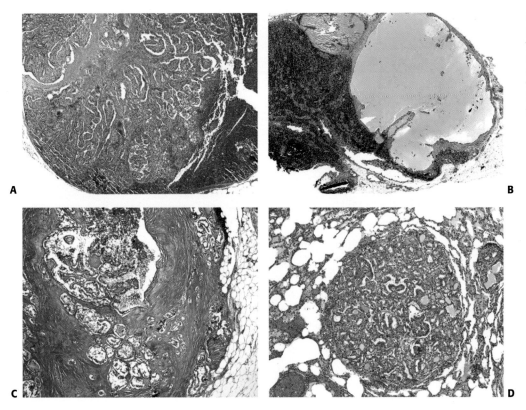

FIGURE 11.21. Papillary carcinoma metastases. A: Tumor metastasis to a lymph node. **B:** Lymph node metastasis with marked cystic change. **C:** Lymph node metastasis with tumor extension through the lymph node capsule. **D:** Tumor metastasis to the lung.

 # GRADING

Papillary carcinomas should not be graded because by definition they are well-differentiated tumors. Emergence of poorly differentiated thyroid carcinoma manifests by a solid, trabecular, or insular growth pattern and loss of characteristic nuclear features, frequently coupled with tumor necrosis and increased mitotic activity.[255]

 # MICROSCOPIC VARIANTS

In addition to classic papillary carcinoma, more than 10 different histologic variants have been described (Table 11.5). Some of them are distinguished solely based on a peculiar microscopic appearance, whereas others appear to have distinct clinical and prognostic characteristics.

Papillary Microcarcinoma

Papillary microcarcinoma is defined by the 2004 WHO classification as a papillary carcinoma that is (1) 1 cm or less in diameter and (2) found incidentally.[256] This definition is more restrictive than those used in many studies where only the size criterion is applied to define this variant. The WHO definition applies to those tumors that were not diagnosed or suspected preoperatively and are true incidental finding in thyroid specimens resected due to a benign disease or during laryngectomy. The purpose of the more restrictive definition is to limit the category to the true "occult" tumors that are common in autopsy series and are unlikely to have a clinical significance.

Papillary microcarcinomas are common and represent the fastest growing group of papillary carcinomas. In surgical thyroidectomies performed for benign thyroid nodules papillary microcarcinomas are found in 5% to 17% of cases.[257–259] Based on the SEER data, papillary carcinomas 1 cm or less in size constituted about 30% of all papillary carcinomas in 1988, and about 40% in 2004 to 2008,[5] making it the most common variant of papillary carcinoma in the United States. Similar trends have

been observed in France[3] and many other countries around the world (reviewed in ref.[260]). This is probably due to the increased use of ultrasonography and other imaging techniques, which can detect 0.2- to 0.3-cm sized tumors. Based on autopsy series, papillary microcarcinomas are found in 6% to 9% of thyroids in patients with no known thyroid disease in many regions on North America, Europe, and South America,[7,261–265] and in 28% to 36% of the glands in Japan and Finland.[8,262]

On gross examination, papillary microcarcinoma can be identified as a small whitish, fibrotic nodule with irregular contours (Fig. 11.22) or as a small ill-defined light-brown nodule. Many microcarcinomas are not seen on gross examination and identified only microscopically.

On microscopic examination, papillary microcarcinomas are sharply demarcated from the surrounding thyroid parenchyma and composed of papillary or follicular structures or a mixture of both (Fig. 11.23). They have either smooth borders with a thin or thick capsule or infiltrative borders and may be associated with significant tumor fibrosis. In 30% to 40% of cases, multiple microcarcinomas are seen.[266,267]

Most papillary microcarcinomas are believed to represent a nonprogressive, clinically innocuous disease. However, some have an aggressive clinical behavior. A meta-analysis of 11 studies that collectively reported 4,432 cases of papillary carcinomas ≤1 cm in size has shown that 7.2% of those had microscopic extrathyroidal extension, 28% had lymph node metastases, and 0.7% had distant metastases, with 5% of patients registering tumor recurrence and 0.3% tumor-related death.[266] Importantly, many of these complications developed in patients with tumors that were diagnosed preoperatively despite their small size.[260,268] These nonincidental tumors constituted up to 80% of all tumors in some studies included in this meta-analysis. The frequency of distant metastases, tumor recurrence or death from disease in tumors meeting strict criteria, that is, true incidental finding, is not clearly established but is likely to be very low.

Factors consistently found to be associated with higher risk of recurrence include tumor multifocality and lymph node metastasis at presentation.[269,270] More recently, *BRAF* V600E mutation was correlated with extrathyroidal extension,[271–274] lymph node

Table 11.5

Microscopic Variants of Papillary Carcinoma

Variant	Diagnostic Criteria	Prevalence among Papillary Carcinomas (%)
Papillary microcarcinoma	Size 1 cm or less Incidental finding	~40
Follicular variant	>50% follicular growth pattern No well-formed papillae	20–30
Tall cell variant	>50% tall columnar cells with height three times their width	5–10
Solid variant	>50% solid, trabecular or insular growth	1–3
Diffuse sclerosing variant	Diffuse tumor growth within gland Abundant fibrosis Extensive lymphocytic infiltration Numerous psammoma bodies Squamous metaplasia	1–2
Columnar cell variant	Columnar cells with nuclear stratification	<1
Oncocytic variant	>50% cells with oncocytic cytoplasm	<1
Warthin-like variant	Dense lymphocytic infiltration in papillary stalks Cells with oncocytic cytoplasm	<1
Clear cell variant	>50% cells with clear cytoplasm	<1
Cribriform-morular variant	Cribriform growth pattern Morules	<1
Papillary carcinoma with prominent hobnail features	>50% cells with hobnail features	<1
Papillary carcinoma with fasciitis-like stroma	Abundant cellular stroma resembling nodular fasciitis	<1

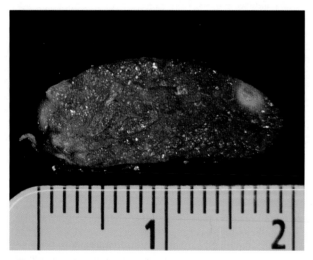

FIGURE 11.22. Gross appearance of papillary microcarcinoma. This 0.2-cm tumor presents as a whitish nodule located immediately under the thyroid capsule.

metastasis,[273,274] and multifocality[274] of microcarcinoma. However, as *BRAF* mutation is found in 24% to 63% of these tumors,[271–274] it is unlikely that most microcarcinomas that carry this mutation have aggressive behavior.

Recently, a molecular-pathologic (MP) scoring system was developed for the risk stratification of papillary microcarcinoma.[275] It involves the combination of *BRAF* mutation status and three histopathologic features: superficial tumor location, intraglandular tumor spread/multifocality, and tumor fibrosis (Fig. 11.24). Criteria for each of these histopathologic features are described in the legend to Figure 11.24. A simple, unweighted MP score utilizes a sum of these features and stratifies papillary microcarcinomas into low (score 0 to 2), moderate (score 3), and high (score 4) risk groups, with the probability of lymph node metastases or tumor recurrence of 0%, 20%, and 60%, respectively.[275]

Follicular Variant

This is a common variant that currently comprises 20% to 30% of all papillary carcinomas.[213,276] Its diagnostic criteria are (1) complete lack of well-formed papillae, (2) exclusively or predominantly a follicular growth pattern, and (3) presence of characteristic nuclear features of papillary carcinoma. A solid, nested, or trabecular architecture can be present as well as scattered abortive, poorly formed papillae, but a follicular pattern should be the predominant pattern (>50%) in a tumor that lacks well-developed papillae (Fig. 11.25).

Historically, all thyroid tumors with follicular growth were diagnosed as follicular carcinomas. The follicular variant of papillary carcinoma was originally described by Lindsay[277] in 1960 and further characterized as a distinct variant by Chen and Rosai,[278]

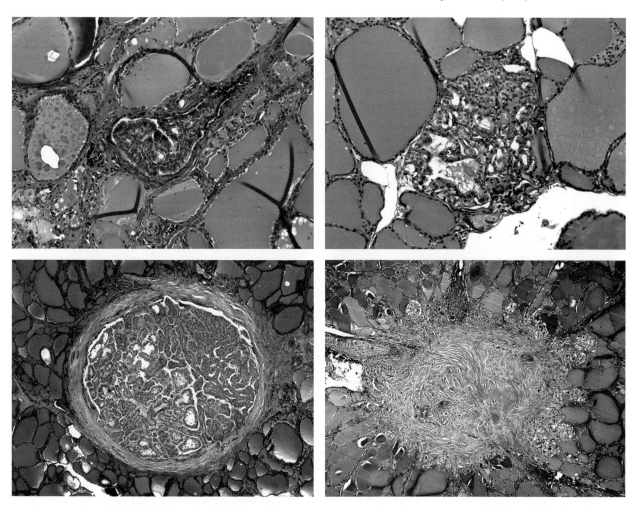

FIGURE 11.23. Microscopic appearance of papillary microcarcinoma. The composite illustrates four different tumors showing a spectrum of sizes, growth patterns, encapsulation, and fibrosis. *(Left upper)* A 0.03-cm tumor with papillary architecture. *(Right upper)* A 0.07-cm tumor with follicular growth pattern. *(Left lower)* A 0.34-cm encapsulated tumor. *(Right lower)* A 0.28-cm tumor with extensive central fibrosis.

who realized that, despite the follicular architecture, tumors with nuclear features of papillary carcinoma have biologic properties of papillary rather than follicular carcinoma. Although generally this is the case and these tumors should undoubtedly be designated as papillary carcinomas, they represent a distinct variant of papillary carcinoma with several characteristic molecular and biologic features, some of which are closer to follicular tumors. Follicular variant papillary carcinomas frequently harbor *RAS* mutations and may also have *BRAF* K601E mutation and *PAX8/PPARγ* rearrangement, which are common in follicular tumors and are rare in classic papillary carcinoma (Table 11.6).[160,161] They reveal a higher frequency of aneuploidy and exhibit patterns of chromosome gains and losses resembling those of follicular tumors[96,279] and show gene expression profiles that are distinct from classic papillary carcinomas.[194]

Grossly, these tumors are frequently well circumscribed (Fig. 11.9 C) and may be encapsulated, whereas they rarely show pronounced cystic changes. Microscopically, the tumors are composed of follicles that may show significant variability in size and shape or be rather monotonous. Elongated, twisted, and irregularly-shaped follicles are common. The colloid frequently, but not always, stains more intensely with eosin and shows focal scalloping at the periphery. Multinucleated giant cells may be seen within the follicles. The cells lining the follicles are typically larger than in nonneoplastic thyroid or in follicular tumors, and their nuclei are unevenly spaced along the basement membrane and show

loss of polarity (Fig. 11.26). Most of the characteristic nuclear features of papillary carcinoma are present, particularly nuclear enlargement, chromatin clearing, and irregularity of nuclear contours. Other nuclear features, particularly nuclear crowding and pseudoinclusions, are typically less abundant than in classic papillary carcinoma. Tumor fibrosis is common and typically found as discrete, acellular fibrotic bands. Single psammoma bodies may be found, but they are significantly less common than in classic papillary carcinoma.

The tumors may have an infiltrative border or a pushing border with smooth outlines and a capsule (Fig. 11.27 A,B). In comparison with classic papillary carcinoma, the follicular variant tumors demonstrate a higher frequency of tumor encapsulation and lower rates of extrathyroid extension and regional lymph node metastases.[160,280–282] When nodal metastases are present, the tumor frequently shows a mixture of papillary and follicular growth with well-formed papillary structures that were not seen in the primary tumor nodule (Fig. 11.27 C). A tendency for slightly higher rates of blood vessel invasion (Fig. 11.27 D) and distant metastases has been noted in some studies.[160,236,245] In addition to lung and bone metastases,[236,283,284] metastatic spread to unusual sites such as skin and kidney have been reported.[285,286] Overall, the clinical behavior of these tumors is similar to classic papillary carcinoma, with the exception of two subtypes, encapsulated follicular variant and diffuse follicular variant.

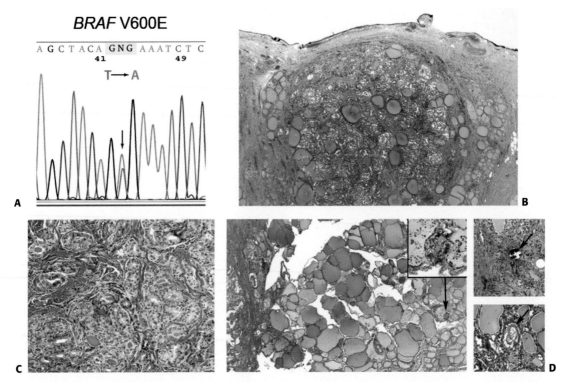

FIGURE 11.24. Prognostic molecular-pathologic (MP) score for papillary microcarcinoma. The score is a sum of four features: (1) positive status for *BRAF* V600E mutation (**A**); (2) superficial tumor location defined as tumor location immediately at the surface of the thyroid (**B**), with or without extrathyroidal extension; (3) significant sclerotic-type tumor fibrosis (**C**); and (4) intraglandular tumor spread/multifocality defined as presence of at least one of the following findings: two or more microcarcinomas, additional small tumor focus separated from the main tumor mass by benign thyroid parenchyma (**D,** *left*), isolated psammoma bodies in the stroma (**D,** *right upper*), or tumor aggregates within a lymphatic channel (**D,** *right lower*).

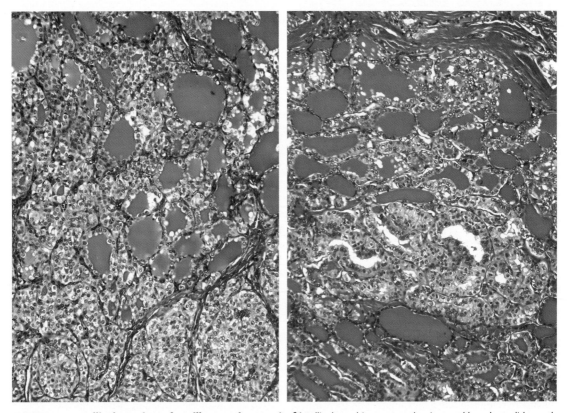

FIGURE 11.25. Follicular variant of papillary carcinoma. *(Left)* Follicular architecture predominates although a solid growth pattern is also seen. *(Right)* Rudimentary papillary structures are present (center), although no well-defined papillae are seen.

Table 11.6

Mutational Profiles of Classic Papillary Carcinoma and Follicular Variant of Papillary Carcinoma

	BRAF V600E (%)	RET/PTC (%)	RAS	BRAF K601E	PAX8/PPARγ
Classical papillary carcinoma	60	25	0	0	0
Follicular variant	10	<5	45%	5%	<5%

Encapsulated Follicular Variant

This subtype of the follicular variant is characterized by total encapsulation (Fig. 11.28). The tumor may show vascular and/or capsular invasion, or reveal no invasion. Since no papillae or psammoma bodies are found, the diagnosis of papillary carcinoma rests solely on the finding of characteristic nuclear features. Whereas in the past, the encapsulated follicular variant was relatively rare, at present time half to two-thirds of all follicular variant papillary carcinomas belong to this type.[282] The increase in the occurrence of this tumor type is mostly due to change in stringency of diagnostic criteria for papillary carcinoma that occurred progressively during the 1990s, which resulted in more frequent diagnosis of malignancy in nodules with partially developed nuclear features of papillary carcinoma.[11-13]

The capsule is complete and moderately thick but can vary from very thick to very thin, formed by a single layer of fibrous tissue. The

diagnostic nuclear features of papillary carcinoma are present either diffusely (Fig. 11.29) or multifocally, intermixed with the areas showing much more flattened cells lacking the nuclear features of papillary carcinoma (Fig. 11.30).[287,288] The reason for such a patchy appearance is not known. However, all areas probably represent the malignant neoplasm, as a similar patchy presence of nuclear features may sometimes be seen in metastatic foci within lymph nodes (Fig. 11.31). By convention, the entire nodule containing multifocal areas diagnostic for papillary carcinoma is considered as a single papillary carcinoma. This should be distinguished from a discrete, well-delineated focus of papillary carcinoma developing within a hyperplastic nodule or a follicular adenoma (Fig. 11.32).

In those cases where nuclear features are only moderately developed, this subtype of the follicular variant poses a significant diagnostic dilemma. At present, there is no consensus on how many nuclear features are sufficient for diagnosis and how

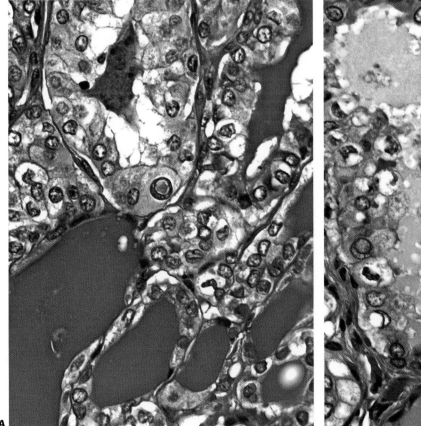
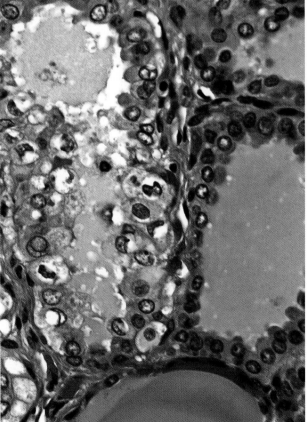

FIGURE 11.26. Follicular variant of papillary carcinoma. A: Neoplastic follicles contain dark eosinophilic colloid and are lined by cells with enlarged nuclei that are haphazardly arranged and show marked irregularity of the contours, nuclear grooves, and pseudoinclusions. **B:** The increased size, irregularity of contours, and uneven spacing of the nuclei in the neoplastic follicle (left) are easily recognizable when compared with the adjacent nonneoplastic cells (right).

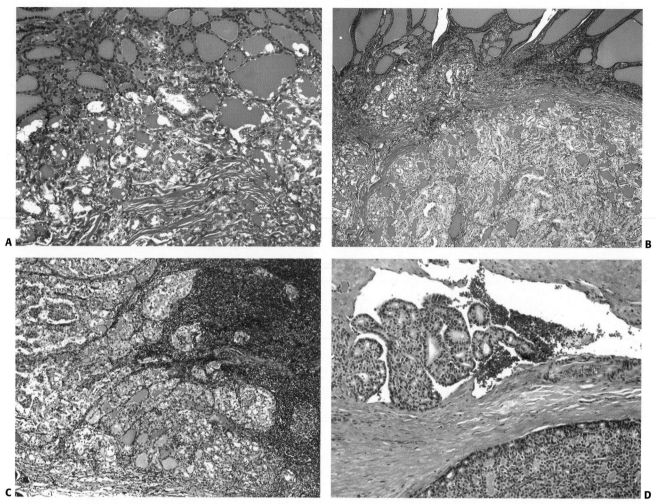

FIGURE 11.27. Follicular variant of papillary carcinoma: invasion and spread. A: This tumor shows an infiltrative border. **B:** This tumor is encapsulated with areas of tumor invasion through the capsule. **C:** Lymph node with a metastatic tumor showing a predominantly follicular architecture, although well-formed papillae can also be seen. **D:** Vascular invasion to a pericapsular vein.

prominent they should be. As a result, high interobserver variability has been reported for these tumors even between experienced endocrine pathologists.[289,290] Whereas some interpret such a variability as inability to arrive at a correct diagnosis even by experienced endocrine pathologists, the more likely explanation is that these tumors progress from an overtly benign to a clearly

malignant phenotype through multiple intermediate stages. When a tumor is removed at one or these intermediate stages of progression, it possesses some but not all nuclear features of papillary carcinoma, causing significant diagnostic challenge.

Of the six main nuclear features discussed earlier in great details, we particularly rely on two features: (1) nuclear enlargement

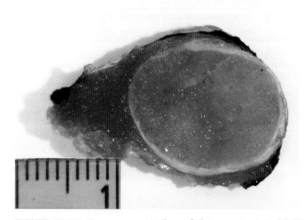

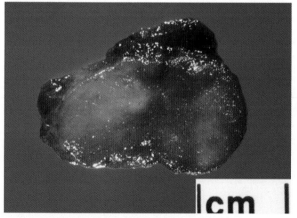

FIGURE 11.28. Gross presentation of the encapsulated follicular variant of papillary carcinoma. The tumor is well circubscribed and have either thick *(left)* or thin *(right)* capsule. The cut surface is frequently dark-brown, corresponding to larger follicles and more abundant colloid, or light-tan to whitish, corresponding to more cellular, microfollicular and solid, architecture.

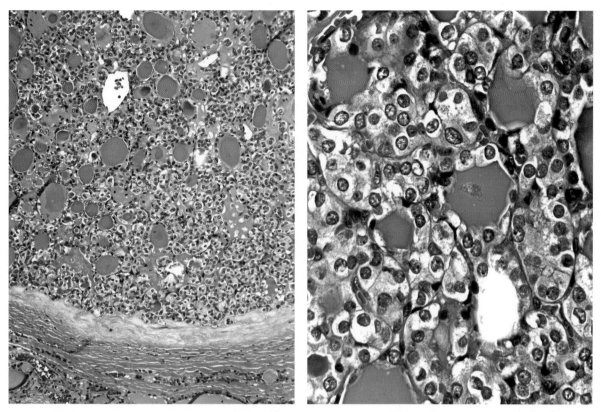

FIGURE 11.29. Encapsulated follicular variant of papillary carcinoma with diffusely present nuclear features of papillary carcinoma.

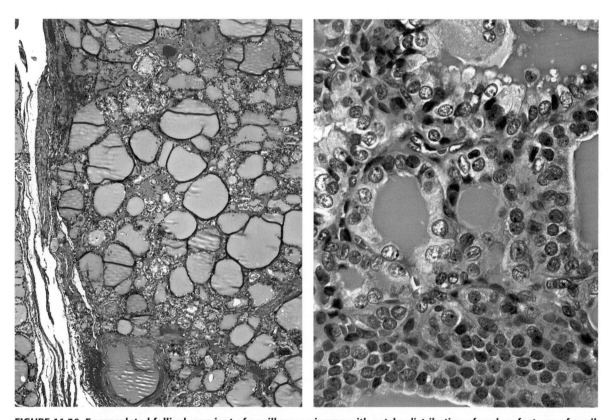

FIGURE 11.30. Encapsulated follicular variant of papillary carcinoma with patchy distribution of nuclear features of papillary carcinoma. *(Left)* A thin capsule demarcates the lesion that contains focal areas with distinct appearance on low power view. ***(Right)*** High-power view shows the area with relatively well-developed nuclear features of papillary carcinoma *(top)* and adjacent area with small, round, hyperchromatic nuclei *(bottom)*.

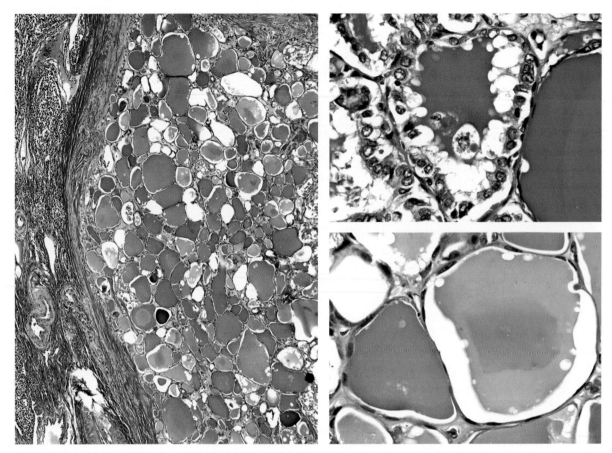

FIGURE 11.31. Patchy distribution of the diagnostic nuclear features in a lymph node metastasis. This metastasis of the follicular variant papillary carcinoma shows a prominent follicular architecture *(left)* with admixture of follicles lined by cells with well-developed nuclear features of papillary carcinoma *(right top)* and follicles lined by cells with flattened hyperchromatic nuclei *(right bottom)*.

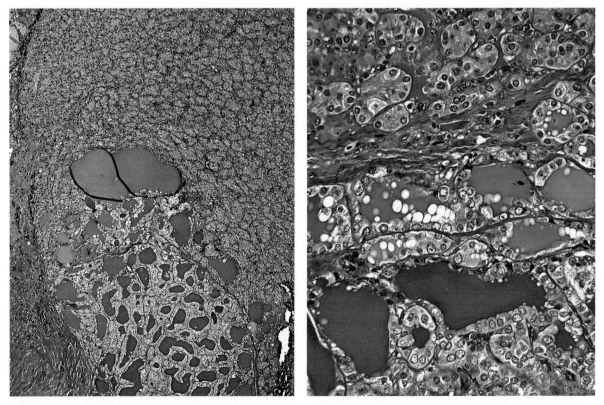

FIGURE 11.32. Papillary carcinoma, follicular variant, developing within a follicular adenoma. The papillary carcinoma *(bottom part of each panel)* presents as a single focus sharply demarcated from the remaining follicular adenoma.

of the tumor cells as compared with adjacent nonneoplastic cells and (2) irregularity of the nuclear contours. Importantly, there should be a sharp border between the tumor nodule composed of cells with large, irregularly-shaped nuclei and the adjacent benign parenchyma, instead of a gradual decrease in the nuclei size and irregularity of the nuclei contours seen in benign reactive lesions. Abundant nuclear grooves and pseudoinclusions are rarely seen in these tumors. Additional,

minor diagnostic features that are helpful and favor papillary carcinoma over a follicular adenoma or hyperplastic nodule are (1) irregular, elongated follicles; (2) abortive papillae; (3) irregularly spaced nuclei showing a lack of polarity and a haphazard nuclear placement; (4) presence of substantial fibrosis within the nodule; (5) densely eosinophilic colloid with peripheral scalloping; and (6) multinucleated giant cells within the lumens of follicles (Fig. 11.33).

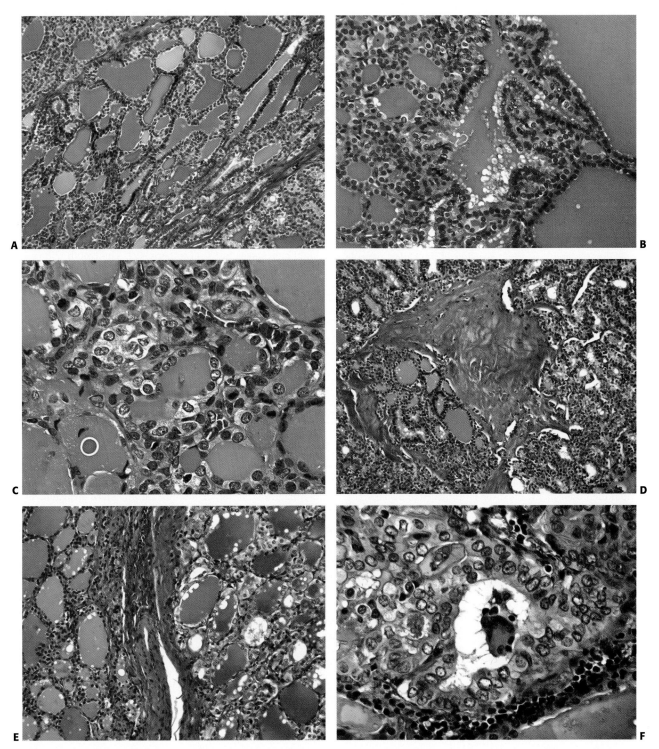

FIGURE 11.33. Minor diagnostic features that favor follicular variant of papillary carcinoma over a follicular adenoma or hyperplastic nodule: elongated, irregularly-shaped follicles **(A)**, small, poorly formed, abortive papillae **(B)**, irregularly spaced nuclei with loss of polarity **(C)**, discrete areas of fibrosis **(D)**, densely eosinophilic colloid with peripheral scalloping **(E,** *right***),** and multinucleated giant cells **(F).**

Immunohistochemical stains (particularly HBME-1) and molecular markers (such as *BRAF*) are diagnostically helpful when positive, as described in more detailed later in the chapter. Despite high specificity, their sensitivity is relatively low,[291] which limits the diagnostic utility of these ancillary methods.

These encapsulated tumors often show no invasion, although in about one-third of cases either tumor capsule invasion or vascular invasion or both invasion types are noted.[288,292]

The behavior of these tumors is indolent. A summary of six studies that reported 107 cases of encapsulated follicular variant, revealed that 25% of patients had lymph node metastases and only 1% had distant metastases.[227] Among these 107 patients, 1 died of disease and 2 were alive with disease, whereas the rest (97%) of patients were alive and well with various follow-up periods. In a study of 61 cases of encapsulated follicular variant, lymph node metastases were observed in 5%, and there was no distant metastasis.[288] With median follow-up of 11 years, only one patient developed tumor recurrence, and the tumor in this case had capsular and vascular invasion. No adverse events were found in any of the encapsulated and noninvasive tumors, including 31 patients treated with lobectomy only. In another study of a cohort of thyroid tumors followed on average for 12 years, none of 66 patients with encapsulated follicular variant of papillary carcinoma died of disease.[292] Despite a low probability, some patients with encapsulated follicular variants may present with distant, particularly bone, metastases or develop metastasis during follow-up.[284,293] Tumors prone to metastatic behavior often have a thick capsule and significant intratumoral fibrosis, and virtually all of them reveal vascular invasion or invasion of the tumor capsule. Therefore, pathologic evaluation of these tumors should include microscopic examination of the entire tumor capsule to rule out invasion, as well as careful evaluation of the tumor to rule out the presence of poorly differentiated carcinoma areas or other unfavorable diagnostic features such as tumor necrosis or high ($\geq$3 per 10 high-power fields) mitotic activity.[294] In the absence of these features, a noninvasive encapsulated follicular variant papillary carcinoma is expected to have an extremely indolent biologic behavior with very low risk of recurrence or extrathyroidal spread, even in patients with lobectomy.

Owing to the difficulty in diagnosing these lesions and low probability of aggressive behavior, it has been proposed to designate these lesions as "well-differentiated tumors of uncertain malignant potential."[295] This terminology, however, is not widely accepted as it is not linked to a defined clinical management for these patients. Instead, it is important to designate these tumors in the diagnostic line as "Encapsulated follicular variant of papillary carcinoma" and state if the tumor has vascular or tumor capsule invasion.

Diffuse (Multinodular) Follicular Variant

This is a rare aggressive subtype of the follicular variant that typically occurs in young females and is characterized by multifocal involvement of one or both thyroid lobes.[296,297] Multiple tumor nodules are found on gross examination, and microscopically they have various degree of encapsulation, frequent infiltrative growth, and a follicular architecture with normal to small size follicles, although areas of solid, trabecular, and macrofollicular growth may also be seen (Fig. 11.34). In some cases, the tumor diffusely involves the gland. Nuclear features of papillary carcinoma are present, but fibrosis and psammoma bodies are uncommon. Vascular invasion and extrathyroidal extension are typically found, and lymph node and distant metastases are very common. The metastases tend to preserve the follicular architecture and rarely show well-formed papillae.

Macrofollicular Variant

This rarest subtype of the follicular variant is characterized by a very large size of tumor follicles (Fig. 11.35).[298,299] The macrofollicles (>200 μm in diameter) constitute >50% of the tumor and may be admixed with smaller size follicular structures. The cells lining the follicles exhibit characteristic nuclear features of papillary carcinoma, although they may be spotty, with some follicles lined by cells with dark nuclei characteristic of follicular lesions. The tumors are frequently of large size, and encapsulation is common. Based on the meta-analysis of 51 published cases, lymph node metastases are present in 20% of tumors, and distant, typically lung, metastases in 6% of tumors.[300,299] The lymph node metastases tend to preserve a macrofollicular growth pattern. Recently, two cases of the macrofollicular variant with disseminated bone metastases have been reported.[300] The importance of recognizing this subtype is two-fold. In preoperative FNA samples, it represents a common source of false negative cytology due to abundant colloid and focal nature of nuclear features of papillary carcinoma.[301-303] In the surgical samples, it resembles nodular goiter or macrofollicular adenoma macroscopically and on low power microscopic examination, and it can be misdiagnosed as a benign lesion if nuclear characteristics are not carefully sought.[300,304]

Tall Cell Variant

Tall cell variant is characterized by predominance (>50%) of tall columnar tumor cells whose height is at least three times their width. The requirement for the height being three times the width was introduced in the 2004 WHO classification[256] to make the diagnostic criterion for this variant more stringent. Previous

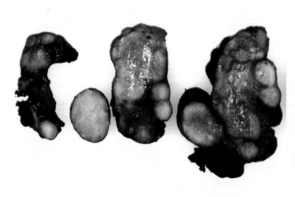
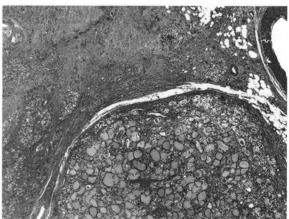

FIGURE 11.34. Diffuse (multinodular) follicular variant of papillary carcinoma. (Left) On gross examination, the tumor shows multiple well- to ill-defined light-tan nodules some of which extend beyond the thyroid capsule. **(Right)** Microscopically, the tumor nodules have the normofollicular architecture and various degree of encapsulation, with tumor extension into perithyroidal adipose tissue.

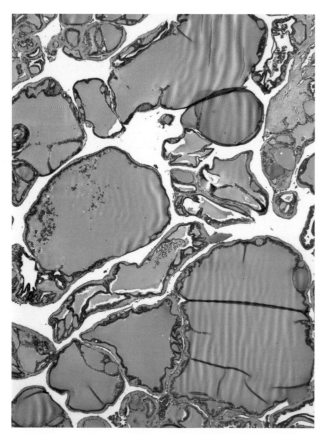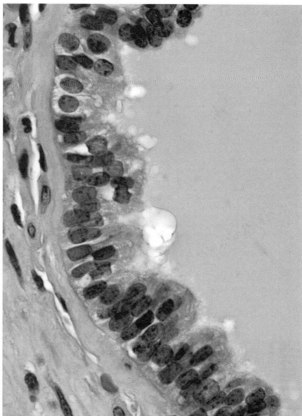

FIGURE 11.35. Macrofollicular subtype of the follicular variant of papillary carcinoma.

publications, including those by Hawk and Hazard[218] who described this variant in 1976, required the cell height to be two times the width. Tall cell variant comprises 5% to 10% of all papillary carcinomas.[218,239,276,305,306] It is exceedingly rare among pediatric tumors and seen with lower frequency in young patients. *BRAF* V600E mutation is very common and found in about 80% of these tumors.[121,122] Some reports suggest that *TP53* immunoreactivity is often seen in these tumors in contrast to the classic papillary carcinoma.[307]

In addition to the increased height of cells, other microscopic features of this variant include prominent cell borders, large amount of dense eosinophilic cytoplasm, and a somewhat distinct architectural pattern with thin elongated follicles and closely packed papillae with delicate branching and thin (delicate) fibrovascular cores giving impression of the trabecular growth (Fig. 11.36). Nuclear features of papillary carcinoma are very prominent, particularly nuclear grooves and pseudoinclusions that are found in abundance, whereas chromatin clearing may not be pronounced. Dense eosinophilia of the cytoplasm is likely due to increased mitochondria, which are seen ultramicroscopically, although mitochondria are still less abundant as compared with oncocytic cells and they lack structural abnormalities.[308]

In most studies, the tall cell variant tumors present at an older age, have larger tumor size, show more common extrathyroidal extension, and develop distant metastases more often than classic papillary carcinoma.[218,309–311] In addition, several reports have shown that this variant is associated with a higher recurrence rate and increased tumor-related mortality (22% to 25%).[218,306,309,311,312] Whereas in part the poorer prognosis is due to a typically older patient age and high tumor stage at presentation, some studies have shown that even when matched by age and tumor size/stage with the classic papillary cancer, the tall cell variant shows a significantly higher rate of lymph node and distant metastases[313] and lower 5-year disease-specific survival.[314]

Tall cell variant papillary carcinomas are prone to dedifferentiation. They are often found as a well-differentiated component within anaplastic (undifferentiated) carcinomas and poorly differentiated thyroid carcinomas.[121,315] This may also influence the shorter survival.

Owing to its association with less favorable prognosis, it is important to recognize the tall cell variant during microscopic examination and mention it in the pathology report. Currently, this variant appears to be underdiagnosed in a significant proportion of cases.[316] On the other hand, it is important to avoid overdiagnosing this variant. The tall cell variant should be distinguished from the Warthin-like variant, which shows dense lymphocytic infiltration of tumor stroma and is rarely infiltrative, and from the oncocytic variant, which is composed of cells that are rarely very tall, show no distinct cell borders, and have prominent nucleoli.

Tumors that contain less than 50% of cells with tall cell characteristics should not be assigned to this variant but designated as "papillary carcinoma with tall cell features." The influence of a minor tall cell component on tumor behavior is uncertain at this time and awaits systematic studies, but some experts believe that these tumors may have more frequent metastases or recurrence.[317] In our experience, classic papillary carcinomas with a minor tall cell component are more frequently positive for *BRAF* V600E mutation, a marker of more aggressive behavior of papillary carcinoma, than tumors with no tall cell features.

Solid Variant

These papillary carcinomas have exclusively or predominantly (>50%) a solid, trabecular, or nested (insular) growth pattern. The most common growth pattern is solid with sheets and nests of cells separated by fibrous stroma (Fig. 11.37 A,B). The stroma ranges from thin and delicate fibrous bands to thick with

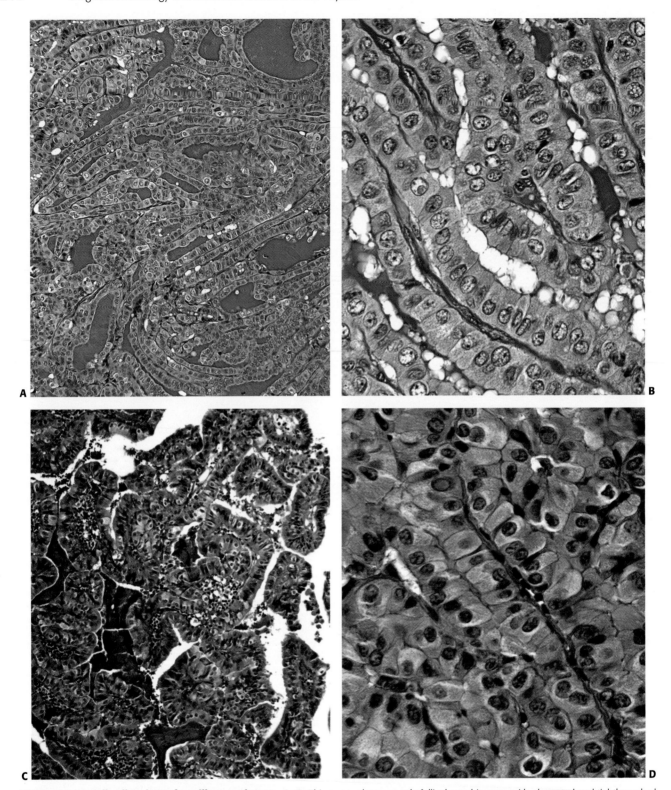

FIGURE 11.36. Tall cell variant of papillary carcinoma. A, B: This tumor shows mostly follicular architecture with elongated and tightly packed follicles lined by tall cells with pronounced nuclear features of papillary carcinoma. **C, D:** This tumor is composed predominantly of papillae, many of which are also closely packed and show delicate branching.

abundant fibrosis. The trabecular pattern consists of curvilinear anatomosing bands of tumor (Fig. 11.37 C,D). The insular or nested pattern is a variation of the solid pattern with more defined tumor nests surrounded by fibrovascular stroma with a separation artifact (Fig. 11.37 E,F). The solid areas are frequently admixed with a minor component represented by microfollicular structures. Larger size follicles and abortive papillae may also be seen. Well-formed papillary structures may be present, although typically they are difficult to find. The cells have a moderate amount of cytoplasm and nuclei with well-developed nuclear features of papillary carcinoma. Scattered psammoma bodies may be found.

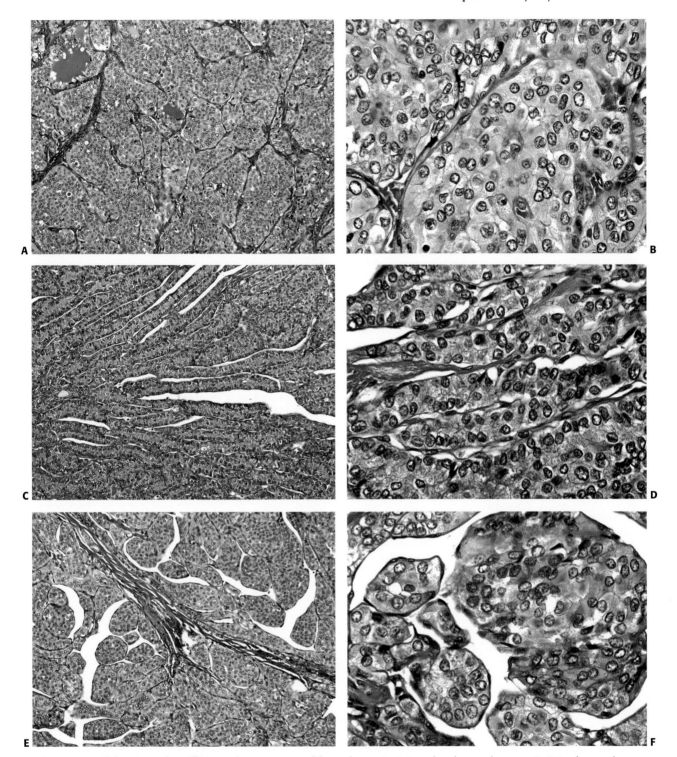

FIGURE 11.37. Solid variant of papillary carcinoma. A, B: Solid growth pattern. **C, D:** Trabecular growth pattern. **E, F:** Insular growth patern.

In large series, the solid variant constitutes 1% to 3% of adult papillary carcinomas.[276,318] The prevalence of the solid variant is higher in young patients, particularly among children exposed to ionizing radiation. For example, in pediatric papillary carcinomas developed after the Chernobyl nuclear accident, solid variant comprised 30% to 35% of all papillary carcinomas.[35,319] In this population, most (80%) of the solid variant papillary carcinomas had *RET/PTC3* rearrangement.[38] However, this association is probably restricted to pedictric or radiation-associated tumors, as

RET/PTC3 rearrangement was rare in solid variant tumors from the general, mostly adult population.[318]

The prognosis for this tumor variant in adults is slightly less favorable. These tumors appear to be more frequently associated with distant metastases (typically to lung), which develop in about 15% of cases, and with a slightly higher mortality rate, which was 10% and 12% in two studies with 10 and 19 years mean follow-up.[318,320] Whether this slightly more aggressive behavior is also expected for tumors diagnosed in children is not known. Among children with post-Chernobyl papillary carcinomas, many of which had a solid variant morphology, the mortality was very low (<1%) during the first decade of follow-up.[23,33] Similarly, it remains unclear if the prognosis is altered in tumors with a minor solid component.

The solid variant papillary carcinoma should be distinguished from poorly differentiated thyroid carcinoma, with which it shares the solid, trabecular, and insular growth patterns. The distinction is based primarily on the preservation of nuclear features and lack of necrosis and high mitotic activity in the solid variant,[255] as described in more detail in Chapter 12.

Diffuse Sclerosing Variant

This variant is typically found in children and young adults and is characterized by diffuse involvement of one or both thyroid lobes by the tumor. It constitutes 1% to 2% of papillary carcinomas,[276,321,322] has strong female predominance, and is much more common in young patients. The mean age at diagnosis is in the range of 18 to 29 years in most series with 10 or more cases.[321-327] It can occur in patients with a history of radiation exposure.[35,36] Tumors belonging to this variant frequently reveal *RET/PTC* rearrangement, whereas *BRAF* mutation is rarely found.[113,328]

Grossly, these tumors present with diffuse enlargement of one or both thyroid lobes with no discrete tumor mass or an ill-defined dominant mass recognizable on gross examination (Fig. 11.38). The cut surface shows a patchy, reticulated whitish-gray and gritty appearance.

Microscopically, this variant is characterized by the following five features (Fig. 11.39):

(1) diffuse gland involvement by the tumor
(2) dense, sclerotic fibrosis
(3) extensive lymphocytic infiltration
(4) numerous psammoma bodies
(5) frequent squamous metaplasia

The tumor foci are frequently found within lymphatic channels and have mixed solid and papillary architecture with common squamous morules. Extrathyroid extension is common. Lymph node metastases are found in about 80% of cases and often affect many lymph nodes and on both sides of the neck. The metastatic tumor is frequently composed of a mixture of solid and papillary areas with abundant psammoma bodies and occasional foci of squamous metaplasia. The frequency of distant, predominantly lung, metastases varies significantly between the reported series and is 10% to 15% based on almost 100 published cases summarized by Lam et al.[325] in 2006 and several more recent reports.[321,322,329]

The prognostic implication of this variant remain controversial. Some authors believe that this variant represents a more aggressive tumor type as it presents with massive involvement of the thyroid gland and has a higher rate of local and distant metastases at presentation. The disease-free survival is lower than in classic papillary carcinoma.[321,329,330] Nevertheless, the overall mortality appears to be low, with a disease-specific survival of approximately 93% at 10 years of follow-up.[325] The favorable outcome may be due to the young age of the patients. Rare cases of transformation of squamous metaplasia into highly aggressive squamous carcinoma have been described in older patients with this variant.[327]

Columnar Cell Variant

This rare variant of papillary carcinoma is characterized by predominance of columnar cells with pronounced nuclear stratification (Fig. 11.40).[331] It constitutes about 0.2% of all papillary carcinomas.[332] The cytoplasm is eosinophilic or clear, and in some tumors, shows prominent subnuclear vacuoles resembling early secretory endometrium.[333] The cytoplasmic vacuoles may also be located in a supranuclear cell compartment. The nuclei are elongated, frequently with dark chromatin, and with characteristic nuclear features of papillary carcinoma present focally and not nearly as pronounced as in classic papillary carcinoma. The tumor may show a papillary, follicular, solid, or cribriform growth pattern or a combination of those. Elongated follicular structures and slender papillae that are tightly packed resembling a cribriform architectural pattern are common. Areas of spindle cell growth and foci of squamous metaplasia can be found. Rare psammoma bodies may be seen. The cells preserve TTF1 immunoreactivity, whereas thyroglobulin staining is typically patchy and weak.[334,335] TP53 immunostaining can be found in most cases, but it is typically weak.[332] *BRAF* V600E mutation is found in one-third of cases.[332] Several cases of a mixed tall cell and columnar cell papillary carcinoma have been described.[336,337]

The columnar cell variant was initially reported as an invariably aggressive variant with extrathyroidal extension, distant metastases, and death from disease.[331] More recently, several encapsulated tumors or tumors lacking extrathyroidal extension have been described, and those patients had an excellent prognosis.[335,338] In a series of 16 cases reported by Wenig et al.,[335] 13 (81%) patients with tumors confined to the thyroid had either no

FIGURE 11.38. Diffuse sclerosing variant of papillary carcinoma. Gross photograph shows a cross-section of two thyroid lobes with multiple interdigitating whitish streaks and no definitive tumor mass, and enlarged bilateral lymph nodes with metastases.

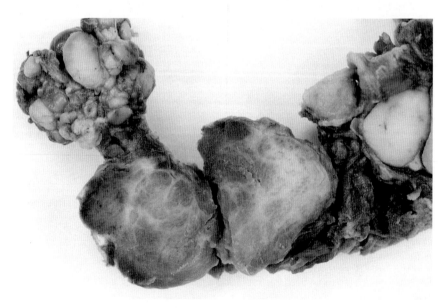

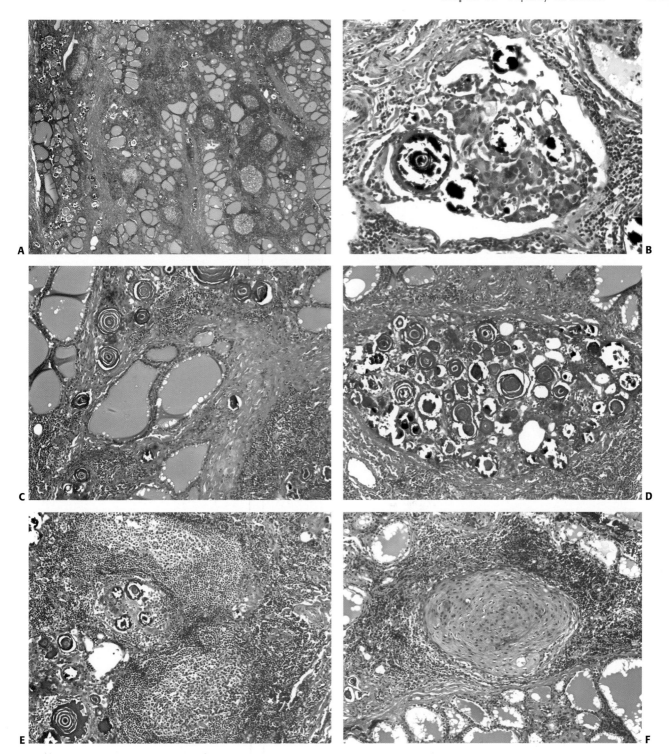

FIGURE 11.39. Microscopic features of the diffuse sclerosing variant of papillary carcinoma. A, B: Diffuse tumor growth with tumor aggregates frequently located within lymphatic channels. **C:** Extensive fibrosis. **D:** Abundant psammoma bodies. **E:** Marked lymphocytic infiltration. **F:** Squamous metaplasia.

evidence of disease (69%) or develop recurrence (12%) during an average follow-up of 5.8 years, whereas 2 (12%) patients had aggressive tumors with lung metastases. The latter patients had large tumors with infiltrative growth and extrathyroidal extension at presentation. In another study, the risk of death from disease was associated with large, locally invasive and metastatic tumors arising in older male patients, whereas small intrathyroidal tumors

in younger females had no complications on follow-up.[332] This suggests that unfavorable prognosis is not a uniform feature of this variant and is generally limited to patients with an advanced disease at presentation.

The unusual appearance of the columnar cell variant may mimic a metastatic adenocarcinoma from other primary sites. This can be resolved using immunohistochemistry.

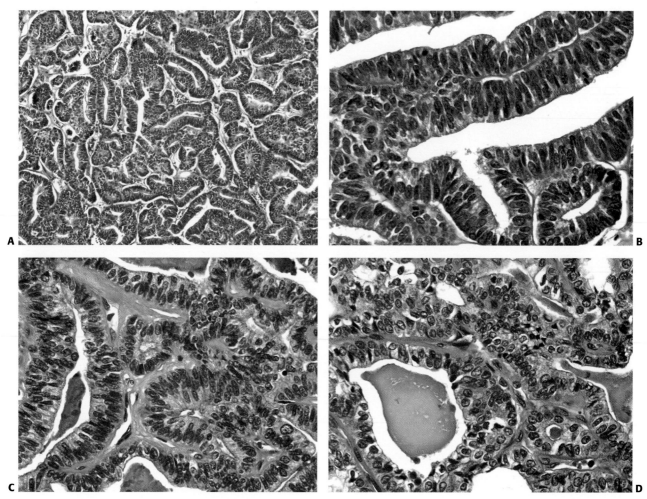

FIGURE 11.40. Columnar cell variant of papillary carcinoma. A, B: This tumor is composed of elongated tightly packed follicles lined by cells with marked nuclear stratification. The nuclei are elongated with dark chromatin and show no nuclear features of papillary carcinoma. **C, D:** In this tumor, some areas reveal elongated nuclei with pronounced stratification **(C)** and other areas show nuclei with less pronounced stratification and better developed nuclear features of papillary carcinoma.

Oncocytic (Hürthle Cell) Variant

The oncocytic variant of papillary carcinoma is rare. The cells have indistinct cell borders and reveal abundant, dense eosinophilic, granular, opaque cytoplasm characteristic of oncocytic (Hürthle) cells and the nuclear features of papillary carcinoma. These nuclear features should be diffuse and well developed, as some degree of chromatin clearing and nuclear contour irregularity is a common feature of oncocytic thyroid cells, and these limited features alone are insufficient for this diagnosis. The predominant pattern of growth is papillary (Fig. 11.41), although it can also be follicular (Fig. 11.42) or solid. The nuclei may show an apical polarization. Nucleoli are typically seen, although they may be less prominent than in oncocytic follicular adenoma and carcinoma. Psammoma bodies may be found. Electron microscopy demonstrates abundant mitochondria similar to other oncocytic tumors.[308,339]

Local lymph node metastases occur in 5% to 40% of cases.[340–342] Although some studies revealed a slightly higher recurrence and mortality associated with this variant, most reports have shown a prognosis similar to conventional papillary carcinoma.[339,341,342]

BRAF mutation is found in about half of these tumors.[343] Somatic and germ-line mutations of the *GRIM-19* gene involved in mitochondrial metabolism and cell death pathways have been found in 3 out of 10 oncocytic papillary carcinomas.[187] A high

prevalence of *RET/PTC* rearrangement has also been found, although it was detected using highly sensitive techniques.[188–190] The significance of this finding is not clear as these ultrasensitive techniques also led to *RET/PTC* detection in most oncocytic follicular adenomas and carcinomas.

Chronic lymphocytic (Hashimoto) thyroiditis is found in the background of 38% to 87% of thyroid glands with oncocytic papillary carcinomas and was suggested to be involved in pathogenesis of these tumors.[339,341]

Warthin-Like Variant

This rare variant may be considered as a subtype of oncocytic papillary carcinoma. It is characterized by cells with oncocytic cytoplasm and nuclear features of papillary carcinoma lining papillary structures with dense lymphocytic infiltration in the stalks (Fig. 11.43).[344] This microscopic appearance resembles Warthin tumor of salivary glands, which yields the tumor name. Warthin-like variant of papillary carcinoma has a strong female predominance (10:1).[344–346] Most cases, but not all of them, are associated with chronic lymphocytic (Hashimoto) thyroiditis. The tumors are usually well circumscribed and solid, although some may have prominent central cystic changes. The cells infiltrating the papillary stalk are a mixture of T lymphocytes, B lymphocytes, and

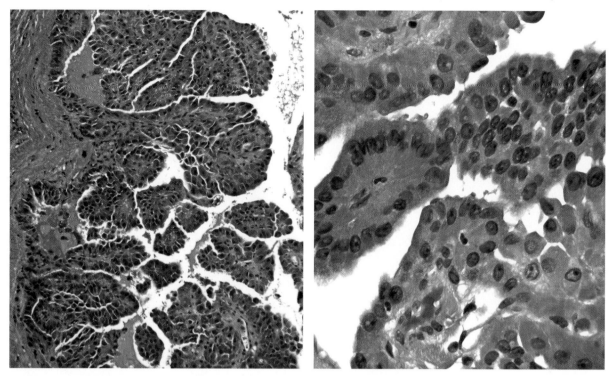

FIGURE 11.41. Oncocytic variant of papillary carcinoma with a papillary growth pattern.

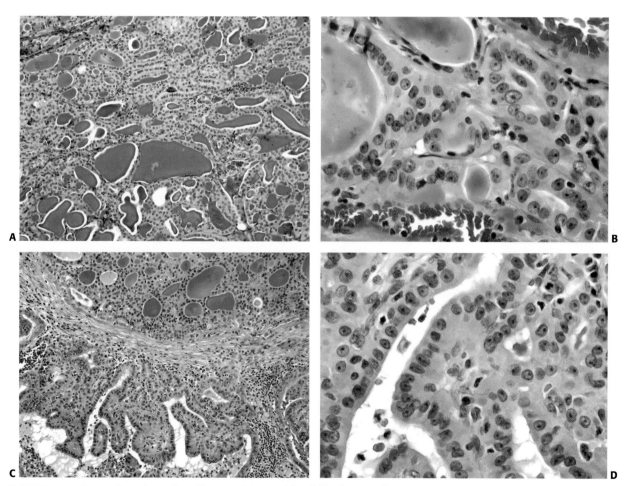

FIGURE 11.42. Oncocytic variant of papillary carcinoma with a follicular growth pattern. Follicular architecture is seen in the primary tumor nodule **(A, B)**, whereas a mixture of follicular and papillary growth was found in the lymph node metastasis **(C, D).**

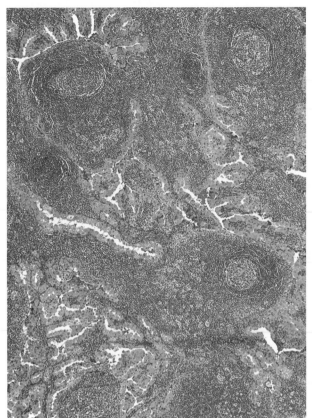 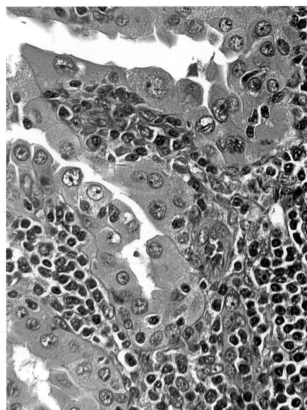

FIGURE 11.43. Warthin-like variant of papillary carcinoma.

plasma cells.[344] Germinal centers can be seen. The inflammatory infiltrate frequently spills into the adjacent thyroid parenchyma.

Most of these tumors are confined to the thyroid gland at presentation. Lymph node metastases may occur, although distant metastases are rare and prognosis is not different from conventional papillary carcinomas.[344,345] A single case of Warthin-like variant of papillary carcinoma with an area of dedifferentiation has been reported.[347]

Clear Cell Variant

This rare variant of papillary carcinoma is composed predominantly (>50%) of cells showing clear cytoplasm and nuclear features of papillary carcinoma (Fig. 11.44). This quality of cytoplasm can be due to the accumulation of glycogen, lipid, thyroglobulin, or distended mitochondria.[250] The nuclear features of papillary carcinoma are well developed. A papillary, follicular, or solid architecture can be seen. The tumors are composed entirely of clear cells or may contain small areas of cells with plain eosinophilic cytoplasm or granular cytoplasm of an oncocytic type. The cells retain thyroglobulin and TTF1 immunoreactivity, although thyroglobulin staining is frequently weak and patchy. In some cases, the cytoplasm is PAS positive and diastase sensitive, which reflects the accumulation of glycogen.[250] These tumors behave similarly to classic papillary carcinoma.[348]

The clear appearance of cytoplasm may mimic metastatic carcinomas, particularly from the kidney. These tumors should also be distinguished from clear cell medullary carcinoma and parathyroid tumors. The distinction relies on finding the nuclear features of papillary carcinoma and pertinent immunohistochemical studies.

Cribriform-Morular Variant

This distinct variant of papillary carcinoma was first described in patients with familial adenomatous polyposis (FAP).[349] It typically

presents with multiple, well-demarcated or encapsulated tumor nodules showing a mixture of cribriform, trabecular, solid, papillary, and follicular growth patterns and characteristic whorls or morules composed of spindle cells (Fig. 11.45). The morular cells show no evidence of keratinization. Prominent cribriform architecture and morules are the most distinct features of this variant, although in some tumors morules are not find. Microfollicular structures can be present, although colloid is rarely seen in the lumens. The cells have cuboidal or tall shape and may have oncocytic cytoplasm. Nuclear features of papillary carcinoma are found, although they may be well developed only focally. Some cells have nuclei with peculiar chromatin clearing probably due to the accumulation of biotin-like substances (Fig. 11.46), which is more often seen within morular structures.[350] Psammoma bodies are rare. The cells preserve strong immunoreactivity for cytokeratins and TTF1, and typically show only focal and weak staining for thyroglobulin. Lymph node metastases develop in 10% to 20% of patients, and survival is not different than in classic papillary carcinoma.[349,351]

This variant is rare and constitutes less than 0.5% of all papillary carcinomas.[352,353] It is invariably found in young women (mean age, 25 to 27 years), many of whom have clinical evidence of FAP and germline mutation in the adenomatous polyposis coli (*APC*) gene, which frequently affects exon 15.[354] However, this variant is also seen in patients with no FAP.[350] Those patients are typically also young females and although they do not carry a germline APC mutation, the tumors frequently reveal somatic mutation in the *APC* gene or in the *CTNNB1* gene coding for β-catenin.[355–357] *BRAF* mutations are not found.[358,359] In large series of patients with this variant of papillary carcinoma, approximately 40% of patients are found to have FAP, whereas the rest have no evidence of familial disease.[353,360] Patient age, tumor size, and microscopic tumor appearance cannot distinguish between familial and sporadic disease, although the presence of multiple

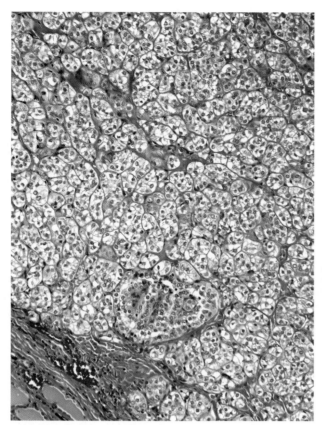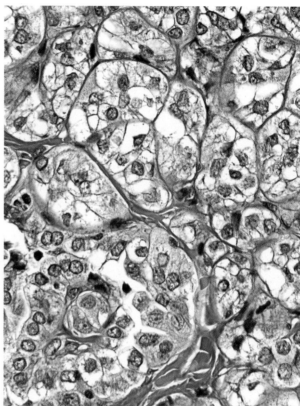

FIGURE 11.44. Clear cell variant of papillary carcinoma.

tumor nodules as opposed to a solitary nodule is a strong indicator of a familial disease.[353,360]

Both, inactivating mutation of the *APC* tumor suppressor gene and activating mutation of the *CTNNB1* gene, result in the prevention of cytoplasmic degradation of β-catenin, leading to its accumulation in the cytoplasm and translocation to the nucleus. This can be identified by immunohistochemistry, which demonstrates a change in β-catenin expression from the membranous pattern found in normal thyroid cells, to the cytoplasmic and nuclear staining in tumor cells (Fig. 11.47).[353,358,361] Although not entirely specific for this variant, the presence of aberrant β-catenin immunoreactivity provides strong evidence for the cribriform-morular variant of papillary carcinoma, particularly in a tumor with suspicious microscopic features.

As many patients with cribriform-morular variant have FAP and thyroid cancer can precede clinically detectable colonic abnormalities in 40% of patients,[360] recognizing this variant is important as it should raise the possibility of a familial disease and prompt colonic examination and possibly genetic testing for germline *APC* mutation.

Papillary Carcinoma with Prominent Hobnail Features

This recently described variant comprises approximately 0.2% of papillary carcinomas.[362] It is characterized by the predominance of cells with a hobnail appearance (Fig. 11.48). The tumors typically occur in older patients (mean age, 58 years) with female predominance typical of all papillary carcinomas.[362] The pattern of growth is usually papillary or papillary-follicular, with predominance of complex, micropapillary structures lined by cuboidal to more elongated cells with high nuclear:cytoplasmic ratio and apically placed nuclei with bulging of the apical surface that gives a hobnail appearance (Fig. 11.48). Characteristic nuclear features are present, although they may be less prominent as in classic papillary carcinoma. Mitotic

figures are common (≥3 per 10 HPFs) and atypical mitoses can be seen.[362] No necrosis is found. Psammoma bodies are occasionally seen. Extrathyroidal extension and wide vascular invasion are common. The tumor cells preserve immunoreactivity for thyroglobulin and TTF1, and typically show strong nuclear staining for TP53.[362,363] *BRAF* V600E mutation is found in more than half of these tumors, whereas *RET/PTC* rearrangement is typically absent.[362]

In the largest series reported to date,[362] this variant was defined based on the presence of at least 30% of cells with hobnail features. However, only one out of eight cases in this series had only 30% of cells with these features, whereas all other tumors had 50% to 100% cells with such an appearance.

This variant of papillary carcinoma appears to be associated with a more aggressive tumor behavior. In a series of eight cases reported by Asioli et al.,[362] five patients had metastases involving lung and typically other distant sites and four patients died of disease. Incidentally, the only tumor in this series that had only 30% of cells with hobnail features was diagnosed in a young patient (28-year old female) who had no metastases or other complications after 10 years of follow-up.

Papillary Carcinoma with Fasciitis-Like Stroma

This rare variant is characterized by the presence of abundant cellular stroma that resembles nodular fasciitis.[364] To date, less than 20 cases have been reported.[364–372] The stroma is composed of fascicles of spindle cells intermingled with epithelial islands of papillary carcinoma (Fig. 11.49). In addition to a cellular, fascicular growth, a more loose arrangement of spindle cells with myxoid matrix and areas of dense, keloid-like collagen may also be seen. Importantly, the elongated nuclei of the stromal cells are bland, with fine chromatin and small nucleoli. Mitotic figures are

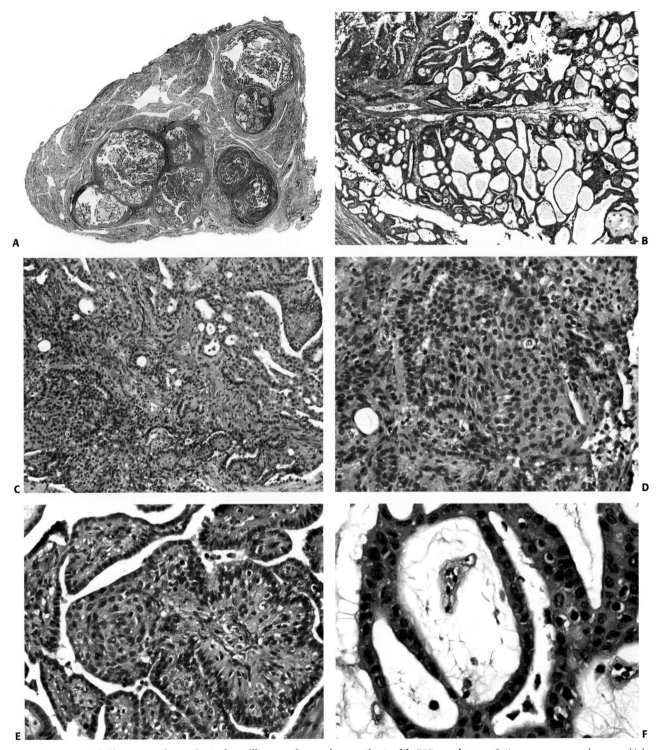

FIGURE 11.45. Cribriform-morular variant of papillary carcinoma in a patient with FAP syndrome. A: Low power scan shows multiple discrete and encapsulated tumor nodules in thyroid lobe. Cribriform **(B, F)**, solid **(C, D)** and papillary **(E)** architecture is seen as well as morular structures **(D, E)**. (Case courtesy of Dr. Vânia Nosé.)

rare. The spindle cells reveal immunoreactivity for vimentin and muscle-specific actin, consistent with myofibroblastic origin.[364,366] The proportion of the stromal component varies but should be significant, and microscopic areas entirely devoid of the epithelial elements must be seen in order to qualify for this variant.

The behavior of these tumors appears to be similar to classic papillary carcinoma, with about 25% of reported cases having lymph node metastases but no death from disease based on a limited follow-up in several reported cases.[367]

The importance of this variant is primarily two-fold. First, it should not be mistaken for a benign reactive fibrosis. This may occur when the papillary carcinoma component is not sufficiently sampled and the majority of the nodule is composed of stroma. Second, the presence of spindle cells adjacent to typical papillary carcinoma may be mistaken for tumor transformation into anaplastic thyroid carcinoma with a spindle cell pattern. The distinction is important as it leads to different therapeutic approaches and yields a sharply different prognosis. The separation relies on the lack of

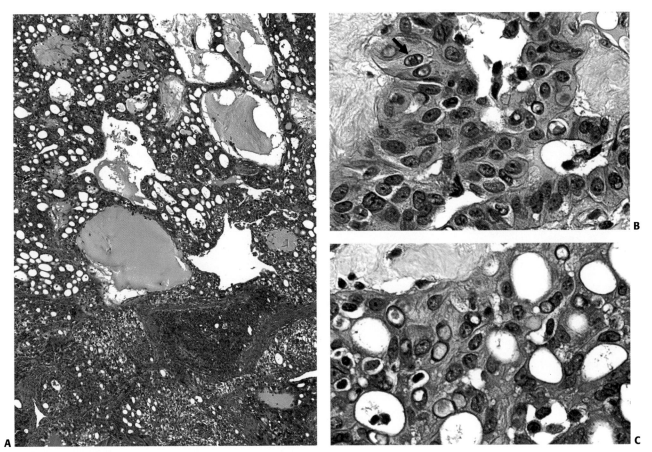

FIGURE 11.46. Cribriform-morular variant of papillary carcinoma. A: This case shows a mixture of cribriform and solid architecture. **B:** The tumor cells show some irregularity of nuclear contours and occasional nuclear grooves *(arrow)*, although nuclear features of papillary carcinoma are overall poorly developed. **C:** Focally, the tumor cell nuclei show homogeneous, light eosinophilic to clear appearance, which is different from classic optically clear nuclei of papillary carcinoma.

highly pleomorphic nuclei, high mitotic activity, and necrosis, which all are easily found in anaplastic carcinoma. Other fibroproliferative lesions can be excluded by finding the foci of papillary carcinoma.

Other variants of papillary carcinoma

Some papillary carcinomas with pure papillary growth or a mixture of a papillary and follicular architecture have a complete capsule. The papillae have well-developed fibrovascular stalks and show abundant nuclear features of papillary carcinoma. These distinguish encapsulated papillary carcinoma from follicular adenoma with papillary hyperplasia (see Chapter 8). These encapsulated papillary carcinomas show less frequent lymph node metastases, and their biologic behavior is even more indolent than those of typical, invasive papillary carcinoma, with rare distant metastases and no cancer-related deaths documented.[213,373–376]

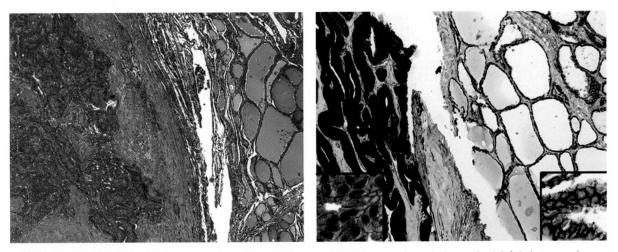

FIGURE 11.47. Cribriform-morular variant of papillary carcinoma. *(Left)* The tumor has a thick capsule. *(Right)* The tumor shows a characteristic cytoplasmic and nuclear pattern of β-catenin immunostaining, in contrast to a membranous pattern of staining seen in normal thyroid cells. In both panels, the tumor is on the left and normal thyroid on the right.

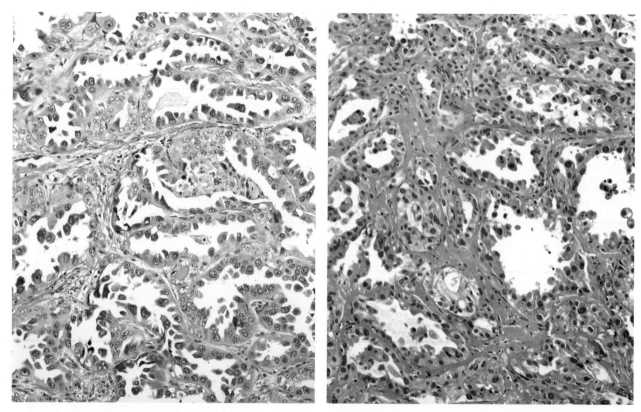

FIGURE 11.48. Papillary carcinoma with prominent hobnail features. *(Left)* The tumor shows a micropapillary architecture and dyscohesive cells with loss of polarity and large nuclei with distinct nucleoli. *(Right)* The tumor shows a more follicular growth pattern with occasional micropapillae. (Images cortesy of Dr. Ricardo V. Lloyd.)

Historically, some of these tumors were designated as "papillary adenoma," the term that is no longer in use and is misleading as these tumors are malignant.

Papillary carcinomas may contain small or larger amount of mature adipose tissue[377] (Fig. 11.50) or reveal mucin production,[378] which carries no diagnostic or prognostic significance.

The coexistence of papillary carcinoma with foci of poorly differentiated thyroid carcinoma, anaplastic (undifferentiated) carcinoma, or squamous cell carcinoma[256] does not represent a variant of papillary carcinoma, as a diagnosis of one of these more aggressive carcinomas has to be made in these cases. Information on the coexisting papillary carcinoma may be incorporated as an additional, secondary diagnostic line or be placed in the comment section of the diagnosis. Mixed medullary-papillary carcinomas of the thyroid are discussed in Chapter 14.

IMMUNOHISTOCHEMICAL FEATURES

The diagnosis of papillary carcinoma is typically made based on microscopic examination alone. However, some cases may benefit from immunohistochemical studies, which are typically performed either (1) to establish the follicular cell origin of metastases and thyroid tumors with unusual appearance or (2) to assist the diagnosis of malignancy.

Markers of thyroid follicular cells

Thyroglobulin is produced exclusively by thyroid follicular cells and is therefore the most specific marker for thyroid follicular cell origin. The reactivity is seen in the luminal colloid and cell cytoplasm and is typically diffuse, although it may be more focal and of moderate to weak intensity in tumors with no obvious colloid accumulation (Fig. 11.51 A,B). TTF1, a nuclear transcription factor, shows strong and diffuse nuclear reactivity in virtually all cases (Fig. 11.51 C). The nuclear pattern and strong intensity of staining makes it a robust and reliable diagnostic marker, although TTF1 is not specific for thyroid follicular cells and also stains lung tumors, small cell carcinomas from different locations, medullary thyroid carcinoma, and tumors of the diencephalon.[379,380]

Two other thyroid transcription factors, PAX8 (Fig. 11.51 D) and TTF2, show strong diffuse nuclear reactivity in papillary carcinoma and may also be used to support the follicular cell origin.[381] PAX8 immunoreactivity has been well characterized, showing strong uniform staining in thyroid follicular cells and exceedingly rare weak reactivity in lung carcinomas.[381-383] However, PAX8 expression is not specific for thyroid follicular cells and is also seen in tumors of kidney, ovary, and endometrium, lymphoid cells, and in about half of medullary thyroid carcinomas.[381-384]

A pattern of reactivity for cytokeratins in papillary carcinomas is identical to those seen in normal thyroid cells. They are positive for CK7, CAM 5.2, and AE1/AE3, and negative for CK20.[385,386] Immunoreactivity for vimentin is almost always present. Important negative markers are calcitonin, CEA, and neuroendocrine markers.

Diagnostic Immunohistochemical Markers

Several immunostains can be used to aid the differential diagnosis between papillary carcinoma and benign thyroid lesions. Among those, most experience has been accumulated for galectin-3, HBME-1, CK19, and CITED1 antibodies.

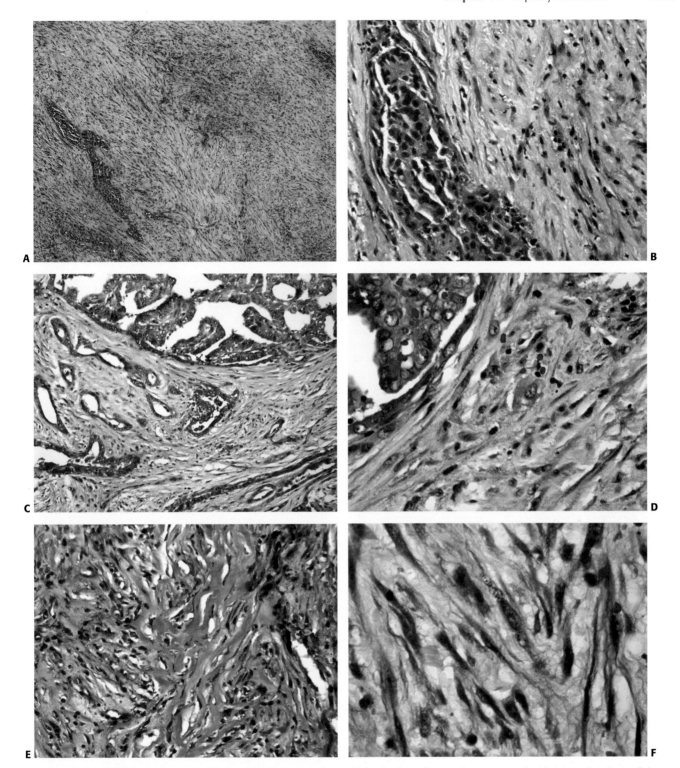

FIGURE 11.49. Papillary carcinoma with fasciitis-like stroma. Small islands of papillary carcinoma are embedded into abundant cellular stroma **(A–E)**. In some areas of the tumor, the stroma is dense, kelloid-like **(E)**, and in other areas it is loose, nodular fasciitis like **(F)**. The spindle cells of the stroma are bland. (Case courtesy of Dr. Ricardo V. Lloyd.)

Galectin-3, a β-galactoside-binding lectin that regulates cell adhesion and other cell functions, is detected by immunohistochemistry in most papillary carcinomas but not in nonneoplastic thyroid cells.[387] Importantly, the protein is expressed in the nucleus and cytoplasm and therefore a positive result should include staining in both of these cell compartments (Fig. 11.52). Cytoplasmic staining only, frequently coarsely granular, is common

in cells with oncocytic cytoplasm and should be disregarded (Fig. 11.53 A). Positive staining is found in almost all classic papillary carcinomas (Table 11.7). In the follicular variant, the frequency of staining is lower, and it is usually focal and of moderate to weak intensity (Fig. 11.52 C,D). Galectin-3 immunoreactivity is not restricted to papillary carcinoma and is also seen in follicular thyroid carcinoma as well as in 6% to 30% of follicular

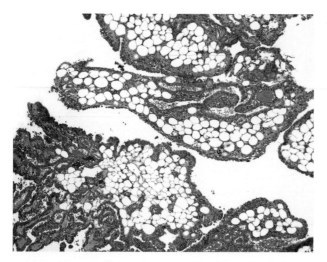

FIGURE 11.50. Papillary carcinoma with abundant adipose tissue in the stroma.

adenomas.[388–391] Areas of Hashimoto thyroiditis may also show focal reactivity, typically restricted to epithelial cells in the areas of dense lymphocytic infiltration (Fig. 11.53 B). Strong staining

is seen in macrophages within the follicular lumens or germinal centers and in some endothelial cells (Fig. 11.53 C-E).

HBME-1 antibody has been generated against the microvillous surface of mesothelial cells,[392] although a specific antigen is not known. Reactivity is seen along the cell membranes with accentuation at the apical surface (Fig. 11.54). Staining of the cytoplasm and luminal colloid should not be scored as positive. HBME-1 immunoreactivity is found in almost all classic papillary carcinomas[393,394] and with lower frequency in the follicular variant (Table 11.7). The staining has higher specificity as compared with galectin-3, as it is seen in a smaller fraction of benign nodules. HBME-1 is more specific than galectin-3 and CK19 in distinction between papillary carcinoma and benign papillary hyperplasia.[395]

Overexpression of CITED1, a nuclear protein that participates in the regulation of transcription, was first found in papillary carcinomas by cDNA expression array and then by immunohistochemistry.[193,391] The staining should be seen in the nucleus and cytoplasm (Fig. 11.55), as the reactivity limited to the cytoplasm is nonspecific. This stain is less sensitive and is typically found in approximately two-thirds of classic papillary carcinomas and in half of the follicular variants (Table 11.7). In our experience, it is a valuable addition to a diagnostic panel as it occasionally highlights papillary carcinomas that are negative for galectin-3 and HBME-1.

Keratin CK19 has a cytoplasmic and membranous distribution and has been considered as a helpful marker of thyroid

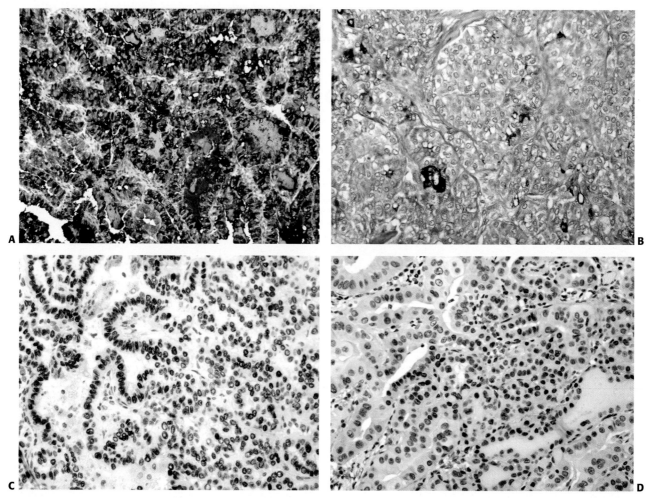

FIGURE 11.51. Immunohistochemical features of papillary carcinoma. A: Strong and diffuse thyroglobulin staining in classic papillary carcinoma. **B:** Thyroglobulin staining is focal in the solid variant of papillary carcinoma. **C:** Diffuse nuclear reactivity for TTF1. **D:** Diffuse nuclear reactivity for PAX8.

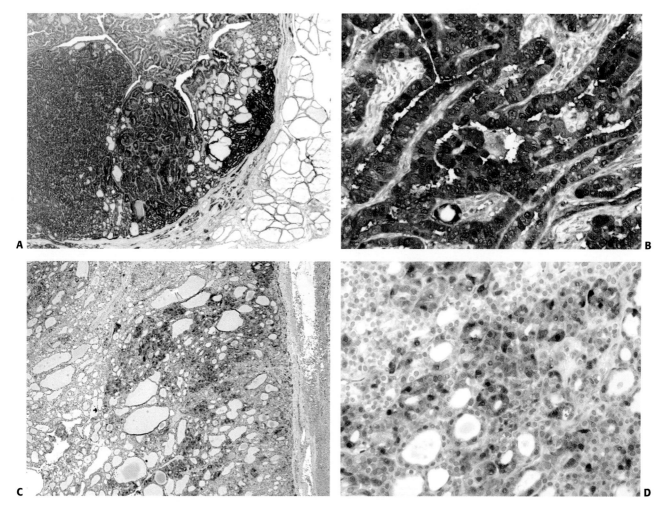

FIGURE 11.52. Immunostaining of papillary carcinoma for galectin-3. A, B: Diffuse and strong staining, both cytoplasmic and nuclear, in classic papillary carcinoma. **C, D:** The staining of the follicular variant of papillary carcinoma is more focal and of less intensity.

malignancy.[396] Although the overexpression of this gene in thyroid tumors has been confirmed using molecular techniques, the immunostaining has low specificity.[397] In addition to frequent immunoreactivity in follicular adenomas, 10% to 50% of normal thyroid tissues and hyperplastic nodules are also positive for CK19.[388,391,398,399] Paradoxically, in some cases we have observed a reverse pattern of reactivity for CK19, that is, positive staining of normal thyroid tissue and negative staining of tumor.

These immunostains can be used in isolation or as a panel, and their performance characteristics should be defined in each individual laboratory. Some investigators find a relatively low specificity of individual antibodies but high specificity and sensitivity of papillary carcinoma detection when a combination of antibodies is used, such as galectin-3/HBME-1/CK19.[389,391,399] Our panel for diagnostically challenging cases includes HBME-1, galectin-3, and CITED1, and we find one or two of these stains positive in <10% of follicular adenomas. We consider the presence of strong diffuse immunoreactivity for more than one of these antibodies (Fig. 11.56) as compelling evidence for carcinoma, and strong diffuse reactivity for one of these antibodies (particularly HBME-1) or focal reactivity for two or more antibodies as a substantial evidence for malignancy. Importantly, in our experience[400] and as reported by others,[394] virtually 100% of metastatic papillary carcinomas, irrespective of the tumor variant, show strong and diffuse immunoreactivity for galectin-3 and HBME-1.

RET immunostain using antibodies against the C-terminal domain (only C terminus of the RET protein is expressed as a result

of *RET/PTC* rearrangement) has been explored as a surrogate marker of a *RET/PTC* rearrangement. In our experience, staining using the existing commercial antibodies has low correlation with the presence of *RET/PTC* and is not helpful diagnostically.

Proliferative index detected by Ki-67 immunostaining in papillary carcinomas[388,401] is typically less than 5%. Most papillary carcinomas reveal no TP53 staining.

Other immunohistochemical markers that have been explored for the diagnosis of papillary carcinoma include TPO, fibronectin-1, S100A4, cyclin D1, and p27, among others.[402] Although many of these proteins have altered expression in papillary carcinoma, the diagnostic usefulness of these antibodies has not been well established.

 # MOLECULAR DIAGNOSTICS

Several mutational markers may assist the diagnosis of papillary carcinoma. Their potential use in surgical samples is discussed below, whereas the role of mutational markers in the diagnosis of papillary carcinoma and other types of thyroid cancer in thyroid FNA samples is discussed in Chapter 21.

BRAF

BRAF mutation is a reliable marker of papillary carcinoma or associated malignancy. The V600E *BRAF* mutation, which constitutes

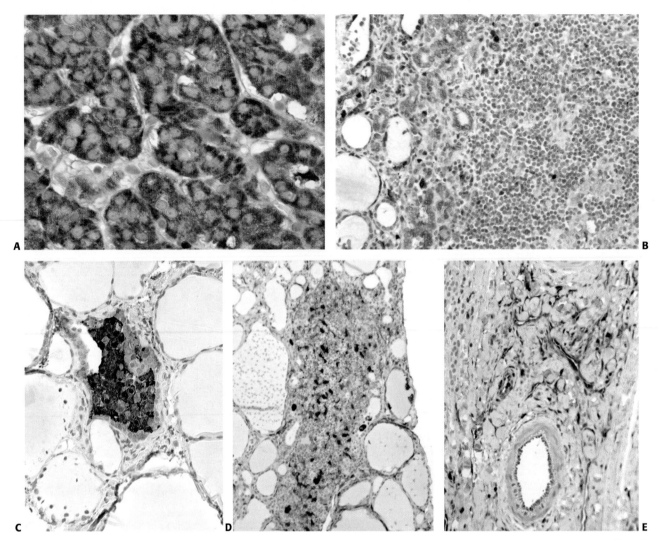

FIGURE 11.53. Challenges and pitfalls in interpreting galectin-3 immunostaining. A: Non-specific cytoplasmic reactivity in oncocytic cells of follicular adenoma. **B:** Positive staining in scattered epithelial cells in Hashimoto thyroiditis. Positive staining is also seen in macrophages located within thyroid follicles **(C)** and in germinal centers **(D)**, and in reactive endothelial cells **(E).**

the vast majority of all *BRAF* alterations detected in the thyroid, is found in approximately 45% of papillary carcinomas and with lower frequency in poorly differentiated and anaplastic carcinomas arising from papillary carcinoma.[110,114,121,126,403] This mutation has not been found in any of the over 500 benign thyroid tumors studied by various groups,[122] and therefore V600E *BRAF* detection is virtually diagnostic for malignancy. Most tumors carrying this mutation are classic papillary carcinomas and tall cell variants. Those tumors rarely pose diagnostic difficulty in the surgical material. However, 10% to 15% of tumors with this mutation belong to the follicular variant,[121,122,282] where the diagnosis may not be straightforward by microscopy (Fig. 11.57). Moreover, testing for this mutation may be needed for better risk stratification and postsurgical management of patients with papillary carcinoma. As discussed later in the chapter, *BRAF* V600E is associated with higher probability of tumor recurrence[240,404–406] and tumor-related mortality.[407,408]

Table 11.7

Frequency of Positive Immunostaining in Papillary Carcinoma and Other Thyroid Lesions[a]

	Galectin-3 (%)	HBME-1 (%)	CITED1 (%)	CK19 (%)
Papillary carcinoma, classic papillary	95–100	90–100	50–90	95–100
Papillary carcinoma, follicular variant	65–100	65–100	45–80	90–100
Follicular carcinoma	50–90	40–90	15–20	40–70
Follicular adenoma	5–35	5–20	5–15	5–45
Normal thyroid/hyperplastic nodule	0–1	0–1	0	5–40

[a]Based on the reports by Nakamura et al,[388] Scognamiglio et al,[389] Saggiorato et al,[390] Prasad et al,[391] Barut et al.,[399] and our own experience.

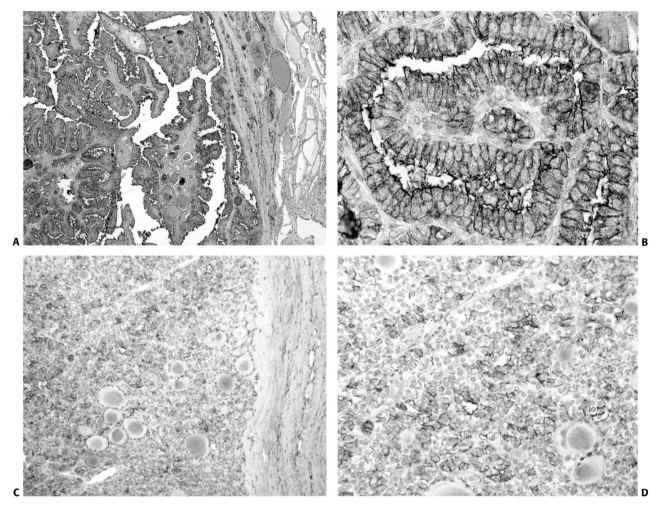

FIGURE 11.54. Immunostaining of papillary carcinoma for HBME-1. A, B: Classic papillary carcinoma. **C, D:** Follicular variant of papillary carcinoma.

Another *BRAF* mutation, K601E, has been reported with low frequency (1%) in papillary carcinomas and in a single case of follicular adenoma.[409] Most papillary carcinomas carrying K601E mutation are of the follicular variant.[115,118,119] In our experience with 15 *BRAF* K601E-positive thyroid nodules, all were papillary carcinomas, either the follicular variant (14) or solid variant (1). were papillary carcinomas, either the follicular variant (14) or solid variant (1). Other mutations in *BRAF*, including small insertions or deletions surrounding codon 600,[115–117,410] and chromosomal rearrangements resulting in *BRAF* fusion to other genes[37] are very rare and appear to be specific for papillary carcinoma.

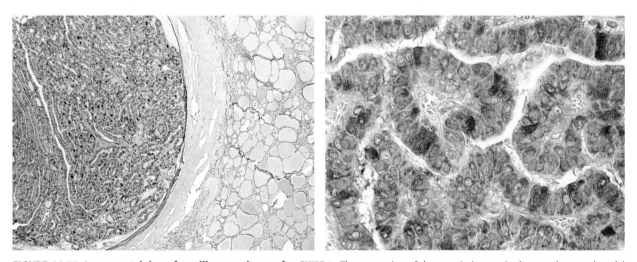

FIGURE 11.55. Immunostaining of papillary carcinoma for CITED1. The expression of the protein is seen in the cytoplasm and nuclei of the tumor cells.

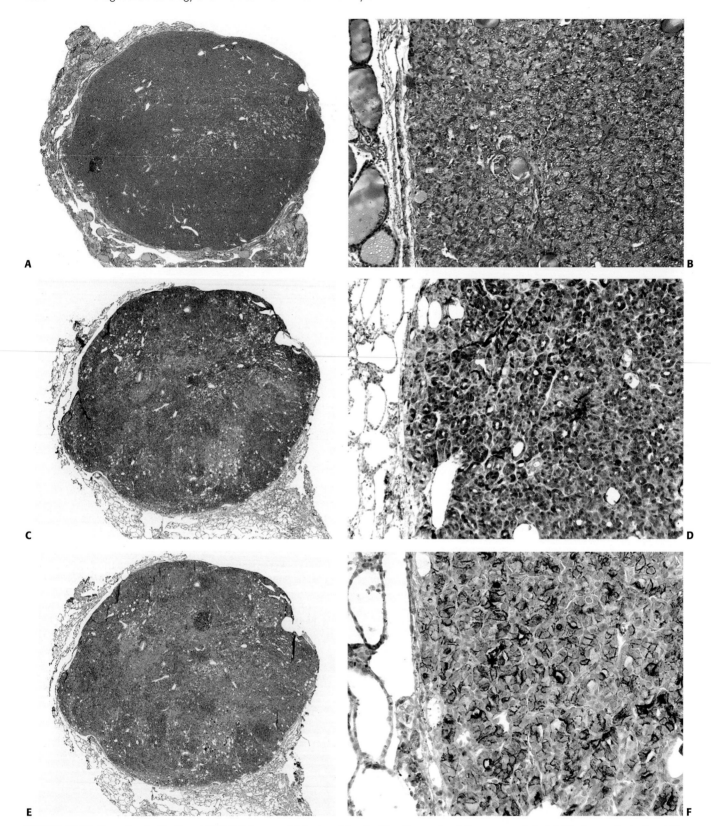

FIGURE 11.56. Use of galectin-3 and HBME-1 immunohistochemistry for the diagnosis of the encapsulated follicular variant of papillary carcinoma. This encapsulated tumor shows diffuse but moderately expressed nuclear features of papillary carcinoma **(A, B).** Immunostained sections show diffuse and strong reactivity for galectin-3 **(C, D)** and HBME-1 **(E, F)**, strongly supporting the diagnosis.

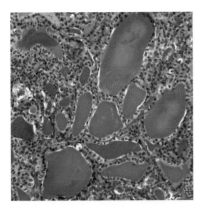
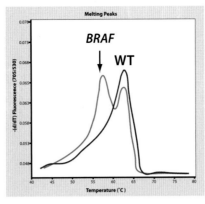
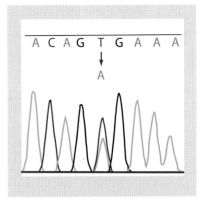

FIGURE 11.57. Use of mutational analysis to assist the diagnosis of papillary carcinoma. This follicular variant papillary carcinoma had moderately developed nuclei features of papillary carcinoma **(left)**, but was found positive for *BRAF* mutation by LightCycler PCR and fluorescence melting curve analysis **(middle)** and confirmed to have a V600E mutation by sequencing **(right)**, confirming the diagnosis.

RET/PTC

RET/PTC rearrangement can serve as another diagnostic marker of papillary carcinoma. However, the detection of this alteration is more difficult, and the interpretation of the results is confounded by the fact that distribution of *RET/PTC* rearrangement within the tumor may be quite heterogeneous and vary from involving a significant proportion of tumor cells (clonal *RET/PTC*) to being detected only in single or few tumor cells (nonclonal *RET/PTC*).[147,149] This circumstance, coupled with a significant geographic variability in the prevalence of *RET/PTC*, accounts for high variability in the reported frequency of *RET/PTC* in papillary carcinomas and in the reported specificity of *RET/PTC* detection.[146,148] Whereas many studies have found *RET/PTC* restricted to papillary carcinomas,[151,159,411,412] other studies using highly sensitive detection techniques have detected this rearrangement in many adenomas and even in nonneoplastic thyroid lesions.[63,413–415]

In practical terms, it can be assumed that clonal *RET/PTC*, which is found in more than 1% of cells within the tumor by a reliable diagnostic method, is generally specific for papillary carcinoma (Table 11.8). The choice of the detection method for *RET/PTC* is dictated by the type of sample available (see also Chapter 20). In snap-frozen or freshly collected tumor samples, the testing can be reliably performed by reverse transcriptase PCR (RT-PCR) in a conventional or real-time mode (Fig. 11.58).[416] The sensitivity of *RET/PTC* detection should remain above 1% of tumor cells (i.e., should not detect the rearrangement present in less than 1% of cells tested) to avoid detecting a nonclonal rearrangement, which has no diagnostic implications. When formalin-fixed and

paraffin-embedded tissue is available for testing, FISH is the assay of choice (Fig. 11.58, right panel) The FISH assay should be validated to have an appropriate cut-off level, which generally should be no less than 7% of cells with the rearrangement pattern.[150,417] The test should be able to detect two most common types of *RET/PTC*, which are *RET/PTC1* and *RET/PTC3*.

Testing for *RET/PTC* rearrangements can be diagnostically helpful, as detection of a clonal *RET/PTC* rearrangement using a clinically validated method is virtually diagnostic for papillary carcinoma. In surgical material, however, the diagnostic utility of *RET/PTC* is relatively limited because most tumors carrying this mutation are classic papillary carcinomas or tumors of the diffuse sclerosing variant,[113] and their histologic diagnosis is rarely problematic.

RAS

RAS mutations are not restricted to papillary carcinoma and also found in other malignant and benign thyroid neoplasms. In thyroid tumors, *NRAS* codon 61 and *HRAS* codon 61 mutations are most common and testing for these two hot spots may be sufficient to detect the majority of *RAS* mutations. Among papillary carcinomas, these mutations are found almost exclusively in the follicular variant (Fig. 11.59); the frequency of *RAS* mutation is about 45% in this tumor variant.[160,418] In addition, about 45% of conventional type follicular carcinomas and 30% of conventional type follicular adenomas carry this mutation. Some studies have reported *RAS* mutations in hyperplastic nodules, although these lesions by virtue of carrying a clonal mutation are tumors and

Table 11.8		
Clinical Significance of *RET/PTC* Rearrangement Based on the Level of Detection		
	Clonal *RET/PTC* (Found in >1% of tumor cells)	Non-clonal *RET/PTC* (Found in <1% of tumor cells)
Detection techniques	• Standard RT-PCR • FISH with appropriate cut-off levels • Southern blot analysis	Ultra-sensitive RT-PCR (nested PCR with two rounds of amplification)
Prevalence in thyroid papillary carcinomas	10–20%*	>40%
Specificity	Specific for papillary carcinoma	Non-specific finding in various thyroid lesions
Suitability for clinical diagnostic use	Yes	No

*The prevalence is higher in pediatric populations and in papillary carcinomas associated with exposure to ionizing radiation.

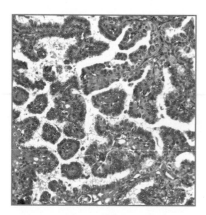
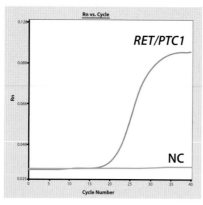
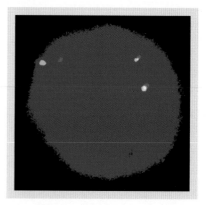

FIGURE 11.58. Detection of *RET/PTC* rearrangement. This case of classic papillary carcinoma *(left)* was positive for *RET/PTC1* rearrangement detected by LightCycler PCR amplification *(middle)* and by FISH using probes corresponding to the RET (green color) and H4 (red color) genes *(right)*.

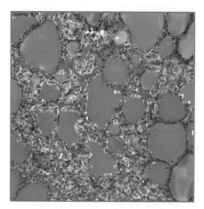
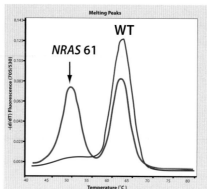
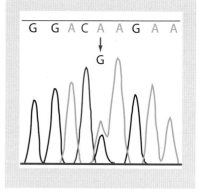

FIGURE 11.59. Detection of *RAS* mutation. This case of the follicular variant of papillary carcinoma *(left)* was positive for *NRAS* codon 61 mutation by LightCycler PCR and fluorescence melting curve analysis *(middle)* and confirmed to have a CAA CGA (Q61R) mutation by sequencing *(right)*.

therefore should be designated as follicular adenomas. Overall, the detection of *RAS* mutation indicates the presence of a tumor, although it does not establish the diagnosis of malignancy.

Other Potential Diagnostic Markers

TRK rearrangements, which involve the *NTRK1* gene, are found in less than 5% of papillary carcinomas,[174,175] although some studies from Italy and Germany have found this rearrangement in 10% to 15% of papillary carcinomas.[167,176,177] At least three fusion types exist. The diagnostic utility of testing for *TRK* rearrangement has not been widely explored.

Expression of various miRNAs appears to differ between papillary carcinomas and benign thyroid lesions and potentially may be used diagnostically in surgical and FNA samples.[198–200,203] Highly overexpressed miRNAs have been identified, such as miRNA-221 and miRNA-222, and more extensive validation of these and other miRNAs is needed to determine their specificity as a diagnostic marker of papillary carcinoma.

A large number of genes with altered expression in papillary carcinomas have been detected using array-type techniques, and some of them may be of potential diagnostic use.[191,193,194] Some of the markers, such as HMGA2 and IMP3, have been further validated by RT-PCR,[419,420] although their diagnostic use at this time is limited.

 ULTRASTRUCTURAL FEATURES

Ultrastructurally, papillary carcinoma cells show cuboidal, columnar, or polygonal shape, are linked by desmosomes and tight junctions, and rest on a basal lamina that is often irregular and multilayered (Fig. 11.60).[222,421,422] Numerous microvilli and single cilia are present at the apical pole of most cells. The most characteristic finding is marked irregularity of nuclear membrane with numerous folds and indentations. Some nuclei are divided by indentations into lobules connected with each other only by thin channels of the nuclear substance. Single deep invaginations give rise to nuclear grooves seen on light microscopy. Nuclear pseudoinclusions are formed by invaginations that have a more round shape and contain significant amount of the cytoplasm. They are surrounded by a rim of nuclear membrane and often contain recognizable cytoplasmic organelles. Connection to the main body of cell cytoplasm may be seen. Most nuclei have finely dispersed chromatin with condensation along the nuclear membrane. Nucleoli are frequently seen. Some nuclei contain true nuclear inclusions or nuclear bodies.[222,423,424] They appear as spherules containing dense homogeneous, granular, or fibrillar material or a combination of those and are sometimes surrounded by a clear halo (Fig. 11.61). At least some of these inclusions are made of ribonucleoproteins, and they may be derived from nucleoli.[424,425]

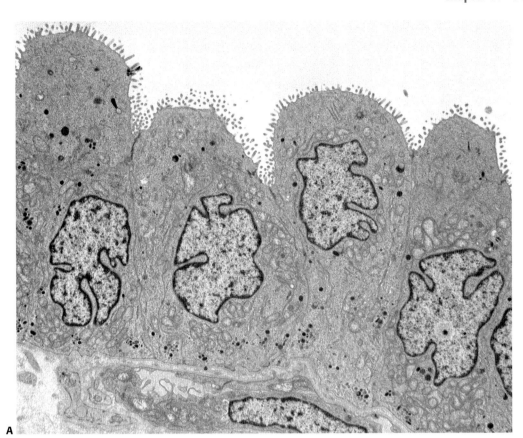

A

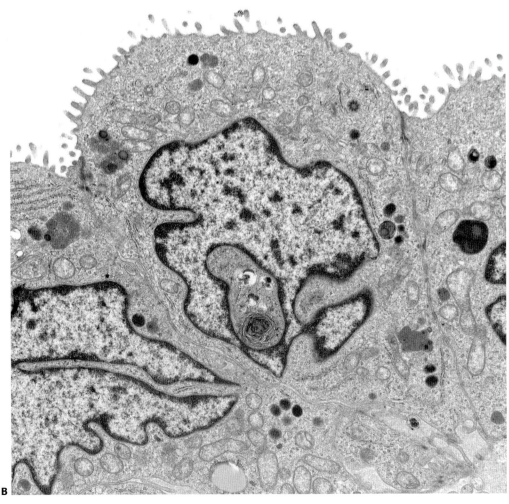

B

FIGURE 11.60. Ultrastructural features of papillary carcinoma. A: Cells rest on a continuous basal lamina that separates them from a capillary vessel. The nuclei show highly irregular contours with condensation of heterochromatin among the nuclear membrane. Microvilli are seen on the apical surface. **B:** Cell in the center of the field contains a nuclear pseudoinclusion and one to the left shows a nuclear groove. Both of these intranuclear structures are rimmed by a nuclear membrane and contain cytoplasmic organelles.

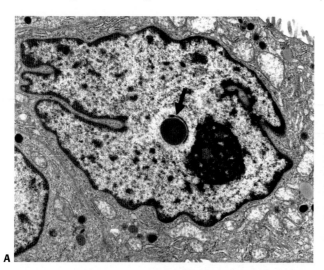
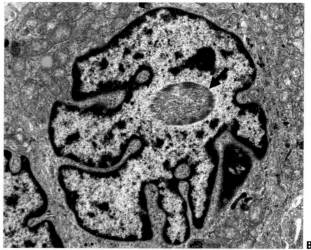

FIGURE 11.61. Nuclear inclusions seen in papillary carcinoma cells by electron microscopy. A: This inclusion has a dense homogeneous core surrounded by a zone of chromatin clearing. The nucleolus in located in the vicinity. **B:** This true nuclear inclusion has a granular and filamentous core.

The cytoplasm contains usual organelles, including well-developed granular endoplasmic reticulum, mitochondria, and Golgi complex. The mitochondria are particularly abundant in the oncocytic variant of papillary carcinoma. Dense exocytotic vesicles and large phagolysosomal bodies are often seen.

Psammoma bodies can be found within the stroma of papillary stalks or within lymphatic vessels, and electron microscopy further highlights the concentric layers of mineralization (Fig. 11.62). Psammoma bodies may reveal an amorphous, granular core or contain electron-dense crystals in the core. In some psammoma bodies, the layers of calcium deposition may be seen centered around a necrotic cell.[230]

 # CYTOLOGIC FEATURES

The cytologic diagnosis of papillary carcinoma primarily rests on nuclear features. Overall, FNA cytology is very useful in identifying patients who are at risk for papillary carcinoma. When the diagnostic cytologic features are present, the test is highly specific. However, the aspirated material may not show all the features, and some papillary carcinomas, especially the follicular variant, may demonstrate overlapping features with other thyroid lesions.

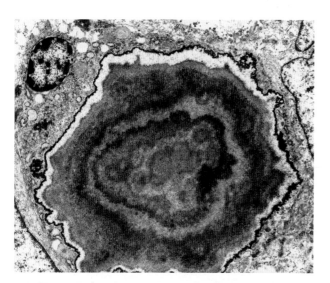

FIGURE 11.62. Ultramicroscopic image of a psammoma body showing concentric layers of mineralization.

The aspirate of conventional papillary carcinoma is cellular with a relatively small amount of thick ("bubble gum") colloid. In occasional cases, psammoma bodies and multinucleated histiocytic giant cells are identified. The aspirated neoplastic cell population is arranged in round clusters, sheets, microfollicles, or papillary structures. In contrast to benign thyroid follicular cells that demonstrate a honeycomb pattern with evenly spaced round uniform nuclei, papillary carcinoma cells show nuclear enlargement, loss of organization, and crowding. The individual neoplastic cells are cuboidal, columnar, polygonal, oval, or round. Some cells demonstrate "squamoid" type of dense cytoplasm. Most of the nuclei of the neoplastic cells are enlarged and oval. The chromatin pattern is "powdery" and nucleoli tend to be small and eccentrically placed. In contrast to histologic preparations, cytologic specimens do not show nuclear clearing. The hallmark cytologic features are nuclear membrane irregularities, nuclear grooves, and intranuclear pseudoinclusions, although they may be present only focally (Fig. 11.63).[426,427] In the absence of nuclear pseudoinclusions, the presence of nuclear grooves in >20% of neoplastic cells is highly suggestive of papillary carcinoma.[428,429] Cases with fewer percentage of nuclear grooves lack specificity and one should include other benign lesions in the differential diagnosis.

It is important to distinguish the true nuclear features of papillary carcinoma from nonspecific artifacts. For example, the nuclear grooves should be oriented along the longitudinal axis of the elongated nuclei, and the intranuclear pseudoinclusions should appear "punched out" with a rim of dense chromatin at the outer edge of the pseudoinclusion.

The current Bethesda System for Reporting Thyroid Cytopathology (BSRTC) recognizes six diagnostic categories of reporting thyroid FNA samples (Table 11.9).[430,431] Using this reporting system, most papillary carcinomas, particularly those of classic papillary type, are reported as "malignant" or "suspicious for malignancy." The risk of malignancy for cases diagnosed as "malignant" is 97% to 99% (Table 11.10).[430,431] The rare false positive cases are due to benign processes that show exuberant reactive changes resulting in nuclear features overlapping with those of papillary carcinoma. The types of lesions mimicking papillary carcinoma include chronic lymphocytic (Hashimoto) thyroiditis with oncocytic metaplasia, Graves disease, and dyshormonogenetic goiter. Some tumors, particularly follicular variants, may be reported as "atypia of undetermined significance"/"follicular lesion of undetermined significance" or "follicular neoplasm"/"suspicious for follicular neoplasm" based on BSRTC.

FNA of the variants of papillary carcinoma may yield features that deviate from the classic papillary carcinoma. The follicular variant typically reveals a cellular population of epithelial cells

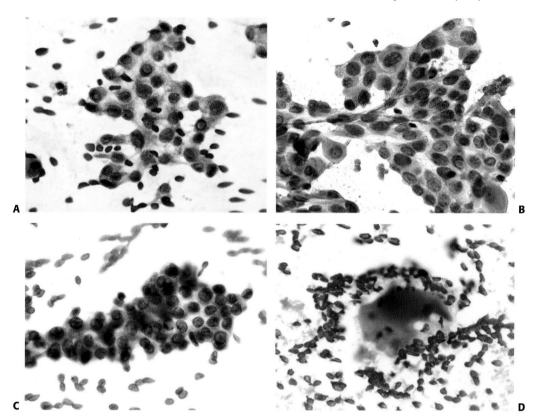

FIGURE 11.63. Cytologic features of classic papillary carcinoma. A: The diagnostic areas of conventional papillary carcinoma of thyroid show nuclear grooves and intranuclear pseudoinclusions (Papanicolaou stain). **B:** Papillary cluster showing cells with nuclear enlargement, disorganization, crowding, contour irregularities, and pseudoinclusions (Papanicolaou stain). **C:** Well-developed intranuclear pseudoinclusions and nuclear membrane irregularities are present in this papillary cluster (Papanicolaou stain). **D:** Dense, thick colloid is often seen in association with papillary carcinoma (Papanicolaou stain).

arranged in sheets and small microfollicles. There is general agreement that microfollicles are circular structures composed of <15 cells.[432] Colloid, when present, tends to be dense and not abundant. The architectural features of the follicular variant overlap with other entities such as follicular adenoma, follicular carcinoma, and hyperplastic nodule. Approximately one-third of the cases of follicular variant show sufficient nuclear features of papillary carcinoma, allowing the prospective diagnosis using FNA cytology (Fig. 11.64 A).[433–435] The remaining cases are given indeterminate diagnoses (follicular neoplasm, atypia of undetermined significance, or suspicious) (Fig. 11.64 B). The inability to render a definitive diagnosis is often due to the incomplete manifestation of architectural and nuclear features of the typical papillary carcinoma (papillary fragments, nuclear grooves, intranuclear pseudoinclusions, and powdery chromatin). Papillary carcinoma with predominance of follicular pattern and a minor or absent papillary architectural component often yields cytologic material with relatively bland nuclear features. The nuclei of these follicular variants are frequently round. Nuclear grooves and nuclear membrane irregularities are subtle, and intranuclear pseudoinclusions are often lacking. When the typical cytologic features of papillary carcinoma are not present, the most sensitive finding may be the presence of syncytial clusters of epithelial cells with nuclear enlargement, elevation of nuclear-cytoplasmic ratio, crowding, and absence of the honeycomb pattern of benign colloid nodules. These syncytial clusters, however, are not specific for the follicular variant of papillary carcinoma and may be encountered in other follicular lesions such as follicular adenoma, follicular carcinoma, and cellular hyperplastic nodules.

The macrofollicular subtype of the follicular variant shows a predominance of large follicles and abundant colloid. Fine needle aspirates yield relatively hypocellular specimens with watery colloid and epithelial cells with variable cytologic appearance. Aspirates from large neoplastic follicles yield flat sheets, and the nuclear changes may be subtle. Features of papillary carcinoma are often only focally present and therefore, these tumors represent a relatively common source of false negative cytology diagnoses.[301]

Cytologic preparation from a typical case of tall cell variant demonstrates elongated, tall cells with abundant cytoplasm, distinct cell borders, "soap-bubble"-like intranuclear pseudoinclusions, and intraepithelial neutrophils.[436,437] The tall appearance in cytology preparations may not be appreciated when the neoplastic cells are not oriented properly in a cell cluster (Fig. 11.65).

The oncocytic (Hürthle cell) variant is characterized by cellular specimens with sheets and papillary clusters of large round to slightly oval cells with abundant granular cytoplasm in a background showing a variable amount of thick and thin colloid. The nuclear features are those of papillary carcinoma—the nuclei are round to oval with nuclear grooves and pseudoinclusions. Prominent nucleoli are rarely seen. The absence of nucleoli and presence of colloid are helpful in distinguishing the oncocytic variant papillary carcinoma from oncocytic adenoma or carcinoma.[438]

FNA of diffuse sclerosing variant of papillary carcinoma demonstrates neoplastic cells with the typical nuclear features of papillary carcinoma. However, this variant also shows some unusual features. Numerous psammoma bodies, metaplastic squamous cells, lymphocytes, and multinucleated giant cells are typically found, and the metaplastic squamous cells may occasionally show marked atypia.[439,440] In the absence of the diagnostic papillary carcinoma cells, the presence of numerous psammoma bodies, lymphocytes, and metaplastic squamous cells is highly suggestive of the diffuse sclerosing variant.

Cytologic samples of the columnar cell variant are typically cellular and composed of monolayer sheets and syncytial aggregates

Table 11.9

Bethesda System for Reporting Thyroid Cytopathology: Diagnostic Categories, Cytologic Features, and Estimated Incidence of Each Category

Diagnostic Category[a]	Cytologic Features[a]	Estimated Incidence (%)[b]
Unsatisfactory/nondiagnostic	• Hypocellular • Poor fixation/preservation	5–24

Benign	Sparse to moderately cellular specimen with:
	  • follicular cells
	  • oncocytic (Hürthle) cells
	  • macrophages
	  • lymphocytes
	  • colloid
		54–77

Atypia of undetermined significance/follicular lesion of undetermined significance (AUS/FLUS)	Heterogeneous group with:
	  • focal architectural or cytologic (nuclear) atypia
	  • not sufficient for the other categories below
	Contributing factors:
	  • well-differentiated nature of the neoplasm
	  • compromised nature of specimens
		3–18

Follicular neoplasm/suspicious for follicular neoplasm (FN/SFN)	• Cellular specimen with microfollicular groups • Subtle atypical features (e.g., nuclear membrane irregularities) may be present	1.5–10
Suspicious for malignant cells	• Sparse sampling of highly atypical cells • Cellular sample with most but not all malignant criteria fulfilled	2–4
Malignant	• Fulfills criteria for malignant neoplasm (most commonly papillary carcinoma)	2–7

[a]As reported in refs.[430,431].
[b]As reported in refs.[488–493].

of neoplastic cells. The nuclei tend to be elongated, stratified, crowded, and hyperchromatic. Nuclear grooves and intranuclear pseudoinclusions are rare or absent.[441,442] Given the lack of the typical cytologic features of papillary carcinoma, a precise prospective FNA diagnosis may be difficult.

As noted above, several thyroid lesions have the potential of mimicking papillary carcinoma in the aspiration material. Graves disease and its treatment with radioactive iodine can produce significant nuclear atypia causing concern for neoplasia, especially

papillary carcinoma.[443–445] Striking changes including nuclear enlargement, anisonucleosis, hyperchromasia, and cytoplasmic enlargement and vacuolization may be encountered. However, they tend to be randomly distributed, and the typical nuclear features of papillary carcinoma are not well developed. Similarly, dyshormonogenetic goiter can produce cellular cytologic specimens with microfollicular pattern of epithelial cells with round to oval nuclei showing uniform chromatin and inconspicuous nucleoli. Nuclear membrane irregularities and grooves are not readily identified.

Table 11.10

Bethesda System for Reporting Thyroid Cytopathology: Diagnostic Categories, Risk of Malignancy, and Recommended Management[a]

Diagnostic Category	Risk of Malignancy	Recommended Management
Unsatisfactory/non-diagnostic	N/A	Repeat FNA
Benign	0–3%	Clinical follow-up
Atypia of undetermined significance/follicular lesion of undetermined significance	5–15%	Repeat FNA
Follicular neoplasm/suspicious for follicular neoplasm	15–30%	Thyroid lobectomy
Suspicious for malignant cells	60–75%	Thyroid lobectomy or total thyroidectomy
Malignant	97–99%	Total thyroidectomy

[a]As reported in refs.[430,431].

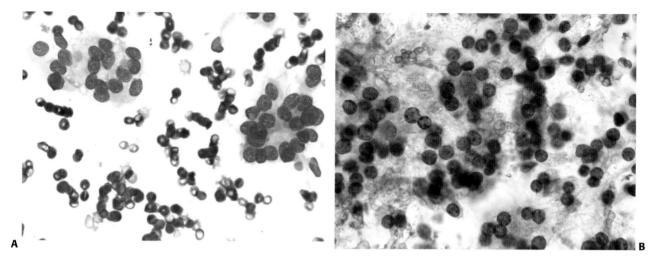

FIGURE 11.64. Cytology of the follicular variant of papillary carcinoma. A: Two clusters of neoplastic cells with microfollicular architecture. Nuclear features of papillary carcinoma are moderately developed and suspicious for malignancy (Diff-Quik stain). **B:** Despite numerous microfollicular clusters, the cells are bland and mimic a follicular neoplasm (Papanicolaou stain).

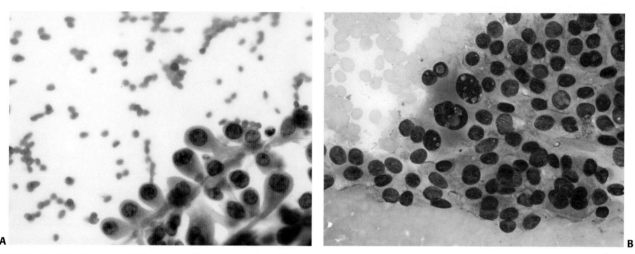

FIGURE 11.65. Cytology of the tall cell variant of papillary carcinoma. A: The elongated neoplastic cells are seen with abundant cytoplasm and sharply demarcated cell borders (Papanicolaou stain). **B:** In this cell cluster, the nuclei are large with multiple "soap bubble" type pseudoinclusions, but the cells are not "tall" (Diff-Quik stain).

Nonetheless, these features overlap with those of follicular variant papillary carcinoma.[446]

Immunohistochemical stains may be applied to cytology specimens, especially when cell block material is available. As discussed earlier in this chapter, immunohistochemical stains for galectin-3, HBME-1, CITED1, and CK19 are potentially useful markers in distinguishing papillary carcinoma from benign nodules.[447–449] In particular, HBME-1 demonstrates relatively high specificity when cytoplasmic membranous staining is present (Fig. 11.66). However, immunohistochemical markers in cytology samples must be used with caution and correlated with cytomorphologic and other features.

Recently, mutational and other molecular markers have been introduced as a helpful diagnostic adjunct to thyroid cytology. Their use is described in detail in Chapter 21.

 DIFFERENTIAL DIAGNOSIS

The differential diagnosis of papillary carcinoma is discussed throughout the chapter, particularly when pertinent to a

specific tumor variant, and is summarized in Table 11.11. In practice, classic papillary carcinoma seldom imposes diagnostic difficulty due to a characteristic papillary pattern which is rarely seen in other thyroid tumors and nonneoplastic lesions. Papillary carcinomas that lack papillary architecture can be more challenging to diagnose, and they have to be distinguished from other lesions that share similar nonpapillary growth patterns.

Tumors with Papillary Architecture

Classic papillary carcinoma is diagnosed based on the prominent papillary growth and characteristic nuclear features of papillary carcinoma. Papillae may also be found in follicular adenomas and nonneoplastic hyperplasia, although those are delicate, nonarborizing papillae with no well-developed fibrovascular stalks. Moreover, these benign papillary structures are lined by epithelial cells with basally located, small, round nuclei with smooth contours and dark chromatin.

Papillary architecture may also be seen in metastatic carcinomas of papillary type, but these are rare. The most common sites

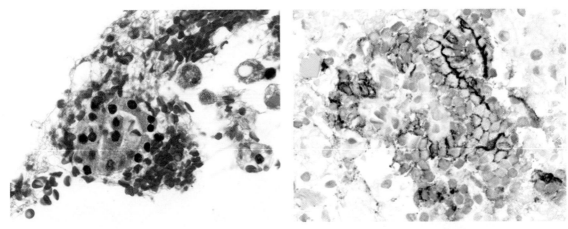

FIGURE 11.66. HBME-1 immunostaining in cytologic samples from the follicular variant of papillary carcinoma. (Left) A cluster of epithelial cells shows nuclei with slight contour irregularities (Hematoxylin and Eosin stain). **(Right)** Immunohistochemical stain for HBME-1 demonstrates discrete membranous staining. This feature is often associated with papillary carcinoma. Both images are from cell block sections.

Table 11.11

Differential Diagnosis of Papillary Thyroid Carcinoma

Prevalent Growth Pattern or Cell Type	Major Differential Diagnosis
Classic papillary growth pattern	Follicular adenoma with papillary hyperplasia Hyperplastic nodule with papillae Papillary hyperplasia in treated Graves disease Metastatic carcinoma (papillary renal cell, lung, breast carcinoma)
Follicular growth pattern	Follicular adenoma Hyperplastic nodule Follicular carcinoma Metastatic renal cell carcinoma
Solid growth pattern	Poorly differentiated carcinoma Medullary carcinoma
Papillary carcinoma with extensive fibrosis	Anaplastic carcinoma Riedel thyroiditis
Clear cell type	Medullary carcinoma Parathyroid tissue or tumor Metastatic renal cell carcinoma
Columnar cell type	Metastatic adenocarcinoma

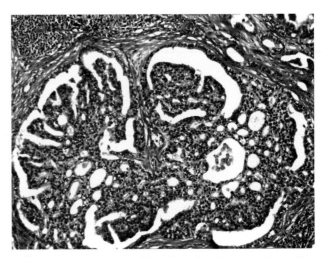

FIGURE 11.67. Level IV neck lymph node with metastatic papillary carcinoma from the lung primary.

Tumors with Follicular Architecture

Follicular variant papillary carcinomas, particularly when encapsulated, frequently pose a significant diagnostic challenge as they need to be distinguished from a follicular adenoma or a hyperplastic nodule. Follicular carcinoma may be considered when the tumor reveals capsular or vascular invasion. The differential diagnosis rests on the identification of characteristic nuclear features of papillary carcinoma. If they are not well developed, the diagnosis may be difficult. A set of minor diagnostic features may be applied in the borderline cases, as discussed and illustrated earlier in the chapter (see Section "Encapsulated Follicular Variant"). In addition, immunostains may offer some help. Positive staining for galectin-3, HBME-1, and CITED1, particularly when strong and diffuse (Fig. 11.56), strongly supports a malignant diagnosis, although it does not distinguish between papillary carcinoma and follicular carcinoma. Detection of *BRAF* V600E mutation or clonal *RET/PTC* rearrangement is virtually diagnostic of papillary carcinoma, although both mutations are relatively infrequent in the follicular variant tumors. *RAS* mutations, and less commonly *BRAF* K601E and *PAX8/PPARγ* mutations, are found in the follicular variant papillary carcinomas and indicate the presence of a neoplasm but are not diagnostic of this disease because they can be also seen in follicular carcinomas and adenomas.

of origin are kidney, lung, and breast (Chapter 18). Metastatic carcinoma should be considered when the tumor is bilateral, multifocal, makes no colloid, and shows no psammoma bodies. If metastatic tumor is suspected, immunohistochemical stains are helpful, particularly thyroglobulin, TTF1, and PAX8, although only thyroglobulin is entirely specific for thyroid follicular cells. Other immunohistochemical and molecular markers that may be used to establish the tumor origin are discussed and illustrated in Chapter 18. When papillary carcinoma is found in the neck lymph nodes and no obvious thyroid nodularity is noted, the other most common tumor sites metastasizing to this region are lung (Fig. 11.67) and breast.

Metastatic renal cell carcinoma of conventional type may enter the differential diagnosis due to a pseudofollicular architecture. The presence of characteristic nuclear features of papillary carcinoma and colloid formation typically rule out this possibility, and in more challenging cases a panel of immunohistochemical and molecular markers can be used (Chapter 18).

Tumors with Solid, Trabecular, or Insular Architecture

Solid variant papillary carcinomas should be distinguished from a poorly differentiated thyroid carcinoma. Both tumor types share solid, trabecular, and nested (insular) growth patterns, but they have substantially different biologic behavior and prognosis. The separation is based on the preservation of nuclear features and lack of necrosis and high mitotic activity ($\geq$3/10 HPF) in papillary carcinomas.[255]

Medullary carcinoma should be considered, particularly when a tumor with this architecture also shows clear cells. Immunostains for thyroglobulin and calcitonin are usually sufficient to establish the diagnosis. Importantly, when reviewing the thyroglobilin staining, immunoreactivity of entrapped thyroid follicles should not be misinterpreted as evidence for the *follicular* cell origin of the tumor nodule.[250]

Tumors with Extensive Fibrosis

Tumors with extensive fibrosis, such as seen in papillary carcinoma with fasciitis-like stroma, have to be distinguished from anaplastic (undifferentiated) thyroid carcinoma with spindle cell pattern (Chapter 13). The distinction relies on the lack of marked nuclear atypia, necrosis, and high mitotic activity in spindle cells adjacent to the foci of papillary carcinoma. Riedel thyroiditis and other fibroproliferative lesions such as fibromatosis can be excluded by finding the foci of papillary carcinoma.

 TREATMENT AND PROGNOSIS

Treatment

Papillary carcinoma is treated by surgery. Most patients diagnosed on preoperative FNA cytology undergo total or near-total thyroidectomy.[450,451] Dissection of central compartment lymph nodes may be performed.[452] When a definitive diagnosis of malignancy is not established preoperatively, the typical initial surgical approach is lobectomy with an intraoperative frozen section consultation. If the latter yields the diagnosis of papillary carcinoma, the surgery is expanded to total or near-total thyroidectomy. If the diagnosis of malignancy is established only with permanent sections, a second surgery to remove the remaining lobe is typically performed, except for small (<1 cm), intrathyroidal, unifocal, low-risk tumors.[453] The goal of completion thyroidectomy is to prevent tumor growth in the remaining lobe and to allow for radioactive iodine therapy and long-term disease monitoring.

Postoperative[131]I ablation is typically administered to patients with stages II–IV disease, where it leads to the reduction in tumor recurrence, distant metastases, and tumor-related mortality.[454,455] Among patients with stage I tumors, particularly with tumors <1 cm in size, the radioiodine treatment is restricted to those with multifocal disease, vascular invasion, nodal metastases, and other unfavorable tumor characteristics.[453] The ^{131}I therapy relies on relatively specific uptake of radioiodine by differentiated thyroid cells, and it aims to destroy the remaining nonneoplastic thyroid tissue and tumor cells in the thyroid bed and at metastatic sites. The treatment is carried out either following withdrawal of thyroid hormone replacement therapy or using stimulation by recombinant TSH to increase the avidity of thyroid cells for

radioiodine.[456] Dose of ^{131}I is typically between 30 to 100 mCi and can be higher (100 to 200 mCi) in high-risk patients. One of the complications of radioiodine therapy is a modest increase in the risk of secondary cancers.[457,458]

Adjuvant external beam radiation therapy may be used when complete tumor resection is not possible. Most recently, new therapies that target specific molecular alterations in papillary carcinoma have been developed; those are discussed below.

Disease Monitoring

Long-term disease monitoring is achieved by measuring serum thyroglobulin and by neck ultrasound, and less commonly by whole-body radioiodine scanning and other anatomic imaging (CT and MRI) and functional imaging (FDG-PET) procedures. The highest sensitivity (95% to 100%) of the detection of persistent or recurrent disease is achieved by measuring serum thyroglobulin following recombinant TSH stimulation in combination with neck ultrasound.[459–461]

Prognosis

Papillary carcinomas as a group are indolent tumors and have the best survival out of all types of thyroid cancer. In the United States, the 5-year survival was 96% and 10-year survival was 93% for patients diagnosed in 1985 to 1990.[462] However, the prognosis is strongly influenced by the extent of the disease, as the 10-year survival is 99.8% in patients with AJCC/UICC stage I and only 40.7% in those with stage IV disease.[463]

Tumor recurrence may be the first sign of unfavorable outcome. Overall, recurrence occurs in 15% to 35% of patients and manifests either locally in the thyroid bed or neck lymph nodes (two-thirds of cases) or at distant sites (one-third of cases).[211,212] At the time of death, half or more of patients have local tumor recurrence and about 80% have distant metastases, most frequently to the lung.[464,465] Death typically occurs from respiratory failure due to pulmonary metastases or uncontrolled local disease with suffocation from airway obstruction or compression of large blood vessels of the neck and mediastinum.[464,465]

Independent risk factors for tumor-related mortality include patient age at diagnosis, tumor size, extrathyroidal extension, and distant metastases (Table 11.12).[212,466–469] Older age at diagnosis is the strongest risk factor, although the age of onset of the increased risk varies between different studies and was found to be 40, 45, or 50 years, and every decade thereafter entails higher risk of dying from the disease. The AJCC/UICC staging uses a threshold of 45 years (Chapter 7). Larger tumor size is associated

Table 11.12

Risk Factors Associate with Mortality from Papillary Carcinoma

Independent Risk Factors	Other Potential Risk Factors*
Patient age	Gender
Tumor size	Lymph node metastases
Extrathyroidal extension	Tumor multicentricity
Distant metastases	Completeness of resection
BRAF V600E (?)*	Specific histologic variants (columnar cell, tall cell, solid, diffuse sclerosing variants)

*Found in several but not all studies and/or only on univariate analysis.
*Found as an independent risk factor of death from disease in one study,[407] pending additional confirmation.

with proportional decrease in survival, although some find significantly increased risk mostly in tumors >3.0 or 4.0 cm.[466,469] Extrathyroidal extension is a commonly identifiable prognostic factor, although some studies suggest that only extensive extrathyroidal invasion, and not minimal extrathyroidal extension, correlates with poor prognosis.[247,248]

Other potential prognostic factors include male gender, lymph node metastases, tumor multicentricity, vascular invasion, completeness of resection, and specific histologic variants (Table 11.9). Many, but not all, studies have found that male patients have a higher risk of dying from papillary carcinoma than do females despite a higher incidence of papillary carcinoma in the latter.[249,466-468] The presence of lymph node metastases in most studies was associated with higher rate of tumor recurrence but not with decreased survival.[249,469,470] Some authors have reported that higher histologic grade defined by tumor necrosis, vascular invasion, or marked nuclear atypia was associated with significantly shorter survival.[239,471] However, this approach can leads to the inclusion of papillary carcinomas with either poorly differentiated or anaplastic carcinoma areas, which are known to correlate with a dramatically poorer prognosis.

All major factors determining survival are incorporated in tumor staging and other prognostic scoring systems. The AJCC/UICC staging takes into account tumor size, extrathyroidal extension, distant metastases, and lymph node metastases, which influence the stage in a different way in patients under 45 years of age and in those 45 years and older (see Chapter 7). The staging correlates well with survival.[454,462,463] Several other prognostic scoring systems have been developed to better separate patients who are at higher risk for tumor recurrence and disease-specific mortality.[212,472,473] They are discussed in Chapter 7.

Molecular Prognostic Factors

BRAF

BRAF V600E mutation has emerged as an important prognostic marker for papillary carcinoma. Its association with more aggressive tumor characteristics, such as extrathyroidal extension, advanced tumor stage at presentation, and lymph node or distant metastases, has been found in most studies involving large series of patients (reviewed in ref.[123]). More importantly, *BRAF* V600E has been found to be an independent predictor of tumor recurrence, even in patients with low stage disease,[240,404,405] and an independent risk factor for tumor-related death.[407] The more aggressive behavior of *BRAF* V600E positive tumors may be due to the fact that this mutation leads to the alteration of function of sodium iodide symporter (*NIS*) and other genes metabolizing iodide, decreasing the ability of tumors to trap radioiodine, predisposing to treatment failure of the recurrent disease.[404,474-476] Therefore, a higher dose of radioiodine has been suggested for initial postoperative treatment of patients with *BRAF*-positive cancer.[477] These patients may also benefit from lower levels of suppression of TSH and closer postsurgical follow-up.[477]

The association between *BRAF* V600E and more aggressive disease characteristics has been also reported in small size, low-stage tumors[119,404] and in papillary microcarcinomas.[271-274,478,479] A recent analysis of a large series of T1 papillary carcinomas has demonstrated that *BRAF* V600E remains strongly associated with extrathyroidal extension and lymph node metastases in this tumor group.[119] This suggests that *BRAF* V600E may potentially be used for risk stratification and more individualized clinical management of patients with microcarcinomas and other small size intrathyroidal papillary carcinomas.

However, the use of *BRAF* alone for risk stratification of these tumors remains controversial, particularly taking into account the fact that it affects approximately 45% of papillary carcinomas, whereas only 10% to 15% of these tumors are known to have a more aggressive clinical behavior. Recently, it has been shown that *BRAF* association with tumor recurrence may be limited to older (≥65 years) patients.[480] In addition, as discussed earlier in the chapter, the more accurate risk stratification of thyroid microcarcinomas may be achieved by combining the *BRAF* status with several specific histopathologic tumor features (Fig. 11.24).[275] Therefore, it is likely that *BRAF* V600E will be used in combination with other clinical or histopathologic parameters to accurately define a subset of tumors with potentially unfavorable outcome.

It is important to note that the association with tumor aggressiveness is limited to the *BRAF* V600E mutation and is not found for K601E or other rare types of *BRAF* mutation.

Other Molecular Markers

Association between other mutational markers and prognosis is based on limited findings and needs further confirmation. One study reported the association between *RAS* mutation and a higher frequency of distant metastases.[165] In another study, the presence of *TRK* rearrangement correlated with a higher rate of local recurrence rate and tumor-related mortality.[177] Some data suggest that *RET/PTC* rearrangement, particularly *RET/PTC1*, may serve as a marker of more indolent tumor behavior.[146]

Several upregulated (miR-146b, miR-221, and miR-222) and downregulated (miR-34b and miR-130b) miRNAs have been found to be dysregulated at higher levels in papillary carcinomas with recurrence or distant metastases,[205] or in advanced stage tumors,[206] suggesting that they may serve as prognostic markers.

Association between aneuploidy and death from papillary carcinoma was observed in some studies[481] but was not confirmed in other reports.[95] More aggressive tumors appear to have a higher total number of chromosomal alterations detected by CGH, and gain of 1q and amplification of 1q correlated with distant metastases and disease-specific survival in some observations.[103,104]

Targeted Therapies

Clinical trials using molecular inhibitors directed against specific activated pathways or gene products are available for patients with locally advanced and/or radioiodine-refractory papillary carcinomas (www.ClinicalTrials.gov). Most agents are tyrosine kinase inhibitors of angiogenesis (VEGFR) and MAPK signaling. The early published results of phase II trials of sorafenib, sunitinib, axitinib, and other agents showed partial response in 10% to 30% of patients with papillary cancer, and stable disease in 30% to 60% of patients, with total clinical benefit seen in up to 80% of patients with papillary cancer.[482-486] It remains to be found if specific mutations (*BRAF*, etc.) can predict tumor response to these and other agents, such as the *BRAF*-specific inhibitor PLX4032.[487]

REFERENCES

1. Burgess JR. Temporal trends for thyroid carcinoma in Australia: an increasing incidence of papillary thyroid carcinoma (1982–1997). *Thyroid.* 2002;12:141–149.
2. Davies L, Welch HG. Increasing incidence of thyroid cancer in the United States, 1973–2002. *Jama.* 2006;295:2164–2167.
3. Leenhardt L, Grosclaude P, Cherie-Challine L. Increased incidence of thyroid carcinoma in France: a true epidemic or thyroid nodule management effects? Report from the French Thyroid Cancer Committee. *Thyroid.* 2004;14:1056–1060.
4. Akslen LA, Haldorsen T, Thoresen SO, et al. Incidence of thyroid cancer in Norway 1970–1985. Population review on time trend, sex, age, histological type and tumour stage in 2625 cases. *Apmis.* 1990;98:549–558.
5. Howlader N, Noone AM, Krapcho M, et al. SEER Cancer Statistics Review, 1975–2008, National Cancer Institute. Bethesda, MD, http://seer.cancer.gov/csr/1975_2008/, based on November 2010 SEER data submission, posted to the SEER Web site, 2011.
6. Parkin DM, Bray F, Ferlay J, et al. Global cancer statistics, 2002. *CA Cancer J Clin.* 2005;55:74–108.
7. Bisi H, Fernandes VS, de Camargo RY, et al. The prevalence of unsuspected thyroid pathology in 300 sequential autopsies, with special reference to the incidental carcinoma. *Cancer.* 1989;64:1888–1893.

8. Harach HR, Franssila KO, Wasenius VM. Occult papillary carcinoma of the thyroid. A "normal" finding in Finland. A systematic autopsy study. *Cancer.* 1985,56.531–538.
9. Albores-Saavedra J, Henson DE, Glazer E, et al. Changing patterns in the incidence and survival of thyroid cancer with follicular phenotype—papillary, follicular, and anaplastic: a morphological and epidemiological study. *Endocr Pathol.* 2007;18:1–7.
10. Burgess JR, Tucker P. Incidence trends for papillary thyroid carcinoma and their correlation with thyroid surgery and thyroid fine-needle aspirate cytology. *Thyroid.* 2006;16:47–53.
11. Suster S. Thyroid tumors with a follicular growth pattern: problems in differential diagnosis. *Arch Pathol Lab Med.* 2006;130:984–988.
12. Widder S, Guggisberg K, Khalil M, et al. A pathologic re-review of follicular thyroid neoplasms: the impact of changing the threshold for the diagnosis of the follicular variant of papillary thyroid carcinoma. *Surgery.* 2008;144:80–85.
13. Rosai J. The encapsulated follicular variant of papillary thyroid carcinoma: back to the drawing board. *Endocr Pathol.* 2010;21:7–11.
14. Mathur A, Moses W, Rahbari R, et al. Higher rate of BRAF mutation in papillary thyroid cancer over time: A single-institution study. *Cancer.* 2011;117:4390–4395.
15. Sykorova V, Dvorakova S, Ryska A, et al. BRAFV600E mutation in the pathogenesis of a large series of papillary thyroid carcinoma in Czech Republic. *J Endocrinol Invest.* 2010;33:318–324.
16. Ronckers CM, Ron E. Thyroid cancer. In: Freedman LS, Edwards BK, Ries LAG, et al., eds. *Cancer Incidence in Four Member Countries (Cyprus, Egypt, Israel, and Jordan) of the Middle East Cancer Consortium (MECC) Compared with US SEER.* 2006; Bethesda, MD: National Cancer Institute; NIH Pub. No. 06-5873.
17. Shapiro NL, Bhattacharyya N. Population-based outcomes for pediatric thyroid carcinoma. *Laryngoscope.* 2005;115:337–340.
18. Ron E, Lubin JH, Shore RE, et al. Thyroid cancer after exposure to external radiation: a pooled analysis of seven studies. *Radiat Res.* 1995;141:259–277.
19. Winship T, Rosvoll RV. Cancer of the thyroid in children. *Proc Natl Cancer Conf.* 1970;6:677–681.
20. Hundahl SA, Cady B, Cunningham MP, et al. Initial results from a prospective cohort study of 5583 cases of thyroid carcinoma treated in the United States during 1996. U.S. and German Thyroid Cancer Study Group. An American College of Surgeons Commission on Cancer Patient Care Evaluation study. *Cancer.* 2000;89:202–217.
21. Ron E, Kleinerman RA, Boice JD Jr, et al. A population-based case-control study of thyroid cancer. *J Natl Cancer Inst.* 1987;79:1–12.
22. Chernobyl's Legacy: Health, Envorinmental and Socio-Economic Impacts: The Chernobyl Forum 2003–2005; 2005.
23. Cardis E, Howe G, Ron E, et al. Cancer consequences of the Chernobyl accident: 20 years on. *J Radiol Prot.* 2006;26:127–140.
24. Tronko M, Bogdanova T, Voskoboynyk L, et al. Radiation induced thyroid cancer: fundamental and applied aspects. *Exp Oncol.* 2010;32:200–204.
25. Holm LE, Hall P, Wiklund K, et al. Cancer risk after iodine-131 therapy for hyperthyroidism. *J Natl Cancer Inst.* 1991;83:1072–1077.
26. Cardis E, Kesminiene A, Ivanov V, et al. Risk of thyroid cancer after exposure to 131I in childhood. *J Natl Cancer Inst.* 2005;97:724–732.
27. Zablotska LB, Ron E, Rozhko AV, et al. Thyroid cancer risk in Belarus among children and adolescents exposed to radioiodine after the Chornobyl accident. *Br J Cancer.* 2011;104:181–187.
28. Tronko MD, Howe GR, Bogdanova TI, et al. A cohort study of thyroid cancer and other thyroid diseases after the Chornobyl accident: thyroid cancer in Ukraine detected during first screening. *J Natl Cancer Inst.* 2006;98:897–903.
29. Jacob P, Bogdanova TI, Buglova E, et al. Thyroid cancer among Ukrainians and Belarusians who were children or adolescents at the time of the Chernobyl accident. *J Radiol Prot.* 2006;26:51–67.
30. Davis S, Stepanenko V, Rivkind N, et al. Risk of thyroid cancer in the Bryansk Oblast of the Russian Federation after the Chernobyl Power Station accident. *Radiat Res.* 2004;162:241–248.
31. Cardis E, Hatch M. The Chernobyl accident—an epidemiological perspective. *Clin Oncol (R Coll Radiol).* 2011;23:251–260.
32. Schneider AB, Ron E, Lubin J, et al. Dose-response relationships for radiation-induced thyroid cancer and thyroid nodules: evidence for the prolonged effects of radiation on the thyroid. *J Clin Endocrinol Metab.* 1993;77:362–369.
33. Nikiforov YE. Radiation-induced thyroid cancer: what we have learned from Chernobyl. *Endocr Pathol.* 2006;17:307–317.
34. Adams MJ, Shore RE, Dozier A, et al. Thyroid cancer risk 40+ years after irradiation for an enlarged thymus: an update of the Hempelmann cohort. *Radiat Res.* 2010;174:753–762.
35. Nikiforov Y, Gnepp DR. Pediatric thyroid cancer after the Chernobyl disaster: pathomorphologic study of 84 cases (1991–1992) from the Republic of Belarus. *Cancer.* 1994;74:748–766.
36. LiVolsi VA, Abrosimov AA, Bogdanova T, et al. The Chernobyl thyroid cancer experience: pathology. *Clin Oncol (R Coll Radiol).* 2011;23:261–267.
37. Ciampi R, Knauf JA, Kerler R, et al. Oncogenic AKAP9-BRAF fusion is a novel mechanism of MAPK pathway activation in thyroid cancer. *J Clin Invest.* 2005;115:94–101.
38. Nikiforov YE, Rowland JM, Bove KE, et al. Distinct pattern of ret oncogene rearrangements in morphological variants of radiation-induced and sporadic thyroid papillary carcinomas in children. *Cancer Res.* 1997;57:1690–1694.
39. Franceschi S, Boyle P, Maisonneuve P, et al. The epidemiology of thyroid carcinoma. *Crit Rev Oncog.* 1993;4:25–52.
40. Goodman MT, Yoshizawa CN, Kolonel LN. Descriptive epidemiology of thyroid cancer in Hawaii. *Cancer.* 1988;61:1272–1281.
41. Lind P, Langsteger W, Molnar M, et al. Epidemiology of thyroid diseases in iodine sufficiency. *Thyroid.* 1998;8:1179–1183.
42. Harach HR, Escalante DA, Day ES. Thyroid cancer and thyroiditis in Salta, Argentina: a 40-yr study in relation to iodine prophylaxis. *Endocr Pathol.* 2002;13-175–181.
43. Williams ED, Doniach I, Bjarnason O, et al. Thyroid cancer in an iodide rich area: a histopathological study. *Cancer.* 1977;39:215–222.
44. Pettersson B, Coleman MP, Ron E, et al. Iodine supplementation in Sweden and regional trends in thyroid cancer incidence by histopathologic type. *Int J Cancer.* 1996;65:13–19.
45. Guan H, Ji M, Bao R, et al. Association of high iodine intake with the T1799A BRAF mutation in papillary thyroid cancer. *J Clin Endocrinol Metab.* 2009;94:1612–1617.
46. Pellegriti G, De Vathaire F, Scollo C, et al. Papillary thyroid cancer incidence in the volcanic area of Sicily. *J Natl Cancer Inst.* 2009;101:1575–1583.
47. D'Avanzo B, La Vecchia C, Franceschi S,et al. History of thyroid diseases and subsequent thyroid cancer risk. *Cancer Epidemiol Biomarkers Prev.* 1995;4:193–199.
48. Franceschi S, Preston-Martin S, Dal Maso L, et al. A pooled analysis of case-control studies of thyroid cancer. IV. Benign thyroid diseases. *Cancer Causes Control.* 1999;10:583–595.
49. Fagin JA. Minireview: branded from the start-distinct oncogenic initiating events may determine tumor fate in the thyroid. *Mol Endocrinol.* 2002;16:903–911.
50. Williams ED. Mechanisms and pathogenesis of thyroid cancer in animals and man. *Mutat Res.* 1995;333:123–129.
51. Boelaert K, Horacek J, Holder RL, et al. Serum thyrotropin concentration as a novel predictor of malignancy in thyroid nodules investigated by fine-needle aspiration. *J Clin Endocrinol Metab.* 2006;91:4295–4301.
52. Fiore E, Rago T, Provenzale MA, et al. Lower levels of TSH are associated with a lower risk of papillary thyroid cancer in patients with thyroid nodular disease: thyroid autonomy may play a protective role. *Endocr Relat Cancer.* 2009;16:1251–1260.
53. Haymart MR, Glinberg SL, Liu J, et al. Higher serum TSH in thyroid cancer patients occurs independent of age and correlates with extrathyroidal extension. *Clin Endocrinol (Oxf).* 2009;71:434–439.
54. Franco AT, Malaguarnera R, Refetoff S, et al. Thyrotrophin receptor signaling dependence of Braf-induced thyroid tumor initiation in mice. *Proc Natl Acad Sci U S A.* 2011;108:1615–1620.
55. Walker RP, Paloyan E. The relationship between Hashimoto's thyroiditis, thyroid neoplasia, and primary hyperparathyroidism. *Otolaryngol Clin North Am.* 1990;23:291–302.
56. Mazzaferri EL. Thyroid cancer and Graves' disease. *J Clin Endocrinol Metab.* 1990;70:826–829.
57. Holm LE, Blomgren H, Lowhagen T. Cancer risks in patients with chronic lymphocytic thyroiditis. *N Engl J Med.* 1985;312:601–604.
58. Dobyns BM, Sheline GE, Workman JB, et al. Malignant and benign neoplasms of the thyroid in patients treated for hyperthyroidism: a report of the cooperative thyrotoxicosis therapy follow-up study. *J Clin Endocrinol Metab.* 1974;38:976–998.
59. Crile G Jr. Struma lymphomatosa and carcinoma of the thyroid. *Surg Gynecol Obstet.* 1978;147:350–352.
60. Goldman MB, Monson RR, Maloof F. Cancer mortality in women with thyroid disease. *Cancer Res.* 1990;50:2283–2289.
61. Mazokopakis EE, Tzortzinis AA, Dalieraki-Ott EI, et al. Coexistence of Hashimoto's thyroiditis with papillary thyroid carcinoma. A retrospective study. *Hormones (Athens).* 2010;9:312–317.
62. Anil C, Goksel S, Gursoy A. Hashimoto's thyroiditis is not associated with increased risk of thyroid cancer in patients with thyroid nodules: a single-center prospective study. *Thyroid.* 2010;20:601–606.
63. Wirtschafter A, Schmidt R, Rosen D, et al. Expression of the RET/PTC fusion gene as a marker for papillary carcinoma in Hashimoto's thyroiditis. *Laryngoscope.* 1997;107:95–100.
64. Sheils OM, O'Eary JJ, Uhlmann V, et al. RET/PTC-1 activation in Hashimoto thyroiditis. *Int J Surg Pathol.* 2000;8:185–189.
65. Cyniak-Magierska A, Wojciechowska-Durczynska K, Krawczyk-Rusiecka K, et al. Assessment of RET/PTC1 and RET/PTC3 rearrangements in fine-needle aspiration biopsy specimens collected from patients with Hashimoto's thyroiditis. *Thyroid Res.* 2011;4:5.
66. Sadow PM, Heinrich MC, Corless CL, et al. Absence of BRAF, NRAS, KRAS, HRAS mutations, and RET/PTC gene rearrangements distinguishes dominant nodules in Hashimoto thyroiditis from papillary thyroid carcinoma. *Endocr Pathol.* 2010;21:73–79.
67. Nikiforov YE. RET/PTC rearrangement—a link between Hashimoto's thyroiditis and thyroid cancer ... or not. *J Clin Endocrinol Metab.* 2006;91:2040–2042.
68. Negri E, Dal Maso L, Ron E, et al. A pooled analysis of case-control studies of thyroid cancer. II. Menstrual and reproductive factors. *Cancer Causes Control.* 1999;10:143–155.
69. Kolonel LN, Hankin JH, Wilkens LR, et al. An epidemiologic study of thyroid cancer in Hawaii. *Cancer Causes Control.* 1990;1:223–234.
70. Mijovic T, How J, Payne RJ. Obesity and thyroid cancer. *Front Biosci (Schol Ed).* 2011;3:555–564.
71. Renehan AG, Tyson M, Egger M, et al. Body-mass index and incidence of cancer: a systematic review and meta-analysis of prospective observational studies. *Lancet.* 2008;371:569–578.
72. Hemminki K, Eng C, Chen B. Familial risks for nonmedullary thyroid cancer. *J Clin Endocrinol Metab.* 2005;90:5747–5753.
73. Harach HR. Familial nonmedullary thyroid neoplasia. *Endocr Pathol.* 2001;12:97–112.
74. Iwama T, Mishima Y, Utsunomiya J. The impact of familial adenomatous polyposis on the tumorigenesis and mortality at the several organs. Its rational treatment. *Ann Surg.* 1993;217:101–108.

75. Foulkes WD, Kloos RT, Harach HR, et al. Familial non-medullary thyroid cancer. In: DeLellis RA, Lloyd RV, Heitz PU, et al., eds. *Pathology and Genetics of Tumours of Endocrine Organs. World Health Organization Classification of Tumours.* Lyon, France: IARC Press; 2004:257–261.
76. Plail RO, Bussey HJ, Glazer G, et al. Adenomatous polyposis: an association with carcinoma of the thyroid. *Br J Surg.* 1987;74:377–380.
77. Bulow S, Holm NV, Mellemgaard A. Papillary thyroid carcinoma in Danish patients with familial adenomatous polyposis. *Int J Colorectal Dis.* 1988;3:29–31.
78. Boikos SA, Stratakis CA. Carney complex: pathology and molecular genetics. *Neuroendocrinology.* 2006;83:189–199.
79. Ishikawa Y, Sugano H, Matsumoto T, et al. Unusual features of thyroid carcinomas in Japanese patients with Werner syndrome and possible genotype-phenotype relations to cell type and race. *Cancer.* 1999;85:1345–1352.
80. Charkes ND. On the prevalence of familial nonmedullary thyroid cancer. *Thyroid.* 1998;8:857–858.
81. Charkes ND. On the prevalence of familial nonmedullary thyroid cancer in multiply affected kindreds. *Thyroid.* 2006;16:181–186.
82. Malchoff CD, Malchoff DM. Familial nonmedullary thyroid carcinoma. *Cancer Control.* 2006;13:106–110.
83. Burgess JR, Duffield A, Wilkinson SJ, et al. Two families with an autosomal dominant inheritance pattern for papillary carcinoma of the thyroid. *J Clin Endocrinol Metab.* 1997;82:345–348.
84. Uchino S, Noguchi S, Kawamoto H, et al. Familial nonmedullary thyroid carcinoma characterized by multifocality and a high recurrence rate in a large study population. *World J Surg.* 2002;26:897–902.
85. Bevan S, Pal T, Greenberg CR, et al. A comprehensive analysis of MNG1, TCO1, fPTC, PTEN, TSHR, and TRKA in familial nonmedullary thyroid cancer: confirmation of linkage to TCO1. *J Clin Endocrinol Metab.* 2001;86:3701–3704.
86. Canzian F, Amati P, Harach HR, et al. A gene predisposing to familial thyroid tumors with cell oxyphilia maps to chromosome 19p13.2. *Am J Hum Genet.* 1998;63:1743–1748.
87. Malchoff CD, Sarfarazi M, Tendler B, et al. Papillary thyroid carcinoma associated with papillary renal neoplasia: genetic linkage analysis of a distinct heritable tumor syndrome. *J Clin Endocrinol Metab.* 2000;85:1758–1764.
88. McKay JD, Lesueur F, Jonard L, et al. Localization of a susceptibility gene for familial nonmedullary thyroid carcinoma to chromosome 2q21. *Am J Hum Genet.* 2001;69:440–446.
89. Kim H, Piao Z, Park C, et al. Clinical significance of clonality in thyroid nodules. *Br J Surg.* 1998;85:1125–1128.
90. Shattuck TM, Westra WH, Ladenson PW, et al. Independent clonal origins of distinct tumor foci in multifocal papillary thyroid carcinoma. *N Engl J Med.* 2005;352:2406–2412.
91. Sugg SL, Ezzat S, Rosen IB, et al. Distinct multiple RET/PTC gene rearrangements in multifocal papillary thyroid neoplasia. *J Clin Endocrinol Metab.* 1998;83:4116–4122.
92. Giannini R, Ugolini C, Lupi C, et al. The heterogeneous distribution of BRAF mutation supports the independent clonal origin of distinct tumor foci in multifocal papillary thyroid carcinoma. *J Clin Endocrinol Metab.* 2007;92:3511–3516.
93. Park SY, Park YJ, Lee YJ, et al. Analysis of differential BRAF(V600E) mutational status in multifocal papillary thyroid carcinoma: evidence of independent clonal origin in distinct tumor foci. *Cancer.* 2006;107:1831–1838.
94. Schelfhout LJ, Cornelisse CJ, Goslings BM, et al. Frequency and degree of aneuploidy in benign and malignant thyroid neoplasms. *Int J Cancer.* 1990;45:16–20.
95. Jonasson JG, Hrafnkelsson J. Nuclear DNA analysis and prognosis in carcinoma of the thyroid gland. A nationwide study in Iceland on carcinomas diagnosed 1955–1990. *Virchows Arch.* 1994;425:349–355.
96. Wreesmann VB, Ghossein RA, Hezel M, et al. Follicular variant of papillary thyroid carcinoma: genome-wide appraisal of a controversial entity. *Genes Chromosomes Cancer.* 2004;40:355–364.
97. Herrmann MA, Hay ID, Bartelt DH, Jr, et al. Cytogenetic and molecular genetic studies of follicular and papillary thyroid cancers. *J Clin Invest.* 1991;88:1596–1604.
98. Roque L, Nunes VM, Ribeiro C, et al. Karyotypic characterization of papillary thyroid carcinomas. *Cancer.* 2001;92:2529–2538.
99. Frau DV, Lai ML, Caria P, et al. Trisomy 17 as a marker for a subset of noninvasive thyroid nodules with focal features of papillary carcinoma: cytogenetic and molecular analysis of 62 cases and correlation with histologic findings. *J Clin Endocrinol Metab.* 2008;93:177–181.
100. Jenkins RB, Hay ID, Herath JF, et al. Frequent occurrence of cytogenetic abnormalities in sporadic nonmedullary thyroid carcinoma. *Cancer.* 1990;66:1213–1220.
101. Teyssier JR, Liautaud-Roger F, Ferre D, et al. Chromosomal changes in thyroid tumors. Relation with DNA content, karyotypic features, and clinical data. *Cancer Genet Cytogenet.* 1990;50:249–263.
102. Zitzelsberger H, Lehmann L, Hieber L, et al. Cytogenetic changes in radiation-induced tumors of the thyroid. *Cancer Res.* 1999;59:135–140.
103. Kjellman P, Lagercrantz S, Hoog A, et al. Gain of 1q and loss of 9q21.3-q32 are associated with a less favorable prognosis in papillary thyroid carcinoma. *Genes Chromosomes Cancer.* 2001;32:43–49.
104. Wreesmann VB, Sieczka EM, Socci ND, et al. Genome-wide profiling of papillary thyroid cancer identifies MUC1 as an independent prognostic marker. *Cancer Res.* 2004;64:3780–3789.
105. Rodrigues R, Roque L, Espadinha C, et al. Comparative genomic hybridization, BRAF, RAS, RET, and oligo-array analysis in aneuploid papillary thyroid carcinomas. *Oncol Rep.* 2007;18:917–926.
106. Ward LS, Brenta G, Medvedovic M, et al. Studies of allelic loss in thyroid tumors reveal major differences in chromosomal instability between papillary and follicular carcinomas. *J Clin Endocrinol Metab.* 1998;83:525–530.
107. Gillespie JW, Nasir A, Kaiser HE. Loss of heterozygosity in papillary and follicular thyroid carcinoma: a mini review. *In Vivo.* 2000;14:139–140.
108. Hunt JL, Fowler M, Lomago D, et al. Tumor suppressor gene allelic loss profiles of the variants of papillary thyroid carcinoma. *Diagn Mol Pathol.* 2004;13:41–46.
109. Robinson MJ, Cobb MH. Mitogen-activated protein kinase pathways. *Curr Opin Cell Biol.* 1997;9:180–186.
110. Kimura ET, Nikiforova MN, Zhu Z, et al. High prevalence of BRAF mutations in thyroid cancer: genetic evidence for constitutive activation of the RET/PTC-RAS-BRAF signaling pathway in papillary thyroid carcinoma. *Cancer Res.* 2003;63:1454–1457.
111. Soares P, Trovisco V, Rocha AS, et al. BRAF mutations and RET/PTC rearrangements are alternative events in the etiopathogenesis of PTC. *Oncogene.* 2003;22:4578–4580.
112. Frattini M, Ferrario C, Bressan P, et al. Alternative mutations of BRAF, RET and NTRK1 are associated with similar but distinct gene expression patterns in papillary thyroid cancer. *Oncogene.* 2004;23:7436–7440.
113. Adeniran AJ, Zhu Z, Gandhi M, et al. Correlation between genetic alterations and microscopic features, clinical manifestations, and prognostic characteristics of thyroid papillary carcinomas. *Am J Surg Pathol.* 2006;30:216–222.
114. Cohen Y, Xing M, Mambo E, et al. BRAF mutation in papillary thyroid carcinoma. *J Natl Cancer Inst.* 2003;95:625–627.
115. Trovisco V, Vieira de Castro I, Soares P, et al. BRAF mutations are associated with some histological types of papillary thyroid carcinoma. *J Pathol.* 2004;202:247–251.
116. Carta C, Moretti S, Passeri L, et al. Genotyping of an Italian papillary thyroid carcinoma cohort revealed high prevalence of BRAF mutations, absence of RAS mutations and allowed the detection of a new mutation of BRAF oncoprotein (BRAF(V599lns)). *Clin Endocrinol (Oxf).* 2006;64:105–109.
117. Hou P, Liu D, Xing M. Functional characterization of the T1799-1801del and A1799-1816ins BRAF mutations in papillary thyroid cancer. *Cell Cycle.* 2007;6:377–379.
118. Chiosea S, Nikiforova M, Zuo H, et al. A novel complex BRAF mutation detected in a solid variant of papillary thyroid carcinoma. *Endocr Pathol.* 2009;20:122–126.
119. Basolo F, Torregrossa L, Giannini R, et al. Correlation between the BRAF V600E mutation and tumor invasiveness in papillary thyroid carcinomas smaller than 20 millimeters: analysis of 1060 cases. *J Clin Endocrinol Metab.* 2010;95:4197–4205.
120. Knauf JA, Ma X, Smith EP, et al. Targeted expression of BRAFV600E in thyroid cells of transgenic mice results in papillary thyroid cancers that undergo dedifferentiation. *Cancer Res.* 2005;65:4238–4245.
121. Nikiforova MN, Kimura ET, Gandhi M, et al. BRAF mutations in thyroid tumors are restricted to papillary carcinomas and anaplastic or poorly differentiated carcinomas arising from papillary carcinomas. *J Clin Endocrinol Metab.* 2003;88:5399–5404.
122. Xing M. BRAF mutation in thyroid cancer. *Endocr Relat Cancer.* 2005;12:245–262.
123. Xing M. BRAF mutation in papillary thyroid cancer: pathogenic role, molecular bases, and clinical implications. *Endocr Rev.* 2007;28:742–762.
124. Palona I, Namba H, Mitsutake N, et al. BRAFV600E promotes invasiveness of thyroid cancer cells through nuclear factor kappaB activation. *Endocrinology.* 2006;147:5699–5707.
125. Jo YS, Li S, Song JH, et al. Influence of the BRAF V600E mutation on expression of vascular endothelial growth factor in papillary thyroid cancer. *J Clin Endocrinol Metab.* 2006;91:3667–3670.
126. Namba H, Nakashima M, Hayashi T, et al. Clinical implication of hot spot BRAF mutation, V599E, in papillary thyroid cancers. *J Clin Endocrinol Metab.* 2003;88:4393–4397.
127. Knauf JA, Sartor MA, Medvedovic M, et al. Progression of BRAF-induced thyroid cancer is associated with epithelial-mesenchymal transition requiring concomitant MAP kinase and TGFbeta signaling. *Oncogene.* 2011;30:3513–3562.
128. Vasko V, Espinosa AV, Scouten W, et al. Gene expression and functional evidence of epithelial-to-mesenchymal transition in papillary thyroid carcinoma invasion. *Proc Natl Acad Sci U S A.* 2007;104:2803–2808.
129. Grieco M, Santoro M, Berlingieri MT, et al. PTC is a novel rearranged form of the ret proto-oncogene and is frequently detected in vivo in human thyroid papillary carcinomas. *Cell.* 1990;60:557–563.
130. Santoro M, Dathan NA, Berlingieri MT, et al. Molecular characterization of RET/PTC3; a novel rearranged version of the RETproto-oncogene in a human thyroid papillary carcinoma. *Oncogene.* 1994;9:509–516.
131. Bongarzone I, Butti MG, Coronelli S, et al. Frequent activation of ret protooncogene by fusion with a new activating gene in papillary thyroid carcinomas. *Cancer Res.* 1994;54:2979–2985.
132. Fugazzola L, Pierotti MA, Vigano E, et al. Molecular and biochemical analysis of RET/PTC4, a novel oncogenic rearrangement between RET and ELE1 genes, in a post-Chernobyl papillary thyroid cancer. *Oncogene.* 1996;13:1093–1097.
133. Bongarzone I, Monzini N, Borrello MG, et al. Molecular characterization of a thyroid tumor-specific transforming sequence formed by the fusion of ret tyrosine kinase and the regulatory subunit RI alpha of cyclic AMP-dependent protein kinase A. *Mol Cell Biol.* 1993;13:358–366.
134. Klugbauer S, Demidchik EP, Lengfelder E, et al. Detection of a novel type of RET rearrangement (PTC5) in thyroid carcinomas after Chernobyl and analysis of the involved RET-fused gene RFG5. *Cancer Res.* 1998;58:198–203.
135. Klugbauer S, Rabes HM. The transcription coactivator HTIF1 and a related protein are fused to the RET receptor tyrosine kinase in childhood papillary thyroid carcinomas. *Oncogene.* 1999;18:4388–4393.
136. Klugbauer S, Jauch A, Lengfelder E, et al. A novel type of RET rearrangement (PTC8) in childhood papillary thyroid carcinomas and characterization of the involved gene (RFG8). *Cancer Res.* 2000;60:7028–7032.
137. Salassidis K, Bruch J, Zitzelsberger H, et al. Translocation t(10;14)(q11.2:q22.1) fusing the kinetin to the RET gene creates a novel rearranged

form (PTC8) of the RET proto-oncogene in radiation-induced childhood papillary thyroid carcinoma. *Cancer Res.* 2000;60:2786–2789.

138. Corvi R, Berger N, Balczon R, et al. RET/PCM-1: a novel fusion gene in papillary thyroid carcinoma. *Oncogene.* 2000;19:4236–4242.

139. Saenko V, Rogounovitch T, Shimizu-Yoshida Y, et al. Novel tumorigenic rearrangement, Delta rfp/ret, in a papillary thyroid carcinoma from externally irradiated patient. *Mutat Res.* 2003;527:81–90.

140. Nakata T, Kitamura Y, Shimizu K, et al. Fusion of a novel gene, ELKS, to RET due to translocation t(10;12)(q11;p13) in a papillary thyroid carcinoma. *Genes Chromosomes Cancer.* 1999;25:97–103.

141. Ciampi R, Giordano TJ, Wikenheiser-Brokamp K, et al. HOOK3-RET: a novel type of RET/PTC rearrangement in papillary thyroid carcinoma. *Endocr Relat Cancer.* 2007;14:445–452.

142. Santoro M, Melillo RM, Grieco M, et al. The TRK and RET tyrosine kinase oncogenes cooperate with ras in the neoplastic transformation of a rat thyroid epithelial cell line. *Cell Growth Differ.* 1993;4:77–84.

143. Jhiang SM, Sagartz JE, Tong Q, et al. Targeted expression of the ret/PTC1 oncogene induces papillary thyroid carcinomas. *Endocrinology.* 1996;137:375–378.

144. Santoro M, Chiappetta G, Cerrato A, et al. Development of thyroid papillary carcinomas secondary to tissue-specific expression of the RET/PTC1 oncogene in transgenic mice. *Oncogene.* 1996;12:1821–1826.

145. Powell DJ, Jr., Russell J, Nibu K, et al. The RET/PTC3 oncogene: metastatic solid-type papillary carcinomas in murine thyroids. *Cancer Res.* 1998;58:5523–5528.

146. Nikiforov YE. RET/PTC Rearrangement in thyroid tumors. *Endocr Pathol.* 2002;13:3–16.

147. Zhu Z, Ciampi R, Nikiforova MN, et al. Prevalence of RET/PTC rearrangements in thyroid papillary carcinomas: effects of the detection methods and genetic heterogeneity. *J Clin Endocrinol Metab.* 2006;91:3603–3610.

148. Tallini G, Asa SL. RET oncogene activation in papillary thyroid carcinoma. *Adv Anat Pathol.* 2001;8:345–354.

149. Unger K, Zitzelsberger H, Salvatore G, et al. Heterogeneity in the distribution of RET/PTC rearrangements within individual post-Chernobyl papillary thyroid carcinomas. *J Clin Endocrinol Metab.* 2004;89:4272–4279.

150. Zhu Z, Ciampi R, Nikiforova MN, et al. Prevalence of RET/PTC rearrangements in thyroid papillary carcinomas: effects of the detection methods and genetic heterogeneity. *J Clin Endocrinol Metab.* 2006;91:3603–3610.

151. Santoro M, Carlomagno F, Hay ID, et al. Ret oncogene activation in human thyroid neoplasms is restricted to the papillary cancer subtype. *J Clin Invest.* 1992;89:1517–1522.

152. Rabes HM, Demidchik EP, Sidorow JD, et al. Pattern of radiation-induced RET and NTRK1 rearrangements in 191 post-Chernobyl papillary thyroid carcinomas: biological, phenotypic, and clinical implications. *Clin Cancer Res.* 2000;6:1093–1103.

153. Bounacer A, Wicker R, Caillou B, et al. High prevalence of activating ret proto-oncogene rearrangements, in thyroid tumors from patients who had received external radiation. *Oncogene.* 1997;15:1263–1273.

154. Mizuno T, Iwamoto KS, Kyoizumi S, et al. Preferential induction of RET/PTC1 rearrangement by X-ray irradiation. *Oncogene.* 2000;19:438–443.

155. Caudill CM, Zhu Z, Ciampi R, et al. Dose-dependent generation of RET/PTC in human thyroid cells after in vitro exposure to gamma-radiation: a model of carcinogenic chromosomal rearrangement induced by ionizing radiation. *J Clin Endocrinol Metab.* 2005;90:2364–2369.

156. Nikiforova MN, Stringer JR, Blough R, et al. Proximity of chromosomal loci that participate in radiation-induced rearrangements in human cells. *Science.* 2000;290:138–141.

157. Gandhi M, Medvedovic M, Stringer JR, et al. Interphase chromosome folding determines spatial proximity of genes participating in carcinogenic RET/PTC rearrangements. *Oncogene.* 2006;25:2360–2366.

158. Smida J, Salassidis K, Hieber L, et al. Distinct frequency of ret rearrangements in papillary thyroid carcinomas of children and adults from Belarus. *Int J Cancer.* 1999;80:32–38.

159. Tallini G, Santoro M, Helie M, et al. RET/PTC oncogene activation defines a subset of papillary thyroid carcinomas lacking evidence of progression to poorly differentiated or undifferentiated tumor phenotypes. *Clin Cancer Res.* 1998;4:287–294.

160. Zhu Z, Gandhi M, Nikiforova MN, et al. Molecular profile and clinical-pathologic features of the follicular variant of papillary thyroid carcinoma. An unusually high prevalence of ras mutations. *Am J Clin Pathol.* 2003;120:71–77.

161. Di Cristofaro J, Marcy M, Vasko V, et al. Molecular genetic study comparing follicular variant versus classic papillary thyroid carcinomas: association of N-ras mutation in codon 61 with follicular variant. *Hum Pathol.* 2006;37:824–830.

162. Namba H, Rubin SA, Fagin JA. Point mutations of ras oncogenes are an early event in thyroid tumorigenesis. *Mol Endocrinol.* 1990;4:1474–1479.

163. Ezzat S, Zheng L, Kolenda J, et al. Prevalence of activating ras mutations in morphologically characterized thyroid nodules. *Thyroid.* 1996;6:409–416.

164. Vasko VV, Gaudart J, Allasia C, et al. Thyroid follicular adenomas may display features of follicular carcinoma and follicular variant of papillary carcinoma. *Eur J Endocrinol.* 2004;151:779–786.

165. Hara H, Fulton N, Yashiro T, et al. N-ras mutation: an independent prognostic factor for aggressiveness of papillary thyroid carcinoma. *Surgery.* 1994;116:1010–1016.

166. Barbacid M, Lamballe F, Pulido D, et al. The trk family of tyrosine protein kinase receptors. *Biochim Biophys Acta.* 1991;1072:115–127.

167. Pierotti MA, Bongarzone I, Borello MG, et al. Cytogenetics and molecular genetics of carcinomas arising from thyroid epithelial follicular cells. *Genes Chromosomes Cancer.* 1996;16:1–14.

168. Martin-Zanca D, Hughes SH, Barbacid M. A human oncogene formed by the fusion of truncated tropomyosin and protein tyrosine kinase sequences. *Nature.* 1986;319:743–748.

169. Radice P, Sozzi G, Miozzo M, et al. The human tropomyosin gene involved in the generation of the TRK oncogene maps to chromosome 1q31. *Oncogene.* 1991;6:2145–2148.

170. Greco A, Pierotti MA, Bongarzone I, et al. TRK-T1 is a novel oncogene formed by the fusion of TPR and TRK genes in human papillary thyroid carcinomas. *Oncogene.* 1992;7:237–242.

171. Miranda C, Minoletti F, Greco A, et al. Refined localization of the human TPR gene to chromosome 1q25 by in situ hybridization. *Genomics.* 1994;23:714–715.

172. Greco A, Mariani C, Miranda C, et al. The DNA rearrangement that generates the TRK-T3 oncogene involves a novel gene on chromosome 3 whose product has a potential coiled-coil domain. *Mol Cell Biol.* 1995;15:6118–6127.

173. Russell JP, Powell DJ, Cunnane M, et al. The TRK-T1 fusion protein induces neoplastic transformation of thyroid epithelium. *Oncogene.* 2000;19:5729–5735.

174. Delvincourt C, Patey M, Flament JB, et al. Ret and trk proto-oncogene activation in thyroid papillary carcinomas in French patients from the Champagne-Ardenne region. *Clin Biochem.* 1996;29:267–271.

175. Wajjwalku W, Nakamura S, Hasegawa Y, et al. Low frequency of rearrangements of the ret and trk proto-oncogenes in Japanese thyroid papillary carcinomas. *Jpn J Cancer Res.* 1992;83:671–675.

176. Bongarzone I, Vigneri P, Mariani L, et al. RET/NTRK1 rearrangements in thyroid gland tumors of the papillary carcinoma family: correlation with clinicopathological features. *Clin Cancer Res.* 1998;4:223–228.

177. Musholt TJ, Musholt PB, Khaladj N, et al. Prognostic significance of RET and NTRK1 rearrangements in sporadic papillary thyroid carcinoma. *Surgery.* 2000;128:984–993.

178. Beimfohr C, Klugbauer S, Demidchik EP, et al. NTRK1 re-arrangement in papillary thyroid carcinomas of children after the Chernobyl reactor accident. *Int J Cancer.* 1999;80:842–847.

179. French CA, Alexander EK, Cibas ES, et al. Genetic and biological subgroups of low-stage follicular thyroid cancer. *Am J Pathol.* 2003;162:1053–1060.

180. Castro P, Rebocho AP, Soares RJ, et al. PAX8-PPARgamma rearrangement is frequently detected in the follicular variant of papillary thyroid carcinoma. *J Clin Endocrinol Metab.* 2006;91:213–220.

181. Hou P, Liu D, Shan Y, et al. Genetic alterations and their relationship in the phosphatidylinositol 3-kinase/Akt pathway in thyroid cancer. *Clin Cancer Res.* 2007;13:1161–1170.

182. Wu G, Mambo E, Guo Z, et al. Uncommon mutation, but common amplifications, of the PIK3CA gene in thyroid tumors. *J Clin Endocrinol Metab.* 2005;90:4688–4693.

183. Dahia PL, Marsh DJ, Zheng Z, et al. Somatic deletions and mutations in the Cowden disease gene, PTEN, in sporadic thyroid tumors. *Cancer Res.* 1997;57:4710–4713.

184. Maximo V, Sobrinho-Simoes M. Hurthle cell tumours of the thyroid. A review with emphasis on mitochondrial abnormalities with clinical relevance. *Virchows Arch.* 2000;437:107–115.

185. Tallini G. Oncocytic tumours. *Virchows Arch.* 1998;433:5–12.

186. Katoh R, Harach HR, Williams ED. Solitary, multiple, and familial oxyphil tumours of the thyroid gland. *J Pathol.* 1998;186:292–299.

187. Maximo V, Botelho T, Capela J, et al. Somatic and germline mutation in GRIM-19, a dual function gene involved in mitochondrial metabolism and cell death, is linked to mitochondrion-rich (Hurthle cell) tumours of the thyroid. *Br J Cancer.* 2005;92:1892–1898.

188. Cheung CC, Ezzat S, Ramyar L, et al. Molecular basis off Hurthle cell papillary thyroid carcinoma. *J Clin Endocrinol Metab.* 2000;85:878–882.

189. Chiappetta G, Toti P, Cetta F, et al. The RET/PTC oncogene is frequently activated in oncocytic thyroid tumors (Hurthle cell adenomas and carcinomas), but not in oncocytic hyperplastic lesions. *J Clin Endocrinol Metab.* 2002;87:364–369.

190. Musholt PB, Imkamp F, von Wasielewski R, et al. RET rearrangements in archival oxyphilic thyroid tumors: new insights in tumorigenesis and classification of Hurthle cell carcinomas? *Surgery.* 2003;134:881–889; discussion 889.

191. Chevillard S, Ugolin N, Vielh P, et al. Gene expression profiling of differentiated thyroid neoplasms: diagnostic and clinical implications. *Clin Cancer Res.* 2004;10:6586–6597.

192. Finley DJ, Arora N, Zhu B, et al. Molecular profiling distinguishes papillary carcinoma from benign thyroid nodules. *J Clin Endocrinol Metab.* 2004;89:3214–3223.

193. Huang Y, Prasad M, Lemon WJ, et al. Gene expression in papillary thyroid carcinoma reveals highly consistent profiles. *Proc Natl Acad Sci U S A.* 2001;98:15044–15049.

194. Giordano TJ, Kuick R, Thomas DG, et al. Molecular classification of papillary thyroid carcinoma: distinct BRAF, RAS, and RET/PTC mutation-specific gene expression profiles discovered by DNA microarray analysis. *Oncogene.* 2005;24:6646–6656.

195. Frattini M, Ferrario C, Bressan P, et al. Alternative mutations of BRAF, RET and NTRK1 are associated with similar but distinct gene expression patterns in papillary thyroid cancer. *Oncogene.* 2004;23:7436–7440.

196. Bartel DP. MicroRNAs: genomics, biogenesis, mechanism, and function. *Cell.* 2004;116:281–297.

197. Ambros V. The functions of animal microRNAs. *Nature.* 2004;431:350–355.

198. Nikiforova MN, Tseng GC, Steward D, et al. MicroRNA expression profiling of thyroid tumors: biological significance and diagnostic utility. *J Clin Endocrinol Metab.* 2008;93:1600–1608.

199. Pallante P, Visone R, Ferracin M, et al. MicroRNA deregulation in human thyroid papillary carcinomas. *Endocr Relat Cancer.* 2006;13:497–508.

200. He H, Jazdzewski K, Li W, et al. The role of microRNA genes in papillary thyroid carcinoma. *Proc Natl Acad Sci U S A.* 2005;102:19075–19080.

201. Jazdzewski K, Boguslawska J, Jendrzejewski J, et al. Thyroid hormone receptor beta (THRB) is a major target gene for microRNAs deregulated in papillary thyroid carcinoma (PTC). *J Clin Endocrinol Metab;*96:E546–E553.

202. Visone R, Russo L, Pallante P, et al. MicroRNAs (miR)-221 and miR-222, both overexpressed in human thyroid papillary carcinomas, regulate p27Kip1 protein levels and cell cycle. *Endocr Relat Cancer.* 2007;14:791–798.

203. Tetzlaff MT, Liu A, Xu X, et al. Differential expression of miRNAs in papillary thyroid carcinoma compared to multinodular goiter using formalin fixed paraffin embedded tissues. *Endocr Pathol.* 2007;18:163–173.

204. Nikiforova MN, Chiosea SI, Nikiforov YE. MicroRNA expression profiles in thyroid tumors. *Endocr Pathol.* 2009;20:85–91.

205. Yip L, Kelly L, Shuai Y, et al. MicroRNA signature distinguishes the degree of aggressiveness of papillary thyroid carcinoma. *Ann Surg Oncol.* 2011;18:2035–2041.

206. Chou CK, Chen RF, Chou FF, et al. miR-146b is highly expressed in adult papillary thyroid carcinomas with high risk features including extrathyroidal invasion and the BRAF(V600E) mutation. *Thyroid*;20:489–494.

207. Kim TS, Asato R, Akamizu T, et al. A rare case of hyperfunctioning papillary carcinoma of the thyroid gland. *Acta Otolaryngol Suppl.* 2007:55–57.

208. Solbiati L, Cioffi V, Ballarati E. Ultrasonography of the neck. *Radiol Clin North Am.* 1992;30:941–954.

209. Ahuja AT, Ying M, Yuen HY, et al. Power Doppler sonography of metastatic nodes from papillary carcinoma of the thyroid. *Clin Radiol.* 2001;56:284–288.

210. Hwang J, Shin JH, Han BK, et al. Papillary thyroid carcinoma with BRAFV600E mutation: sonographic prediction. *AJR Am J Roentgenol*;194:W425–W430.

211. Hay ID. Papillary thyroid carcinoma. *Endocrinol Metab Clin North Am.* 1990;19:545–576.

212. Mazzaferri EL, Kloos RT. Clinical review 128: current approaches to primary therapy for papillary and follicular thyroid cancer. *J Clin Endocrinol Metab.* 2001;86:1447–1463.

213. Carcangiu ML, Zampi G, Pupi A, et al. Papillary carcinoma of the thyroid. A clinicopathologic study of 241 cases treated at the University of Florence, Italy. *Cancer.* 1985;55:805–828.

214. Kirillov VA, Yuschenko YP, Paplevka AA, et al. Thyroid carcinoma diagnosis based on a set of karyometric parameters of follicular cells. *Cancer.* 2001;92:1818–1827.

215. Rout P, Shariff S. Diagnostic value of qualitative and quantitative variables in thyroid lesions. *Cytopathology.* 1999;10:171–179.

216. Rosai J, Carcangiu ML, DeLellis RA. *Tumors of the Thyroid Gland.* 3rd ed. Washington, DC: Armed Forces Institute of Pathology; 1992.

217. Hapke MR, Dehner LP. The optically clear nucleus. A reliable sign of papillary carcinoma of the thyroid? *Am J Surg Pathol.* 1979;3:31–38.

218. Hawk WA, Hazard JB. The many appearances of papillary carcinoma of the thyroid. *Cleve Clin Q.* 1976;43:207–215.

219. Echeverria OM, Hernandez-Pando R, Vazquez-Nin GH. Ultrastructural, cytochemical, and immunocytochemical study of nuclei and cytoskeleton of thyroid papillary carcinoma cells. *Ultrastruct Pathol.* 1998;22:185–197.

220. Sobrinho-Simoes MA, Goncalves V. Nucleolar abnormalities in human papillary thyroid carcinomas. *Arch Pathol Lab Med.* 1978;102:635–638.

221. Chan JK, Saw D. The grooved nucleus: A useful diagnostic criterion of papillary carcinoma of the thyroid. *Am J Surg Pathol.* 1986;10:672–679.

222. Albores-Saavedra J, Altamirano-Dimas M, Alcorta-Anguizola B, et al. Fine structure of human papillary thyroid carcinoma. *Cancer.* 1971;28:763–774.

223. Gould VE, Gould NS, Benditt EP. Ultrastructural aspects of papillary and sclerosing carcinoma of the thyroid. *Cancer.* 1972;29:1613–1625.

224. Chan JK. Papillary carcinoma of thyroid: classical and variants. *Histol Histopathol.* 1990;5:241–257.

225. Ip YT, Dias Filho MA, Chan JK. Nuclear inclusions and pseudoinclusions: friends or foes of the surgical pathologist? *Int J Surg Pathol*;18:465–481.

226. Oyama T. A histopathological, immunohistochemical and ultrastructural study of intranuclear cytoplasmic inclusions in thyroid papillary carcinoma. *Virchows Arch A Pathol Anat Histopathol.* 1989;414:91–104.

227. Chan JK. Strict criteria should be applied in the diagnosis of encapsulated follicular variant of papillary thyroid carcinoma. *Am J Clin Pathol.* 2002;117:16–18.

228. Rosai J, Carcangiu ML. Pitfalls in the diagnosis of thyroid neoplasms. *Pathol Res Pract.* 1987;182:169–179.

229. Vickery AL, Jr., Carcangiu ML, Johannessen JV, et al. Papillary carcinoma. *Semin Diagn Pathol.* 1985;2:90–100.

230. Johannessen JV, Sobrinho-Simoes M. The origin and significance of thyroid psammoma bodies. *Lab Invest.* 1980;43:287–296.

231. Klinck GH, Winship T. Psammoma bodies and thyroid cancer. *Cancer.* 1959;12:656–662.

232. Tunio GM, Hirota S, Nomura S, et al. Possible relation of osteopontin to development of psammoma bodies in human papillary thyroid cancer. *Arch Pathol Lab Med.* 1998;122:1087–1090.

233. Fiorella RM, Isley W, Miller LK, et al. Multinodular goiter of the thyroid mimicking malignancy: diagnostic pitfalls in fine-needle aspiration biopsy. *Diagn Cytopathol.* 1993;9:351–355; discussion 355–357.

234. Hunt JL, Barnes EL. Non-tumor-associated psammoma bodies in the thyroid. *Am J Clin Pathol.* 2003;119:90–94.

235. Isarangkul W. Dense fibrosis. Another diagnostic criterion for papillary thyroid carcinoma. *Arch Pathol Lab Med.* 1993;117:645–646.

236. Rosai J, Zampi G, Carcangiu ML. Papillary carcinoma of the thyroid. A discussion of its several morphologic expressions, with particular emphasis on the follicular variant. *Am J Surg Pathol.* 1983;7:809–817.

237. Park SH, Suh EH, Chi JG. A histopathologic study on 1,095 surgically resected thyroid specimens. *Jpn J Clin Oncol.* 1988;18:297–302.

238. Lee TK, Myers RT, Marshall RB, et al. The significance of mitotic rate: a retrospective study of 127 thyroid carcinomas. *Hum Pathol.* 1985;16:1042–1046.

239. Akslen LA, LiVolsi VA. Prognostic significance of histologic grading compared with subclassification of papillary thyroid carcinoma. *Cancer.* 2000;88:1902–1908.

240. Kebebew E, Weng J, Bauer J, et al. The prevalence and prognostic value of BRAF mutation in thyroid cancer. *Ann Surg.* 2007;246:466–470; discussion 470–461.

241. Iida F, Yonekura M, Miyakawa M. Study of intraglandular dissemination of thyroid cancer. *Cancer.* 1969;24:764–771.

242. Katoh R, Sasaki J, Kurihara H, et al. Multiple thyroid involvement (intraglandular metastasis) in papillary thyroid carcinoma. A clinicopathologic study of 105 consecutive patients. *Cancer.* 1992;70:1585–1590.

243. Falvo L, Catania A, D'Andrea V, et al. Prognostic importance of histologic vascular invasion in papillary thyroid carcinoma. *Ann Surg.* 2005;241:640–646.

244. Gardner RE, Tuttle RM, Burman KD, et al. Prognostic importance of vascular invasion in papillary thyroid carcinoma. *Arch Otolaryngol Head Neck Surg.* 2000;126:309–312.

245. Mete O, Asa SL. Pathological definition and clinical significance of vascular invasion in thyroid carcinomas of follicular epithelial derivation. *Mod Pathol.* 2011;12:1545–1552.

246. Edge SB, Byrd DR, Compton CC, et al. e. *AJCC Cancer Staging Manual, Seventh Edition.* 7th ed. New York, NY: Springer; 2010.

247. Ito Y, Tomoda C, Uruno T, et al. Prognostic significance of extrathyroid extension of papillary thyroid carcinoma: massive but not minimal extension affects the relapse-free survival. *World J Surg.* 2006;30:780–786.

248. Rivera M, Ricarte-Filho J, Tuttle RM, et al. Molecular, morphologic, and outcome analysis of thyroid carcinomas according to degree of extrathyroid extension. *Thyroid.* 2010;20:1085–1093.

249. Mazzaferri EL, Jhiang SM. Long-term impact of initial surgical and medical therapy on papillary and follicular thyroid cancer. *Am J Med.* 1994;97:418–428.

250. Carcangiu ML, Zampi G, Rosai J. Papillary thyroid carcinoma: a study of its many morphologic expressions and clinical correlates. *Pathol Annu.* 1985;20(pt 1):1–44.

251. Yamashita H, Noguchi S, Murakami N, et al. Extracapsular invasion of lymph node metastasis is an indicator of distant metastasis and poor prognosis in patients with thyroid papillary carcinoma. *Cancer.* 1997;80:2268–2272.

252. Hoie J, Stenwig AE, Kullmann G, et al. Distant metastases in papillary thyroid cancer. A review of 91 patients. *Cancer.* 1988;61:1–6.

253. Dinneen SF, Valimaki MJ, Bergstralh EJ, et al. Distant metastases in papillary thyroid carcinoma: 100 cases observed at one institution during 5 decades. *J Clin Endocrinol Metab.* 1995;80:2041–2045.

254. Xu YH, Song HJ, Qiu ZL, et al. Brain metastases with exceptional features from papillary thyroid carcinoma: report of three cases. *Hell J Nucl Med.* 2011;14:56–59.

255. Volante M, Collini P, Nikiforov YE, et al. Poorly differentiated thyroid carcinoma: the Turin proposal for the use of uniform diagnostic criteria and an algorithmic diagnostic approach. *Am J Surg Pathol.* 2007;31:1256–1264.

256. DeLellis RA, Lloyd RV, Heitz PU, et al, eds. *World Health Organization Classification of Tumours. Pathology and Genetics of Tumours of Endocrine Organs.* Lyon, France: IARC Press; 2004.

257. Fink A, Tomlinson G, Freeman JL, et al. Occult micropapillary carcinoma associated with benign follicular thyroid disease and unrelated thyroid neoplasms. *Mod Pathol.* 1996;9:816–820.

258. Pelizzo MR, Piotto A, Rubello D, et al. High prevalence of occult papillary thyroid carcinoma in a surgical series for benign thyroid disease. *Tumori.* 1990;76:255–257.

259. Yamashita H, Nakayama I, Noguchi S, et al. Thyroid carcinoma in benign thyroid diseases. An analysis from minute carcinoma. *Acta Pathol Jpn.* 1985;35:781–788.

260. Roti E, Rossi R, Trasforini G, et al. Clinical and histological characteristics of papillary thyroid microcarcinoma: results of a retrospective study in 243 patients. *J Clin Endocrinol Metab.* 2006;91:2171–2178.

261. Bondeson L, Ljungberg O. Occult papillary thyroid carcinoma in the young and the aged. *Cancer.* 1984;53:1790–1792.

262. Fukunaga FH, Yatani R. Geographic pathology of occult thyroid carcinomas. *Cancer.* 1975;36:1095–1099.

263. Neuhold N, Kaiser H, Kaserer K. Latent carcinoma of the thyroid in Austria: a systematic autopsy study. *Endocr Pathol.* 2001;12:23–31.

264. Sampson RJ, Woolner LB, Bahn RC, et al. Occult thyroid carcinoma in Olmsted County, Minnesota: prevalence at autopsy compared with that in Hiroshima and Nagasaki, Japan. *Cancer.* 1974;34:2072–2076.

265. Sobrinho-Simoes MA, Sambade MC, Goncalves V. Latent thyroid carcinoma at autopsy: a study from Oporto, Portugal. *Cancer.* 1979;43:1702–1706.

266. Mazzaferri EL. Management of low-risk differentiated thyroid cancer. *Endocr Pract.* 2007;13:498–512.

267. Rassael H, Thompson LD, Heffess CS. A rationale for conservative management of microscopic papillary carcinoma of the thyroid gland: a clinicopathologic correlation of 90 cases. *Eur Arch Otorhinolaryngol.* 1998;255:462–467.

268. Chow SM, Law SC, Chan JK, et al. Papillary microcarcinoma of the thyroid—prognostic significance of lymph node metastasis and multifocality. *Cancer.* 2003;98:31–40.

269. Roti E, degli Uberti EC, Bondanelli M, et al. Thyroid papillary microcarcinoma: a descriptive and meta-analysis study. *Eur J Endocrinol.* 2008;159:659–673.

270. Baudin E, Travagli JP, Ropers J, et al. Microcarcinoma of the thyroid gland: the Gustave-Roussy Institute experience. *Cancer.* 1998;83:553–559.

271. Frasca F, Nucera C, Pellegriti G, et al. BRAF(V600E) mutation and the biology of papillary thyroid cancer. *Endocr Relat Cancer.* 2008;15:191–205.

272. Kwak JY, Kim EK, Chung WY, et al. Association of BRAFV600E mutation with poor clinical prognostic factors and US features in Korean patients with papillary thyroid microcarcinoma. *Radiology.* 2009;253:854–860.

273. Lee X, Gao M, Ji Y, et al. Analysis of differential BRAF(V600E) mutational status in high aggressive papillary thyroid microcarcinoma. *Ann Surg Oncol.* 2009;16:240–245.

274. Lin KL, Wang OC, Zhang XH, et al. The BRAF mutation is predictive of aggressive clinicopathological characteristics in papillary thyroid microcarcinoma. *Ann Surg Oncol.* 2010; 17:3294–3300.

275. Niemeier LA, Akatsu HK, Song C, et al. A combined molecular-pathological score improves risk stratification of thyroid papillary microcarcinoma. *Cancer.* (in press).

276. Lam AK, Lo CY, Lam KS. Papillary carcinoma of thyroid: a 30-yr clinicopathological review of the histological variants. *Endocr Pathol.* 2005;16:323–330.

277. Lindsay S. *Carcinoma of the Thyroid Gland: A Clinical and Pathologic Study of 293 Patients at the University of California Hospital.* Springfield, IL: Charles C Thomas; 1960.

278. Chen KT, Rosai J. Follicular variant of thyroid papillary carcinoma: a clinicopathologic study of six cases. *Am J Surg Pathol.* 1977;1:123–130.

279. Perissel B, Coupier I, De Latour M, et al. Structural and numerical aberrations of chromosome 22 in a case of follicular variant of papillary thyroid carcinoma revealed by conventional and molecular cytogenetics. *Cancer Genet Cytogenet.* 2000;121:33–37.

280. Tielens ET, Sherman SI, Hruban RH, et al. Follicular variant of papillary thyroid carcinoma. A clinicopathologic study. *Cancer.* 1994;73:424–431.

281. Jain M, Khan A, Patwardhan N, et al. Follicular variant of papillary thyroid carcinoma: a comparative study of histopathologic features and cytology results in 141 patients. *Endocr Pract.* 2001;7:79–84.

282. Proietti A, Giannini R, Ugolini C, et al. BRAF status of follicular variant of papillary thyroid carcinoma and its relationship to its clinical and cytological features. *Thyroid.* 2010;20:1263–1270.

283. Tickoo SK, Pittas AG, Adler M, et al. Bone metastases from thyroid carcinoma: a histopathologic study with clinical correlates. *Arch Pathol Lab Med.* 2000;124:1440–1447.

284. Baloch ZW, LiVolsi VA. Encapsulated follicular variant of papillary thyroid carcinoma with bone metastases. *Mod Pathol.* 2000;13:861–865.

285. Smallridge RC, Castro MR, Morris JC, et al. Renal metastases from thyroid papillary carcinoma: study of sodium iodide symporter expression. *Thyroid.* 2001;11:795–804.

286. Loureiro MM, Leite VH, Boavida JM, et al. An unusual case of papillary carcinoma of the thyroid with cutaneous and breast metastases only. *Eur J Endocrinol.* 1997;137:267–269.

287. LiVolsi VA, Baloch ZW. Follicular neoplasms of the thyroid: view, biases, and experiences. *Adv Anat Pathol.* 2004;11:279–287.

288. Liu J, Singh B, Tallini G, et al. Follicular variant of papillary thyroid carcinoma: a clinicopathologic study of a problematic entity. *Cancer.* 2006;107:1255–1264.

289. Lloyd RV, Erickson LA, Casey MB, et al. Observer variation in the diagnosis of follicular variant of papillary thyroid carcinoma. *Am J Surg Pathol.* 2004;28:1336–1340.

290. Elsheikh TM, Asa SL, Chan JK, et al. Interobserver and intraobserver variation among experts in the diagnosis of thyroid follicular lesions with borderline nuclear features of papillary carcinoma. *Am J Clin Pathol.* 2008;130:736–744.

291. Wallander M, Layfield LJ, Jarboe E, et al. Follicular variant of papillary carcinoma: reproducibility of histologic diagnosis and utility of HBME-1 immunohistochemistry and BRAF mutational analysis as diagnostic adjuncts. *Appl Immunohistochem Mol Morphol.* 2010;18:231–235.

292. Piana S, Frasoldati A, Di Felice E, et al. Encapsulated well-differentiated follicular-patterned thyroid carcinomas do not play a significant role in the fatality rates from thyroid carcinoma. *Am J Surg Pathol.* 2010;34:868–872.

293. Hunt JL, Dacic S, Barnes EL, et al. Encapsulated follicular variant of papillary thyroid carcinoma. *Am J Clin Pathol.* 2002;118:602–603; author reply 605–606.

294. Rivera M, Ricarte-Filho J, Patel S, et al. Encapsulated thyroid tumors of follicular cell origin with high grade features (high mitotic rate/tumor necrosis): a clinicopathologic and molecular study. *Hum Pathol.* 2010;41:172–180.

295. Williams ED. Guest editorial: two proposals regarding the terminology of thyroid tumors. *Int J Surg Pathol.* 2000;8:181–183.

296. Sobrinho-Simoes M, Soares J, Carneiro F, et al. Diffuse follicular variant of papillary carcinoma of the thyroid: report of eight cases of a distinct aggressive type of thyroid tumor. *Surg Pathol.* 1990;3:189–203.

297. Ivanova R, Soares P, Castro P, et al. Diffuse (or multinodular) follicular variant of papillary thyroid carcinoma: a clinicopathologic and immunohistochemical analysis of ten cases of an aggressive form of differentiated thyroid carcinoma. *Virchows Arch.* 2002;440:418–424.

298. Albores-Saavedra J, Gould E, Vardaman C, et al. The macrofollicular variant of papillary thyroid carcinoma: a study of 17 cases. *Hum Pathol.* 1991;22:1195–1205.

299. Albores-Saavedra J, Housini I, Vuitch F, et al. Macrofollicular variant of papillary thyroid carcinoma with minor insular component. *Cancer.* 1997;80:1110–1116.

300. Cardenas MG, Kini S, Wisgerhof M. Two patients with highly aggressive macrofollicular variant of papillary thyroid carcinoma. *Thyroid.* 2009;19:413–416.

301. Chung D, Ghossein RA, Lin O. Macrofollicular variant of papillary carcinoma: a potential thyroid FNA pitfall. *Diagn Cytopathol.* 2007;35:560–564.

302. Fadda G, Fiorino MC, Mule A, et al. Macrofollicular encapsulated variant of papillary thyroid carcinoma as a potential pitfall in histologic and cytologic diagnosis. A report of three cases. *Acta Cytol.* 2002;46:555–559.

303. Mesonero CE, Jugle JE, Wilbur DC, et al. Fine-needle aspiration of the macrofollicular and microfollicular subtypes of the follicular variant of papillary carcinoma of the thyroid. *Cancer.* 1998;84:235–244.

304. Gamboa-Dominguez A, Vieitez-Martinez I, Barredo-Prieto BA, et al. Macrofollicular variant of papillary thyroid carcinoma: a case and control analysis. *Endocr Pathol.* 1996;7:303–308.

305. Ito Y, Hirokawa M, Fukushima M, et al. Prevalence and prognostic significance of poor differentiation and tall cell variant in papillary carcinoma in Japan. *World J Surg.* 2008;32:1535–1543.

306. Michels JJ, Jacques M, Henry-Amar M, et al. Prevalence and prognostic significance of tall cell variant of papillary thyroid carcinoma. *Hum Pathol.* 2007;38:212–219.

307. Ruter A, Dreifus J, Jones M, et al. Overexpression of p53 in tall cell variants of papillary thyroid carcinoma. *Surgery.* 1996;120:1046–1050.

308. Sobrinho-Simoes MA, Nesland JM, Holm R, et al. Hurthle cell and mitochondrion-rich papillary carcinomas of the thyroid gland: an ultrastructural and immunocytochemical study. *Ultrastruct Pathol.* 1985;8:131–142.

309. Moreno Egea A, Rodriguez Gonzalez JM, Sola Perez J, et al. Prognostic value of the tall cell variety of papillary cancer of the thyroid. *Eur J Surg Oncol.* 1993;19:517–521.

310. Ostrowski ML, Merino MJ. Tall cell variant of papillary thyroid carcinoma: a reassessment and immunohistochemical study with comparison to the usual type of papillary carcinoma of the thyroid. *Am J Surg Pathol.* 1996;20:964–974.

311. Leung AK, Chow SM, Law SC. Clinical features and outcome of the tall cell variant of papillary thyroid carcinoma. *Laryngoscope.* 2008;118:32–38.

312. Johnson TL, Lloyd RV, Thompson NW, et al. Prognostic implications of the tall cell variant of papillary thyroid carcinoma. *Am J Surg Pathol.* 1988;12:22–27.

313. Ghossein RA, Leboeuf R, Patel KN, et al. Tall cell variant of papillary thyroid carcinoma without extrathyroid extension: biologic behavior and clinical implications. *Thyroid.* 2007;17:655–661.

314. Morris LG, Shaha AR, Tuttle RM, et al. Tall-cell variant of papillary thyroid carcinoma: a matched-pair analysis of survival. *Thyroid.* 2010;20:153–158.

315. Bronner MP, LiVolsi VA. Spindle cell squamous carcinoma of the thyroid: an unusual anaplastic tumor associated with tall cell papillary cancer. *Mod Pathol.* 1991;4:637–643.

316. LiVolsi VA. Papillary thyroid carcinoma: an update. *Mod Pathol.* 2011;24 (suppl 2):S1–S9.

317. LiVolsi VA. Papillary carcinoma tall cell variant (TCV): a review. *Endocr Pathol.* 2010;21:12–15.

318. Nikiforov YE, Erickson LA, Nikiforova MN, et al. Solid variant of papillary thyroid carcinoma: incidence, clinical-pathologic characteristics, molecular analysis, and biologic behavior. *Am J Surg Pathol.* 2001;25:1478–1484.

319. Tronko MD, Bogdanova TI, Komissarenko IV, et al. Thyroid carcinoma in children and adolescents in Ukraine after the Chernobyl nuclear accident: statistical data and clinicomorphologic characteristics. *Cancer.* 1999;86:149–156.

320. Mizukami Y, Noguchi M, Michigishi T, et al. Papillary thyroid carcinoma in Kanazawa, Japan: prognostic significance of histological subtypes. *Histopathology.* 1992;20:243–250.

321. Fukushima M, Ito Y, Hirokawa M, et al. Clinicopathologic characteristics and prognosis of diffuse sclerosing variant of papillary thyroid carcinoma in Japan: an 18-year experience at a single institution. *World J Surg.* 2009;33:958–962.

322. Koo JS, Shin E, Hong SW. Immunohistochemical characteristics of diffuse sclerosing variant of papillary carcinoma: comparison with conventional papillary carcinoma. *Apmis.* 2010;118:744–752.

323. Carcangiu ML, Bianchi S. Diffuse sclerosing variant of papillary thyroid carcinoma. Clinicopathologic study of 15 cases. *Am J Surg Pathol.* 1989;13:1041–1049.

324. Fujimoto Y, Obara T, Ito Y, et al. Diffuse sclerosing variant of papillary carcinoma of the thyroid. Clinical importance, surgical treatment, and follow-up study. *Cancer.* 1990;66:2306–2312.

325. Lam AK, Lo CY. Diffuse sclerosing variant of papillary carcinoma of the thyroid: a 35-year comparative study at a single institution. *Ann Surg Oncol.* 2006;13:176–181.

326. Soares J, Limbert E, Sobrinho-Simoes M. Diffuse sclerosing variant of papillary thyroid carcinoma. A clinicopathologic study of 10 cases. *Pathol Res Pract.* 1989;185:200–206.

327. Thompson LD, Wieneke JA, Heffess CS. Diffuse sclerosing variant of papillary thyroid carcinoma: a clinicopathologic and immunophenotypic analysis of 22 cases. *Endocr Pathol.* 2005;16:331–348.

328. Sheu SY, Schwertheim S, Worm K, et al. Diffuse sclerosing variant of papillary thyroid carcinoma: lack of BRAF mutation but occurrence of RET/PTC rearrangements. *Mod Pathol.* 2007;20:779–787.

329. Koo JS, Hong S, Park CS. Diffuse sclerosing variant is a major subtype of papillary thyroid carcinoma in the young. *Thyroid.* 2009;19:1225–1231.

330. Regalbuto C, Malandrino P, Tumminia A, et al. A diffuse sclerosing variant of papillary thyroid carcinoma: clinical and pathologic features and outcomes of 34 consecutive cases. *Thyroid.* 2011;21:383–389.

331. Evans HL. Columnar-cell carcinoma of the thyroid. A report of two cases of an aggressive variant of thyroid carcinoma. *Am J Clin Pathol.* 1986;85:77–80.

332. Chen JH, Faquin WC, Lloyd RV, et al. Clinicopathological and molecular characterization of nine cases of columnar cell variant of papillary thyroid carcinoma. *Mod Pathol.* 2011;24:739–749.

333. LiVolsi VA. *Surgical Pathology of the Thyroid.* Philadelphia, PA: WB Saunders; 1990.

334. Ferreiro JA, Hay ID, Lloyd RV. Columnar cell carcinoma of the thyroid: report of three additional cases. *Hum Pathol.* 1996;27:1156–1160.

335. Wenig BM, Thompson LD, Adair CF, et al. Thyroid papillary carcinoma of columnar cell type: a clinicopathologic study of 16 cases. *Cancer.* 1998;82:740–753.

336. Akslen LA, Varhaug JE. Thyroid carcinoma with mixed tall-cell and columnar-cell features. *Am J Clin Pathol.* 1990;94:442–445.

337. Putti TC, Bhuiya TA. Mixed columnar cell and tall cell variant of papillary carcinoma of thyroid: a case report and review of the literature. *Pathology.* 2000;32:286–289.

338. Evans HL. Encapsulated columnar-cell neoplasms of the thyroid. A report of four cases suggesting a favorable prognosis. *Am J Surg Pathol.* 1996;20:1205–1211.

339. Berho M, Suster S. The oncocytic variant of papillary carcinoma of the thyroid: a clinicopathologic study of 15 cases. *Hum Pathol.* 1997;28:47–53.

340. Herrera MF, Hay ID, Wu PS, et al. Hurthle cell (oxyphilic) papillary thyroid carcinoma: a variant with more aggressive biologic behavior. *World J Surg.* 1992;16:669–674; discussion 774–665.

341. Beckner ME, Heffess CS, Oertel JE. Oxyphilic papillary thyroid carcinomas. *Am J Clin Pathol.* 1995;103:280–287.

342. Gross M, Eliashar R, Ben-Yaakov A, et al. Clinicopathologic features and outcome of the oncocytic variant of papillary thyroid carcinoma. *Ann Otol Rhinol Laryngol.* 2009;118:374–381.

343. Trovisco V, Soares P, Preto A, et al. Type and prevalence of BRAF mutations are closely associated with papillary thyroid carcinoma histotype and patients' age but not with tumour aggressiveness. *Virchows Arch.* 2005;446;589–595.

344. Apel RL, Asa SL, LiVolsi VA. Papillary Hurthle cell carcinoma with lymphocytic stroma. "Warthin-like tumor" of the thyroid. *Am J Surg Pathol.* 1995;19:810–814.

345. Baloch ZW, LiVolsi VA. Warthin-like papillary carcinoma of the thyroid. *Arch Pathol Lab Med.* 2000;124:1192–1195.

346. Ludvikova M, Ryska A, Korabecna M, et al. Oncocytic papillary carcinoma with lymphoid stroma (Warthin-like tumour) of the thyroid: a distinct entity with favourable prognosis. *Histopathology.* 2001;39:17–24.

347. Amico P, Lanzafame S, Li Destri G, et al. Warthin tumor-like papillary thyroid carcinoma with a minor dedifferentiated component: report of a case with clinicopathologic considerations. *Case Report Med.* 2010;2010:495281.

348. Schroder S, Bocker W. Clear-cell carcinomas of thyroid gland: a clinicopathological study of 13 cases. *Histopathology.* 1986;10:75–89.

349. Harach HR, Williams GT, Williams ED. Familial adenomatous polyposis associated thyroid carcinoma: a distinct type of follicular cell neoplasm. *Histopathology.* 1994;25:549–561.

350. Cameselle-Teijeiro J, Chan JK. Cribriform-morular variant of papillary carcinoma: a distinctive variant representing the sporadic counterpart of familial adenomatous polyposis-associated thyroid carcinoma? *Mod Pathol.* 1999;12:400–411.

351. Perrier ND, van Heerden JA, Goellner JR, et al. Thyroid cancer in patients with familial adenomatous polyposis. *World J Surg.* 1998;22:738–742; discussion 743.

352. Tomoda C, Miyauchi A, Uruno T, et al. Cribriform-morular variant of papillary thyroid carcinoma: clue to early detection of familial adenomatous polyposis-associated colon cancer. *World J Surg.* 2004;28:886–889.

353. Hirokawa M, Maekawa M, Kuma S, et al. Cribriform-morular variant of papillary thyroid carcinoma—cytological and immunocytochemical findings of 18 cases. *Diagn Cytopathol.* 2010;38:890–896.

354. Cetta F, Montalto G, Gori M, et al. Germline mutations of the APC gene in patients with familial adenomatous polyposis-associated thyroid carcinoma: results from a European cooperative study. *J Clin Endocrinol Metab.* 2000;85:286–292.

355. Cameselle-Teijeiro J, Ruiz-Ponte C, Loidi L, et al. Somatic but not germline mutation of the APC gene in a case of cribriform-morular variant of papillary thyroid carcinoma. *Am J Clin Pathol.* 2001;115:486–493.

356. Xu B, Yoshimoto K, Miyauchi A, et al. Cribriform-morular variant of papillary thyroid carcinoma: a pathological and molecular genetic study with evidence of frequent somatic mutations in exon 3 of the beta-catenin gene. *J Pathol.* 2003;199:58–67.

357. Kameyama K, Mukai M, Takami H, et al. Cribriform-morular variant of papillary thyroid carcinoma: ultrastructural study and somatic/germline mutation analysis of the APC gene. *Ultrastruct Pathol.* 2004;28:97–102.

358. Jung CK, Choi YJ, Lee KY, et al. The cytological, clinical, and pathological features of the cribriform-morular variant of papillary thyroid carcinoma and mutation analysis of CTNNB1 and BRAF genes. *Thyroid.* 2009;19:905–913.

359. Schuetze D, Hoschar AP, Seethala RR, et al. The T1799A BRAF mutation is absent in cribriform-morular variant of papillary carcinoma. *Arch Pathol Lab Med.* 2009;133:803–805.

360. Ito Y, Miyauchi A, Ishikawa H, et al. Our experience of treatment of cribriform morular variant of papillary thyroid carcinoma; difference in clinicopathological features of FAP-associated and sporadic patients. *Endocr J.* 2011;58:685–689.

361. Koo JS, Jung W, Hong SW. Cytologic characteristics and beta-catenin immunocytochemistry on smear slide of cribriform-morular variant of papillary thyroid carcinoma. *Acta Cytol.* 2011;55:13–18.

362. Asioli S, Erickson LA, Sebo TJ, et al. Papillary thyroid carcinoma with prominent hobnail features: a new aggressive variant of moderately differentiated papillary carcinoma. A clinicopathologic, immunohistochemical, and molecular study of eight cases. *Am J Surg Pathol.* 2010;34:44–52.

363. Motosugi U, Murata S, Nagata K, et al. Thyroid papillary carcinoma with micropapillary and hobnail growth pattern: a histological variant with intermediate malignancy? *Thyroid.* 2009;19:535–537.

364. Chan JK, Carcangiu ML, Rosai J. Papillary carcinoma of thyroid with exuberant nodular fasciitis-like stroma. Report of three cases. *Am J Clin Pathol.* 1991;95:309–314.

365. Lee YS, Nam KH, Hong SW, et al. Papillary thyroid carcinoma with nodular fasciitis-like stroma. *Thyroid.* 2008;18:577–578.

366. Leal, II, Carneiro FP, Basilio-de-Oliveira CA, et al. Papillary carcinoma with nodular fasciitis-like stroma—a case report in pregnancy. *Diagn Cytopathol.* 2008;36:139–141.

367. Basu S, Nair N, Shet T, et al. Papillary thyroid carcinoma with exuberant nodular fasciitis-like stroma: treatment outcome and prognosis. *J Laryngol Otol.* 2006;120:338–342.

368. Yang YJ, LiVolsi VA, Khurana KK. Papillary thyroid carcinoma with nodular fasciitis-like stroma. Pitfalls in fine-needle aspiration cytology. *Arch Pathol Lab Med.* 1999;123:838–841.

369. Us-Krasovec M, Golouh R. Papillary thyroid carcinoma with exuberant nodular fasciitis-like stroma in a fine needle aspirate. A case report. *Acta Cytol.* 1999;43:1101–1104.

370. Toti P, Tanganelli P, Schurfeld K, et al. Scarring in papillary carcinoma of the thyroid: report of two new cases with exuberant nodular fasciitis-like stroma. *Histopathology.* 1999;35:418–422.

371. Terayama K, Toda S, Yonemitsu N, et al. Papillary carcinoma of the thyroid with exuberant nodular fasciitis-like stroma. *Virchows Arch.* 1997;431:291–295.

372. Michal M, Chlumska A, Fakan F. Papillary carcinoma of thyroid with exuberant nodular fasciitis-like stroma. *Histopathology.* 1992;21:577–579.

373. Schroder S, Bocker W, Dralle H, et al. The encapsulated papillary carcinoma of the thyroid. A morphologic subtype of the papillary thyroid carcinoma. *Cancer.* 1984;54:90–93.

374. Evans HL. Encapsulated papillary neoplasms of the thyroid. A study of 14 cases followed for a minimum of 10 years. *Am J Surg Pathol.* 1987;11:592–597.

375. Ito Y, Hirokawa M, Uruno T, et al. Biological behavior and prognosis of encapsulated papillary carcinoma of the thyroid: experience of a Japanese hospital for thyroid care. *World J Surg.* 2008;32:1789–1794.

376. Baloch ZW, Shafique K, Flannagan M, et al. Encapsulated classic and follicular variants of papillary thyroid carcinoma: comparative clinicopathologic study. *Endocr Pract.* 2010;16:952–959.

377. Gnepp DR, Ogorzalek JM, Heffess CS. Fat-containing lesions of the thyroid gland. *Am J Surg Pathol.* 1989;13:605–612.

378. Chan JK, Tse CC. Mucin production in metastatic papillary carcinoma of the thyroid. *Hum Pathol.* 1988;19:195–200.

379. Katoh R, Miyagi E, Nakamura N, et al. Expression of thyroid transcription factor-1 (TTF-1) in human C cells and medullary thyroid carcinomas. *Hum Pathol.* 2000;31:386–393.

380. Lau SK, Luthringer DJ, Eisen RN. Thyroid transcription factor-1: a review. *Appl Immunohistochem Mol Morphol.* 2002;10:97–102.

381. Nonaka D, Tang Y, Chiriboga L, et al. Diagnostic utility of thyroid transcription factors Pax8 and TTF-2 (FoxE1) in thyroid epithelial neoplasms. *Mod Pathol.* 2008;21:192–200.

382. Laury AR, Perets R, Piao H, et al. A comprehensive analysis of PAX8 expression in human epithelial tumors. *Am J Surg Pathol.* 2011;35:816–826.

383. Tacha D, Zhou D, Cheng L. Expression of PAX8 in normal and neoplastic tissues: a comprehensive immunohistochemical study. *Appl Immunohistochem Mol Morphol.* 2011;19:293–299.

384. Ozcan A, Shen SS, Hamilton C, et al. PAX 8 expression in non-neoplastic tissues, primary tumors, and metastatic tumors: a comprehensive immunohistochemical study. *Mod Pathol.* 2011;24:751–764.

385. Bejarano PA, Nikiforov YE, Swenson ES, et al. Thyroid transcription factor 1, thyroglobulin, cytokeratin 7, and cytokeratin 20 in thyroid neoplasms. *Appl Immunohistochem Mol Morphol.* 2000;8:189–194.

386. Wilson NW, Pambakian H, Richardson TC, et al. Epithelial markers in thyroid carcinoma: an immunoperoxidase study. *Histopathology.* 1986;10:815–829.

387. Bartolazzi A, Gasbarri A, Papotti M, et al. Application of an immunodiagnostic method for improving preoperative diagnosis of nodular thyroid lesions. *Lancet.* 2001;357:1644–1650.

388. Nakamura N, Erickson LA, Jin L, et al. Immunohistochemical separation of follicular variant of papillary thyroid carcinoma from follicular adenoma. *Endocr Pathol.* 2006;17:213–223.

389. Scognamiglio T, Hyjek E, Kao J, et al. Diagnostic usefulness of HBME1, galectin-3, CK19, and CITED1 and evaluation of their expression in encapsulated lesions with questionable features of papillary thyroid carcinoma. *Am J Clin Pathol.* 2006;126:700–708.

390. Saggiorato E, De Pompa R, Volante M, et al. Characterization of thyroid 'follicular neoplasms' in fine-needle aspiration cytological specimens using a panel of immunohistochemical markers: a proposal for clinical application. *Endocr Relat Cancer.* 2005;12:305–317.

391. Prasad ML, Pellegata NS, Huang Y, et al. Galectin-3, fibronectin-1, CITED-1, HBME1 and cytokeratin-19 immunohistochemistry is useful for the differential diagnosis of thyroid tumors. *Mod Pathol.* 2005;18:48–57.

392. Sack MJ, Astengo-Osuna C, Lin BT, et al. HBME-1 immunostaining in thyroid fine-needle aspirations: a useful marker in the diagnosis of carcinoma. *Mod Pathol.* 1997;10:668–674.

393. Miettinen M, Karkkainen P. Differential reactivity of HBME-1 and CD15 antibodies in benign and malignant thyroid tumours. Preferential reactivity with malignant tumours. *Virchows Arch.* 1996;429:213–219.

394. Torregrossa L, Faviana P, Camacci T, et al. Galectin-3 is highly expressed in nonencapsulated papillary thyroid carcinoma but weakly expressed in encapsulated type; comparison with Hector Battifora mesothelial cell 1 immunoreactivity. *Hum Pathol.* 2007;38:1482–1488.

395. Casey MB, Lohse CM, Lloyd RV. Distinction between papillary thyroid hyperplasia and papillary thyroid carcinoma by immunohistochemical staining for cytokeratin 19, galectin-3, and HBME-1. *Endocr Pathol.* 2003;14:55–60.

396. Schelfhout LJ, Van Muijen GN, Fleuren GJ. Expression of keratin 19 distinguishes papillary thyroid carcinoma from follicular carcinomas and follicular thyroid adenoma. *Am J Clin Pathol.* 1989;92:654–658.

397. Sahoo S, Hoda SA, Rosai J, et al. Cytokeratin 19 immunoreactivity in the diagnosis of papillary thyroid carcinoma: a note of caution. *Am J Clin Pathol.* 2001;116:696–702.

398. Cheung CC, Ezzat S, Freeman JL, et al. Immunohistochemical diagnosis of papillary thyroid carcinoma. *Mod Pathol.* 2001;14:338–342.

399. Barut F, Onak Kandemir N, Bektas S, et al. Universal markers of thyroid malignancies: galectin-3, HBME-1, and cytokeratin-19. *Endocr Pathol.* 2010;21:80–89.

400. Saad AG, Biddinger PW, Lloyd RV, et al. Thyroid tissue within cervical lymph nodes: benign thyroid inclusions or metastasis from occult thyroid cancer? *Mod Pathol.* 2005;18:94A.

401. Kjellman P, Wallin G, Hoog A, et al. MIB-1 index in thyroid tumors: a predictor of the clinical course in papillary thyroid carcinoma. *Thyroid.* 2003;13:371–380.

402. Asa SL. The role of immunohistochemical markers in the diagnosis of follicular-patterned lesions of the thyroid. *Endocr Pathol.* 2005;16:295–309.

403. Begum S, Rosenbaum E, Henrique R, et al. BRAF mutations in anaplastic thyroid carcinoma: implications for tumor origin, diagnosis and treatment. *Mod Pathol.* 2004;17:1359–1363.

404. Xing M, Westra WH, Tufano RP, et al. BRAF mutation predicts a poorer clinical prognosis for papillary thyroid cancer. *J Clin Endocrinol Metab.* 2005;90:6373–6379.

405. Kim TY, Kim WB, Rhee YS, et al. The BRAF mutation is useful for prediction of clinical recurrence in low-risk patients with conventional papillary thyroid carcinoma. *Clin Endocrinol (Oxf)*. 2006;65:364–368.
406. Xing M, Clark D, Guan H, et al. BRAF mutation testing of thyroid fine-needle aspiration biopsy specimens for preoperative risk stratification in papillary thyroid cancer. *J Clin Oncol*. 2009;27:2977–2982.
407. Elisei R, Ugolini C, Viola D, et al. BRAF(V600E) mutation and outcome of patients with papillary thyroid carcinoma: a 15-year median follow-up study. *J Clin Endocrinol Metab*. 2008;93:3943–3949.
408. O'Neill CJ, Bullock M, Chou A, et al. BRAF(V600E) mutation is associated with an increased risk of nodal recurrence requiring reoperative surgery in patients with papillary thyroid cancer. *Surgery*. 2010;148:1139–1145; discussion 1145–1136.
409. Trovisco V, Soares P, Sobrinho-Simoes M. B-RAF mutations in the etiopathogenesis, diagnosis, and prognosis of thyroid carcinomas. *Hum Pathol*. 2006;37:781–786.
410. Moretti S, Macchiarulo A, De Falco V, et al. Biochemical and molecular characterization of the novel BRAF(V599Ins) mutation detected in a classic papillary thyroid carcinoma. *Oncogene*. 2006;25:4235–4240.
411. Nikiforova MN, Caudill CM, Biddinger P, et al. Prevalence of RET/PTC rearrangements in Hashimoto's thyroiditis and papillary thyroid carcinomas. *Int J Surg Pathol*. 2002;10:15–22.
412. Jhiang SM, Caruso DR, Gilmore E, et al. Detection of the PTC/retTPC oncogene in human thyroid cancers. *Oncogene*. 1992;7:1331–1337.
413. Elisei R, Romei C, Vorontsova T, et al. RET/PTC rearrangements in thyroid nodules: studies in irradiated and not irradiated, malignant and benign thyroid lesions in children and adults. *J Clin Endocrinol Metab*. 2001;86:3211–3216.
414. Ishizaka Y, Kobayashi S, Ushijima T, et al. Detection of retTPC/PTC transcripts in thyroid adenomas and adenomatous goiter by an RT-PCR method. *Oncogene*. 1991;6:1667–1672.
415. Sheils O, Smyth P, Finn S, et al. RET/PTC rearrangements in Hashimoto's thyroiditis. *Int J Surg Pathol*. 2002;10:167–168; author reply 168–169.
416. Nikiforova MN. Principles of molecular diagnostics in thyroid samples. In: Nikiforov YE, Biddinger PW, Thompson LDR, eds. *Diagnostic Pathology and Molecular Genetics of the Thyroid*. Philadelphia, PA: Lippincott Williams & Wilkins; 2009:363–375.
417. Hieber L, Huber R, Bauer V, et al. Chromosomal rearrangements in post-Chernobyl papillary thyroid carcinomas: evaluation by spectral karyotyping and automated interphase FISH. *J Biomed Biotechnol*. 2011;2011:7.
418. Kondo T, Ezzat S, Asa SL. Pathogenetic mechanisms in thyroid follicular-cell neoplasia. *Nat Rev Cancer*. 2006;6:292–306.
419. Jin L, Seys AR, Zhang S, et al. Diagnostic utility of IMP3 expression in thyroid neoplasms: a quantitative RT-PCR study. *Diagn Mol Pathol*. 2010;19:63–69.
420. Lappinga PJ, Kip NS, Jin L, et al. HMGA2 gene expression analysis performed on cytologic smears to distinguish benign from malignant thyroid nodules. *Cancer Cytopathol*. 2010;118:287–297.
421. Beaumont A, Ben Othman S, Fragu P. The fine structure of papillary carcinoma of the thyroid. *Histopathology*. 1981;5:377–388.
422. Johannessen JV, Gould VE, Jao W. The fine structure of human thyroid cancer. *Hum Pathol*. 1978;9:385–400.
423. Tonietti G, Baschieri L, Salabe G. Papillary and microfollicular carcinoma of human thyroid. An ultrastructural study. *Arch Pathol*. 1967;84:601–614.
424. Sobrinho-Simoes MA, Goncalves V. Nuclear bodies in papillary carcinomas of the human thyroid gland. *Arch Pathol*. 1974;98:94–99.
425. Dupuy-Coin AM, Kalifat SR, Bouteille M. Nuclear bodies as proteinaceous structures containing ribonucleoproteins. *J Ultrastruct Res*. 1972;38:174–187.
426. Christ ML, Haja J. Intranuclear cytoplasmic inclusions (invaginations) in thyroid aspirations. Frequency and specificity. *Acta Cytol*. 1979;23:327–331.
427. Shurbaji MS, Gupta PK, Frost JK. Nuclear grooves: a useful criterion in the cytopathologic diagnosis of papillary thyroid carcinoma. *Diagn Cytopathol*. 1988;4:91–94.
428. Francis IM, Das DK, Sheikh ZA, et al. Role of nuclear grooves in the diagnosis of papillary thyroid carcinoma. A quantitative assessment on fine needle aspiration smears. *Acta Cytol*. 1995;39:409–415.
429. Yang YJ, Demirci SS. Evaluating the diagnostic significance of nuclear grooves in thyroid fine needle aspirates with a semiquantitative approach. *Acta Cytol*. 2003;47:563–570.
430. Baloch ZW, LiVolsi VA, Asa SL, et al. Diagnostic terminology and morphologic criteria for cytologic diagnosis of thyroid lesions: a synopsis of the National Cancer Institute Thyroid Fine-Needle Aspiration State of the Science Conference. *Diagn Cytopathol*. 2008;36:425–437.
431. Ali SZ, Cibas ES. *The Bethesda System for Reporting Thyroid Cytopathology*. New York, NY: Springer; 2010.
432. Renshaw AA, Wang E, Wilbur D, et al. Interobserver agreement on microfollicles in thyroid fine-needle aspirates. *Arch Pathol Lab Med*. 2006;130:148–152.
433. Wu HH, Jones JN, Grzybicki DM, et al. Sensitive cytologic criteria for the identification of follicular variant of papillary thyroid carcinoma in fine-needle aspiration biopsy. *Diagn Cytopathol*. 2003;29:262–266.
434. Baloch ZW, Gupta PK, Yu GH, et al. Follicular variant of papillary carcinoma. Cytologic and histologic correlation. *Am J Clin Pathol*. 1999;111:216–222.
435. Chen H, Zeiger MA, Clark DP, et al. Papillary carcinoma of the thyroid: can operative management be based solely on fine-needle aspiration? *J Am Coll Surg*. 1997;184:605–610.
436. Solomon A, Gupta PK, LiVolsi VA, et al. Distinguishing tall cell variant of papillary thyroid carcinoma from usual variant of papillary thyroid carcinoma in cytologic specimens. *Diagn Cytopathol*. 2002;27:143–148.
437. Ohori NP, Schoedel KE. Response to baloch and liVolsi. *Diagn Cytopathol*. 1999;21:303.
438. Moreira AL, Waisman J, Cangiarella JF. Aspiration cytology of the oncocytic variant of papillary adenocarcinoma of the thyroid gland. *Acta Cytol*. 2004;48:137–141.
439. Lee JY, Shin JH, Han BK, et al. Diffuse sclerosing variant of papillary carcinoma of the thyroid: imaging and cytologic findings. *Thyroid*. 2007;17:567–573.
440. Odashiro DN, Nguyen GK. Diffuse sclerosing variant papillary carcinoma of the thyroid: report of four cases with fine-needle aspirations. *Diagn Cytopathol*. 2006;34:247–249.
441. Perez F, Llobet M, Garijo G, et al. Fine-needle aspiration cytology of columnar-cell carcinoma of the thyroid: report of two cases with cytohistologic correlation. *Diagn Cytopathol*. 1998;18:352 356.
442. Ylagan LR, Dehner LP, Huettner PC, et al. Columnar cell variant of papillary thyroid carcinoma. Report of a case with cytologic findings. *Acta Cytol*. 2004;48:73–77.
443. Anderson SR, Mandel S, LiVolsi VA, et al. Can cytomorphology differentiate between benign nodules and tumors arising in Graves' disease? *Diagn Cytopathol*. 2004;31:64–67.
444. Centeno BA, Szyfelbein WM, Daniels GH, et al. Fine needle aspiration biopsy of the thyroid gland in patients with prior Graves' disease treated with radioactive iodine. Morphologic findings and potential pitfalls. *Acta Cytol*. 1996;40:1189–1197.
445. Sturgis CD. Radioactive iodine-associated cytomorphologic alterations in thyroid follicular epithelium: is recognition possible in fine-needle aspiration specimens? *Diagn Cytopathol*. 1999;21:207–210.
446. Deshpande AH, Bobhate SK. Cytological features of dyshormonogenetic goiter: case report and review of the literature. *Diagn Cytopathol*. 2005;33:252–254.
447. Asioli S, Maletta F, Pacchioni D, et al. Cytological detection of papillary thyroid carcinomas by nuclear membrane decoration with emerin staining. *Virchows Arch*. 2010;457:43–51.
448. Nga ME, Lim GS, Soh CH, et al. HBME-1 and CK19 are highly discriminatory in the cytological diagnosis of papillary thyroid carcinoma. *Diagn Cytopathol*. 2008;36:550–556.
449. Schmitt AC, Cohen C, Siddiqui MT. Paired box gene 8, HBME-1, and cytokeratin 19 expression in preoperative fine-needle aspiration of papillary thyroid carcinoma: diagnostic utility. *Cancer Cytopathol*. 2010;118:196–202.
450. Cooper DS, Doherty GM, Haugen BR, et al. Management guidelines for patients with thyroid nodules and differentiated thyroid cancer. *Thyroid*. 2006;16:109–142.
451. Pacini F, Schlumberger M, Dralle H, et al. European consensus for the management of patients with differentiated thyroid carcinoma of the follicular epithelium. *Eur J Endocrinol*. 2006;154:787–803.
452. White ML, Gauger PG, Doherty GM. Central lymph node dissection in differentiated thyroid cancer. *World J Surg*. 2007;31:895–904.
453. Cooper DS, Doherty GM, Haugen BR, et al. Revised American Thyroid Association management guidelines for patients with thyroid nodules and differentiated thyroid cancer. *Thyroid*. 2009;19:1167–1214.
454. Jonklaas J, Sarlis NJ, Litofsky D, et al. Outcomes of patients with differentiated thyroid carcinoma following initial therapy. *Thyroid*. 2006;16:1229–1242.
455. Sawka AM, Prebtani AP, Thabane L, et al. A systematic review of the literature examining the diagnostic efficacy of measurement of fractionated plasma free metanephrines in the biochemical diagnosis of pheochromocytoma. *BMC Endocr Disord*. 2004;4:2.
456. Pacini F, Ladenson PW, Schlumberger M, et al. Radioiodine ablation of thyroid remnants after preparation with recombinant human thyrotropin in differentiated thyroid carcinoma: results of an international, randomized, controlled study. *J Clin Endocrinol Metab*. 2006;91:926–932.
457. Rubino C, de Vathaire F, Dottorini ME, et al. Second primary malignancies in thyroid cancer patients. *Br J Cancer*. 2003;89:1638–1644.
458. Brown AP, Chen J, Hitchcock YJ, et al. The risk of second primary malignancies up to three decades after the treatment of differentiated thyroid cancer. *J Clin Endocrinol Metab*. 2008;93:504–515.
459. Pacini F, Molinaro E, Castagna MG, et al. Recombinant human thyrotropin-stimulated serum thyroglobulin combined with neck ultrasonography has the highest sensitivity in monitoring differentiated thyroid carcinoma. *J Clin Endocrinol Metab*. 2003;88:3668–3673.
460. Haugen BR, Pacini F, Reiners C, et al. A comparison of recombinant human thyrotropin and thyroid hormone withdrawal for the detection of thyroid remnant or cancer. *J Clin Endocrinol Metab*. 1999;84:3877–3885.
461. Torlontano M, Crocetti U, D'Aloiso L, et al. Serum thyroglobulin and 131I whole body scan after recombinant human TSH stimulation in the follow-up of low-risk patients with differentiated thyroid cancer. *Eur J Endocrinol*. 2003;148:19–24.
462. Hundahl SA, Fleming ID, Fremgen AM, et al. A National Cancer Data Base report on 53,856 cases of thyroid carcinoma treated in the U.S., 1985–1995 (see commetns). *Cancer*. 1998;83:2638–2648.
463. Kosary CL. Cancer of the thyroid. In: Ries LAG, Young JL, Keel GE,et al., eds. *SEER Survival Monograph: Cancer Survival Among Adults: U.S. SEER Program, 1988–2001, Patient and Tumor Characteristics. National Cancer Institute, SEER Program, NIH Pub. No. 07-6215*. Bethesda, MD; 2007:217–225.
464. Kitamura Y, Shimizu K, Nagahama M, et al. Immediate causes of death in thyroid carcinoma: clinicopathological analysis of 161 fatal cases. *J Clin Endocrinol Metab*. 1999;84:4043–4049.
465. Smith SA, Hay ID, Goellner JR, et al. Mortality from papillary thyroid carcinoma. A case-control study of 56 lethal cases. *Cancer*. 1988;62:1381–1388.
466. Shaha AR, Shah JP, Loree TR. Risk group stratification and prognostic factors in papillary carcinoma of thyroid. *Ann Surg Oncol*. 1996;3:534–538.
467. Hay ID, Bergstralh EJ, Goellner JR, et al. Predicting outcome in papillary thyroid carcinoma: development of a reliable prognostic scoring system in a cohort of 1779 patients surgically treated at one institution during 1940 through 1989. *Surgery*. 1993;114:1050–1057; discussion 1057–1058.
468. Salvesen H, Njolstad PR, Akslen LA, et al. Papillary thyroid carcinoma: a multivariate analysis of prognostic factors including an evaluation of the p-TNM staging system. *Eur J Surg*. 1992;158:583–589.

469. DeGroot LJ, Kaplan EL, McCormick M, et al. Natural history, treatment, and course of papillary thyroid carcinoma. *J Clin Endocrinol Metab.* 1990;71:414–424.

470. Grebe SK, Hay ID. Thyroid cancer nodal metastases: biologic significance and therapeutic considerations. *Surg Oncol Clin N Am.* 1996;5:43–63.

471. Akslen LA. Prognostic importance of histologic grading in papillary thyroid carcinoma. *Cancer.* 1993;72:2680–2685.

472. Wartofsky L. Staging of thyroid cancer. In: Wartofsky L, Van Nostrand D, eds. *Thyroid Cancer: A Comprehensive Guide to Clinical Management.* 2nd ed. Totowa, NJ: Humana Press; 2006:87–95.

473. Dean DS, Hay ID. Prognostic indicators in differentiated thyroid carcinoma. *Cancer Control.* 2000;7:229–239.

474. Riesco-Eizaguirre G, Gutierrez-Martinez P, Garcia-Cabezas MA, et al. The oncogene BRAF V600E is associated with a high risk of recurrence and less differentiated papillary thyroid carcinoma due to the impairment of Na+/I-targeting to the membrane. *Endocr Relat Cancer.* 2006;13:257–269.

475. Ricarte-Filho JC, Ryder M, Chitale DA, et al. Mutational profile of advanced primary and metastatic radioactive iodine-refractory thyroid cancers reveals distinct pathogenetic roles for BRAF, PIK3CA, and AKT1. *Cancer Res.* 2009;69:4885–4893.

476. Durante C, Puxeddu E, Ferretti E, et al. BRAF mutations in papillary thyroid carcinomas inhibit genes involved in iodine metabolism. *J Clin Endocrinol Metab.* 2007;92:2840–2843.

477. Xing M. Prognostic utility of BRAF mutation in papillary thyroid cancer. *Mol Cell Endocrinol.* 2010;321:86–93.

478. Rodolico V, Cabibi D, Pizzolanti G, et al. BRAF V600E mutation and p27 kip1 expression in papillary carcinomas of the thyroid <or=1 cm and their paired lymph node metastases. *Cancer.* 2007;110:1218–1226.

479. Lupi C, Giannini R, Ugolini C, et al. Association of BRAF V600E mutation with poor clinicopathological outcomes in 500 consecutive cases of papillary thyroid carcinoma. *J Clin Endocrinol Metab.* 2007;92:4085–4090.

480. Howell GM, Carty SE, Armstrong MJ, et al. Both BRAF V600E mutation and older age (≥65 years) are associated with recurrent papillary thyroid cancer. *Ann Surg Oncol.* 2011;18:3566–3571.

481. Sturgis CD, Caraway NP, Johnston DA, et al. Image analysis of papillary thyroid carcinoma fine-needle aspirates: significant association between aneuploidy and death from disease. *Cancer.* 1999;87:155–160.

482. Cohen EE, Rosen LS, Vokes EE, et al. Axitinib is an active treatment for all histologic subtypes of advanced thyroid cancer: results from a phase II study. *J Clin Oncol.* 2008;26:4708–4713.

483. Gupta-Abramson V, Troxel AB, Nellore A, et al. Phase II trial of sorafenib in advanced thyroid cancer. *J Clin Oncol.* 2008;26:4714–4719.

484. Kloos RT, Ringel MD, Knopp MV, et al. Phase II trial of sorafenib in metastatic thyroid cancer. *J Clin Oncol.* 2009;27:1675–1684.

485. Pennell NA, Daniels GH, Haddad RI, et al. A phase II study of gefitinib in patients with advanced thyroid cancer. *Thyroid.* 2008;18:317–323.

486. Cabanillas ME, Waguespack SG, Bronstein Y, et al. Treatment with tyrosine kinase inhibitors for patients with differentiated thyroid cancer: the M. D. Anderson experience. *J Clin Endocrinol Metab.* 2010;95:2588–2595.

487. Xing J, Liu R, Xing M, et al The BRAFT1799A mutation confers sensitivity of thyroid cancer cells to the BRAFV600E inhibitor PLX4032 (RG7204). *Biochem Biophys Res Commun.* 2010;404:958–962.

488. Marchevsky AM, Walts AE, Bose S, et al. Evidence-based evaluation of the risks of malignancy predicted by thyroid fine-needle aspiration biopsies. *Diagn Cytopathol.* 2010;38:252–259.

489. Nayar R, Ivanovic M. The indeterminate thyroid fine-needle aspiration: experience from an academic center using terminology similar to that proposed in the 2007 National Cancer Institute Thyroid Fine Needle Aspiration State of the Science Conference. *Cancer.* 2009;117:195–202.

490. Theoharis CG, Schofield KM, Hammers L, et al. The Bethesda thyroid fine-needle aspiration classification system: year 1 at an academic institution. *Thyroid.* 2009;19:1215–1223.

491. Jo VY, Stelow EB, Dustin SM, et al. Malignancy risk for fine-needle aspiration of thyroid lesions according to the Bethesda System for Reporting Thyroid Cytopathology. *Am J Clin Pathol.* 2010;134:450–456.

492. Luu MH, Fischer AH, Pisharodi L, et al. Improved preoperative definitive diagnosis of papillary thyroid carcinoma in FNAs prepared with both ThinPrep and conventional smears compared with FNAs prepared with ThinPrep alone. *Cancer Cytopathol.* 2011;119:68–73.

493. Renshaw AA. Should "atypical follicular cells" in thyroid fine-needle aspirates be subclassified? *Cancer Cytopathol.* 2010;118:186–189.

Poorly Differentiated Carcinoma

DEFINITION

Poorly differentiated thyroid carcinoma is an aggressive malignant tumor of follicular cell origin that is characterized by a partial loss of thyroid differentiation and occupies morphologically and behaviorally an intermediate position between well-differentiated papillary and follicular carcinomas and fully dedifferentiated anaplastic carcinoma. Another term frequently used to designate this tumor is *insular carcinoma*, although its usage should be discouraged as it places an emphasis on the growth pattern, which is not specific for this tumor type, rather than on the cell morphology.

HISTORICAL COMMENTS AND EVOLUTION OF DIAGNOSTIC CRITERIA

The tumor currently known as *poorly differentiated carcinoma* was first described by Sakamoto and colleagues in 1983[1] and by Carcangiu and colleagues in 1984.[2] In the first report, Sakamoto et al. analyzed a group of 258 thyroid tumors from Japan and found that those with solid, trabecular, or scirrhous (sclerotic) growth pattern demonstrated biologic behavior intermediate between the rest of the papillary and follicular carcinomas on one side and anaplastic thyroid carcinoma on another. They called tumors with this architecture poorly differentiated carcinoma, irrespective of other histologic characteristics of tumor cells. In the article by Carcangiu et al., the authors reported a series of 25 cases of unusual thyroid carcinoma from the University of Florence Medical School in Italy. These tumors formed characteristic solid nests or "insulae" and were characterized by small size and uniformity of cells, significant mitotic activity, capsular and vascular invasion, and tumor necrosis. The authors postulated that morphologically and behaviorally, this tumor occupied an intermediate position between well-differentiated papillary and follicular carcinoma and anaplastic carcinoma and named it poorly differentiated or insular carcinoma. They noted that this tumor resembled one that was described by Langhans in 1907 as "wuchernde Struma" ("proliferating struma"). These two observations established a concept of thyroid tumor of intermediate differentiation and behavior, but offered significantly different histologic criteria for its diagnosis. Sakamoto and colleagues based the diagnosis exclusively on tumor growth pattern, whereas Carcangiu and colleagues described a distinctive growth pattern as well as other morphologic characteristics of tumor cells, albeit with no clear indication of what features are sufficient to establish the diagnosis.

Subsequent reports have used either the more broad Sakamoto criteria, adding other unusual variants of papillary carcinoma, such as columnar cell variant, diffuse sclerosing variant, and even tall cell variant to the category of poorly differentiated carcinoma,[3–5] or the more restrictive Carcangiu criteria, but still emphasizing an insular growth pattern as sufficient criterion alone for inclusion into the category of poorly differentiated

carcinoma.[6–8] As a result, various groups reported series of tumors carrying the same name but, in reality, having quite different morphologic characteristics. For the most part, the criteria used were broad, which resulted in frequent inclusion in this category some well-differentiated carcinomas, such as solid variant of papillary carcinoma. The 2004 World Health Organization classification of thyroid tumors recognized poorly differentiated carcinoma as a specific entity, stating that it is characterized by solid, trabecular, or insular architecture; infiltrative growth; necrosis; and vascular invasion.[9] Although this description included features beyond the growth pattern, it did not specify how many of those were sufficient to establish this diagnosis. Still some authors suggested that poorly differentiated carcinoma has to be defined exclusively based on the presence of necrosis and high mitotic activity, as these features better stratified patients into prognostic categories than a growth pattern.[10]

In 2006, an international working group of thyroid pathologists from Europe, Japan, and the United States, which included the principal authors of the two original publications, offered a set of consensus diagnostic criteria for this tumor, which was developed at a meeting hosted by Dr. Gianni Bussolati in Turin, Italy.[11] The unifying diagnostic criteria included both the architectural pattern and the cytologic features of tumor cells and were developed based on a series of tumors submitted from different countries and reviewed by a panel of 12 thyroid pathologists. These criteria showed good correlation with tumor behavior and are relatively simple and expected to be reproducible between observers. The Turin consensus criteria provide the basis for discussion in this chapter. As these criteria are relatively recent and many observations available in the literature used various selection criteria, this chapter primarily incorporates the results of studies that used either Turin criteria or reasonably restrictive criteria to define poorly differentiated thyroid carcinoma.

INCIDENCE AND EPIDEMIOLOGY

Poorly differentiated thyroid carcinoma is a rare tumor. When defined by the Turin diagnostic criteria, its incidence varies from <1% in Japan[12] to 1.8% in the United States.[13] Some geographic areas, however, may have a higher incidence of this tumor. Specifically, in the Piemonte region of northern Italy, poorly differentiated carcinoma historically accounted for 4% to 7% of all malignant thyroid tumors,[6,14] and the incidence remained at 6.7% when the Turin diagnostic criteria were applied.[13]

Poorly differentiated carcinoma typically presents on average one decade later than well-differentiated carcinomas. In most series, the mean age of patient was between 55 and 63 years.[1,2,6,11,13] Poorly differentiated carcinoma is exceedingly rare in children and young adults, and this diagnosis should be established with great caution in individuals younger than 30 years. The youngest age of patients in most reported series was 33 to 34 years,[2,11] although it was 14.1 years in one recent study.[13] The tumor is more common in females, with a female predilection ranging from 1.6 to 2:1 in large series of patients.[1,2,11,13]

ETIOLOGIC FACTORS

The etiology remains unknown. Some tumors develop from preexisting well-differentiated papillary or follicular carcinoma, whereas others are likely to develop de novo. The association with benign thyroid disease is suspected based on presumably higher prevalence of this tumor in the Piemonte region of Italy located in the Alps, which used to be an area of endemic goiter.[6,14] In this region, most patients with poorly differentiated carcinoma had a history of goiter, which was confirmed in almost all thyroids at surgery. A history of exposure to therapeutic radiation to the neck region was found in 12% of patients in one series,[2] although this association remains unconfirmed.

PATHOGENESIS AND MOLECULAR GENETICS

It is generally accepted that poorly differentiated carcinoma may develop through three pathogenetic pathways: (1) by partial dedifferentiation of papillary carcinoma, (2) by partial dedifferentiation of follicular (including oncocytic type) carcinoma, and (3) de novo, without a preexisting well-differentiated carcinoma precursor (Fig. 12.1). This assumption is supported by frequent finding of a well-differentiated papillary or follicular carcinoma intermixed with poorly differentiated carcinoma areas (Fig. 12.2) and by observations of temporal progression from classic papillary carcinoma to poorly differentiated carcinoma in subsequent tumor recurrences.[15] In a recent series of 152 tumors, 34% of them did not have a well-differentiated component, whereas the rest showed a residual well-differentiated papillary or follicular carcinoma.[13]

Somatic Mutations

Somatic mutations that occur in poorly differentiated carcinoma are summarized in Table 12.1. Generally, they can be divided into two groups: (1) mutations that also occur in the well-differentiated tumor component and therefore represent an *early* event in tumorigenesis, initiating the development of

well-differentiated cancer and predisposing to subsequent additional molecular events that govern tumor dedifferentiation and (2) mutations that are present only in the poorly differentiated tumor component and therefore are *late* events, directly driving the process of dedifferentiation (Fig. 12.1). The first group includes *BRAF* and *RAS* mutations. The second group includes *TP53* and β-catenin (*CTNNB1*) mutations, which occur in poorly differentiated and also anaplastic carcinomas but not in well-differentiated cancers. Mutations in the effectors of the PI3K/PTEN/AKT signaling pathway are more difficult to place in one of these groups, although they are more likely to represent late events. Of note, clonal *RET/PTC* and *PAX8/PPARγ* rearrangements are less commonly found in poorly differentiated (and anaplastic) carcinomas,[16] suggesting that these oncogenes are less likely to create a "molecular environment" that promotes tumor dedifferentiation. Some studies, however, have reported a more common (18%) occurrence of *RET/PTC* rearrangement in poorly differentiated carcinomas defined on the basis of tumor necrosis and high mitotic activity.[17]

RAS Mutations

Activating point mutations of the *RAS* genes are found in 20% to 40% of poorly differentiated carcinomas.[13,17–19] The most commonly affected hot spot is *NRAS* codon 61, followed by *HRAS* codon 61. *RAS* mutations are not restricted to this tumor type because they can also occur in follicular adenomas, follicular carcinomas, and follicular variant of papillary carcinomas. Many poorly differentiated carcinomas with a *RAS* mutation contain an adjacent component of well-differentiated follicular carcinoma or follicular variant of papillary carcinoma. When areas of poorly differentiated carcinoma and well-differentiated carcinoma are microdissected separately for DNA extraction, an identical *RAS* mutation is found in both components, confirming that it is an early event (Fig. 12.3).

Mutant RAS activates various downstream signaling pathways that stimulate cell proliferation and survival, most important of which in thyroid cells are mitogen-activated protein kinase (MAPK) and PI3K/AKT pathways. Some experimental data suggest that mutant RAS may interfere with DNA damage response and promote chromosome instability.[20,21] The increasing instability

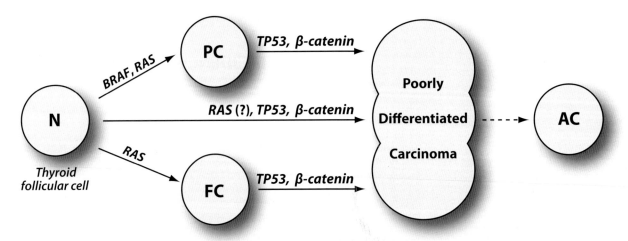

FIGURE 12.1. Poorly differentiated carcinoma may develop by partial dedifferentiation of well-differentiated papillary carcinoma (PC) or follicular carcinoma (FC), or directly, de novo, without a well-differentiated carcinoma stage. The process of dedifferentiation can proceed further and result in transformation to anaplastic carcinoma (AC). *BRAF* and *RAS* mutations are found in both well-differentiated and poorly differentiated carcinomas, indicating that they occur early and confer well-differentiated carcinoma cells with propensity to undergo dedifferentiation, most likely by acquiring additional mutations, such as those of *TP53* and β-catenin (*CTNNB1*) genes. PC, papillary carcinoma; FC, follicular carcinoma; AC, anaplastic carcinoma.

would stimulate the acquisition of additional mutations, which could in turn initiate the process of tumor dedifferentiation. However, *RAS* mutation on its own is unlikely to be sufficient to drive tumor dedifferentiation, as it is common in well-differentiated carcinomas and even in benign thyroid adenomas.

BRAF Mutations

BRAF mutations, which are a characteristic feature of papillary carcinomas, also occur in poorly differentiated carcinomas. The reported incidence of this mutation varies substantially and on average is approximately 15%.[17,19,22,23] Most *BRAF*-positive poorly differentiated carcinomas contain a well-differentiated papillary carcinoma component, typically a tall cell variant (Fig. 12.2A).

Both tumor components reveal a V600E *BRAF* mutation when studied separately, indicating that it occurs early in carcinogenesis.[22] In one study, *BRAF* mutations were found in 12% of the entire series of poorly differentiated carcinoma but in 47% of more aggressive, radioactive iodine refractory and [18F]fluorodeoxyglucose positron emission tomography (FDG-PET) positive poorly differentiated carcinomas.[17]

The oncogenic qualities of *BRAF* V600E mutation are associated with activation of the MAPK signaling pathway. Chronic overstimulation of this pathway by mutant BRAF in thyroid cells of transgenic mice results in the formation of papillary carcinomas that in time undergo progression to poorly differentiated carcinoma.[24] Similar to human poorly differentiated carcinomas, the poorly differentiated foci in these animals showed solid sheets

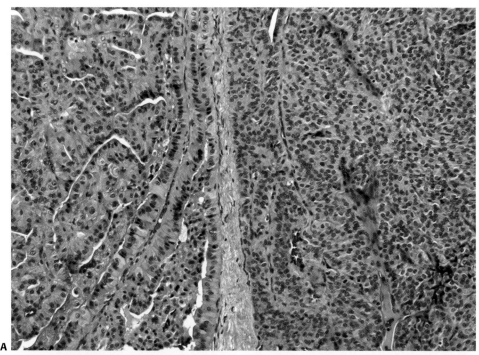

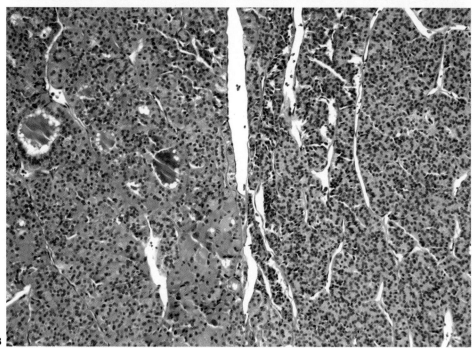

FIGURE 12.2. Poorly differentiated carcinoma (right side of both panels) coexisting with papillary carcinoma, tall cell variant (A), and with oncocytic follicular carcinoma (B).

Table 12.1

Average Prevalence of Mutations in Poorly Differentiated Thyroid Carcinoma and Other Thyroid Carcinomas

Mutated Gene	Papillary Carcinoma	Follicular Carcinoma[a]	Poorly Differentiated Carcinoma	Anaplastic Carcinoma
RAS (%)	10	45	30	50
BRAF (%)	45	0	15	25
RET/PTC (%)	20	0	0[b]	0
PAX8/PPARγ (%)	0–1	35	0	0
TP53 (%)	0	0	30	65
β-Catenin (%)	0	0	25	65

[a] Based on conventional type of follicular carcinoma.
[b] Some studies reported the incidence of 18%,[17] although it remains unclear if it represented clonal RET/PTC.

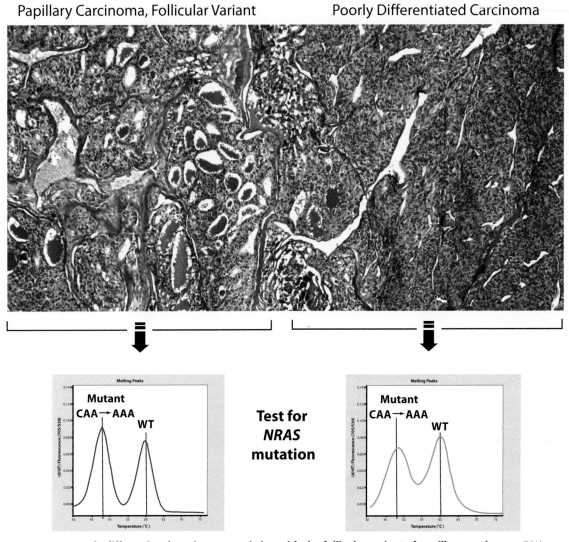

FIGURE 12.3. **Poorly differentiated carcinoma coexisting with the follicular variant of papillary carcinoma.** DNA was isolated separately from the two tumor components and subjected to testing for *RAS* mutations by real-time PCR and post-PCR melting curve analysis on LightCycler, which revealed an identical CAA → AAA *NRAS* mutation at codon 61 in both tumor components.

of cells with more uniform nuclei, scant cytoplasm, and loss of nuclear features of papillary carcinoma (Fig. 12.4). The process of dedifferentiation in the transgenic animals was associated with profound dysregulation of expression of genes involved in cell adhesion and intracellular junction, providing evidence for epithelial–mesenchymal transition in these tumors.[25]

TP53 Mutations

Mutations of the *TP53* tumor suppressor gene occur in about 30% of poorly differentiated carcinomas.[26–28] In contrast to *RAS* and *BRAF*, these mutations are very rare in well-differentiated thyroid carcinomas and represent a late event in thyroid carcinogenesis, being most prevalent in anaplastic thyroid carcinomas.

The *TP53* gene encodes a nuclear transcription factor that plays a central role in the regulation of the cell cycle, DNA repair, and apoptosis. It exerts these functions by its ability to transactivate the expression of genes coding for cell cycle proteins such as p21/WAF1. Mutations typically affect exons 5 to 8 of *TP53* and include inactivating point mutations, small deletions, or insertions. Inactivation of TP53 function results in progressive genome destabilization, accumulation of additional mutations, and emergence of more malignant and less differentiated tumor clones.[29,30] A sharply increased incidence of *TP53* mutations from well-differentiated to poorly differentiated and then to anaplastic carcinomas suggests that TP53 inactivation is crucial for stepwise thyroid cancer progression and plays a direct role in triggering tumor dedifferentiation.

β-Catenin (CTNNB1) Mutations

β-Catenin mutation is another late event potentially involved in tumor dedifferentiation. This cytoplasmic protein, encoded by the *CTNNB1* gene, plays an important role in cell adhesion and signaling along the wingless (Wnt) pathway. Normally, in the absence of Wnt signaling, the protein is located at the inner surface of the cell membrane and at a low level in the cytoplasm, where it is rapidly degraded by the adenomatous polyposis coli (APC) multiprotein complex. Wnt binding stabilizes the protein that accumulates in the cytoplasm and translocates to the nucleus, where it upregulates the transcriptional activity of different genes. Point mutations in exon 3 of *CTNNB1* stabilize the protein by making it insensitive for APC-induced degradation. This results in the accumulation of β-catenin in the nucleus and constitutive activation of the target gene expression.

Point mutations in exon 3 of *CTNNB1* rarely occur in well-differentiated thyroid carcinomas,[31] but they were found in one study in 14 out of 29 (25%) poorly differentiated carcinomas and with a higher frequency in anaplastic carcinomas.[32] Most of the tumors carrying the mutation also demonstrated aberrant nuclear expression of the protein determined by immunohistochemistry with antibodies to β-catenin and an immunofluorescence detection system. Another study, however, found no mutation in exon 3 of *CTNNB1* in 17 poorly differentiated carcinomas.[33] The reason for the discrepant result is not clear but may be because of the different diagnostic criteria used for the selection of cases.

Other Genetic Alterations

The role of the PI3K/PTEN/AKT pathway activation because of mutations in the *PIK3CA* and *PTEN* genes in poorly differentiated carcinomas remains not fully defined. Alterations of the effectors of this signaling pathway appear to be more common in anaplastic carcinomas than in well-differentiated thyroid carcinomas, but they have not been studied extensively in poorly differentiated carcinomas. One study has reported mutations in the *PIK3CA* and *AKT1* genes in some poorly differentiated carcinomas, particularly in those with more aggressive behavior.[17]

Analysis of losses and gains of chromosomal regions by comparative genomic hybridization demonstrated a relatively large number of alterations in poorly differentiated carcinomas.[34,35] The analysis of well-differentiated, poorly differentiated, and anaplastic thyroid carcinomas performed by Wreesmann et al. revealed multiple chromosomal abnormalities that fell into three groups.[35] One group included gains of 5p15, 5q11-13, 8q23, 19p, and 19q and deletions of 8p and 22q that were observed in well-differentiated, poorly differentiated, and anaplastic carcinomas. Another group included gains of 1p34-36, 6p21, 9q34, 17q25, and 20q and deletions of 1p11-31, 2q32-33, 4q11-13, 6q21, and 13q21-31 that were found only in poorly differentiated and anaplastic carcinomas. Finally, gains of 3p13-14 and 11q13 and loss of 5q11-31 were restricted to anaplastic carcinomas. The loss or gain of the same chromosomal regions provides evidence for progression from well-differentiated to poorly differentiated and then

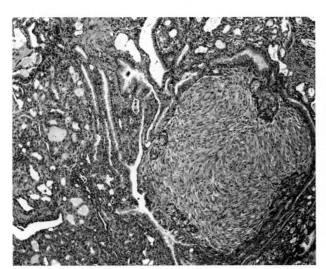
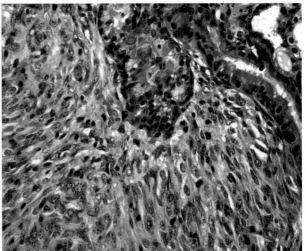

FIGURE 12.4. Microscopic appearance of thyroid tumors developed in transgenic mice with thyroid-specific expression of mutant BRAF V600E. This papillary thyroid carcinoma has tall cell features and focal areas of poorly differentiated carcinoma that are visible as a sharply demarcated solid area showing a uniform population of cells with elongated nuclei and reduced amount of cytoplasm. Based on the data reported by Knauf et al.[24]

to anaplastic carcinoma. The study revealed no losses or gains unique for poorly differentiated carcinomas.

CLINICAL PRESENTATION AND IMAGING

Patients typically present with a solitary thyroid mass, sometimes present for years and recently increased in size.[2] In some cases, symptoms associated with local or distant metastases may be the first presenting signs. The patients are euthyroid. Poorly differentiated carcinomas are typically "cold" on scintigraphy. Ultrasound examination reveals a large solid mass with variable echogenicity and irregular borders. CT may be used to assess the extent of invasion and may show a large mass that infiltrates the surrounding neck structures and encases the trachea.[36] Owing to frequent loss of radioiodine avidity, metastases from the tumor may not be recognizable on the radioactive scan but detected by FDG-PET.

GROSS FEATURES

On gross examination, poorly differentiated carcinoma is typically an overtly infiltrative mass (Fig. 12.5) that often extends beyond the thyroid capsule. Some tumors show partial encapsulation, although a complete and intact capsule is rarely seen. Tumors may range in size from 1 to 10 cm and are most often 4 to 6 cm in size. The cut surface is solid and tan to white-tan in color and frequently demonstrates a variegated appearance with foci of hemorrhage and necrosis. Adjacent areas of uniform, colloid-rich appearance may be noted and correspond to a well-differentiated follicular or papillary carcinoma component (Fig. 12.5B).

MICROSCOPIC FEATURES

Microscopic diagnosis of poorly differentiated carcinoma relies on the detection of evidence of partial tumor dedifferentiation. The consensus Turin diagnostic criteria include the following three features:

1. Solid/trabecular/insular architectural pattern
2. Lack of well-developed nuclear features of papillary carcinoma
3. *One* of the following: 3a—convoluted nuclei, 3b—tumor necrosis, or 3c—three or more mitoses per high-power field (HPF)

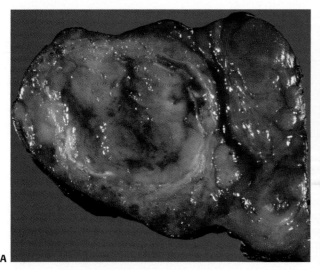

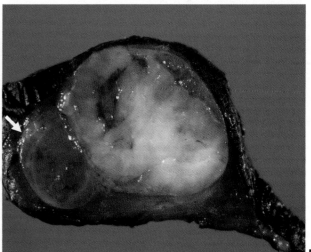

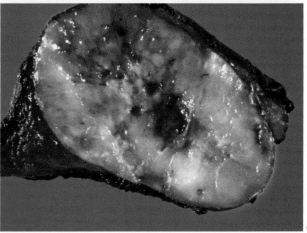

FIGURE 12.5. Gross appearance of poorly differentiated carcinoma. A: The tumor shows an infiltrative growth and friable cut surface with areas of hemorrhage. The remaining fragments of the destroyed capsule are recognizable. **B and C:** This poorly differentiated carcinoma presents as a solid whitish nodule with focal hemorrhage and yellowish spots that probably correspond to the areas of necrosis. A component of well-differentiated follicular variant of papillary carcinoma is seen in **(B)** as a brown, colloid-rich nodule *(arrow)*.

1. Architecture

The tumor shows a solid, trabecular, or insular growth pattern. The solid pattern is seen as sheets of tumor cells with variable amounts of intervening fibrovascular stroma (Fig. 12.6A,B). In some cases, thin bands of fibrosis separate tumor sheets into well-defined nests to yield a nested or insular architecture (Fig. 12.6C,D). The nests may be surrounded by a clear space because of an artifactual retraction of the stroma. The trabecular pattern is formed by

elongated cords or ribbons of tumor cells (Fig. 12.6D,E). The tumor frequently shows a mixture of the three patterns. Small follicular structures may be scattered within the predominantly solid nests of cells, but they are rarely conspicuous and typically contain no or scant colloid. Overall, poorly differentiated carcinoma shows minimal colloid formation. Abundant colloid, if found, typically highlights the foci of residual well-differentiated carcinoma.

Neither an insular nor any of the other two architectural patterns is diagnostic for poorly differentiated carcinoma on

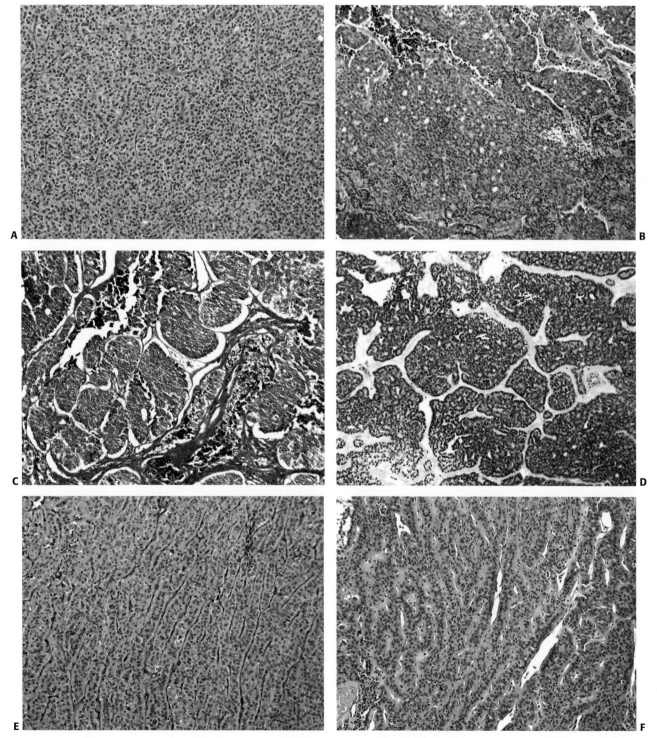

FIGURE 12.6. Characteristic growth patterns of poorly differentiated carcinoma: solid (A and B), insular (C and D), and trabecular (E and F).

its own, and criteria 2 and 3 must be met to establish this diagnosis.

2. Cells

The tumor cells are monotonous, typically of small size, with small, uniform, round, smooth-contoured nuclei with dark, evenly distributed chromatin and inconspicuous nucleoli (Fig. 12.7A,B). Niclear features of papillary carcinoma are not seen.

Despite the small size of the nucleus, the nuclear:cytoplasmic ratio is high because of a decreased volume of cell cytoplasm. Some tumors show a monotonous population of cells with larger nuclei that may show more vesicular chromatin and prominent nucleoli but preserve round configurations and smooth contours (Fig. 12.7C,D). Yet other tumors demonstrate more elongated nuclei with significant irregularity of nuclear contours (so called *convoluted nuclei* as discussed below) (Fig. 12.7E,F). The ir regularity of nuclear outlines in these cells is reminiscent of

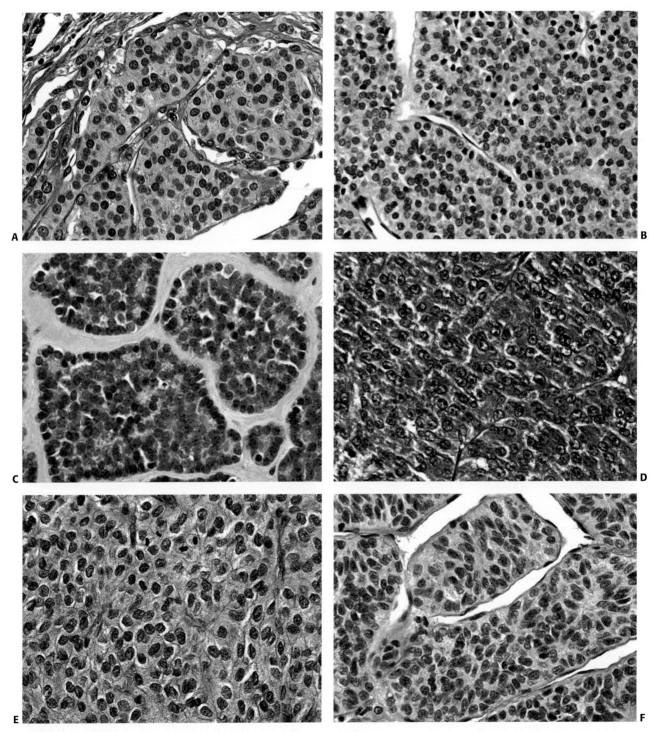

FIGURE 12.7. Cell appearance in poorly differentiated carcinoma. A and B: Small, round, dark, monotonous nuclei. **C and D:** Slightly larger uniform nuclei with smooth contours and either dark chromatin **(C)** or vesicular chromatic and prominent nucleoli **(D)**. **E and F:** Convoluted nuclei. Two mitotic figures are seen in one field **(E).**

papillary carcinoma nuclei. However, no other nuclear features of papillary carcinoma, such as classic optically clear nuclei, nuclear overlapping and crowding, abundant nuclear grooves, and nuclear pseudoinclusions, are noted because those findings would prompt reclassification of the tumor as a solid variant of papillary carcinoma. Some tumors may show more variability in size and shape of nuclei, although really pleomorphic nuclei are rare. No marked nuclear atypia or giant, multinucleated cells should be seen as these are features of anaplastic thyroid carcinoma.

3a. Convoluted Nuclei

Convoluted nuclei are slightly smaller than those of well-differentiated papillary carcinoma and retain some irregularity of the contours, which gives them a raisin-like appearance (Fig. 12.7E,F).[11] However, in contrast to papillary carcinoma nuclei, they are more uniform, have dark and evenly distributed chromatin, and show only scattered nuclear grooves and no nuclear pseudoinclusions. The biologic sense behind this criterion is that the nuclei lose most of the characteristic nuclear features but retain some irregularity of their contours when cells of papillary carcinoma undergo dedifferentiation. Therefore, this serves as morphologic evidence for (1) partial loss of differentiation and (2) tumor origin from a well-differentiated papillary carcinoma. This transition is best appreciated when such nuclei are examined next to the area of well-differentiated papillary carcinoma (Fig. 12.8). Convoluted nuclei, found adjacent to the areas of papillary carcinoma or throughout

the tumor that has no residual well-differentiated component, fulfill the diagnostic criterion #3.

3b. Tumor Necrosis

Because follicular carcinomas never possessed the nuclear features of papillary carcinoma, lack of these nuclear features cannot be used as a criterion for separation of these tumors. Instead, two other criteria can be used, that is, tumor necrosis (criterion 3b) or increased mitotic activity (criterion 3c). Tumor necrosis is a common finding in poorly differentiated carcinomas, including those originating from papillary and follicular carcinomas. It is found in 70% to 97% of these tumors.[11,13] The necrosis is frequently seen as a small, well-defined focus situated in the center of solid nests or insulae (central punctate necrosis) (Fig. 12.9A) or may be more extensive and involve the entire nest or several nests of tumor cells. In some tumors, the necrosis involves large tumor areas but spares zones surrounding blood vessels, producing a so-called *peritheliomatous* appearance (Fig. 12.9B).[2] To meet this criterion, necrosis has to involve a group of tumor cells (single cell necrosis does not count) and should not be secondary to the fine-needle aspiration (FNA) FNA injury.

3c. Increased Mitotic Activity

Generally, poorly differentiated carcinomas reveal higher mitotic count than well-differentiated tumors (Fig. 12.7E). In the series reported by Carcangiu et al.,[2] mitoses were present in all cases

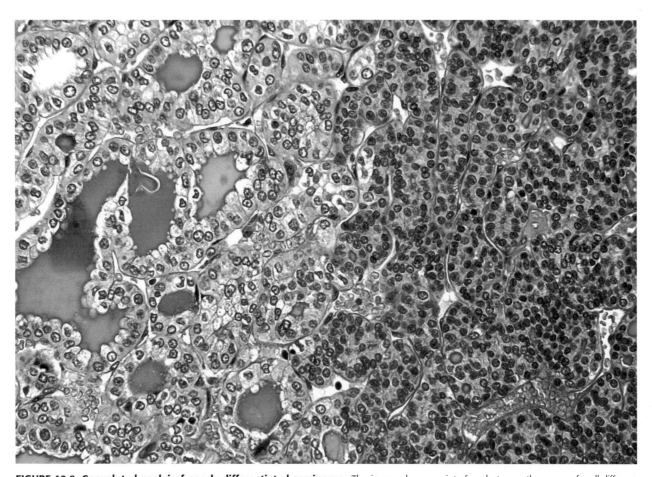

FIGURE 12.8. Convoluted nuclei of poorly differentiated carcinoma. The image shows an interface between the areas of well-differentiated papillary carcinoma, follicular variant *(left),* and poorly differentiated carcinoma *(right)*. Note a clear separation between the nuclei with well-defined features of papillary carcinoma and the convoluted nuclei of poorly differentiated carcinoma which are smaller and more uniform and have darker chromatin but preserve some irregularity of their contours.

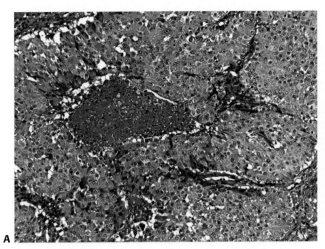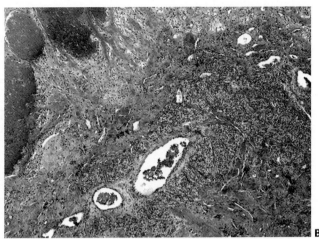

FIGURE 12.9. Tumor necrosis in poorly differentiated carcinoma. A: A well-defined necrotic focus in the center of a cell nest. **B:** Massive necrosis, fresh *(upper left)* and with organization and fibrosis, that spares perivascular areas.

and their count ranged from 1 to 30 per 10 HPFs. To fulfill this criterion, 3 or more mitoses should be found in 10 HPFs (400× magnification: 40× objective combined with 10× eyepiece). This cutoff for mitotic activity was chosen because it correlated well with poor outcome in the Turin series of cases.[11] The increased mitotic activity is found in >90% of cases.[13] Atypical mitoses are found in about 20% of cases.[13]

Subtypes of Poorly Differentiated Carcinoma

On the basis of their putative origin, poorly differentiated carcinomas can be further subdivided into a papillary type, a follicular type, and a not otherwise specified (NOS) type. A papillary origin is obvious when a coexisting well-differentiated papillary carcinoma is found, and it can also be suspected when convoluted nuclei are seen. The follicular origin can be established with certainty only when areas of well-differentiated follicular carcinoma are also seen. Follicular carcinomas of both conventional type and oncocytic type may give rise to poorly differentiated carcinoma.[37] Although the diagnostic criteria for poorly differentiated carcinoma were set up in Turin using a set of non-oncocytic carcinomas,[11] there is no reason to believe that the same criteria cannot be applied to the oncocytic tumors. Poorly differentiated carcinomas of NOS type have round nuclei and reveal no well-differentiated carcinoma component. Most of these tumors are expected to originate from follicular carcinoma or arise de novo. The distinction has no clinical importance as there is no prognostic difference between specific poorly differentiated carcinoma subtypes.[11]

Single case reports of poorly differentiated carcinoma with signet-ring cells,[38] rhabdoid cells,[39,40] and mucin production[41] exist. Similar diagnostic criteria should be applied to tumors with these unusual features. Prognostic implications of these findings are not known.

Tumors with Minor Component of Poorly Differentiated Carcinoma

Poorly differentiated areas typically constitute a significant proportion or a majority of the tumor nodule, but sometimes can be found as a minor component to a well-differentiated papillary or follicular carcinoma. It is not fully understood whether the proportion of poorly differentiated carcinoma areas directly correlate with prognosis. Several studies have reported similarly decreased survival in patients with poorly differentiated carcinoma

constituting >50% of the tumor and in those where it was observed as a minor component.[6,42–44] Because poorly differentiated carcinoma represents a more aggressive tumor type that will most likely determine the overall survival, it should be reported in the first diagnostic line irrespective of its size and proportion within the tumor nodule. However, the proportion of the poorly differentiated component within the tumor nodule should be clearly stated in the report.

 ## SPREAD AND METASTASES

Poorly differentiated carcinomas typically show an irregular infiltrative border or a pushing border with broad-based invasion. Extrathyroidal extension is common. Vascular invasion is found in >90% of cases and is extensive in two-thirds of those cases.[11] About 20% of patients have metastatic disease at presentation, either in cervical lymph nodes or at distant sites.[2]

 ## IMMUNOHISTOCHEMISTRY

Immunohistochemistry can be used to establish the thyroid follicular cell origin of poorly differentiated carcinoma. The tumors frequently retain reactivity for thyroglobulin, although it is typically very focal and limited to small follicular structures containing colloid (Fig. 12.10A). Some authors have found thyroglobulin staining limited to small paranuclear vacuoles.[6,13,14] Strong diffuse reactivity for thyroglobulin is highly unlikely in poorly differentiated carcinoma and it typically highlights the adjacent well-differentiated carcinoma component (Fig. 12.10B).

Reactivity for the nuclear transcription factor TTF1 is diffuse and retained in almost all poorly differentiated carcinomas, but it is frequently of weaker intensity as compared with well-differentiated carcinoma areas (Fig. 12.10C).[45,46] The expression of two other transcription factors, PAX8 and TTF2, is also diffusely present.[45] Expression of cytokeratins (CK7, CAM 5.2, AE1/AE3 cocktail) is strong and diffuse. Overall, the thyroglobulin/TTF1/cytokeratin immunohistochemical profile of poorly differentiated carcinoma is intermediate between well-differentiated carcinomas and anaplastic carcinoma (see for illustration Fig. 13.21 in Chapter 13).

TP53 is expressed by immunohistochemistry in 40% to 70% of cases and can be focal or diffuse.[13,28,47,48] The immunoreactivity is believed to demonstrate the accumulation of the mutant TP53

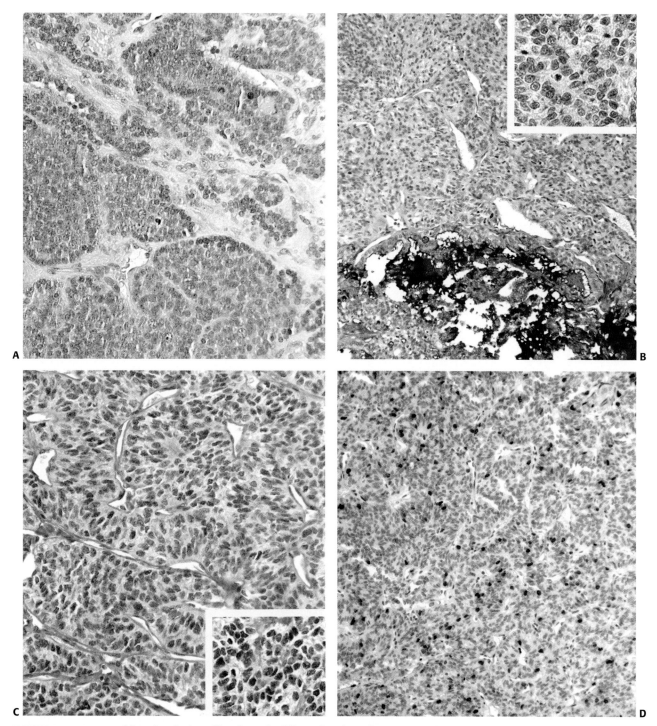

FIGURE 12.10. Immunohistochemical profile of poorly differentiated carcinoma. A and B: Thyroglobulin immunostain reveals very focal positivity limited to small follicular spaces filled with colloid. An area of strong diffuse staining (**B**, *bottom*) corresponds to a well-differentiated papillary carcinoma component. Inset in (**B**) shows high-power view of the poorly differentiated carcinoma. **C:** TTF1 immunostain shows diffuse nuclear staining that is weaker than in the areas of well-differentiated papillary carcinoma *(inset)*. **D:** Staining for Ki-67 using MIB1 antibody showing labeling of 10% of the nuclei.

protein in the nuclei of tumor cells and frequently, but not always, correlates with the molecular detection of *TP53* mutation. Among other cell cycle proteins, loss of expression of cyclin-dependent kinase inhibitors p27 and p21 and overexpression of cyclin D1 has been seen in some poorly differentiated (and more often in anaplastic) carcinomas.[49–51]

A higher proliferation rate of poorly differentiated carcinoma cells can be confirmed using Ki-67 (MIB1) immunostaining

(Fig. 12.10D), which frequently shows a labeling index between 10% and 30%.[9,51]

Immunoreactivity for HBME-1 and galectin-3 is seen in about half of all cases,[13,52] and the staining is typically weaker and more focal than that in well-differentiated cancer. Positive cytoplasmic staining for the insulin-like growth factor mRNA-binding protein 3 (IMP3) has been found in about 60% of poorly differentiated carcinomas and appeared to correlate with worse survival.[13]

MOLECULAR DIAGNOSTICS

Testing for molecular alterations has a limited role in the diagnosis of poorly differentiated carcinoma at the present time owing to the lack of mutations specific for this tumor type. Finding a *TP53* or *β-catenin* mutation would generally favor poorly differentiated carcinoma over well-differentiated carcinoma, although they are frequently seen in anaplastic carcinomas as well. *BRAF* and *RAS* mutations are found in well-differentiated and anaplastic thyroid carcinomas in addition to poorly differentiated carcinoma. *RAS* mutations may also be seen in medullary thyroid carcinoma.

ULTRASTRUCTURAL FEATURES

Ultrastructural features of poorly differentiated carcinoma are not well defined because the diagnostic criteria for this tumor type had not been standardized until recently. The reports on tumors with insular architecture and features that by description meet the current criteria indicate that ultrastructurally poorly differentiated carcinoma cells preserve features of epithelial differentiation.[36] Cells are arranged in sheets with formation of small lumens lined by microvilli. Desmosomes and intermediate and tight junctions are present. Nuclei either have smooth and regular contours or are irregular and reveal deep clefts and pseudoinclusions,[36] the latter likely reflecting the sampling of well-differentiated papillary carcinoma areas. Dense secretory granules may be seen, particularly in those cells that form lumens.

CYTOLOGIC FEATURES

Aspirates of poorly differentiated carcinoma are cellular and may have a necrotic background.[14] Single cells and cell aggregates are seen (Fig. 12.11). The aggregates have a solid, trabecular, or insular/nested cytoarchitecture and may reveal scattered microfollicular structures. The latter may contain dense colloid mimicking the appearance of hyaline globules seen in adenoid cystic carcinoma.[53] The cells have small, round, monotonous nuclei with finely dispersed chromatin and inconspicuous nucleoli. Cytoplasm is scant and cell contours are poorly defined. Intranuclear grooves and pseudoinclusions are typically not seen, and if present, they are likely to derive from the residual well-differentiated papillary carcinoma component. The diagnosis of poorly differentiated carcinoma may be suspected but cannot be established with confidence based on the cytologic evaluation. The most consistently found and diagnostically helpful cytologic features allowing to suggest this diagnosis include the combination of insular, solid, or trabecular pattern; single cells; high nuclear:cytoplasmic ratio; and severe cell crowding.[54,55]

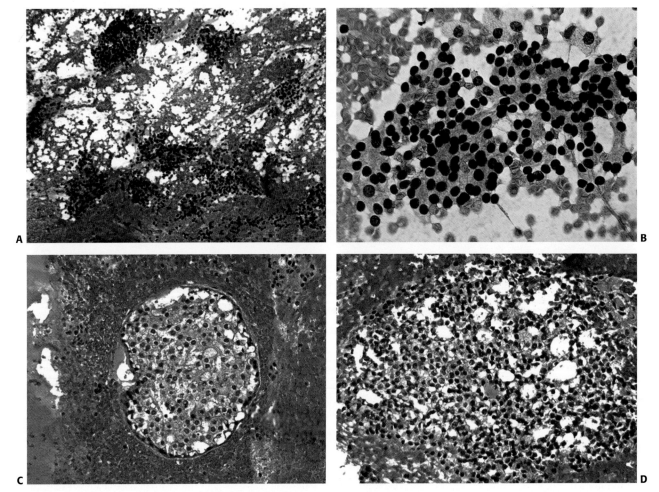

FIGURE 12.11. Cytologic features of poorly differentiated carcinoma. A and B: The smear is cellular and demonstrates multiple groups of cells with deceptively bland nuclei. The cell aggregates have mostly solid configuration with some microfollicular arrangement of the nuclei **(B)** (Papanicolaou stain). **C and D:** Cell block sections showing round shape (almost insular) aggregates of cells with solid and microfollicular architecture and rather monotonous nuclei (Hematoxylin and Eosin stain).

DIFFERENTIAL DIAGNOSIS

The differential diagnosis of poorly differentiated carcinoma includes (1) well-differentiated thyroid carcinomas with solid, trabecular, or insular growth pattern; (2) anaplastic (undifferentiated) thyroid carcinoma; (3) medullary thyroid carcinoma; and (4) metastatic nonthyroid carcinomas.

Distinction from Well-Differentiated Thyroid Carcinoma

The solid variant of papillary carcinoma represents a major diagnostic challenge for poorly differentiated carcinoma of papillary type. The architectural patterns are identical because both tumors share solid, trabecular, and insular architecture (Fig. 12.12). The distinction is made primarily on the basis of the presence or absence of the nuclear features of papillary carcinoma. The solid variant of papillary carcinoma demonstrates cells with enlarged nuclei that lose polarity, show haphazard arrangement within the cell layer, and have highly irregular contours, clear chromatin (ground glass nuclei), and common nuclear grooves and pseudoinclusions. Poorly differentiated carcinoma cells may retain some irregularity of the nuclei contours, but nuclei are smaller and more uniform with dense chromatin and may show occasional grooves but no abundant grooves or pseudoinclusions. In addition, the volume of cytoplasm is substantially reduced with increased nuclear:cytoplasm ratio and more central placement of the nucleus within each cell. The finding of tumor necrosis and/or increased mitotic activity would provide additional support for the diagnosis of poorly differentiated carcinoma but is not required to establish it if convoluted nuclei are found.

Separation from follicular carcinoma of conventional or oncocytic type with solid, trabecular, or insular architecture is based on the finding of tumor necrosis or 3 or more mitoses per 10 HPF.

Distinction from Anaplastic Thyroid Carcinoma

Poorly differentiated carcinoma is distinguished from anaplastic carcinoma by monotonous cell populations and lack of significant nuclear pleomorphism or highly atypical nuclei. In addition, necrosis is less prominent, more frequently involves small areas, and is more punctuate as compared with the geographic distribution in anaplastic carcinomas. Immunohistochemistry can offer additional help, as poorly differentiated carcinomas retain strong and diffuse reactivity for cytokeratins, moderate and diffuse reactivity for TTF1, and at least focal immunoreactivity for thyroglobulin. In

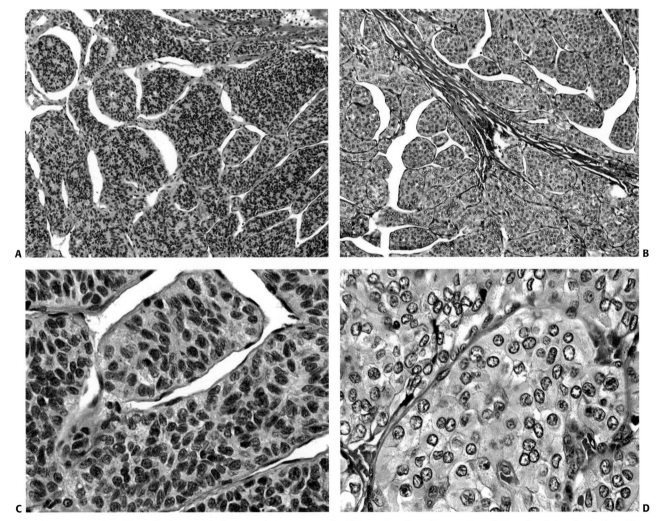

FIGURE 12.12. Comparison of microscopic features between poorly differentiated carcinoma (A and C) and solid variant of papillary carcinoma (B and D). Both tumors may show a prominent insular pattern **(A and B)**, but can be separated based on the lack of the characteristic nuclear features of papillary carcinoma in the poorly differentiated carcinoma cells **(C vs. D)**.

contrast, in anaplastic carcinoma, both thyroglobulin and TTF1 are lost and cytokeratin is retained only focally.

Distinction from Medullary Thyroid Carcinoma

Medullary thyroid carcinoma can enter the differential diagnosis of tumors with a nested growth pattern and monotonous nuclei. Immunostains for thyroglobulin and calcitonin can resolve the issue. TTF1 cannot be used for this purpose as it is also positive in many medullary carcinomas. In addition, detection of a *RET* point mutation is diagnostic of medullary carcinoma, whereas finding a *BRAF* mutation supports the diagnosis of poorly differentiated carcinoma.

Distinction from Nonthyroid Malignancies

Metastatic carcinoma may occasionally be suspected, particularly when no colloid formation is noted in poorly differentiated carcinoma. The presence of a differentiated thyroid carcinoma component rules out this possibility. The thyroid origin can be confirmed by positive staining for thyroglobulin and TTF1, although the latter is not entirely specific for thyroid and also highlights lung tumors and some other tumor types. In addition, PAX8 and TTF2 can be used to support the thyroid origin.[45]

 TREATMENT AND PROGNOSIS

Poorly differentiated thyroid carcinoma is an aggressive thyroid tumor with biologic behavior intermediate between well-differentiated carcinoma and anaplastic carcinoma. This was demonstrated in the two original studies[1,2] and was further confirmed by the Turin consensus study. Among 34 poorly differentiated carcinomas that provided the basis for the Turin criteria, 44% of patients died of disease (mean survival, 57 months), 29% were alive with disease, and 27% had no evidence of disease after a mean follow-up of 9 months.[11] Importantly, in the overall series of 80 thyroid carcinomas reviewed in Turin, *all* of which had solid, trabecular, or insular architecture, the proposed diagnostic criteria made it possible to separate the group of poorly differentiated carcinomas that had significantly

shorter survival as compared with papillary carcinomas and follicular carcinomas with solid, trabecular, or insular growth patterns (Fig. 12.13A). No difference in outcome was found between poorly differentiated carcinomas of papillary type and NOS (including follicular type) (Fig. 12.13B). In a series of 152 patients with poorly differentiated carcinoma diagnosed using the Turin criteria, the 5-year survival rate was 72% and the 10-year survival rate 46%.[13]

Factors found to be associated with worse survival in some studies include patients older than 45 years, larger tumor size (such as ≥4 cm), presence of necrosis and high mitotic activity, *RAS* mutation, and positive IMP3 immunostaining.[13,19,52,56]

Poorly differentiated carcinomas frequently develop recurrence in the residual thyroid or in the thyroid bed and spread to local cervical or mediastinal lymph nodes or distant sites, typically lungs and/or bones.[2] Death occurs as a result of uncontrolled local disease or distant metastases.

The treatment strategies for this tumor have not been standardized. Total thyroidectomy with possible lymph node dissection is the initial approach. The role of postsurgical radioactive iodine therapy and external beam radiotherapy is not fully defined. The existing data on radioiodine therapy are conflicting and probably reflect the variable levels of iodine accumulation by a given tumor.[57–60] However, owing to the high mortality rate and potential for therapeutic benefit, a recent evidence-based review of the topic by a multidisciplinary group of physicians recommended postoperative radioactive iodine therapy for all patients with poorly differentiated carcinoma.[61] In the same review, the authors recommend adjuvant external beam radiation treatment for patients with T3 (>4 cm in size or minimal extrathyroidal extension) tumors without distant metastases, for all patients with T4 (extensive extrathyroidal invasion) tumors, and for all patients with regional lymph node metastases.[61] Other authors recommend external beam radiation therapy for patients with unresectable disease, incompletely excised tumors, and locoregional recurrences.[62] The role of chemotherapy is not well established, although some patients may benefit from it.[63]

Targeted therapies based on the inhibition of BRAF kinase and other effectors of the MAPK and PI3K/AKT signaling pathways and/or TP53 gene therapy may offer a viable therapeutic alternative for patients with poorly differentiated carcinoma in the future.

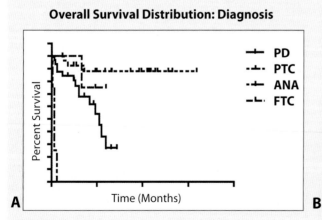

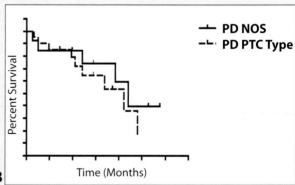

FIGURE 12.13. A: Overall survival of patients with poorly differentiated thyroid carcinoma (PD), papillary thyroid carcinoma (PTC), anaplastic carcinoma (AC), and follicular thyroid carcinoma (FTC) from the Turin series as reported by Volante et al.[11] Note that all of these tumors had a solid, trabecular, or insular architecture. **B:** In the same series of cases, survival was similar for patients with poorly differentiated carcinomas of NOS type (including follicular type) and papillary type (PD PTC type).

REFERENCES

1. Sakamoto A, Kasai N, Sugano H. Poorly differentiated carcinoma of the thyroid. A clinicopathologic entity for a high-risk group of papillary and follicular carcinomas. *Cancer.* 1983;52:1849–1855.
2. Carcangiu ML, Zampi G, Rosai J. Poorly differentiated ("insular") thyroid carcinoma. A reinterpretation of Langhans' "wuchernde Struma". *Am J Surg Pathol.* 1984;8:655–668.
3. Nishida T, Katayama S, Tsujimoto M, et al. Clinicopathological significance of poorly differentiated thyroid carcinoma. *Am J Surg Pathol.* 1999;23:205–211.
4. Pilotti S, Collini P, Manzari A, et al. Poorly differentiated forms of papillary thyroid carcinoma: distinctive entities or morphological patterns? *Semin Diagn Pathol.* 1995;12:249–255.
5. Sobrinho-Simoes M, Nesland JM, Johannessen JV. Columnar-cell carcinoma. Another variant of poorly differentiated carcinoma of the thyroid. *Am J Clin Pathol.* 1988;89:264–267.
6. Papotti M, Botto Micca F, Favero A, et al. Poorly differentiated thyroid carcinomas with primordial cell component. A group of aggressive lesions sharing insular, trabecular, and solid patterns. *Am J Surg Pathol.* 1993;17:291–301.
7. Pilotti S, Collini P, Mariani L, et al. Insular carcinoma: a distinct de novo entity among follicular carcinomas of the thyroid gland. *Am J Surg Pathol.* 1997;21:1466–1473.
8. Ashfaq R, Vuitch F, Delgado R, et al. Papillary and follicular thyroid carcinomas with an insular component. *Cancer.* 1994;73:416–423.
9. DeLellis RA, Lloyd RV, Heitz PU, et al, eds. *World Health Organization Classification of Tumours. Pathology and Genetics of Tumours of Endocrine Organs.* Lyon, France: IARC Press; 2004.
10. Hiltzik D, Carlson DL, Tuttle RM, et al. Poorly differentiated thyroid carcinomas defined on the basis of mitosis and necrosis: a clinicopathologic study of 58 patients. *Cancer.* 2006;106:1286–1295.
11. Volante M, Collini P, Nikiforov YE, et al. Poorly differentiated thyroid carcinoma: the Turin proposal for the use of uniform diagnostic criteria and an algorithmic diagnostic approach. *Am J Surg Pathol.* 2007;31:1256–1264.
12. Ito Y, Hirokawa M, Fukushima M, et al. Prevalence and prognostic significance of poor differentiation and tall cell variant in papillary carcinoma in Japan. *World J Surg.* 2008;32:1535–1543.
13. Asioli S, Erickson LA, Righi A, et al. Poorly differentiated carcinoma of the thyroid: validation of the Turin proposal and analysis of IMP3 expression. *Mod Pathol.* 2010;23:1269–1278.
14. Pietribiasi F, Sapino A, Papotti M, et al. Cytologic features of poorly differentiated "insular" carcinoma of the thyroid, as revealed by fine-needle aspiration biopsy. *Am J Clin Pathol.* 1990;94:687–692.
15. Rosai J, Carcangiu ML, DeLellis RA. *Tumors of the Thyroid Gland.* 3rd ed. Washington, DC: Armed Forces Institute of Pathology; 1992.
16. Nikiforov YE. Genetic alterations involved in the transition from well-differentiated to poorly differentiated and anaplastic thyroid carcinomas. *Endocr Pathol.* 2004;15:319–327.
17. Ricarte-Filho JC, Ryder M, Chitale DA, et al. Mutational profile of advanced primary and metastatic radioactive iodine-refractory thyroid cancers reveals distinct pathogenetic roles for BRAF, PIK3CA, and AKT1. *Cancer Res.* 2009;69:4885–4893.
18. Garcia-Rostan G, Zhao H, Camp RL, et al. Ras mutations are associated with aggressive tumor phenotypes and poor prognosis in thyroid cancer. *J Clin Oncol.* 2003;21:3226–3235.
19. Volante M, Rapa I, Gandhi M, et al. RAS mutations are the predominant molecular alteration in poorly differentiated thyroid carcinomas and bear prognostic impact. *J Clin Endocrinol Metab.* 2009;94:4735–4741.
20. Fagin JA. Minireview: branded from the start-distinct oncogenic initiating events may determine tumor fate in the thyroid. *Mol Endocrinol.* 2002;16:903–911.
21. Saavedra HI, Knauf JA, Shirokawa JM, et al. The RAS oncogene induces genomic instability in thyroid PCCL3 cells via the MAPK pathway. *Oncogene.* 2000;19:3948–3954.
22. Nikiforova MN, Kimura ET, Gandhi M, et al. BRAF mutations in thyroid tumors are restricted to papillary carcinomas and anaplastic or poorly differentiated carcinomas arising from papillary carcinomas. *J Clin Endocrinol Metab.* 2003;88:5399–5404.
23. Costa AM, Herrero A, Fresno MF, et al. BRAF mutation associated with other genetic events identifies a subset of aggressive papillary thyroid carcinoma. *Clin Endocrinol (Oxf).* 2008;68:618–634.
24. Knauf JA, Ma X, Smith EP, et al. Targeted expression of BRAFV600E in thyroid cells of transgenic mice results in papillary thyroid cancers that undergo dedifferentiation. *Cancer Res.* 2005;65:4238–4245.
25. Knauf JA, Sartor MA, Medvedovic M, et al. Progression of BRAF-induced thyroid cancer is associated with epithelial-mesenchymal transition requiring concomitant MAP kinase and TGFbeta signaling. *Oncogene.* 2011;30:3153–3162.
26. Dobashi Y, Sugimura H, Sakamoto A, et al. Stepwise participation of p53 gene mutation during dedifferentiation of human thyroid carcinomas. *Diagn Mol Pathol.* 1994;3:9–14.
27. Donghi R, Longoni A, Pilotti S, et al. Gene p53 mutations are restricted to poorly differentiated and undifferentiated carcinomas of the thyroid gland. *J Clin Invest.* 1993;91:1753–1760.
28. Takeuchi Y, Daa T, Kashima K, et al. Mutations of p53 in thyroid carcinoma with an insular component. *Thyroid.* 1999;9:377–381.
29. La Perle KM, Jhiang SM, Capen CC. Loss of p53 promotes anaplasia and local invasion in ret/PTC1-induced thyroid carcinomas. *Am J Pathol.* 2000;157:671–677.
30. Powell DJ Jr, Russell JP, Li G, et al. Altered gene expression in immunogenic poorly differentiated thyroid carcinomas from RET/PTC3p53−/− mice. *Oncogene.* 2001;20:3235–3246.
31. Miyake N, Maeta H, Horie S, et al. Absence of mutations in the beta-catenin and adenomatous polyposis coli genes in papillary and follicular thyroid carcinomas. *Pathol Int.* 2001;51:680–685.
32. Garcia-Rostan G, Camp RL, Herrero A, et al. Beta-catenin dysregulation in thyroid neoplasms: down-regulation, aberrant nuclear expression, and CTNNB1 exon 3 mutations are markers for aggressive tumor phenotypes and poor prognosis. *Am J Pathol.* 2001;158:987–996.
33. Rocha AS, Soares P, Fonseca E, et al. E-cadherin loss rather than beta-catenin alterations is a common feature of poorly differentiated thyroid carcinomas. *Histopathology.* 2003;42:580–587.
34. Rodrigues RF, Roque L, Rosa-Santos J, et al. Chromosomal imbalances associated with anaplastic transformation of follicular thyroid carcinomas. *Br J Cancer.* 2004;90:492–496.
35. Wreesmann VB, Ghossein RA, Patel SG, et al. Genome-wide appraisal of thyroid cancer progression. *Am J Pathol.* 2002;161:1549–1556.
36. Killeen RM, Barnes L, Watson CG, et al. Poorly differentiated ("insular") thyroid carcinoma. Report of two cases and review of the literature. *Arch Otolaryngol Head Neck Surg.* 1990;116:1082–1086.
37. Papotti M, Torchio B, Grassi L, et al. Poorly differentiated oxyphilic (Hurthle cell) carcinomas of the thyroid. *Am J Surg Pathol.* 1996;20:686–694.
38. Fellegara G, Rosai J. Signet ring cells in a poorly differentiated Hurthle cell carcinoma of the thyroid combined with two papillary microcarcinomas. *Int J Surg Pathol.* 2007;15:388–390.
39. Agrawal AR, Nair N. Unusual metastasis of poorly differentiated thyroid carcinoma to the masticator space. *Clin Nucl Med.* 2007;32:516–518.
40. Albores-Saavedra J, Sharma S. Poorly differentiated follicular thyroid carcinoma with rhabdoid phenotype: a clinicopathologic, immunohistochemical and electron microscopic study of two cases. *Mod Pathol.* 2001;14:98–104.
41. Kondo T, Kato K, Nakazawa T, et al. Mucinous carcinoma (poorly differentiated carcinoma with extensive extracellular mucin deposition) of the thyroid: a case report with immunohistochemical studies. *Hum Pathol.* 2005;36:698–701.
42. Flynn SD, Forman BH, Stewart AF, et al. Poorly differentiated ("insular") carcinoma of the thyroid gland: an aggressive subset of differentiated thyroid neoplasms. *Surgery.* 1988;104:963–970.
43. Decaussin M, Bernard MH, Adeleine P, et al. Thyroid carcinomas with distant metastases: a review of 111 cases with emphasis on the prognostic significance of an insular component. *Am J Surg Pathol.* 2002;26:1007–1015.
44. Sasaki A, Daa T, Kashima K, et al. Insular component as a risk factor of thyroid carcinoma. *Pathol Int.* 1996;46:939–946.
45. Nonaka D, Tang Y, Chiriboga L, et al. Diagnostic utility of thyroid transcription factors Pax8 and TTF-2 (FoxE1) in thyroid epithelial neoplasms. *Mod Pathol.* 2008;21:192–200.
46. Bejarano PA, Nikiforov YE, Swenson ES, et al. Thyroid transcription factor-1, thyroglobulin, cytokeratin 7, and cytokeratin 20 in thyroid neoplasms. *Appl Immunohistochem Mol Morphol.* 2000;8:189–194.
47. Dobashi Y, Sakamoto A, Sugimura H, et al. Overexpression of p53 as a possible prognostic factor in human thyroid carcinoma. *Am J Surg Pathol.* 1993;17:375–381.
48. Pilotti S, Collini P, Del Bo R, et al. A novel panel of antibodies that segregates immunocytochemically poorly differentiated carcinoma from undifferentiated carcinoma of the thyroid gland. *Am J Surg Pathol.* 1994;18:1054–1064.
49. Wang S, Lloyd RV, Hutzler MJ, et al. The role of cell cycle regulatory protein, cyclin D1, in the progression of thyroid cancer. *Mod Pathol.* 2000;13:882–887.
50. Wiseman SM, Masoudi H, Niblock P, et al. Anaplastic thyroid carcinoma: expression profile of targets for therapy offers new insights for disease treatment. *Ann Surg Oncol.* 2007;14:719–729.
51. Tallini G, Garcia-Rostan G, Herrero A, et al. Downregulation of p27KIP1 and Ki67/Mib1 labeling index support the classification of thyroid carcinoma into prognostically relevant categories. *Am J Surg Pathol.* 1999;23:678–685.
52. Pulcrano M, Boukheris H, Talbot M, et al. Poorly differentiated follicular thyroid carcinoma: prognostic factors and relevance of histological classification. *Thyroid.* 2007;17:639–646.
53. Malhotra P, Deewan U, Krishnani N. Poorly differentiated thyroid carcinoma mimicking adenoid cystic carcinoma on aspiration cytology: a case report. *Acta Cytol.* 2009;53:591–593.
54. Bongiovanni M, Bloom L, Krane JF, et al. Cytomorphologic features of poorly differentiated thyroid carcinoma: a multi-institutional analysis of 40 cases. *Cancer.* 2009;117:185–194.
55. Bongiovanni M, Sadow PM, Faquin WC. Poorly differentiated thyroid carcinoma: a cytologic-histologic review. *Adv Anat Pathol.* 2009;16:283–289.
56. Volante M, Landolfi S, Chiusa L, et al. Poorly differentiated carcinomas of the thyroid with trabecular, insular, and solid patterns: a clinicopathologic study of 183 patients. *Cancer.* 2004;100:950–957.
57. Lin JD, Chao TC, Hsueh C. Clinical characteristics of poorly differentiated thyroid carcinomas compared with those of classical papillary thyroid carcinomas. *Clin Endocrinol (Oxf).* 2007;66:224–228.
58. Justin EP, Seabold JE, Robinson RA, et al. Insular carcinoma: a distinct thyroid carcinoma with associated iodine-131 localization. *J Nucl Med.* 1991;32:1358–1363.

59. Lai HW, Lee CH, Chen JY, et al. Insular thyroid carcinoma: collective analysis of clinicohistologic prognostic factors and treatment effect with radioiodine or radiation therapy. *J Am Coll Surg.* 2006;203:715–722.

60. Tuttle RM, Grewal RK, Larson SM. Radioactive iodine therapy in poorly differentiated thyroid cancer. *Nat Clin Pract Oncol.* 2007;4:665–668.

61. Sanders EM Jr, LiVolsi VA, Brierley J, et al. An evidence-based review of poorly differentiated thyroid cancer. *World J Surg.* 2007;31:934–945.

62. Patel KN, Shaha AR. Poorly differentiated and anaplastic thyroid cancer. *Cancer Control.* 2006;13:119–128.

63. Auersperg M, Us-Krasovec M, Petric G, et al. Results of combined modality treatment in poorly differentiated and anaplastic thyroid carcinoma. *Wien Klin Wochenschr.* 1990;102:267–270.

Anaplastic (Undifferentiated) Carcinoma

DEFINITION

Anaplastic carcinoma is a highly aggressive malignant thyroid tumor composed of undifferentiated cells that demonstrate immunohistochemical or ultrastructural features of epithelial differentiation. It is derived from follicular epithelial cells but is characteristically devoid of morphologic and immunophenotypic markers of thyroid origin. Another term frequently used to designate this tumor is *undifferentiated carcinoma*. Other synonyms used in the past include spindle and giant cell carcinoma, sarcomatoid carcinoma, pleomorphic carcinoma, metaplastic carcinoma, and carcinosarcoma.

INCIDENCE AND EPIDEMIOLOGY

Anaplastic carcinoma is a rare type of thyroid cancer comprising 1% to 1.7% of all thyroid malignancies registered in two different United States national databases and 1% to 2% of thyroid cancer cases in many other countries.[1-4] The incidence is higher (up to 8%) in some parts of Europe and in several other countries, particularly in association with iodine-deficiency and endemic goiter areas.[5-8] A higher incidence correlates with low socioeconomic status in some studies, possibly because of a delay of diagnosis of well-differentiated thyroid cancer, a precursor for anaplastic carcinoma.[8] Over the past decades, the incidence of anaplastic carcinoma has remained unchanged or even slightly decreased in many countries. In the United States, the incidence showed a 22% decrease between 1973 and 2003 based on the Surveillance, Epidemiology, and End Results (SEER) database.[9] This decrease may be attributed to eradication of severe iodine deficiency by iodization of food supplies, earlier detection and treatment of well-differentiated thyroid carcinomas, exclusion of medullary carcinomas and lymphomas, and better recognition of poorly differentiated thyroid carcinoma.[10]

Anaplastic carcinoma is typically a tumor of older adults; only 13% to 25% of patients are younger than 60 years at diagnosis.[11-13] The tumors are exceedingly rare before the age of 40, although single cases have been documented.[14-16] The tumor is more common in females, with a female predilection ranging from 1.5:1 to 2.5:1 in large series of patients.[13,17-19]

ETIOLOGIC FACTORS

Preexisting Thyroid Disease

Preexisting thyroid disease, both malignant and benign, is a major etiologic factor for anaplastic carcinoma.

Preexisting Carcinoma

Differentiated thyroid carcinoma affects the risk of anaplastic carcinoma by serving as a direct precursor lesion. Indeed, it is currently believed that many, if not most, anaplastic carcinomas develop through the process of dedifferentiation of a well-differentiated or poorly differentiated thyroid carcinoma. All major types of well-differentiated follicular cell-derived carcinomas can be involved. As anaplastic carcinoma is considered to be a follicular cell-derived neoplasm, cases of "anaplastic transformation" in medullary thyroid carcinoma [20] should not be considered as part of the same disease spectrum.

The existence of anaplastic transformation is strongly supported by the common occurrence of anaplastic carcinoma in patients with a history of previously treated well-differentiated thyroid cancer and by frequent finding of a differentiated component adjacent to the anaplastic carcinoma area on pathologic examination (Fig. 13.1). A review of series with >50 cases and adequate adequate histologic characterization demonstrates the presence of preexisting or coexisting well-differentiated carcinoma in 23% to 78% of cases.[14,17,18,20,21] Papillary carcinoma is the most common coexistent carcinoma and is found in >80% of cases showing both components.[21] Follicular carcinoma is far less frequent in series published subsequent to the description of the follicular variant of papillary carcinoma, and both conventional type and oncocytic (Hürthle cell) follicular carcinoma can be found.[22] Although possibly underdocumented, anaplastic carcinoma is least frequently associated with poorly differentiated carcinomas. Explanations for the underdocumentation may be due to the historical lack of a uniform definition for poorly differentiated carcinoma (see Chapter 12) and low impact of the finding of poorly differentiated carcinoma in those cases where the anaplastic component is detected.

Some cases of anaplastic carcinoma fail to reveal the areas of well-differentiated or poorly differentiated carcinoma. This may be due to the replacement of a less aggressive component by a more malignant tumor, or due to sampling error, or reflect a possibility that some anaplastic carcinomas develop directly, bypassing a stage of more differentiated carcinoma (Fig. 13.2).

Preexisting Benign Thyroid Disease

A history of long-standing goiter is a well-documented risk factor for anaplastic carcinoma development. In a large cohort of thyroid cancer cases from the United States, ~25% of patients had a personal history of goiter.[13] The prevalence of preexisting goiter was even higher in some other series approaching 50%.[20,23] Many patients had a history of goiter present for a very long time, such as for 20 to 60 years.[20] It is not entirely clear whether long-standing goiter predisposes to anaplastic carcinoma by increasing the risk of well-differentiated thyroid cancer or independently, by increasing the rate of cell proliferation, or through other and yet unknown mechanisms.

Iodine Deficiency

A higher incidence of anaplastic carcinoma has been reported in areas of dietary iodine deficiency, particularly among those individuals who lived in these areas for at least 20 years or during childhood.[7,24] Iodine supplementation in the regions of severe iodine deficiency coincided with reduction in the incidence of anaplastic carcinoma.[25,26] It is likely that iodine deficiency influences the rate of anaplastic carcinoma by increasing the incidence of goiter.

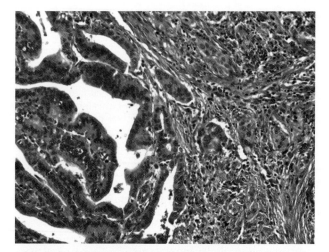

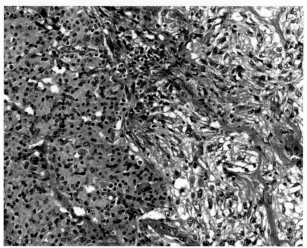

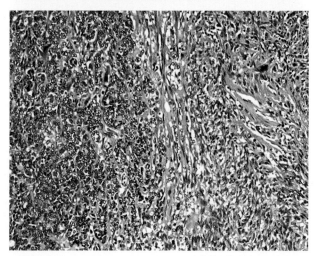

FIGURE 13.1. Anaplastic carcinoma associated with a more differentiated carcinoma component. The latter is a well-differentiated papillary carcinoma **(top)**, well-differentiated oncocytic follicular carcinoma **(middle)**, and poorly differentiated carcinoma **(bottom)**. In each panel, the more differentiated carcinoma component is on the left.

Radiation Exposure

Almost 10% of patient with anaplastic carcinoma have a history of radiation exposure.[13] This suggests the possible role of radiation in tumor development. Studies of large cohorts of patients exposed to ionizing radiation have not found an increase in anaplastic carcinomas, although this may be due to a low overall rate of this tumor occurrence. Ten to twelve percent of patients have a prior history of another malignancy.[13,19] This may reflect a general genetic predisposition to carcinogenesis in these patients or be related to the radiation treatment of the first malignancy.

PATHOGENESIS AND MOLECULAR GENETICS

Clonality

Representing the most undifferentiated neoplasm of the thyroid, clonality is not an issue of debate in anaplastic carcinoma. The rare tumors subjected to X-inactivation–based assays confirm this.[27] The cytogenetic evolution of multiple "subclones" with different chromosomal alterations has been documented, although this should not be construed as true polyclonality.[28]

Cytogenetic Abnormalities

Anaplastic carcinoma typically has a complex karyotype with multiple and diverse numerical and structural chromosomal abnormalities.[29,30] By comparative genomic hybridization, the mean number of chromosomal alterations ranges from 2.4 to 10.[31-33] There is a progressive accumulation of chromosomal alterations when comparing well differentiated carcinomas with poorly differentiated carcinomas and finally anaplastic carcinomas, which is in keeping with the multistep dedifferentiation process.[33,34] Anaplastic carcinomas arising in a background of follicular carcinoma appear to have more chromosomal instability reflected by an increased number of alterations as compared with anaplastic carcinomas arising from papillary carcinoma or those without a differentiated component.[31] This is not surprising in light of a significantly higher frequency of chromosomal instability observed in follicular carcinomas than in papillary carcinomas (see Chapter 10).

The prevalence of specific chromosomal abnormalities varies from study to study, but the most common alterations include gains of chromosome 1p (up to 33%) and 3p (up to 27%), losses of chromosome 5q (up to 33%), and alterations, either gains or losses of chromosome 8 (up to 44%) and 5p (up to 33%).[31-33] Decrease in the frequency of gains at 7p and increase in losses at 7q may coincide with anaplastic transformation of follicular and poorly differentiated carcinomas.[34]

DNA Ploidy

A correlate to the abnormally clumped chromatin and marked nuclear pleomorphism noted in anaplastic carcinomas is the change in DNA ploidy. The tumors are aneuploid in nearly 100% of cases.[35,36]

Loss of Heterozygosity

In correlation with multiple large-scale chromosomal alterations detected cytogenetically, loss of heterozygosity (LOH) is frequent in anaplastic carcinomas. As anaplastic transformation represents an "end-stage" of tumor progression for follicular cell-derived neoplasms, it can be expected that tumors will harbor multiple deletions at known tumor suppressor gene loci. The mean fractional allelic loss (i.e., frequency of LOH at specific

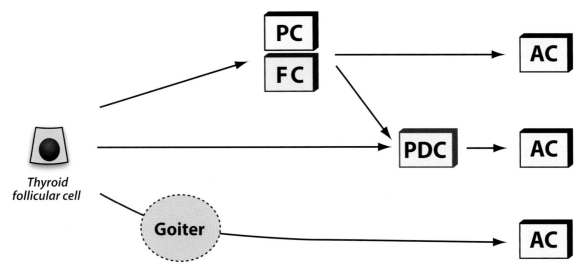

FIGURE 13.2. Putative pathways in the development of anaplastic carcinoma. Current evidence suggests that anaplastic carcinoma may develop by anaplastic transformation of well-differentiated papillary carcinoma well-differentiated follicular carcinoma or poorly differentiated carcinoma or directly from follicular cells, particularly in a setting of a long-standing goiter. AC, anaplastic carcinoma; PC, papillary carcinoma; FC, follicular carcinoma; PDC, poorly differentiated carcinoma.

chromosomal loci) in anaplastic carcinoma is high and ranges from 0.20 to 0.72.[37–39] Among the most frequent regions of LOH are 1q, 9p, 17p, 16p, 17q, and 18q. When there is a differentiated component, a subset of LOH may be common to both components, although the anaplastic carcinoma component has additional losses, providing molecular evidence for anaplastic transformation of well-differentiated tumors.[38,40]

Somatic Mutations

Mutations that occur in anaplastic carcinomas can be divided into two groups. One includes genetic alterations that are found in both anaplastic and well-differentiated carcinomas, such as *BRAF* and *RAS* mutations. The fact that they are present in well-differentiated carcinomas suggests that these mutations are early events in thyroid tumorigenesis and are insufficient alone to induce tumor dedifferentiation. Although insufficient for dedifferentiation, they predispose to acquisition of subsequent events that will govern anaplastic transformation. Of note, other mutations commonly found in well-differentiated papillary and follicular carcinomas, such as *RET/PTC* and *PAX8/PPARγ*, are rare in

anaplastic carcinomas, suggesting that they do not promote tumor dedifferentiation. This is particularly true for *RET/PTC1*, whereas *RET/PTC3* rearrangement has been seen in some papillary carcinomas prone to dedifferentiation.[41,42] The other group includes *TP53* and β-catenin (*CTNNB1*) mutations, which frequently occur in anaplastic carcinomas but not in well-differentiated cancers. These mutations are likely to be directly responsible for anaplastic transformation (Fig. 13.3).

RAS Mutations

Activating point mutations of *RAS* are common in follicular adenomas, follicular carcinomas, and follicular variant of papillary carcinomas (see Chapters 8, 10, and 11). In anaplastic carcinomas, the prevalence of *RAS* mutations ranges from 10% to 60% and is ~30% in the largest reported series.[43–46]

As in well-differentiated tumors, the mutations usually affect *NRAS* codon 61 and *HRAS* codon 61, although other hot spots (codons 12/13 of *NRAS, KRAS,* and *HRAS*) may be occasionally involved. Mutations in codons other than 12, 13, and 61 have been reported, although their functional significance is unclear.[47]

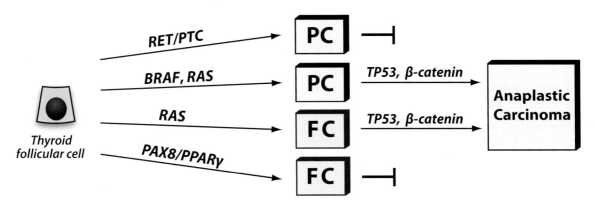

FIGURE 13.3. Gene mutations in the development of anaplastic carcinoma. *BRAF* and *RAS* mutations are found in both well-differentiated and anaplastic carcinomas indicating that they occur early and likely to predispose to anaplastic transformation, which is governed by *TP53* and β-catenin (*CTNNB1*) mutations. Tumors with *RET/PTC* (particularly *RET/PTC1*) and *PAX8/PPARγ* are not prone to anaplastic transformation. Mutations in the *PIK3CA* and *PTEN* genes are also found in anaplastic carcinomas, although their exact placement in the scheme of stepwise progression is not entirely clear.

The differentiated component in these tumors, when present, is typically a follicular carcinoma or follicular variant of papillary carcinoma. An identical *RAS* mutation is found in both tumor components, consistent with being an early event.

The main oncogenic effects of mutant RAS involve the activation of the mitogen-activated protein kinase (MAPK) and PI3K/AKT signaling cascades. Although *RAS* mutations occur early in tumorigenesis, their frequent presence in anaplastic carcinomas suggests that they are likely to confer the tumors with propensity to dedifferentiate. This may be due to the effect of mutant RAS on promoting chromosome instability and interfering with DNA damage response, which have been demonstrated in cultured thyroid cells.[48,49] The increasing instability may predispose the tumor cells to acquire additional mutations, which would in turn initiate anaplastic transformation. The ability of RAS activation to induce the loss of multiple thyroid differentiation markers such as thyroglobulin, thyrotropin-stimulating hormone receptor, sodium/iodide symporter (NIS) and thyroid transcription factor 1 (TTF1) in the cultured thyroid cells[50] is likely to be an in vitro phenomenon. Indeed, the presence of *RAS* mutations in benign thyroid tumors argues strongly against the direct role of RAS activation on the dedifferentiation of human thyroid cells in vivo.

BRAF Mutations

BRAF mutations are common in papillary carcinomas (see Chapter 11) and are found in ~25% of anaplastic carcinomas.[45,51] Many *BRAF*-positive anaplastic carcinomas contain a well-differentiated papillary carcinoma component, frequently tall cell variant, whereas some tumors show no morphologic evidence of a differentiated component. Similar to papillary carcinomas, the mutations in anaplastic carcinomas are also V600E and are found in both papillary carcinoma and anaplastic carcinoma areas, indicating that they occur early in carcinogenesis.[45,52,53]

BRAF V600E mutation leads to constitutive activation of the MAPK signaling pathway, and its expression in transgenic mice results in the formation of papillary carcinomas that undergo progression to poorly differentiated carcinomas.[54] However, the tumors in these animals did not undergo anaplastic transformation, consistent with the requirement for addition mutations to reach a fully undifferentiated phenotype.

PI3K/PTEN/AKT Pathway Mutations

Mutations in the effectors of this signaling pathway occur in 5% to 10% of well-differentiated follicular carcinomas (see Chapter 10). In anaplastic carcinomas, 6% to 23% of tumors demonstrate *PIK3CA* mutations and 6% to 16% *PTEN* mutations.[45,46,51,55,56] Most *PIK3CA* mutations are located at exon 20, the kinase domain, and exon 9, the helical domain, and lead to the activation of this pathway, as demonstrated by the increased phosphorylation of the AKT protein.[45] In addition, an increase in *PIK3CA* gene copy numbers is found in ~40% of anaplastic carcinomas.[51,57] In the *PTEN* gene, point mutations and small frameshift deletions most frequently occur in exons 5 and 7, leading to the loss of function of the PTEN protein and the subsequent activation of AKT.[46]

It remains not fully understood whether *PIK3CA* and *PTEN* mutations represent an early or late event in thyroid carcinogenesis. They are present with a similar or slightly higher prevalence in anaplastic carcinomas as compared with well-differentiated papillary and follicular carcinomas. However, in contrast to *BRAF* and *RAS* mutations, which almost never coexist in the same tumor, *PIK3CA* and other mutations are frequently seen in anaplastic carcinomas coexisting with *BRAF* or *RAS* mutations, suggesting that they may be a late event.[45,51] It has also been suggested that gradual increase in AKT stimulation is required for progression from adenoma to well-differentiated follicular carcinoma and then to anaplastic carcinoma.[46]

TP53 Mutations

TP53 mutations are among the most frequent genetic alterations in anaplastic carcinoma and are typically found in 50% to 80% of tumors.[58–61] The mutational profile is based largely on the screening of exons 5 to 8, where most mutations occur in cancer. The distribution of mutations in thyroid anaplastic carcinomas is similar to that of most other malignancies. The mutation sites are scattered along the evolutionarily conserved domains in these exons. G:C to A:T transitions are the prevalent types of mutation, often in CpG-rich regions, although transversions and small deletions and insertions occur as well.[62]

TP53 is a nuclear transcription factor that plays an important role in cell cycle regulation, DNA repair and apoptosis, functioning as a tumor suppressor gene. Mutations impair TP53 binding to specific DNA sequences and thus inhibit its transcriptional regulation activity. Mutant TP53 accumulates in the nucleus and manifests immunohistochemically as increased staining (see section Immunohistochemistry). *TP53* is commonly altered as a late event in carcinogenesis involving various tumor types. In thyroid cells, *TP53* mutations appear to be crucial for the process of tumor dedifferentiation. As such, they are far more common in anaplastic carcinomas than in poorly differentiated carcinomas and are practically absent in well-differentiated carcinomas. In tumors that contain anaplastic and well-differentiated carcinoma components, *TP53* mutations are detected only in the anaplastic component.[40,63] The best illustration of the multistep tumor progression is provided by a case where a well-differentiated component showed a *RAS*+/*TP53*– genotype, whereas the adjacent anaplastic carcinoma was *RAS*+/*TP53*+.[64]

In mouse models, the loss of TP53 in well-differentiated tumors induces anaplastic transformation.[65] Reintroduction of wild-type TP53 in anaplastic carcinoma cell lines carrying *TP53* mutation results in the reexpression of thyroid specific genes such as TPO and PAX8 and the reacquisition of the ability to respond to thyroid-stimulating hormone stimulation.[66,67] This provides another evidence for the role of TP53 in anaplastic transformation and also points to the restoration of *TP53* function as a potential therapeutic approach for these tumors.

β-Catenin (CTNNB1) Mutations

Mutations in the gene coding for β-catenin represents another event involved in anaplastic transformation. β-Catenin is a cytoplasmic protein encoded by the *CTNNB1* gene and involved in cell adhesion as well as in the wingless (Wnt) signaling pathway.[68,69] In the absence of Wnt signaling, β-catenin is expressed mainly on the cell surface, whereas cytoplasmic protein is rapidly degraded after phosphorylation by a multiprotein complex, which includes the adenomatous polyposis coli (APC) protein. Wnt antagonizes this degradation and allows β-catenin to relocate to the nucleus to stimulate target genes. APC and β-catenin mutations can interfere with degradation, resulting in nuclear localization and gene activation promoting tumorigenesis. Point mutations in exon 3 of β-catenin affect the GSK3β phosphorylation sites required for degradation. These mutations are seen in up to 65% of anaplastic carcinomas and with lower prevalence in poorly differentiated thyroid carcinomas.[70,71] They are not found in well-differentiated thyroid carcinomas, with the exception of the cribriform-morular variant of papillary carcinoma.[72] Unlike this rare variant of papillary carcinoma, β-catenin mutations in anaplastic carcinomas are often multiple, on average 2.4 mutations per case, indicative of the high level of genetic instability.[70,71] Mutational status correlates, although not always, with nuclear immunoexpression of β-catenin.

Other Genetic Alterations

Other components of the Wnt signaling pathway may be altered in anaplastic carcinomas. For instance, *APC* mutations occur in about 10% of cases. On the basis of limited evidence, it appears that these mutations are mutually exclusive with β-catenin mutations.[73] Neither *EGFR* amplification nor mutations at exons 18, 19, and 21 are present in anaplastic carcinomas, although there is a high frequency (50%) of polysomy for chromosome 7, where *EGFR* is located.[74–76] Although loss of TP53 function promotes anaplasia in mice with papillary carcinomas induced by *RET/PTC1*,[65] *RET/PTC1* rearrangement is rarely found in human anaplastic carcinoma suggesting that it is less likely to predispose to tumor dedifferentiation than *RAS* and *BRAF* mutations.[47,77]

Profound alterations in gene expression, microRNA, and protein composition are also found in anaplastic carcinomas,[78] although the relevance of specific genetic events to pathogenesis of this tumor awaits further analyses.

CLINICAL PRESENTATION AND IMAGING

The classic presentation of anaplastic carcinoma is a rapidly growing neck mass, which is noted in nearly all cases.[17] Tumor volume may double as rapidly as in 1 week.[79] The mean tumor size at presentation is about 6 cm.[19] Other frequent presentation symptoms include hoarseness, dysphagia, and vocal cord paralysis. Up to 50% of patients have extrathyroidal extension at presentation. The most commonly invaded structures include extrinsic muscles, trachea, esophagus, larynx, and laryngeal nerves. Some patients may present with weight loss. Distant metastases are found at presentation in ~45% of patients (Fig. 13.4), and a similar proportion of patients have cervical lymphadenopathy.[13,17,19] The most common sites of metastasis are lungs, bones, and brain. Patients are generally euthyroid on presentation, but rare case reports of transient thyrotoxicosis, presumably secondary to destruction of thyroid parenchyma and rapid release of thyroid hormone, have been described.[80–82] Some patients may have leukocytosis as a result of secretion of macrophage colony-stimulating factor.[83,84] Additional rare clinical presentations include venous thrombosis

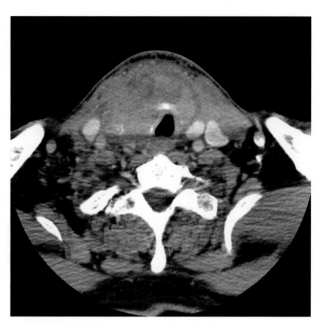

FIGURE 13.5. CT scan of anaplastic carcinoma. It shows an infiltrative heterogeneous mass with thyroid cartilage invasion and encroaching on the adjacent vasculature.

and humoral hypercalcemia of malignancy, the latter due to parathyroid hormone–related protein secretion.[84–86]

CT is the preferred method to characterize disease in the neck, whereas MRI is indicated to assess mediastinal extent.[87] Using either of these diagnostic modalities, anaplastic is typically an infiltrative heterogeneous mass with irregular borders, and necrosis (Fig. 13.5). On MRI, T1-weighted signal intensities vary from low to high, whereas T2-weighted signal intensities are often high.[87] Calcifications are common. Carotid and internal jugular vein involvement is frequently seen. Lymph nodes involved often show rim enhancement on CT.[88,89] Anaplastic carcinoma does not typically have uptake of radioactive iodine, either in primary or in metastatic foci and is "cold" on scintigraphy. In fact, areas of radioiodine uptake would suggest a differentiated component.[12] The role of combined 18F-fluorodeoxyglucose positron emission tomography and CT for preoperative and postoperative disease assessment is not fully defined, although it has been found to be helpful in some cases.[90,91]

GROSS FEATURES

On gross examination, anaplastic carcinoma is typically a widely infiltrative mass that replaces the thyroid gland and extends into the adjacent soft tissue or skeletal muscle (Fig. 13.6). Tumors may range from 1 to 20 cm in size but are typically >5 cm.[92] Fewer than 10% are confined to the thyroid.[19] The cut surface typically demonstrates a friable variegated appearance with multiple foci of hemorrhage and necrosis. Firm or granular tan-brown areas should be sampled for histologic evaluation as they may harbor a residual well-differentiated carcinoma. Very rarely, heterologous elements such as bone or cartilage are grossly identified.[93] The paucicellular variant, however, typically shows a homogeneous, firm, tan-white cut surface, mimicking Riedel thyroiditis.

MICROSCOPIC FEATURES

Anaplastic carcinoma may manifest as a multitude of microscopic appearances, often within the same tumor case or even same

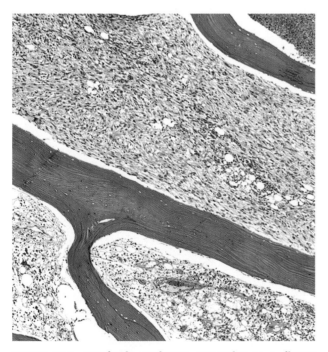

FIGURE 13.4. Anaplastic carcinoma presenting as a distant metastasis to the femur. The tumor is seen on top, permeating between bony trabeculae.

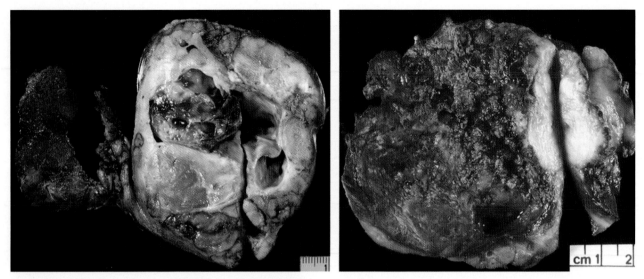

FIGURE 13.6. Gross appearance of anaplastic carcinoma. Left: Tumor replaces the entire right lobe and shows a fleshy, friable cut surface with multiple areas of necrosis and hemorrhage. **Right:** This tumor infiltrates skeletal muscle *(bottom)*.

slide. However, certain features are common to all tumors. They include (1) widely invasive growth, (2) extensive tumor necrosis, (3) marked nuclear pleomorphism, and (4) high mitotic activity. Indeed, the microscopic appearance of anaplastic carcinoma on low-power magnification is almost invariably infiltrative, both within the thyroid parenchyma and in the adjacent tissues. The invasion of perithyroidal fat tissue and skeletal muscle is

common (Fig. 13.7A). The characteristic feature is the permeation or "colonization" of the vessel walls in medium-size veins and arteries (Fig. 13.7B,C). Areas of coagulative necrosis with irregular contours are common (Fig. 13.8A) and may demonstrate tumor cell palisading. All tumor cell types have pleomorphic nuclei with highly irregular nuclear contours and thick coarse chromatin (Fig. 13.8B). The cells are arranged in solid sheets,

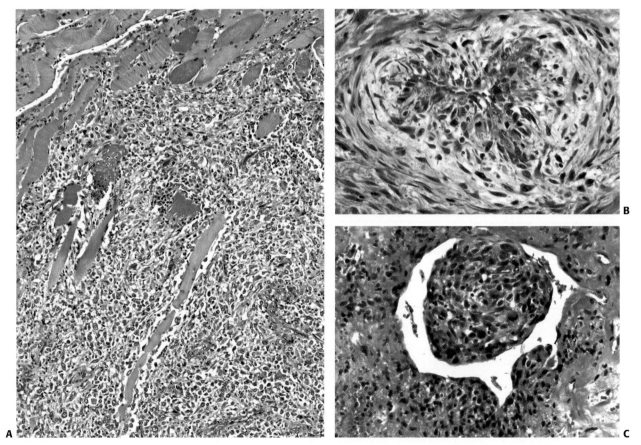

FIGURE 13.7. A: Anaplastic carcinoma infiltrating skeletal muscle. **B and C:** Anaplastic carcinoma permeating and colonizing a medium-sized artery. The vessel in **(C)** also shows an intravascular tumor "thrombus."

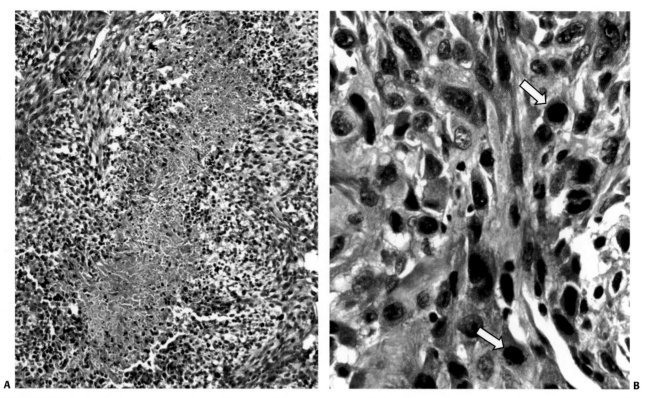

FIGURE 13.8. A: Anaplastic carcinoma demonstrating geographic coagulative necrosis. **B:** Pronounced nuclear atypia in anaplastic carcinoma. The nuclei show marked pleomorphism, hyperchromasia, and thickened, irregular nuclear membranes. Two mitotic figures are seen *(arrows)*.

with no follicle formation or colloid. The latter can be seen in the entrapped nonneoplastic thyroid cells or well-differentiated carcinoma areas.

From a cytologic standpoint, anaplastic carcinoma typically contains a mixture of spindled, epithelioid, and pleomorphic giant cells, as described below. Scattered single necrotic cells with pyknotic nuclei are frequently seen. Mitoses are typically abundant and atypical forms may be present (Fig. 13.8B).

The stroma ranges from hyalinized and sclerotic to fibrocellular and desmoplastic. An inflammatory background is common and usually consists of neutrophilic infiltrates. Occasionally (in about 10%), osteoclast-like giant cells may contribute to this inflammatory milieu (Fig. 13.9).[12,94] These giant cells contain numerous bland nuclei, which are different from the surrounding highly pleomorphic nuclei of carcinoma cells (Fig. 13.9B,C). They show immunohistochemical and ultrastructural features of monocytic/histiocytic lineage and are likely to derive from histiocytoid mononuclear cells through cellular fusion.[95]

A preponderance of one cell type gives rise to the common histologic patterns of anaplastic carcinoma.

Spindle Cell Pattern

This is the most common histologic pattern, predominating in about 50% of cases.[14,17,79] It recapitulates the appearance of a pleomorphic high-grade sarcoma. Cells may be arranged in a storiform pattern reminiscent of a so-called *malignant fibrous histiocytoma*, (Fig. 13.10A,B) particularly the inflammatory or myxoid types, or in "herringbone" patterned long fascicles resembling fibrosarcoma (Fig. 13.10C). Occasionally, the spindle cell pattern in anaplastic carcinoma may contain a branching staghorn or "hemangiopericytoma-like" vasculature (Fig. 13.10D). Rarely, hemorrhage and cell dyshesion resulting in an anastomosing network of blood-filled spaces reminiscent of

angiosarcoma (Fig. 13.11A).[96,97] In <5% of cases, heterologous elements such as malignant bone and cartilage may be seen (Fig. 13.11B,C).[9,12]

Pleomorphic Giant Cell Pattern

This pattern is the second most common, predominating in about 30% to 40% of cases.[14,17] The pleomorphism of cells is even more pronounced than in the other types, with sheets of bizarre cells typically seen. The tumor cells are often multinucleated and show marked nuclear hyperchromasia (Fig. 13.12A). The cytoplasm ranges from amphophilic to eosinophilic. Multiple small intracytoplasmic hyaline globules have been described in this variant.[14] Cell dyshesion is prominent often imparting an alveolar or a pseudoglandular growth pattern (Fig. 13.12B). This variant may also resemble angiosarcoma when these pseudoglandular spaces are filled with blood.

Squamoid Pattern

This is a less common appearance of anaplastic carcinomas, which is seen in <20% of tumors in most series.[14,17,20] The microscopic features resemble those of a nonkeratinizing squamous cell carcinoma of the lung or upper aerodigestive tract. The growth pattern is characteristically nested with either a "back to back" arrangement of squamoid cell nests or their separation by desmoplastic stroma (Fig. 13.13). In some situations, this "stroma" may actually represent an intermingled spindle cell component. The cells show moderate nuclear pleomorphism, and multinucleated giant cells are rare. The cytoplasm is dense and often eosinophilic. There may be evidence of true "squamous" differentiation, including intracytoplasmic bridges and keratinization, although it is rarely prominent. Mucin (usually extracellular) may rarely be demonstrable by histochemical stains.[12,14]

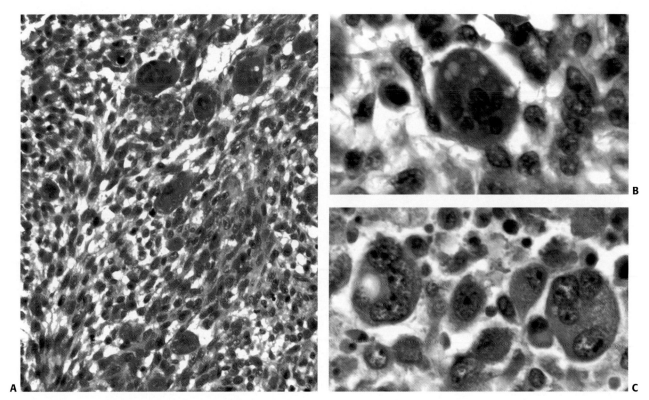

FIGURE 13.9. Osteoclast-like giant cells in anaplastic carcinoma. Multiple osteoclast-like giant cells in this anaplastic carcinoma **(A and B)** can be distinguished from tumor giant cells (shown for comparison in **C**) by their dense retracted cytoplasm and small, monomorphic, benign-appearing nuclei.

 ## MICROSCOPIC VARIANTS

Paucicellular Variant

This is a very rare variant (<1%) that mimics a benign process, particularly Riedel thyroiditis. Although only more recently described as a variant,[98] this pattern was recognized much earlier as part of the spectrum of the spindle cell pattern.[20] Indeed, the tumors with spindled cell pattern may have focal paucicellular areas. The prevailing thought is that these areas represent a healing fibroproliferative response to an earlier phase of necrosis.[99] Histologically, this variant is characterized by a dense infiltrative fibrous stroma with a chronic inflammatory infiltrate (Fig. 13.14). By definition, only scattered tumor cells, typically of a spindle type, are embedded within this stroma. Despite their low density, these cells, when examined singly, are still highly atypical with nuclear features similar to the more conventional patterns. In addition, the areas of coagulative necrosis are often present, albeit without the palisading seen in the more common patterns. Vessel wall infiltration is still commonly seen.

It is important to recognize this variant because it can be diagnostically challenging, may be seen in younger patients and may have a slightly more indolent course.[98,99]

Rhabdoid Variant

This is a rare variant as well. Although a recent series reported the presence of rhabdoid cells in 10% of anaplastic carcinomas and up to a third of poorly differentiated thyroid carcinomas,[21] cases in which this is a prominent pattern are confined to small case series.[100–104] Historically, this variant has been lumped into either poorly differentiated thyroid carcinoma or anaplastic carcinoma, but the abysmal outcome of patients with this variant and the similarities to the more common giant cell pattern of

anaplastic carcinoma with hyaline inclusions suggests that rhabdoid thyroid tumors are more appropriately considered anaplastic carcinomas. This variant is characterized by a proliferation of cells with dense globoid hyaline inclusions that displace the nucleus eccentrically (Fig. 13.15A,B). The rhabdoid inclusions are typically strongly positive for vimentin and in most cases for low molecular weight cytokeratins (Fig. 13.15C,D) but are negative for thyroglobulin.

Small Cell Variant

This variant using modern criteria and immunohistochemistry is likely nonexistent. Even well before the immunohistochemical era, it was recognized that this "variant" behaved differently than other anaplastic carcinomas.[105] With the advent of immunohistochemistry and refinement of histologic definitions, essentially all thyroid "small cell carcinomas" have been reclassified as lymphomas, medullary carcinoma, or poorly differentiated thyroid carcinomas.[14,106,107] Historically, a few small cell neuroendocrine carcinomas of the larynx have been sent in consultation to our institution as possible small cell variants of anaplastic thyroid carcinoma.

 ## ANAPLASTIC CARCINOMA WITH COEXISTING WELL-DIFFERENTIATED OR POORLY DIFFERENTIATED CARCINOMA

Small or larger areas of well-differentiated or poorly differentiated carcinoma are frequently found in the gland affected by anaplastic carcinoma.[14,17,18,20,21,23,108] Coexisting well-differentiated papillary carcinoma is often the tall cell or follicular variant.

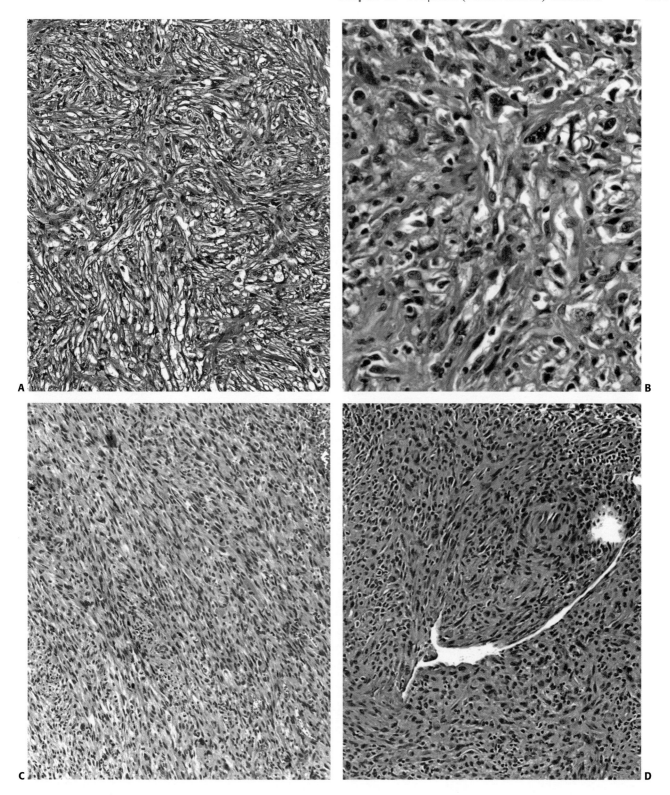

FIGURE 13.10. Spindle cell pattern of anaplastic carcinoma. A: A storiform arrangement of spindled tumor cells. **B:** On higher magnification, the spindle cells contain nuclei that are highly atypical, ranging from elongated to plump with marked hyperchromasia. **C:** Occasionally, there is a long fascicular fibrosarcoma-like arrangement of spindle cells. **D:** Some tumors have branching staghorn-like vessels typical of the so-called *hemangiopericytoma-like* vasculature.

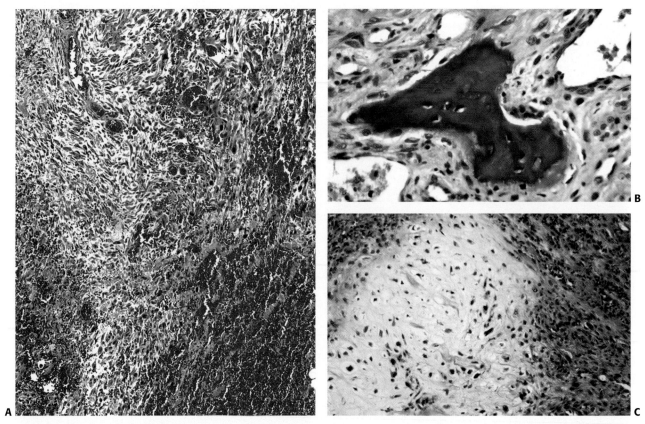

FIGURE 13.11. A: Anaplastic carcinoma showing a "pseudoangiosarcomatous" appearance. Cell dyshesion as a result of extravasated blood and engorged capillaries imparts a resemblance to the anastomosing vascular spaces of angiosarcoma. **B and C:** Anaplastic carcinoma demonstrating the heterologous element of bone **(B)** and hyaline cartilage **(C)**.

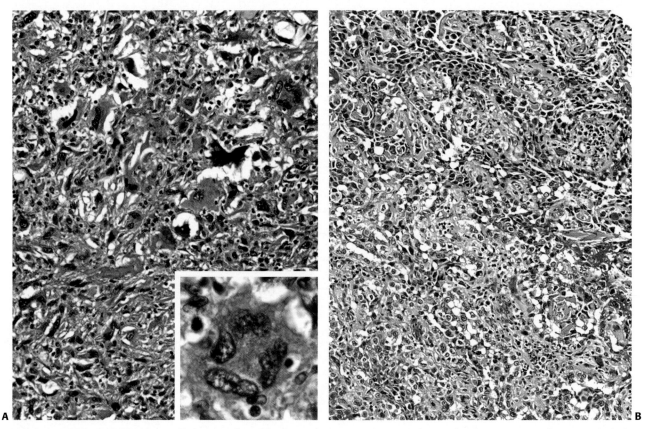

FIGURE 13.12. Pleomorphic giant cell pattern of anaplastic carcinoma. A: Sheets of pleomorphic, bizarre tumor cells, some of which are multinucleated **(inset)**. **B:** Occasional areas may show pseudoglandular spaces.

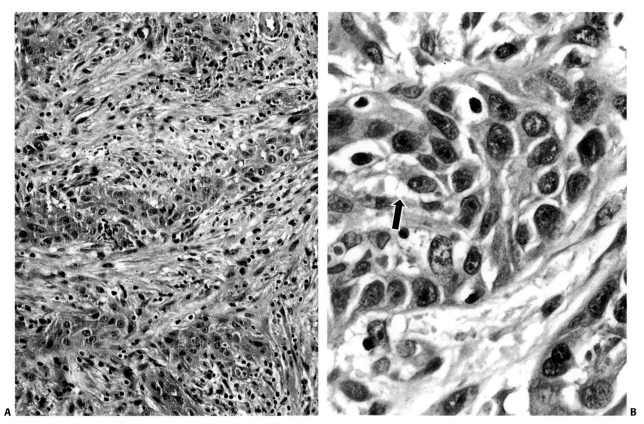

FIGURE 13.13. Squamoid pattern of anaplastic carcinoma. A: Cohesive epithelioid nests with dense eosinophilic cytoplasm intermingled with the spindle cell pattern. **B:** Occasionally, the squamoid areas are focally truly squamous, with more distinct cell borders and even intercellular bridges *(arrow)*.

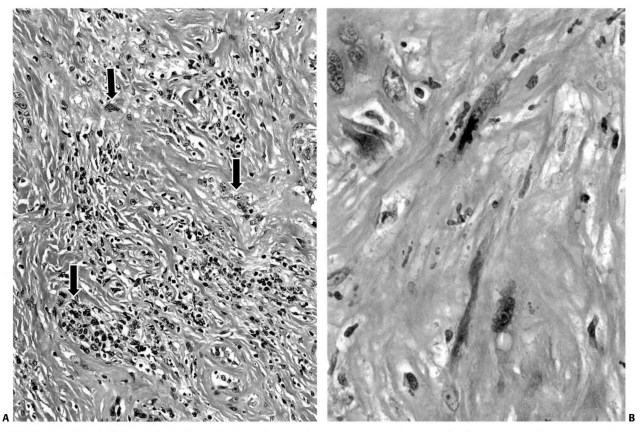

FIGURE 13.14. Paucicellular variant of anaplastic carcinoma. A: Only rare tumor cells and small cell groups *(arrows)* are seen in a dense fibroinflammatory stroma. **B:** On high-power examination, although sparse, these cells are still markedly pleomorphic and hyperchromatic with occasional prominent nucleoli.

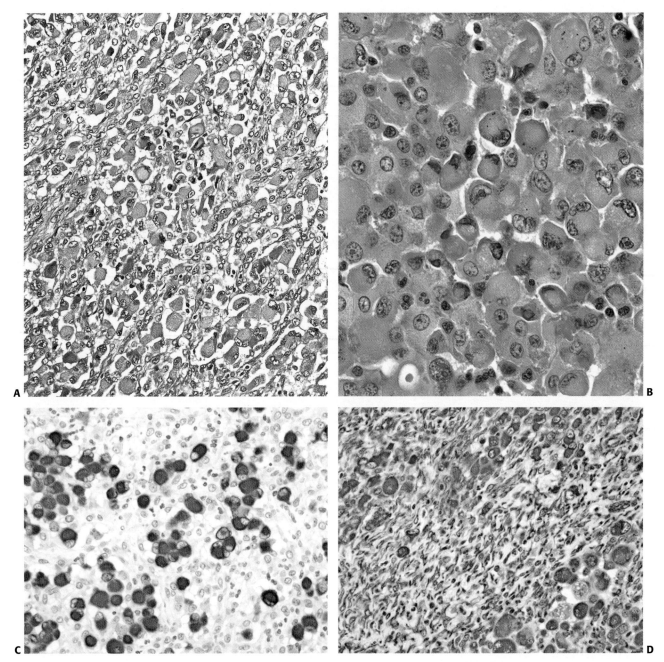

FIGURE 13.15. Rhabdoid variant of anaplastic carcinoma. A: Dyshesive sheets of cells. **B:** Cells contain dense globoid hyaline inclusions that eccentrically displace the nucleus. These inclusions are strongly positive for cytokeratin cocktail AE1/AE3 **(C)** and vimentin **(D)**.

The coexisting well-differentiated or poorly differentiated carcinoma areas can be highlighted by preserved thyroglobulin, TTF1, and PAX8 immunoreactivity. The finding of coexisting well-differentiated or poorly differentiated carcinoma is helpful in establishing a definitive diagnosis of anaplastic thyroid carcinoma by ruling out metastatic carcinoma and nonepithelial malignancy.

The proportion of anaplastic carcinoma in a given tumor may influence prognosis. Although data are limited, survival is likely to be more prolonged in those cases where anaplastic carcinoma comprises only a small component of an otherwise well-differentiated papillary or follicular carcinoma.[23,83,109] Therefore, the proportion of anaplastic carcinoma and coexistent well-differentiated or poorly differentiated carcinoma in a given tumor should be clearly stated in the pathology report.

 IMMUNOHISTOCHEMISTRY

The immunohistochemical profile of anaplastic carcinoma is summarized in Table 13.1.[14,18,110–118] In anaplastic carcinoma, immunostains are commonly used to establish epithelial differentiation. However, negativity for epithelial markers does not exclude the diagnosis of anaplastic carcinoma. Cytokeratins are the most frequently positive epithelial markers in anaplastic carcinomas, although keratin antibody type, method of antigen retrieval, and number of different keratins studied have led to a wide range of reported immunoreactive frequency (45% to 91%, mean 69%).[14,18,110–116] In more recent series, >80% of tumors are positive for cytokeratin (Fig. 13.16A).[18,112,113] Within a given tumor, however, the reactivity is often weak and very focal (Fig. 13.16B). In fact,

Table 13.1

Immunohistochemical Profile of Anaplastic Carcinoma

Antibody	Frequency of Positive Staining[a]	References
CKs (overall)	++	14,18,110–116
EMA	+	18,110,112,116
CEA	+	14,110,116
Thyroglobulin	−[b]	14,110,114–116
TTF1	±	112,117,118
TTF2	±	117
PAX8	++	117,119
P63	++[c]	124,125
TP53	++	108,120,121
P21	+	108,120,121
Cyclin D1	++	120,123
EGFR	+	74,75
Her2/Neu	+	74,75
PDGFR-β	+	74,75

[a] Percentage of cases showing positive staining: "++" corresponds to >50% of cases;, "+" corresponds to 10%–50% of cases, "±" corresponds to 1%–9% of case, and "−" corresponds to no positive cases.
[b] Diffusion from surrounding thyroid excluded.
[c] Small series only.

strong diffuse reactivity is typical of differentiated carcinomas and should raise doubts about the diagnosis of anaplastic carcinoma.

In light of the aforementioned staining heterogeneity, it is recommended that a polyspecific cytokeratin antibody or cocktail of cytokeratin antibodies be used to prove epithelial differentiation. Polyspecific antibodies (such as CAM 5.2, which detects CK8, CK18, and CK19) or cocktails (such as AE1/AE3, which detects CK1 to CK8,

CK10, CK14 to CK16, and CK19) understandably outperform individual keratin antibodies. In our experience, AE1/AE3 is preferred as it stains more intensely, and it is positive in a larger percentage of cells.

The expression of the specific keratin types may vary in different microscopic patterns of anaplastic carcinoma. The squamoid pattern shows the highest frequency and most complex keratin expression profile, often positive for CK7, CK8, CK13, CK14, CK17, CK18, and CK19. In contrast, the spindle cell subtype shows the weakest and lowest frequency of CK positivity, often expressing only CK8, CK7, or CK18. The pleomorphic giant cell subtype has a cytokeratin profile complexity that is in between that of the squamoid and spindle cell subtypes.[112,113]

Epithelial membrane antigen (EMA) is also positive, but often to a lesser degree, ranging in frequency from 20% to 54% (mean 38%).[18,110,112,116] Carcinoembryonic antigen (CEA) is not commonly expressed (range 0% to 13%) and is usually restricted to the squamoid pattern.[14,110,116]

Regarding markers of thyroid differentiation, PAX8 appears to be the most helpful marker. PAX8 immunoreactivity is retained in 76% to 79% of anaplastic carcinomas (Fig. 13.17).[117,119] In most positive cases, the nuclear staining is moderately intense but diffuse. The frequency of retaining the PAX8 immunoreactivity may depend on the predominant growth pattern. In one study of 26 anaplastic carcinomas, positive staining was observed in 100% of tumors with the squamoid pattern, 68% of tumors with the pleomorphic giant cell pattern, and 50% of tumors with the spindle pattern.[119]

The interpretation of thyroglobulin immunoreactivity is controversial. It has been reported to be anywhere from 0% to 50% (mean 18%).[14,110,114–116] However, reactivity is often weak and equivocal, and the prevailing opinion is that rather than true immunopositivity, this reactivity may simply represent (1) components of differentiated carcinoma, (2) entrapped normal follicles, or (3) diffusion of thyroglobulin from surrounding thyroid parenchyma (Fig. 13.18A).[11,12]

TTF1 and TTF2 are only rarely expressed in anaplastic carcinomas (Fig. 13.18B).[112,117,118] Strong TTF1 immunoreactivity typically highlights the areas of well-differentiated carcinoma or entrapped normal thyroid parenchyma.

Cell cycle deregulation in anaplastic carcinomas is common, particularly with regard to TP53 alterations. From a diagnostic standpoint, TP53 is a marker that is useful to separate anaplastic carcinoma from more differentiated thyroid carcinomas (Fig. 13.19A). By immunohistochemistry, TP53 is strongly expressed in 39% to 100% of cases.[108,120–122] The immunoreactivity is believed to demonstrate the accumulation of the mutant TP53

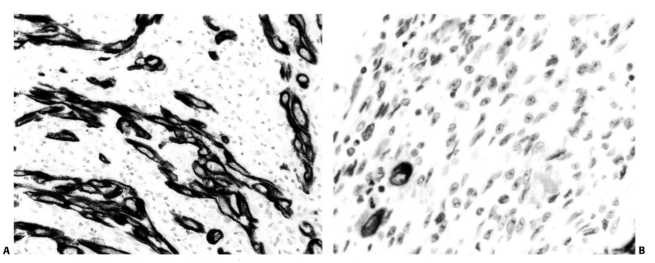

FIGURE 13.16. Cytokeratin immunostaining in anaplastic carcinoma. A: This tumor area shows strong immunoreactivity in about half of cells. However, it is unusual for cases to be strongly positive throughout. Areas of positivity are typically patchy, occasionally showing only rare positive single cells **(B)**. **A,** CAM 5.2 immunostain; **B,** AE1/AE3 immunostain.

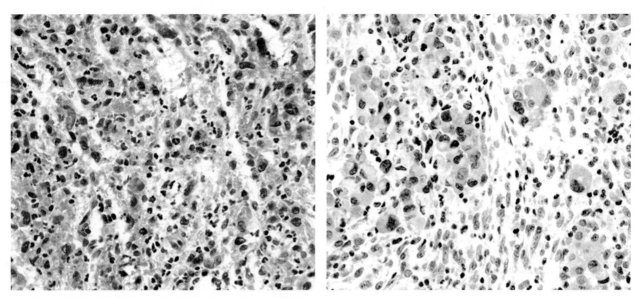

FIGURE 13.17. PAX8 nuclear immunoreactivity in anaplastic carcinoma. PAX8 expression is often retained in anaplastic carcinomas, as illustrated in a spindle cell–patterned anaplastic carcinoma **(left)** and in a rhabdoid anaplastic carcinoma **(right)**.

protein. The cyclin-dependent kinase inhibitor p21 is induced by wild-type TP53. Cyclin D1 has been noted to be strongly expressed by immunohistochemistry in 62% to 77% of anaplastic carcinomas. However, cyclin D1 overexpression is not specific for this tumor type and is seen in other aggressive thyroid carcinomas including tall cell variant of papillary carcinoma and poorly differentiated carcinomas.[120,123]

Interestingly, p63, a marker typically used to support squamous/basal differentiation, is positive in up to 71% of anaplastic

carcinomas, although this is based on small series of tumors (Fig. 13.19B).[124,125]

High proliferative rate of anaplastic carcinoma cells can be confirmed using Ki-67 (MIB1) immunostaining, which typically shows a labeling index of about 50% (range 5% to 100%).[121,122,126–128]

Growth factors of potential therapeutic interest such as EGFR, HER-2/Neu, and PDGFR-β are overexpressed immunohistochemically in 20% to 60% of cases; however, gene amplification has not been noted.[74,75]

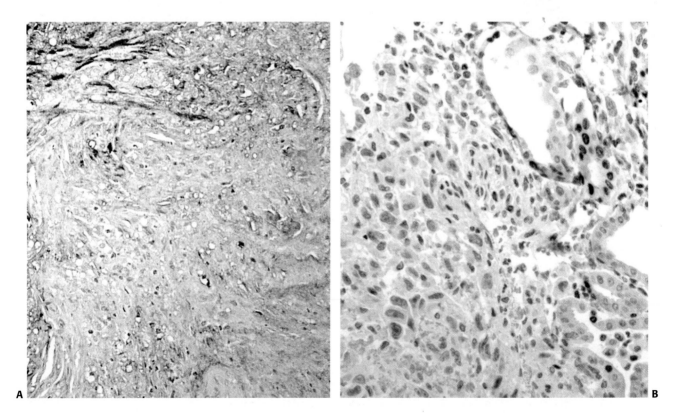

FIGURE 13.18. A: Thyroglobulin background staining of anaplastic carcinoma stroma. This is the result of diffusion from the surrounding thyroid parenchyma and should not be considered positive staining. **B:** TTF1 is negative in this anaplastic carcinoma, whereas a well-differentiated follicular carcinoma component (right) is positive.

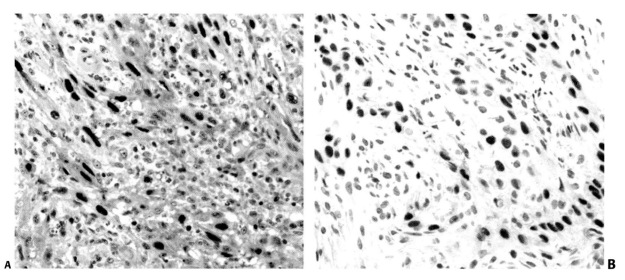

FIGURE 13.19. A: Strong TP53 nuclear reactivity is frequently seen in anaplastic carcinoma. **B:** p63 immunoreactivity may be present in anaplastic carcinoma cells.

MOLECULAR DIAGNOSTICS

The diagnosis of anaplastic carcinoma is made largely by morphology and immunohistochemistry, although testing for molecular alterations may occasionally be used to aid the diagnosis. Although *TP53* and *β*-catenin mutations are common in anaplastic carcinomas, they can occasionally be seen in poorly differentiated carcinomas as well. In addition, immunohistochemistry is a quick and relatively inexpensive surrogate for the alterations in TP53 and *β*-catenin. *BRAF* and *RAS* mutations are not entirely specific for thyroid carcinomas and would not always differentiate anaplastic carcinoma from other high-grade tumors, although they are very rare in sarcomas. Moreover, typical hot spots for *RAS* mutations (*NRAS* codon 61 and *HRAS* codon 61) are exceptionally rare in other tumors except melanomas. Therefore, if a particular site of origin or tumor type is suspected on encountering an undifferentiated tumor, *BRAF* and *RAS* mutational status in conjunction with the gene alterations typically seen at this putative site may provide additional evidence for or against anaplastic carcinoma. The low prevalence of *RET/PTC* and *PAX8/PPARγ* fusions in anaplastic carcinomas precludes its utility in establishing thyroid origin when the differential diagnosis includes other anaplastic tumors, although it would be highly specific if found.

ULTRASTRUCTURAL FEATURES

Ultrastructural examination often shows only rudimentary evidence of epithelial differentiation. Nuclei are often convoluted with dense clumped chromatin and prominent nucleoli. Desmosomes are present but are far less common than those in differentiated thyroid carcinomas. Apical microvilli seen in differentiated thyroid lesions are rare to absent. Unlike differentiated thyroid carcinomas, evidence for secretory activity, namely, prominent rough endoplasmic reticulum and dense secretory granules, is absent. However, nondescript electron-dense granules are commonly seen, likely of lysosomal derivation.[12] Mitochondria may be scattered to abundant but less are than those of oncocytic lesions. Intermediate filaments range from scattered to abundant. They may form whorled structures in the rhabdoid variant of anaplastic carcinoma. These filaments are likely a mixture of keratin and vimentin.[104] Basal lamina is often incomplete to absent, and the cells

will often show complex interdigitations. In the giant cell subtype, the characteristics of the multinucleated tumor cells are similar to those of the mononuclear cells supporting a common origin.[129–131] Very rarely, evidence for true heterologous differentiation such as actin, myosin, and Z-bands can be seen.[132]

CYTOLOGIC FEATURES

On an adequate fine needle aspiration (FNA), anaplastic carcinoma is clearly malignant. However, it is undifferentiated to the point that it is difficult to confirm a thyroid origin. Anaplastic carcinoma is composed of large, pleomorphic cells that range from round or ovoid to spindle shaped (Fig. 13.20). Most aspirates demonstrate more than one cell morphology.[133] Chromatin is coarse and clumped with prominent, often multiple nucleoli. Mitoses may be readily identified even on aspirate smears. Cytoplasm may range from pale and vacuolated to dense and partly keratinized. On an aspirate smear, tumor cells may either appear singly or appear as tissue fragments. These fragments may vary in size and shape but do not form predictable groups as seen in differentiated carcinomas. Aspirates of anaplastic carcinoma do not typically show colloid, and, if present, it is likely derived from the uninvolved thyroid parenchyma. Anaplastic carcinoma aspirates are often accompanied by significant amounts of necrotic debris, mixed inflammatory infiltrates, and hemorrhage, occasionally to the point of obscuring the diagnosis.[134] Abundant neutrophils are found in many cases and may serve as an important diagnostic clue.[133] Rarely, a prominent osteoclast-like giant cell component may be aspirated.[135,136] Occasionally, a differentiated component may be present, imparting a dual population of tumor cells.

The sensitivity of FNA for the diagnosis of malignancy in cases of anaplastic carcinoma ranges from 71% to 97%.[134,137] Common reasons for false negatives include inadequacy, obscuring inflammation, or the prominence of a differentiated component. Anaplastic carcinoma with fibrous spindled component or abundant calcification may not be amenable to aspiration, in which case, core or incisional biopsies may be performed. False-positive cases are rare; however, anaplastic carcinoma may be mistaken for large cell lymphoma or metastatic carcinoma.[138,139] Without clinical history and immunohistochemical studies on cell blocks, the differentiation of anaplastic carcinoma from metastatic carcinoma or lymphoma on FNA may be impossible.

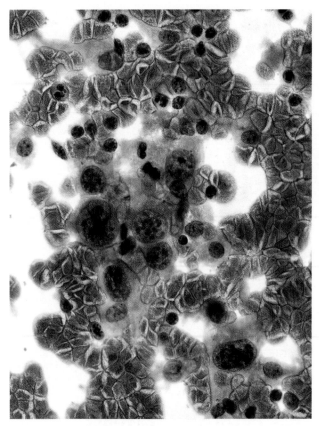

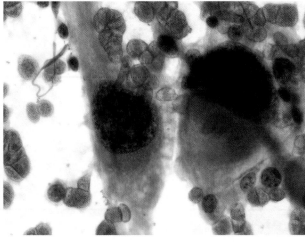

FIGURE 13.20. Cytologic features of anaplastic carcinoma. Left: A smear preparation of an anaplastic carcinoma fine needle aspirate demonstrating a dyshesive nest of tumor cells bordered by single cells in a hemorrhagic background with scattered inflammatory cells (Papanicolaou stain). **Right:** These tumor cells are much larger than the surrounding inflammatory cells and show dense coarse chromatin and thick cytoplasm (Papanicolaou stain).

 DIFFERENTIAL DIAGNOSIS

The differential diagnosis of anaplastic carcinoma is fairly broad because of various patterns encountered in this tumor. As the morphology is nondescript and immunohistochemically, markers of differentiation (thyroglobulin, TTF1, TTF2, and to lesser extent PAX8) are frequently lost, this is a diagnosis that requires incorporation of patients' history and clinical parameters as well. Histologically, differential diagnostic considerations revolve around two broad categories, that is, the distinction from (1) differentiated thyroid carcinomas and nonneoplastic thyroid lesions and (2) nonthyroid malignancies or thyroid nonepithelial tumors with an undifferentiated or spindle cell appearance. The differential diagnosis is summarized in Table 13.2.

Distinction from Thyroid Carcinomas and Benign Lesions

Poorly differentiated thyroid carcinoma is often regarded as an intermediate form between well-differentiated and anaplastic carcinomas, and a gradual morphologic transition from well-differentiated to poorly differentiated and then to anaplastic carcinomas can occasionally be seen. However, it is important to properly separate these tumors because therapeutic approaches and survival are substantially different between anaplastic and poorly differentiated thyroid carcinomas. Poorly differentiated carcinoma is distinguished by its relative cell monomorphism and more defined patterns of growth (solid, trabecular, and insular). Follicles can be seen. Necrosis is less prominent and may be more punctate as compared with the geographic distribution in anaplastic carcinomas.[140,141] The immunophenotype not only conveys the concept of a continuum from well to poorly and then to undifferentiated but also has practical application (Fig. 13.21). Although keratin, thyroglobulin, and TTF1 are strongly expressed in well-differentiated thyroid carcinoma, poorly differentiated carcinomas typically lose thyroglobulin but retain TTF1 and keratin expression, although staining is often less intense, particularly for TTF1. In anaplastic carcinoma, both thyroglobulin and TTF1 are lost, with only keratin being retained, often only focally.

Some well-differentiated carcinomas may show patterns (i.e., squamous or spindle cell metaplasia) or stroma (i.e., fasciitis like) that mimic those of anaplastic carcinoma (see Chapter 11) but will not show the frank nuclear pleomorphism, hyperchromasia, necrosis, and mitotic activity seen in anaplastic carcinoma.[142,143] Here, TTF1 may be useful as well since it will be retained in these mimics of anaplastic carcinoma.

The paucicellular variant of anaplastic carcinoma may mimic Riedel thyroiditis. However, on careful examination, the tumor cells in this variant of anaplastic carcinoma, although sparse, are still atypical. Here strong immunopositivity for TP53 may be useful in highlighting scattered highly atypical cells. This stain should be mostly negative in spindled stromal cells in Riedel thyroiditis.[99]

Medullary thyroid carcinoma can rarely undergo dedifferentiation/anaplastic transformation and lose immunoreactivity for calcitonin and CEA. In such cases, ultrastructural demonstration of neurosecretory granules may help in the diagnosis.[144,145] A high index of suspicion for medullary carcinoma should be maintained if an anaplastic thyroid tumor occurs in a young patient or a patient with multiple endocrine neoplasia (MEN) type 2A or type 2B syndromes. In addition, detection of a *RET* point mutation is diagnostic of medullary carcinoma, whereas finding of a *BRAF* mutation or *RET/PTC* rearrangement confirms the diagnosis of anaplastic carcinoma in this setting.

Other unusual primary thyroid carcinomas may enter the differential diagnosis and are discussed in further detail in Chapter 15. Spindle epithelial tumor with thymus-like differentiation (SETTLE) may be confused with the spindled pattern of anaplastic carcinoma. Carcinoma with thymus-like elements (CASTLE) may enter the differential diagnosis in the squamoid pattern of

Table 13.2

Differential Diagnosis of Anaplastic Carcinoma

Category	Clinical and Morphologic Features that Differentiate from Anaplastic Carcinoma	Ancillary Studies Distinguishing from Anaplastic Carcinoma
Thyroid carcinomas and benign lesions		
Poorly differentiated thyroid carcinoma	Monomorphic cell population Solid, trabecular, or insular growth Necrosis usually less prominent	TTF1 retained, cytokeratin retained and diffuse
PTC with squamous or spindle cell metaplasia and PTC with fasciitis-like stroma	Absence of frank nuclear pleomorphism and hyperchromasia No necrosis Low mitotic activity	TTF1 and thyroglobulin retained, −TP53 low to negative
Riedel thyroiditis (vs. paucicellular anaplastic carcinoma)	Absence of atypical pleomorphic cells No necrosis or vascular permeation	TP53 cytokeratin negative
Anaplastic medullary thyroid carcinoma	Young patient History of multiple endocrine neoplasia type 2A or type 2B	Neurosecretory granules on EM *RET* point mutations
SETTLE	Young patient Monophasic or biphasic with more monomorphic spindle cells	Myoepithelial phenotype (smooth muscle actin)
CASTLE	Nested with tumor lobules separated by stroma Not as pleomorphic cells More vesicular nuclei and syncytial growth	CD5 positive
Nonthyroid tumors and nonepithelial thyroid tumors		
Upper aerodigestive tract squamous cell carcinoma	Epicenter in a mucosal site Squamous dysplasia or in situ carcinoma present Keratinization more prominent Absence of a differentiated thyroid carcinoma component	Lack of *BRAF* or *RAS* mutations
Metastatic poorly differentiated or undifferentiated carcinoma	Epicenter at site of primary with a corresponding pattern of spread Absence of a differentiated thyroid carcinoma component with transition	Lack of *BRAF* or *RAS* mutations Tissue-specific immunostains (i.e., CDX2 for colorectal primary)
Melanoma	Melanin pigment (if present)	S100, tyrosinase, HMB-45, MART-1 positive
Lymphoma	Single cells on cytologic preparation	LCA often positive along with other lymphoid markers
True sarcomas	Absence of a differentiated thyroid carcinoma component except for synovial sarcoma (or glandular malignant peripheral nerve sheath tumor), absence of epithelial differentiation Presence of classic morphology for a given sarcoma entity	Presence of a sarcoma-specific immunophenotype or translocation Lack of *BRAF* or *RAS* mutations

anaplastic carcinoma. SETTLE is distinguished from anaplastic carcinoma by the presence of less pleomorphic and atypical cells and the absence of necrosis. SETTLE is also more commonly seen in younger individuals. In addition, evidence for a myoepithelial phenotype has been reported in SETTLE, and thus, smooth muscle actin reactivity if prominent would favor SETTLE.[146] CASTLE has the appearance of a nonkeratinizing squamous cell carcinoma or lymphoepithelial carcinoma. It is usually nested with lobules separated by fibrous stroma. Although malignant, the nuclei are not very pleomorphic and are composed of vesicular nuclei and a syncytial growth, which is in contrast with the pleomorphism and hyperchromasia of the squamoid pattern of anaplastic carcinoma. Immunohistochemically, CASTLE is often positive for CD5, whereas anaplastic carcinoma is not.[147]

Distinction from Nonthyroid Malignancies and Sarcomas

Anaplastic carcinoma may be confused with various true sarcomas, metastatic carcinomas from other sites, lymphomas, and melanomas. When presented with a biopsy of a tumor that may histologically fit the diagnosis of anaplastic carcinoma, a clinical history of prior malignancy and knowledge of which sites are involved by tumor is very important. Typically, the epicenter of anaplastic carcinoma is in the thyroidal or mediastinal region. Although locoregional extension from a laryngeal squamous cell carcinoma may present as a thyroid mass, it will also show mucosal and submucosal involvement. Even with extensive metastatic disease, the bulk of the tumor volume in anaplastic carcinoma will

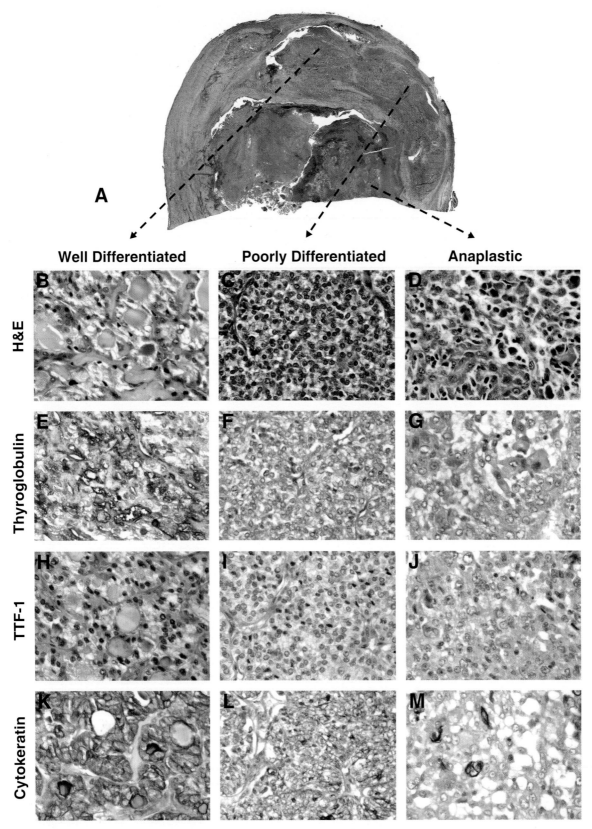

FIGURE 13.21. Change in immunohistochemical profile during progression from well-differentiated carcinoma to anaplastic carcinoma. A: Whole slide scan of a section of a thyroid tumor containing the areas of well-differentiated, poorly differentiated, and anaplastic carcinomas. Higher magnification of the areas of well-differentiated carcinoma (follicular variant of papillary carcinoma) **(B)**, poorly differentiated carcinoma **(C)**, and anaplastic carcinoma **(D)**. The areas of well-differentiated carcinoma strongly express thyroglobulin **(E)**, TTF1 **(H)**, and CK (CAM 5.2) **(K)**. The areas of poorly differentiated carcinoma lose thyroglobulin positivity **(F)** but are still weakly positive for TTF1 **(I)** and moderately positive for CK **(L)**. The areas of anaplastic carcinoma lose immunoexpression of thyroglobulin **(G)** and TTF1 **(J)** and only focally retain expression of cytokeratin (CAM 5.2) **(M)**.

still usually be locoregional. However, in metastases to the thyroid from other sites, the bulk of the disease will tend to be situated at the site of the primary (i.e., lung, kidney).

Although immunophenotype and morphologic features of anaplastic carcinomas can be seen in other undifferentiated tumors, the histologic detection of a focal differentiated component is virtually diagnostic of anaplastic carcinoma. It is ideal, however, to demonstrate a histologic transition from this component to the anaplastic component, since a very rare exception to this rule is the occurrence of a metastasis to a differentiated thyroid tumor (see Chapter 18).

Immunohistochemical staining may also be useful in the separation of anaplastic carcinoma from other tumors. Preserved PAX8 immunoreactivity provides strong support for anaplastic carcinoma, unless the differential diagnosis includes a metastatic carcinoma from the kidney, ovary, or endometrium.[148] Melanomas will be S100 positive along with other melanoma antigens such as HMB-45, Melan-A, and tyrosinase. Lymphomas will typically be positive for LCA and/or other hematopoietic markers. True sarcomas, although rare, can occur in the thyroid. To entertain this possibility, the absence of a differentiated thyroid carcinoma component must be shown. The absence of epithelial differentiation is also required, with the exception of synovial sarcoma (or theoretically, glandular malignant peripheral nerve sheath tumor). If these are absent, the presence of classic morphology for a given entity (i.e., solitary fibrous tumor, liposarcoma) and the documentation of a sarcoma specific immunophenotype (i.e., follicular dendritic cell sarcoma) or a specific translocation (i.e., t(X;18) in synovial sarcoma) would support a true named sarcoma. Selected true sarcomas of the thyroid are discussed in further detail in Chapter 16.

Finding *BRAF* or *RAS* (*NRAS* codon 61, *HRAS* codon 61) point mutations or *RET/PTC* rearrangement strongly supports the diagnosis of anaplastic carcinoma in many cases, with the most notable exception of cutaneous melanoma that is frequently positive for *BRAF* and *NRAS* mutations. In addition, we have recently observed that primary thyroid lymphomas may harbor mutations of the *BRAF* and *RAS* genes, and therefore, these mutations cannot be used to differentiate these tumors.

TREATMENT AND PROGNOSIS

Anaplastic carcinoma is one of the most aggressive tumors known to humans. The prognosis is abysmal with a median survival in most series of only 3 to 6 months.[149] Only 20% of patients survive for 1 year.[149] Age, extrathyroidal spread of the disease, gender, and tumor size >5 cm are predictors of outcome in most series.[17,19,79,105,122,150] A prognostic index incorporating these variables as well as acuteness of presentation and leukocytosis >10,000 per μl has been proposed.[83] A review of the SEER data on 516 patients indicates that age >60 years, extent of disease (local vs. regional vs. distant metastases), and the combined use of radiation and surgery are the only independent prognosticators.[19]

Death is usually a result of local relapse, and it appears in most series that the utilization of a combined approach to adequately control local disease imparts an improved outcome.[18,79,150–152] Long-term survivors do exist. Most patients have disease confined to the thyroid and have only focal anaplastic transformation in an otherwise differentiated tumor. Survival in such patients is often >5 years but still worse than in differentiated tumors without focal anaplasia.[83,109] Regarding histologic subtypes and variants of anaplastic carcinoma, the paucicellular variant may have a more indolent course, but this has not been confirmed in a systematic fashion as it is only rarely the predominant pattern.[99] Otherwise, histologic appearance does not affect prognosis.

The favored therapeutic approach is multimodal, combining surgery, radiation, and chemotherapy.[153] On presentation, most patients have an extensive disease burden that precludes

resectability of disease.[19] Utility of surgery in the treatment of anaplastic carcinoma is mainly for diagnostic and palliative purposes. However, there is some evidence that complete surgical excision has a role in tumors with limited extent. As such, neck dissections are warranted if there is hope of total excision of nodal disease.[79,150,154–156]

Radioactive iodine therapy has no utility in anaplastic carcinomas as this tumor is not iodine avid. However, radiotherapy, classically external beam but now including three-dimensional conformal therapy and intensity modulated radiotherapy, is another commonly used modality of treatment, utilized in more than half of patients in the United States.[19] Most protocols use 30 to 60 Gy doses.[79,150] Anaplastic carcinoma has a rapid doubling rate, and to improve efficacy, hyperfractionation or accelerated dosing regimens in combination with a chemosensitizer such as doxorubicin are favored. However, these regimens must be carefully designed to minimize toxicity.[151,152,155]

Conventional chemotherapy is also commonly used as part of the treatment regime as distant metastases are present in most patients.[157] Doxorubicin is commonly given as a single agent or in combination with cisplatin. As noted above, doxorubicin is often given with hyperfractionated dosing because of its chemosensitizing properties.[79,157] Other regimens have been used with varying results.[158,159] Overall, however, response to chemotherapy is poor. The expression of *MDR-1* and its product P-glycoprotein and multidrug resistance–associated protein in cell lines and actual tumors has been quoted as a possible mechanism for drug resistance in anaplastic carcinomas.[160,161] A phase II trial of Taxol showed a partial response in 47% of patients and a complete response in 5% of patients with anaplastic carcinoma.[159]

Targeted therapies with tyrosine kinase inhibitors such as sorafenib, axitinib, and gefitinib have reached a phase II trial for patients with advanced thyroid cancer including anaplastic carcinoma.[162–165] The early published results showed partial response in some cases, mostly in patients with well-differentiated carcinoma, whereas response in patients with anaplastic carcinoma was generally not seen. However, the number of patients with anaplastic carcinoma enrolled in these studies was low, and some more recent results are more encouraging, showing longer survival in some patients with anaplastic carcinoma treated with sorafenib.[166]

TP53 is inactivated in more than half of anaplastic carcinomas and has also been a candidate for therapeutic intervention. The experimental attempts for adenovirus-mediated *TP53* gene therapy showed some promise in controlling anaplastic carcinoma cells growth,[167] although this therapeutic modality has not been extensively tested in the clinical setting.

REFERENCES

1. Howlader N, Noone AM, Krapcho M, et al. SEER cancer statistics review, 1975–2008. National Cancer Institute. SEER web site. http://seer.cancer.gov/csr/1975_2008/. Accessed July 20, 2011.
2. Hundahl SA, Fleming ID, Fremgen AM, et al. A National Cancer Data Base report on 53,856 cases of thyroid carcinoma treated in the U.S., 1985–1995 [see comments]. *Cancer*. 1998;83:2638–2648.
3. Akslen LA, Haldorsen T, Thoresen SO, et al. Incidence of thyroid cancer in Norway 1970–1985. Population review on time trend, sex, age, histological type and tumour stage in 2625 cases. *APMIS*. 1990;98:549–558.
4. Burgess JR. Temporal trends for thyroid carcinoma in Australia: an increasing incidence of papillary thyroid carcinoma (1982–1997). *Thyroid*. 2002;12:141–149.
5. Ain KB. Anaplastic thyroid carcinoma: behavior, biology, and therapeutic approaches. *Thyroid*. 1998;8:715–726.
6. Pettersson B, Coleman MP, Ron E, et al. Iodine supplementation in Sweden and regional trends in thyroid cancer incidence by histopathologic type. *Int J Cancer*. 1996;65:13–19.
7. Belfiore A, La Rosa GL, Padova G, et al. The frequency of cold thyroid nodules and thyroid malignancies in patients from an iodine-deficient area. *Cancer*. 1987;60:3096–3102.
8. Bakiri F, Djemli FK, Mokrane LA, et al. The relative roles of endemic goiter and socioeconomic development status in the prognosis of thyroid carcinoma. *Cancer*. 1998;82:1146–1153.

9. Albores-Saavedra J, Henson DE, Glazer E, et al. Changing patterns in the incidence and survival of thyroid cancer with follicular phenotype—papillary, follicular, and anaplastic: a morphological and epidemiological study. *Endocr Pathol.* 2007;18:1–7.

10. Green LD, Mack L, Pasieka JL. Anaplastic thyroid cancer and primary thyroid lymphoma: a review of these rare thyroid malignancies. *J Surg Oncol.* 2006;94:725–736.

11. Ordonez N, Baloch Z, Matias-Guiu X, et al. Undifferentiated (anaplastic) carcinoma. In: DeLellis RA, Lloyd RV, Heitz PU, Eng C, eds. *Pathology and Genetics of Tumours of Endocrine Organs.* Vol 8. Lyon, France: IARC; 2004:77–80.

12. Rosai J, Carcangiu ML, DeLellis RA. Undifferentiated (anaplastic) carcinoma. In: Rosai J, Carcangiu ML, DeLellis RA, eds. *Tumors of the Thyroid Gland.* Vol 6. 3rd ed. Washington, DC: Armed Forces Institute of Pathology; 1992: 135–159.

13. Hundahl SA, Cady B, Cunningham MP, et al. Initial results from a prospective cohort study of 5583 cases of thyroid carcinoma treated in the United States during 1996. U.S. and German Thyroid Cancer Study Group. An American College of Surgeons Commission on Cancer Patient Care Evaluation study. *Cancer.* 2000;89:202–217.

14. Carcangiu ML, Steeper T, Zampi G, et al. Anaplastic thyroid carcinoma. A study of 70 cases. *Am J Clin Pathol.* 1985;83:135–158.

15. Schoumacher P, Metz R, Bey P, et al. Anaplastic carcinoma of the thyroid gland. *Eur J Cancer.* 1977;13:381–383.

16. Pichardo-Lowden A, Durvesh S, Douglas S, et al. Anaplastic thyroid carcinoma in a young woman: a rare case of survival. *Thyroid.* 2009;19:775–779.

17. McIver B, Hay ID, Giuffrida DF, et al. Anaplastic thyroid carcinoma: a 50-year experience at a single institution. *Surgery.* 2001;130:1028–1034.

18. Venkatesh YS, Ordonez NG, Schultz PN, et al. Anaplastic carcinoma of the thyroid. A clinicopathologic study of 121 cases. *Cancer.* 1990;66:321–330.

19. Kebebew E, Greenspan FS, Clark OH, et al. Anaplastic thyroid carcinoma. Treatment outcome and prognostic factors. *Cancer.* 2005;103:1330–1335.

20. Nishiyama RH, Dunn EL, Thompson NW. Anaplastic spindle-cell and giant-cell tumors of the thyroid gland. *Cancer.* 1972;30:113–127.

21. Albores-Saavedra J, Hernandez M, Sanchez-Sosa S, et al. Histologic variants of papillary and follicular carcinomas associated with anaplastic spindle and giant cell carcinomas of the thyroid: an analysis of rhabdoid and thyroglobulin inclusions. *Am J Surg Pathol.* 2007;31:729–736.

22. Chem KT, Rosai J. Follicular variant of thyroid papillary carcinoma: a clinico-pathologic study of six cases. *Am J Surg Pathol.* 1977;1:123–130.

23. Aldinger KA, Samaan NA, Ibanez M, et al. Anaplastic carcinoma of the thyroid: a review of 84 cases of spindle and giant cell carcinoma of the thyroid. *Cancer.* 1978;41:2267–2275.

24. Zivaljevic V, Vlajinac H, Jankovic R, et al. Case-control study of female thyroid cancer—menstrual, reproductive and hormonal factors. *Eur J Cancer Prev.* 2003;12:63–66.

25. Harach HR, Escalante DA, Day ES. Thyroid cancer and thyroiditis in Salta, Argentina: a 40-yr study in relation to iodine prophylaxis. *Endocr Pathol.* 2002;13:175–181.

26. Bacher-Stier C, Riccabona G, Totsch M, et al. Incidence and clinical characteristics of thyroid carcinoma after iodine prophylaxis in an endemic goiter country. *Thyroid.* 1997;7:733–741.

27. Namba H, Matsuo K, Fagin JA. Clonal composition of benign and malignant human thyroid tumors. *J Clin Invest.* 1990;86:120–125.

28. Bol S, Belge G, Thode B, et al. Cytogenetic tetraclonality in a rare spindle cell variant of an anaplastic carcinoma of the thyroid. *Cancer Genet Cytogenet.* 2001;125:163–166.

29. Roque L, Soares J, Castedo S. Cytogenetic and fluorescence in situ hybridization studies in a case of anaplastic thyroid carcinoma. *Cancer Genet Cytogenet.* 1998;103:7–10.

30. Jenkins RB, Hay ID, Herath JF, et al. Frequent occurrence of cytogenetic abnormalities in sporadic nonmedullary thyroid carcinoma. *Cancer.* 1990;66:1213–1220.

31. Miura D, Wada N, Chin K, et al. Anaplastic thyroid cancer: cytogenetic patterns by comparative genomic hybridization. *Thyroid.* 2003;13:283–290.

32. Wilkens L, Benten D, Tchinda J, et al. Aberrations of chromosomes 5 and 8 as recurrent cytogenetic events in anaplastic carcinoma of the thyroid as detected by fluorescence in situ hybridisation and comparative genomic hybridisation. *Virchows Arch.* 2000;436:312–318.

33. Wreesmann VB, Ghossein RA, Patel SG, et al. Genome-wide appraisal of thyroid cancer progression. *Am J Pathol.* 2002;161:1549–1556.

34. Rodrigues RF, Roque L, Rosa-Santos J, et al. Chromosomal imbalances associated with anaplastic transformation of follicular thyroid carcinomas. *Br J Cancer.* 2004;90:492–496.

35. Ekman ET, Wallin G, Backdahl M, et al. Nuclear DNA content in anaplastic giant-cell thyroid carcinoma. *Am J Clin Oncol.* 1989;12:442–446.

36. Klemi PJ, Joensuu H, Eerola E. DNA aneuploidy in anaplastic carcinoma of the thyroid gland. *Am J Clin Pathol.* 1988;89:154–159.

37. Kitamura Y, Shimizu K, Tanaka S, et al. Allelotyping of anaplastic thyroid carcinoma: frequent allelic losses on 1q, 9p, 11, 17, 19p, and 22q. *Genes Chromosomes Cancer.* 2000;27:244–251.

38. Hunt JL, Tometsko M, LiVolsi VA, et al. Molecular evidence of anaplastic transformation in coexisting well-differentiated and anaplastic carcinomas of the thyroid. *Am J Surg Pathol.* 2003;27:1559–1564.

39. Kadota M, Tamaki Y, Sekimoto M, et al. Loss of heterozygosity on chromosome 16p and 18q in anaplastic thyroid carcinoma. *Oncol Rep.* 2003;10:35–38.

40. Ito T, Seyama T, Mizuno T, et al. Genetic alterations in thyroid tumor progression: association with *p53* gene mutations. *Jpn J Cancer Res.* 1993;84: 526–531.

41. Mochizuki K, Kondo T, Nakazawa T, et al. RET rearrangements and *BRAF* mutation in undifferentiated thyroid carcinomas having papillary carcinoma components. *Histopathology.* 2010;57:444–450.

42. Sugg SL, Ezzat S, Zheng L, et al. Oncogene profile of papillary thyroid carcinoma. *Surgery.* 1999;125:46–52.

43. Wang HM, Huang YW, Huang JS, et al. Anaplastic carcinoma of the thyroid arising more often from follicular carcinoma than papillary carcinoma. *Ann Surg Oncol.* 2007;14:3011–3018.

44. Lemoine NR, Mayall ES, Wyllie FS, et al. High frequency of *ras* oncogene activation in all stages of human thyroid tumorigenesis. *Oncogene.* 1989;4: 159–164.

45. Garcia-Rostan G, Costa AM, Pereira-Castro I, et al. Mutation of the *PIK3CA* gene in anaplastic thyroid cancer. *Cancer Res.* 2005;65:10199–10207.

46. Hou P, Liu D, Shan Y, et al. Genetic alterations and their relationship in the phosphatidylinositol 3-kinase/Akt pathway in thyroid cancer. *Clin Cancer Res.* 2007;13:1161–1170.

47. Quiros RM, Ding HG, Gattuso P, et al. Evidence that one subset of anaplastic thyroid carcinomas are derived from papillary carcinomas due to *BRAF* and *p53* mutations. *Cancer.* 2005;103:2261–2268.

48. Fagin JA. Minireview: branded from the start-distinct oncogenic initiating events may determine tumor fate in the thyroid. *Mol Endocrinol.* 2002;16:903–911.

49. Saavedra HI, Knauf JA, Shirokawa JM, et al. The *RAS* oncogene induces genomic instability in thyroid PCCL3 cells via the MAPK pathway. *Oncogene.* 2000;19:3948–3954.

50. De Vita G, Bauer L, da Costa VM, et al. Dose-dependent inhibition of thyroid differentiation by *RAS* oncogenes. *Mol Endocrinol.* 2005;19:76–89.

51. Santarpia L, El-Naggar AK, Cote GJ, et al. Phosphatidylinositol 3-kinase/akt and ras/raf-mitogen-activated protein kinase pathway mutations in anaplastic thyroid cancer. *J Clin Endocrinol Metab.* 2008;93:278–284.

52. Namba H, Nakashima M, Hayashi T, et al. Clinical implication of hot spot *BRAF* mutation, V599E, in papillary thyroid cancers. *J Clin Endocrinol Metab.* 2003;88:4393–4397.

53. Nikiforova MN, Kimura ET, Gandhi M, et al. *BRAF* mutations in thyroid tumors are restricted to papillary carcinomas and anaplastic or poorly differentiated carcinomas arising from papillary carcinomas. *J Clin Endocrinol Metab.* 2003;88:5399–5404.

54. Knauf JA, Ma X, Smith EP, et al. Targeted expression of *BRAF*V600E in thyroid cells of transgenic mice results in papillary thyroid cancers that undergo dedifferentiation. *Cancer Res.* 2005;65:4238–4245.

55. Dahia PL, Marsh DJ, Zheng Z, et al. Somatic deletions and mutations in the Cowden disease gene, *PTEN*, in sporadic thyroid tumors. *Cancer Res.* 1997;57:4710–4713.

56. Ricarte-Filho JC, Ryder M, Chitale DA, et al. Mutational profile of advanced primary and metastatic radioactive iodine-refractory thyroid cancers reveals distinct pathogenetic roles for *BRAF, PIK3CA,* and *AKT1. Cancer Res.* 2009;69:4885–4893.

57. Wang Y, Hou P, Yu H, et al. High prevalence and mutual exclusivity of genetic alterations in the phosphatidylinositol-3-kinase/akt pathway in thyroid tumors. *J Clin Endocrinol Metab.* 2007;92:2387–2390.

58. Fagin JA, Matsuo K, Karmakar A, et al. High prevalence of mutations of the *p53* gene in poorly differentiated human thyroid carcinomas. *J Clin Invest.* 1993;91:179–184.

59. Donghi R, Longoni A, Pilotti S, et al. Gene *p53* mutations are restricted to poorly differentiated and undifferentiated carcinomas of the thyroid gland. *J Clin Invest.* 1993;91:1753–1760.

60. Dobashi Y, Sugimura H, Sakamoto A, et al. Stepwise participation of *p53* gene mutation during dedifferentiation of human thyroid carcinomas. *Diagn Mol Pathol.* 1994;3:9–14.

61. Ito T, Seyama T, Mizuno T, et al. Unique association of *p53* mutations with undifferentiated but not with differentiated carcinomas of the thyroid gland. *Cancer Res.* 1992;52:1369–1371.

62. Shahedian B, Shi Y, Zou M, et al. Thyroid carcinoma is characterized by genomic instability: evidence from *p53* mutations. *Mol Genet Metab.* 2001;72:155–163.

63. Nakamura T, Yana I, Kobayashi T, et al. *p53* gene mutations associated with anaplastic transformation of human thyroid carcinomas. *Jpn J Cancer Res.* 1992;83:1293–1298.

64. Asakawa H, Kobayashi T. Multistep carcinogenesis in anaplastic thyroid carcinoma: a case report. *Pathology.* 2002;34:94–97.

65. La Perle KM, Jhiang SM, Capen CC. Loss of *p53* promotes anaplasia and local invasion in *ret/PTC1*-induced thyroid carcinomas. *Am J Pathol.* 2000;157:671–677.

66. Moretti F, Farsetti A, Soddu S, et al. *p53* re-expression inhibits proliferation and restores differentiation of human thyroid anaplastic carcinoma cells. *Oncogene.* 1997;14:729–740.

67. Fagin JA, Tang SH, Zeki K, et al. Reexpression of thyroid peroxidase in a derivative of an undifferentiated thyroid carcinoma cell line by introduction of wild-type *p53. Cancer Res.* 1996;56:765–771.

68. Kraus C, Liehr T, Hulsken J, et al. Localization of the human beta-catenin gene (*CTNNB1*) to 3p21: a region implicated in tumor development. *Genomics.* 1994;23:272–274.

69. van Hengel J, Nollet F, Berx G, et al. Assignment of the human beta-catenin gene (*CTNNB1*) to 3p22-->p21.3 by fluorescence in situ hybridization. *Cytogenet Cell Genet.* 1995;70:68–70.

70. Garcia-Rostan G, Camp RL, Herrero A, et al. Beta-catenin dysregulation in thyroid neoplasms: down-regulation, aberrant nuclear expression, and *CTNNB1* exon 3 mutations are markers for aggressive tumor phenotypes and poor prognosis. *Am J Pathol.* 2001;158:987–996.

71. Garcia-Rostan G, Tallini G, Herrero A, et al. Frequent mutation and nuclear localization of beta-catenin in anaplastic thyroid carcinoma. *Cancer Res.* 1999;59:1811–1815.

72. Xu B, Yoshimoto K, Miyauchi A, et al. Cribriform-morular variant of papillary thyroid carcinoma: a pathological and molecular genetic study with evidence

of frequent somatic mutations in exon 3 of the beta-catenin gene. *J Pathol.* 2003;199:58–67.

73. Kurihara T, Ikeda S, Ishizaki Y, et al. Immunohistochemical and sequencing analyses of the Wnt signaling components in Japanese anaplastic thyroid cancers. *Thyroid.* 2004;14:1020–1029.
74. Elliott DD, Sherman SI, Busaidy NL, et al. Growth factor receptors expression in anaplastic thyroid carcinoma: potential markers for therapeutic stratification. *Hum Pathol.* 2008;39:15–20.
75. Lee DH, Lee GK, Kong SY, et al. Epidermal growth factor receptor status in anaplastic thyroid carcinoma. *J Clin Pathol.* 2007;60:881–884.
76. Ricarte-Filho JC, Matsuse M, Lau C, et al. Absence of common activating mutations of the epidermal growth factor receptor gene in thyroid cancers from American and Japanese patients. *Int J Cancer.* 2011 Jun 29. doi: 10.1002/ijc.26267. [Epub ahead of print].
77. Tallini G, Santoro M, Helie M, et al. *RET/PTC* oncogene activation defines a subset of papillary thyroid carcinomas lacking evidence of progression to poorly differentiated or undifferentiated tumor phenotypes. *Clin Cancer Res.* 1998;4:287–294.
78. Smallridge RC, Marlow LA, Copland JA. Anaplastic thyroid cancer: molecular pathogenesis and emerging therapies. *Endocr Relat Cancer.* 2009;16:17–44.
79. Are C, Shaha AR. Anaplastic thyroid carcinoma: biology, pathogenesis, prognostic factors, and treatment approaches. *Ann Surg Oncol.* 2006;13:453–464.
80. Mangla JC, Rastogi GK, Pathak IC. Anaplastic carcinoma of the thyroid complicating severe thyrotoxicosis. *J Indian Med Assoc.* 1967;49:286 passim.
81. Basaria S, Udelsman R, Tejedor-Sojo J, et al. Anaplastic pseudothyroiditis. *Clin Endocrinol (Oxf).* 2002;56:553–555.
82. Oppenheim A, Miller M, Anderson GH Jr, et al. Anaplastic thyroid cancer presenting with hyperthyroidism. *Am J Med.* 1983;75:702–704.
83. Sugitani I, Kasai N, Fujimoto Y, et al. Prognostic factors and therapeutic strategy for anaplastic carcinoma of the thyroid. *World J Surg.* 2001;25:617–622.
84. Yazawa S, Toshimori H, Nakatsuru K, et al. Thyroid anaplastic carcinoma producing granulocyte-colony-stimulating factor and parathyroid hormone-related protein. *Intern Med.* 1995;34:584–588.
85. Panzironi G, Rainaldi R, Ricci F, et al. Gray-scale and color Doppler findings in bilateral internal jugular vein thrombosis caused by anaplastic carcinoma of the thyroid. *J Clin Ultrasound.* 2003;31:111–115.
86. Dackiw A, Pan J, Xu G, et al. Modulation of parathyroid hormone-related protein levels (PTHrP) in anaplastic thyroid cancer. *Surgery.* 2005;138:456–463.
87. Weber AL, Randolph G, Aksoy FG. The thyroid and parathyroid glands. CT and MR imaging and correlation with pathology and clinical findings. *Radiol Clin North Am.* 2000;38:1105–1129.
88. Ishikawa H, Tamaki Y, Takahashi M, et al. Comparison of primary thyroid lymphoma with anaplastic thyroid carcinoma on computed tomographic imaging. *Radiat Med.* 2002;20:9–15.
89. Takashima S, Morimoto S, Ikezoe J, et al. CT evaluation of anaplastic thyroid carcinoma. *AJR Am J Roentgenol.* 1990;154:1079–1085.
90. Nguyen BD, Ram PC. PET/CT staging and posttherapeutic monitoring of anaplastic thyroid carcinoma. *Clin Nucl Med.* 2007;32:145–149.
91. McDougall IR, Davidson J, Segall GM. Positron emission tomography of the thyroid, with an emphasis on thyroid cancer. *Nucl Med Commun.* 2001;22:485–492.
92. Haigh PI. Anaplastic thyroid carcinoma. *Curr Treat Options Oncol.* 2000;1:353–357.
93. Donnell CA, Pollock WJ, Sybers WA. Thyroid carcinosarcoma. *Arch Pathol Lab Med.* 1987;111:1169–1172.
94. Hashimoto H, Koga S, Watanabe H, et al. Unidifferentiated carcinoma of the thyroid gland with osteoclast-like giant cells. *Acta Pathol Jpn.* 1980;30: 323–334.
95. Gaffey MJ, Lack EE, Christ ML, et al. Anaplastic thyroid carcinoma with osteoclast-like giant cells. A clinicopathologic, immunohistochemical, and ultrastructural study. *Am J Surg Pathol.* 1991;15:160–168.
96. Mills SE, Stallings RG, Austin MB. Angiomatoid carcinoma of the thyroid gland. Anaplastic carcinoma with follicular and medullary features mimicking angiosarcoma. *Am J Clin Pathol.* 1986;86:674–678.
97. Bisceglia M, Vairo M, Tardio G, et al. [Primary angiosarcoma of the thyroid. Presentation of a case (epithelioid type) and nosological problems]. *Pathologica.* 1995;87:154–161.
98. Wan SK, Chan JK, Tang SK. Paucicellular variant of anaplastic thyroid carcinoma. A mimic of Reidel's thyroiditis. *Am J Clin Pathol.* 1996;105: 388–393.
99. Canos JC, Serrano A, Matias-Guiu X. Paucicellular variant of anaplastic thyroid carcinoma: report of two cases. *Endocr Pathol.* 2001;12:157–161.
100. Chetty R, Govender D. Follicular thyroid carcinoma with rhabdoid phenotype. *Virchows Arch.* 1999;435:133–136.
101. Albores-Saavedra J, Sharma S. Poorly differentiated follicular thyroid carcinoma with rhabdoid phenotype: a clinicopathologic, immunohistochemical and electron microscopic study of two cases. *Mod Pathol.* 2001;14:98–104.
102. Sumida T, Hamakawa H, Imaoka M, et al. A case of submandibular malignant rhabdoid tumor transformed from papillary thyroid carcinoma. *J Oral Pathol Med.* 2001;30:443–447.
103. Lai ML, Faa G, Serra S, et al. Rhabdoid tumor of the thyroid gland: a variant of anaplastic carcinoma. *Arch Pathol Lab Med.* 2005;129:e55–e57.
104. Sato K, Waseda R, Tatsuzawa Y, et al. Papillary thyroid carcinoma with anaplastic transformation showing a rhabdoid phenotype solely in the cervical lymph node metastasis. *Pathol Res Pract.* 2006;202:55–59.
105. Rafla S. Anaplastic tumors of the thyroid. *Cancer.* 1969;23:668–677.
106. Tobler A, Maurer R, Hedinger CE. Undifferentiated thyroid tumors of diffuse small cell type. Histological and immunohistochemical evidence for their lymphomatous nature. *Virchows Arch A Pathol Anat Histopathol.* 1984;404:117–126.
107. Mambo NC, Irwin SM. Anaplastic small cell neoplasms of the thyroid: an immunoperoxidase study. *Hum Pathol.* 1984;15:55–60.
108. Lam KY, Lo CY, Chan KW, et al. Insular and anaplastic carcinoma of the thyroid: a 45-year comparative study at a single institution and a review of the significance of *p53* and *p21*. *Ann Surg.* 2000;231:329–338.
109. van den Brekel MW, Hekkenberg RJ, Asa SL, et al. Prognostic features in tall cell papillary carcinoma and insular thyroid carcinoma. *Laryngoscope.* 1997;107:254–259.
110. Wilson NW, Pambakian H, Richardson TC, et al. Epithelial markers in thyroid carcinoma: an immunoperoxidase study. *Histopathology.* 1986;10:815–829.
111. Schroder S, Wodzynski A, Padberg B. [Cytokeratin expression of benign and malignant epithelial thyroid gland tumors. An immunohistologic study of 154 neoplasms using 8 different monoclonal cytokeratin antibodies] *Pathologe.* 1996;17:425–432.
112. Miettinen M, Franssila KO. Variable expression of keratins and nearly uniform lack of thyroid transcription factor 1 in thyroid anaplastic carcinoma. *Hum Pathol.* 2000;31:1139–1145.
113. Lam KY, Lui MC, Lo CY. Cytokeratin expression profiles in thyroid carcinomas. *Eur J Surg Oncol.* 2001;27:631–635.
114. LiVolsi VA, Brooks JJ, Arendash-Durand B. Anaplastic thyroid tumors. Immunohistology. *Am J Clin Pathol.* 1987;87:434–442.
115. Hurlimann J, Gardiol D, Scazziga B. Immunohistology of anaplastic thyroid carcinoma. A study of 43 cases. *Histopathology.* 1987;11:567–580.
116. Ordonez NG, El-Naggar AK, Hickey RC, et al. Anaplastic thyroid carcinoma. Immunocytochemical study of 32 cases. *Am J Clin Pathol.* 1991;96:15–24.
117. Nonaka D, Tang Y, Chiriboga L, et al. Diagnostic utility of thyroid transcription factors Pax8 and TTF-2 (FoxE1) in thyroid epithelial neoplasms. *Mod Pathol.* 2008;21:192–200.
118. Bejarano PA, Nikiforov YE, Swenson ES, et al. Thyroid transcription factor-1, thyroglobulin, cytokeratin 7, and cytokeratin 20 in thyroid neoplasms. *Appl Immunohistochem Mol Morphol.* 2000;8:189–194.
119. Bishop JA, Sharma R, Westra WH. PAX8 immunostaining of anaplastic thyroid carcinoma: a reliable means of discerning thyroid origin for undifferentiated tumors of the head and neck. *Hum Pathol.* 2011;42:1873–1877.
120. Wiseman SM, Masoudi H, Niblock P, et al. Anaplastic thyroid carcinoma: expression profile of targets for therapy offers new insights for disease treatment. *Ann Surg Oncol.* 2007;14:719–729.
121. Saltman B, Singh B, Hedvat CV, et al. Patterns of expression of cell cycle/apoptosis genes along the spectrum of thyroid carcinoma progression. *Surgery.* 2006;140:899–905; discussion 905–896.
122. Siironen P, Hagstrom J, Maenpaa HO, et al. Anaplastic and poorly differentiated thyroid carcinoma: therapeutic strategies and treatment outcome of 52 consecutive patients. *Oncology.* 2010;79:400–408.
123. Wang S, Lloyd RV, Hutzler MJ, et al. The role of cell cycle regulatory protein, cyclin D1, in the progression of thyroid cancer. *Mod Pathol.* 2000;13:882–887.
124. Preto A, Reis-Filho JS, Ricardo S, et al. *P63* expression in papillary and anaplastic carcinomas of the thyroid gland: lack of an oncogenetic role in tumorigenesis and progression. *Pathol Res Pract.* 2002;198:449–454.
125. Kim YW, Do IG, Park YK. Expression of the GLUT1 glucose transporter, p63 and p53 in thyroid carcinomas. *Pathol Res Pract.* 2006;202:759–765.
126. Tallini G, Garcia-Rostan G, Herrero A, et al. Downregulation of p27KIP1 and Ki67/Mib1 labeling index support the classification of thyroid carcinoma into prognostically relevant categories. *Am J Surg Pathol.* 1999;23:678–685.
127. Nakamura N, Erickson LA, Jin L, et al. Immunohistochemical separation of follicular variant of papillary thyroid carcinoma from follicular adenoma. *Endocr Pathol.* 2006;17:213–223.
128. Erickson LA, Jin L, Wollan PC, et al. Expression of p27kip1 and Ki-67 in benign and malignant thyroid tumors. *Mod Pathol.* 1998;11:169–174.
129. Dumitriu L, Stefaneanu L, Tasca C. The anaplastic transformation of differentiated thyroid carcinoma. An ultrastructural study. *Endocrinologie.* 1984;22:91–96.
130. Stefaneanu L, Tasca C. An electron-microscopic study of human thyroid cancer. *Endocrinologie.* 1979;17:233–239.
131. Jao W, Gould VE. Ultrastructure of anaplastic (spindle and giant cell) carcinoma of the thyroid. *Cancer.* 1975;35:1280–1292.
132. Carda C, Ferrer J, Vilanova M, et al. Anaplastic carcinoma of the thyroid with rhabdomyosarcomatous differentiation: a report of two cases. *Virchows Arch.* 2005;446:46–51.
133. Rivera M, Sang C, Gerhard R, et al. Anaplastic thyroid carcinoma: morphologic findings and PAX-8 expression in cytology specimens. *Acta Cytol.* 2010;54:668–672.
134. Us-Krasovec M, Golouh R, Auersperg M, et al. Anaplastic thyroid carcinoma in fine needle aspirates. *Acta Cytol.* 1996;40:953–958.
135. Lee JS, Lee MC, Park CS, et al. Fine needle aspiration cytology of anaplastic carcinoma with osteoclastlike giant cells of the thyroid. A case report. *Acta Cytol.* 1996;40:1309–1312.
136. Mehdi G, Ansari HA, Siddiqui SA. Cytology of anaplastic giant cell carcinoma of the thyroid with osteoclast-like giant cells—a case report. *Diagn Cytopathol.* 2007;35:111–112.
137. Giard RW, Hermans J. Use and accuracy of fine-needle aspiration cytology in histologically proven thyroid carcinoma: an audit using a national nathology database. *Cancer.* 2000;90:330–334.
138. Daneshbod Y, Omidvari S, Daneshbod K, et al. Diffuse large B cell lymphoma of thyroid as a masquerader of anaplastic carcinoma of thyroid, diagnosed by FNA: a case report. *Cytojournal.* 2006;3:23.
139. Lu JY, Lin CW, Chang TC, et al. Diagnostic pitfalls of fine-needle aspiration cytology and prognostic impact of chemotherapy in thyroid lymphoma. *J Formos Med Assoc.* 2001;100:519–525.
140. Carcangiu ML, Zampi G, Rosai J. Poorly differentiated ("insular") thyroid carcinoma. A reinterpretation of Langhans' "wuchernde Struma". *Am J Surg Pathol.* 1984;8:655–668.
141. Volante M, Collini P, Nikiforov YE, et al. Poorly differentiated thyroid carcinoma: the Turin proposal for the use of uniform diagnostic criteria and an algorithmic diagnostic approach. *Am J Surg Pathol.* 2007;31:1256–1264.

142. Chan JK, Carcangiu ML, Rosai J. Papillary carcinoma of thyroid with exuberant nodular fasciitis-like stroma. Report of three cases. *Am J Clin Pathol.* 1991;95:309–314.

143. Vergilio J, Baloch ZW, LiVolsi VA. Spindle cell metaplasia of the thyroid arising in association with papillary carcinoma and follicular adenoma. *Am J Clin Pathol.* 2002;117:199–204.

144. Osaka M, Soga J, Tamiya Y, et al. Dedifferentiation of neoplastic cells in medullary thyroid carcinoma: report of a case. *Surg Today.* 1999;29:1189–1194.

145. Zeman V, Nemec J, Platil A, et al. Anaplastic transformation of medullary thyroid cancer. *Neoplasma.* 1978;25:249–255.

146. Xu B, Hirokawa M, Yoshimoto K, et al. Spindle epithelial tumor with thymus-like differentiation: a case report with pathological and molecular genetics study. *Hum Pathol.* 2003;34:190–193.

147. Reimann JD, Dorfman DM, Nose V. Carcinoma showing thymus-like differentiation of the thyroid (CASTLE): a comparative study: evidence of thymic differentiation and solid cell nest origin. *Am J Surg Pathol.* 2006;30:994–1001.

148. Tacha D, Zhou D, Cheng L. Expression of PAX8 in normal and neoplastic tissues: a comprehensive immunohistochemical study. *Appl Immunohistochem Mol Morphol.* 2011;19:293–299.

149. Smallridge RC, Copland JA. Anaplastic thyroid carcinoma: pathogenesis and emerging therapies. *Clin Oncol (R Coll Radiol).* 2010,22.486–497.

150. Junor EJ, Paul J, Reed NS. Anaplastic thyroid carcinoma: 91 patients treated by surgery and radiotherapy. *Eur J Surg Oncol.* 1992;18:83–88.

151. Tennvall J, Lundell G, Hallquist A, et al. Combined doxorubicin, hyperfractionated radiotherapy, and surgery in anaplastic thyroid carcinoma. Report on two protocols. The Swedish Anaplastic Thyroid Cancer Group. *Cancer.* 1994;74·1348–1354

152. Tennvall J, Lundell G, Wahlberg P, et al. Anaplastic thyroid carcinoma: three protocols combining doxorubicin, hyperfractionated radiotherapy and surgery. *Br J Cancer.* 2002;86:1848–1853.

153. Brignardello E, Gallo M, Baldi I, et al. Anaplastic thyroid carcinoma: clinical outcome of 30 consecutive patients referred to a single institution in the past 5 years. *Eur J Endocrinol.* 2007;156:425–430.

154. Nilsson O, Lindeberg J, Zedenius J, et al. Anaplastic giant cell carcinoma of the thyroid gland: treatment and survival over a 25-year period. *World J Surg.* 1998;22:725–730.

155. Lang BH, Lo CY. Surgical options in undifferentiated thyroid carcinoma. *World J Surg.* 2007;31:969–977.

156. Haigh PI, Ituarte PH, Wu HS, et al. Completely resected anaplastic thyroid carcinoma combined with adjuvant chemotherapy and irradiation is associated with prolonged survival. *Cancer.* 2001;91:2335–2342.

157. Pudney D, Lau H, Ruether JD, et al. Clinical experience of the multimodality management of anaplastic thyroid cancer and literature review. *Thyroid.* 2007;17:1243–1250.

158. Haddad R, Mahadevan A, Posner MR, et al. Long term survival with adjuvant carboplatin, paclitaxel, and radiation therapy in anaplastic thyroid cancer. *Am J Clin Oncol.* 2005;28:104.

159. Ain KB, Egorin MJ, DeSimone PA. Treatment of anaplastic thyroid carcinoma with paclitaxel: phase 2 trial using ninety-six-hour infusion. Collaborative Anaplastic Thyroid Cancer Health Intervention Trials (CATCHIT) Group. *Thyroid.* 2000;10:587–594.

160. Yamashita T, Watanabe M, Onodera M, et al. Multidrug resistance gene and P-glycoprotein expression in anaplastic carcinoma of the thyroid. *Cancer Detect Prev.* 1994;18:407–413.

161. Sugawara I, Arai T, Yamashita T, et al. Expression of multidrug resistance-associated protein (MRP) in anaplastic carcinoma of the thyroid. *Cancer Lett.* 1994;82:185–188.

162. Cohen EE, Rosen LS, Vokes EE, et al. Axitinib is an active treatment for all histologic subtypes of advanced thyroid cancer: results from a phase II study. *J Clin Oncol.* 2008;26:4708–4713.

163. Gupta-Abramson V, Troxel AB, Nellore A, et al. Phase II trial of sorafenib in advanced thyroid cancer. *J Clin Oncol.* 2008;26:4714–4719.

164. Kloos RT, Ringel MD, Knopp MV, et al. Phase II trial of sorafenib in metastatic thyroid cancer. *J Clin Oncol.* 2009;27:1675–1684.

165. Pennell NA, Daniels GH, Haddad RI, et al. A phase II study of gefitinib in patients with advanced thyroid cancer. *Thyroid.* 2008;18:317–323.

166. Ho AL, Sherman E. Clinical development of kinase inhibitors for the treatment of differentiated thyroid cancer. *Clin Adv Hematol Oncol.* 2011;9:32–41.

167. Nagayama Y, Yokoi H, Takeda K, et al. Adenovirus-mediated tumor suppressor *p53* gene therapy for anaplastic thyroid carcinoma in vitro and in vivo. *J Clin Endocrinol Metab.* 2000;85:4081–4086.

14

Paul W. Biddinger

Medullary Carcinoma

DEFINITION

Medullary thyroid carcinoma is a malignant tumor of the thyroid gland that exhibits C-cell differentiation. Synonyms include C-cell carcinoma, solid carcinoma, solid amyloidotic carcinoma, solid carcinoma with amyloid stroma, compact cell carcinoma, and neuroendocrine carcinoma of the thyroid.

HISTORICAL COMMENTS

The term *medullary carcinoma of the thyroid* was first used in reports published in 1955 and 1959 by Hazard and colleagues.[1,2] They distinguished this carcinoma by its solid nonfollicular pattern, amyloid stroma, and biologic behavior intermediate that of papillary and anaplastic thyroid carcinomas. They chose the term *medullary* because of the discrete gross appearance and sheetlike histologic pattern that seemed similar to medullary carcinoma of the breast.[3] Although Hazard et al. coined the term *medullary thyroid carcinoma* and were the first to define it as a distinct clinicopathologic entity, earlier reports appear to have described the same tumor (Fig. 14.1).[4–6]

In 1966, Williams[7] suggested that medullary carcinomas derived from the C (parafollicular) cell, noting that this origin would resolve the discrepancy between its undifferentiated appearance and relatively good prognosis. Meyer and Abdel-Bari[8] in 1968 reported calcitonin-like activity in an extract of medullary carcinoma. In the following year, Bussolati et al.[9] demonstrated calcitonin in histologic sections of medullary carcinoma by means of immunofluorescent staining. Immunohistochemical stains for calcitonin and other components of medullary carcinoma have become part of the standard clinical repertory over the last four decades, expanding our appreciation for medullary thyroid carcinoma's range of morphologic and clinical expression.

In 1961, Sipple[10] reported a case of pheochromocytoma associated with thyroid carcinoma and reviewed five others from the literature. None of the cases carried the specific diagnosis of medullary thyroid carcinoma, but this is not surprising given that they were reported before or only shortly after the establishment of this diagnostic term. Sipple syndrome has since become the eponymous name for multiple endocrine neoplasia type 2A (MEN2A).

Schimke and Hartmann[11] documented the association of medullary thyroid carcinoma and pheochromocytoma and its autosomal dominant inheritance in 1965. In 1968, Steiner et al.[12] described a large kinship with medullary carcinoma, pheochromocytoma, and hyperparathyroidism, affirming the autosomal dominant inheritance with high penetrance and variable expressivity. They proposed the term *multiple endocrine neoplasia type 2* to distinguish it from the established entity of multiple endocrine adenomatosis involving the pituitary, parathyroids, and pancreas, which is now designated multiple endocrine neoplasia type 1.

Williams and Pollock[13] reported the association of multiple mucosal neuromata with medullary thyroid carcinoma and pheochromocytoma in 1966. Subsequent reports by Schimke et al.[14] and Gorlin et al.[15] in 1968 confirmed this association as a distinct clinicopathologic entity, which we now recognize as multiple endocrine neoplasia type 2B (MEN2B). MEN2B is also known as Wagenmann–Froboese syndrome, an infrequently used eponym that recognizes case reports from the 1920s of individuals who had facial characteristics of MEN2B.[16,17] In 1986, Farndon et al.[18] recognized a familial form of medullary thyroid carcinoma without extrathyroidal manifestations. Their observation of hereditary medullary carcinoma distinct from MEN2A and MEN2B has been verified by subsequent studies and is now designated familial medullary thyroid carcinoma (FMTC).

INCIDENCE AND EPIDEMIOLOGY

In the United States, medullary carcinoma accounts for approximately 2% to 4% of thyroid malignancies.[19–21] The incidence of medullary carcinoma in the United States was 0.21 per 100,000 population in 2005 to 2006.[22] It occurs on both a sporadic and a hereditary basis. Most cases are sporadic and have a peak incidence in the fifth or sixth decade.[23] The pattern of inheritance is autosomal dominant. In most studies, the male to female ratio is about equal, although a slight female predominance has been reported for sporadic disease.[23,24]

Internationally, the reported rates for medullary carcinoma vary approximately from 0.02 to 0.35 per 100,000 person-years, with medullary carcinoma being the third most frequent type of thyroid malignancy after papillary and follicular carcinomas.[25] The international rates of medullary carcinoma among males tend to be higher compared with that for females.

The prevalence of occult medullary carcinoma in thyroidectomy specimens is approximately 0.3%.[26] A meta-analysis of autopsy studies revealed a prevalence between 0.1% to 0.2%, with most tumors being <1 cm in diameter.[27] The prevalence of occult medullary carcinoma is approximately 0.4% in autopsy series in which the thyroid was completely submitted for histologic examination and immunostained for calcitonin.[28,29]

Hereditary Medullary Thyroid Carcinoma

Hereditary forms of medullary thyroid carcinoma account for 15% to 30% of total cases.[23,24,30,31] The three subtypes are MEN2A, MEN2B, and FMTC. MEN2A is the most common of the three subtypes, accounting for about 75% to 90% of familial cases.[23,32,33] FMTC and MEN2B account for about 15% and 5% of cases, respectively.[32]

Hereditary cases of medullary carcinoma have a frequency of about 1 in 30,000.[32] Affected individuals generally present at a younger age, typically in the third decade or earlier depending on the particular mutation. Significant numbers of hereditary cases are now detected and treated at early ages owing to the availability of molecular testing for *RET* germline mutations. However, medullary thyroid carcinoma is still the most common cause of death of individuals with MEN2A, MEN2B, and FMTC.[32]

Fig. 1.

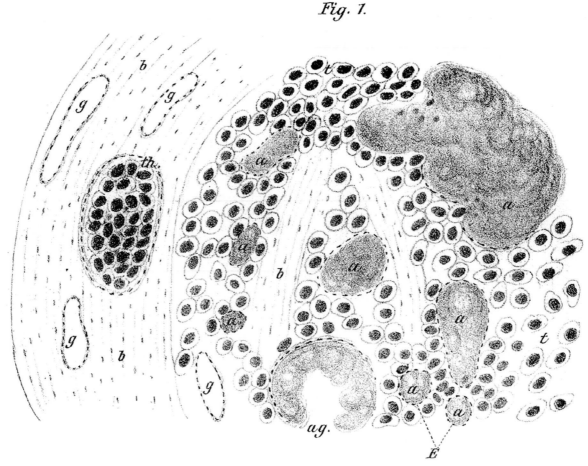

FIGURE 14.1. Drawing from Jaquet's 1906 publication regarding an apparent case of medullary thyroid carcinoma. The drawing depicts a metastatic lesion in the mediastinum with a uniform population of tumor cells and deposits of amyloid. The letter key to his diagram is as follows: a, amyloid; t, tumor cells; g, blood vessels; th, tumor thrombus in blood vessel; b, connective tissue; ag, blood vessel transformed by amyloid; E, endothelial membrane. (From Jacquet J. Ein Fall von metastasierenden Amyloidtumoren (Lymphosarkom). *Virchows Arch Pathol Anat.* 1906;185:251–268.)

Multiple Endocrine Neoplasia Type 2A

Multiple endocrine neoplasia type 2A (MEN2A) is characterized by medullary thyroid carcinoma, pheochromocytoma, and primary parathyroid hyperplasia (Fig. 14.2A). Cutaneous lichen amyloidosis or Hirschsprung disease is associated with rare cases of MEN2A.[33,34] Medullary carcinoma is usually the first clinical manifestation of MEN2A. The penetrance of medullary carcinoma is 90% to 100% within affected families, and the age at presentation is usually in the third or fourth decade of life.[21,33,34] Approximately 50% of individuals affected with MEN2A also develop pheochromocytoma, and about 10% to 30% experience hyperparathyroidism because of parathyroid hyperplasia.[32–36] Rare families with features of MEN2A do not have an identifiable *RET* mutation. In such cases, a clinical diagnosis of MEN2A can be made if at least two of the three classic features are present.[21]

Multiple Endocrine Neoplasia Type 2B

Individuals with multiple endocrine neoplasia type 2B (MEN2B) have a 100% risk of developing medullary thyroid carcinoma and,

in about 50% of cases, pheochromocytoma (Fig. 14.2B).[34] MEN2B kindred is also characterized by marfanoid habitus, mucosal neuromas (Fig. 14.3), gastrointestinal ganglioneuromatosis, and abnormal thickening of the corneal nerves.[37] Parathyroid hyperplasia rarely occurs in affected individuals. Medullary carcinoma usually presents before the age of 10. MEN2B is the most ominous form of hereditary medullary carcinoma because of its early development and rapid progression to metastatic disease.

Familial Medullary Thyroid Carcinoma

Familial medullary thyroid carcinoma (FMTC) is characterized by medullary thyroid carcinoma alone. FMTC usually manifests during the fifth to sixth decade of life, and these medullary carcinomas tend to have indolent clinical courses.[32] Rigorous criteria have been developed for the diagnosis of FMTC to help prevent small MEN2A kindreds from being categorized incorrectly. The criteria are (1) >10 carriers in a kindred, (2) multiple carriers or affected family members older than 50, and (3) no evidence of pheochromocytoma or hyperparathyroidism in family members affected by or at risk for medullary carcinoma.[32,33] These criteria may incorrectly place small FMTC kindreds in the MEN2A

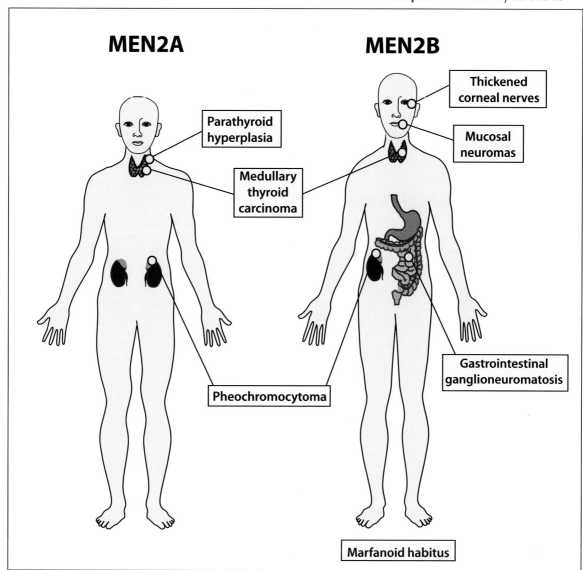

FIGURE 14.2. Characteristic abnormalities associated with MEN2A and MEN2B.

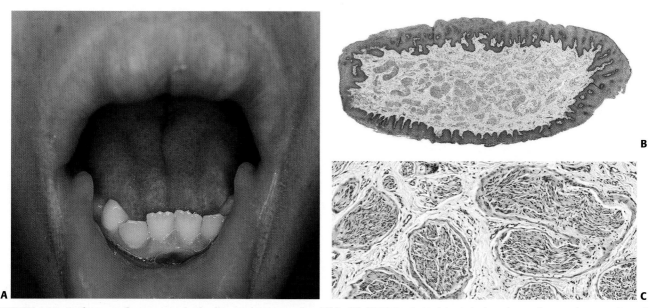

FIGURE 14.3. Oral mucosal neuromas in the lips and tongue of a child with MEN2B. A: Nodules in both oral commissures, the upper lip and the tip of the tongue. **B and C:** Low-power **(B)** and medium-power **(C)** photomicrographs of a biopsy showing numerous, irregular nerve bundles.

category, but this error is offset by the reduced likelihood of overlooking a pheochromocytoma.

The American Thyroid Association (ATA) currently views FMTC as a variant of MEN2A that has decreased penetrance for pheochromocytoma and primary hyperparathyroidism. The ATA criteria for FMTC are (1) absence of pheochromocytoma or primary hyperparathyroidism in two or more generations of a family or (2) a *RET* mutation that only has been identified in FMTC kindreds.[21] The ATA advises caution in diagnosing FMTC in small kindreds or a single affected generation because of the potential that these cases may prove to be MEN2A with a risk of pheochromocytoma.

Sporadic Medullary Thyroid Carcinoma

Sporadic medullary thyroid carcinoma is defined by the lack of a family history of medullary carcinoma and other disorders associated with the multiple endocrine neoplasia syndromes. Sporadic cases are more common than their hereditary counterparts, accounting for 70% to 85% of all cases of medullary carcinoma.[24,30,31,38] Although most cases are due to acquired somatic mutations, 1% to 10% or possibly more of apparent sporadic cases show germline *RET* mutations.[32,39–41] The presence of a germline mutation changes the diagnosis to a hereditary form of medullary carcinoma. Many of these individuals have de novo germline mutations and thus represent the initial appearance of hereditary medullary thyroid carcinoma in a kindred.

 ETIOLOGIC FACTORS

The etiology of familial medullary carcinoma is primarily due to a germline mutation of the *RET* gene as will be discussed below in the next section. A point mutation is identifiable in almost all individuals with clinical, pathologic, and/or historical findings characteristic of hereditary disease.[41] The specific cause of the germline mutations is unknown.

About one- to two-thirds of sporadic medullary carcinomas have somatic *RET* mutations, and as with hereditary cases, the cause of these *RET* mutations is unknown. Mounting evidence suggests that other genetic mutations and/or epigenetic events contribute to the development of sporadic and possibly hereditary medullary carcinoma as discussed below. Specific etiologic factors for other mutations or epigenetic changes have not been identified.

 PATHOGENESIS AND MOLECULAR GENETICS

Germline RET Mutations

Familial medullary carcinomas are associated with gain-of-function mutations in the *RET* gene. A 1985 study of a cell line transfected with human lymphoma DNA revealed a novel transforming gene.[42] This proved to be a fusion gene containing a portion of a gene that coded for a tyrosine kinase domain. This tyrosine kinase gene became known as *RET*, its name a contraction acronym of *RE*arranged during *T*ransfection. Genetic linkage analysis localized the MEN2A locus to the centromeric region of chromosome 10 in 1987.[43] Subsequent studies revealed that *RET* mapped to chromosome 10q11.2 and that germline mutations of *RET* were the primary cause of MEN2A, MEN2B, and FMTC.[44–46] Most germline mutations are point mutations. *RET* is the gene associated with both MEN2/FMTC disorders and Hirschsprung disease, but the sets of germline mutations are different. In contrast to activating mutations in hereditary medullary carcinoma, loss-of-function mutations are responsible for Hirschsprung disease.[36] Of

note, *RET* is also involved in the pathogenesis of papillary thyroid carcinoma, where a portion of the gene is fused and activated as a result of chromosomal rearrangement known as *RET/PTC* (see Chapter 11).

RET has 21 exons and approximately 55,000 base pairs.[47] It codes for a protein (RET) that is a member of the receptor tyrosine kinase superfamily. The receptor comprises an extracellular domain with calcium-dependent cell adhesion (cadherin) and cysteine-rich regions, a transmembrane domain, and an intracellular domain with regions of tyrosine kinase activity (Fig. 14.4).[34]

The RET receptor is activated when a complex ligand binds to the extracellular domain. Glial cell line–derived neurotrophic factor (GDNF) binds to GDNF family receptor $\alpha 1$, a glycosylphosphatidylinositol protein located on the cell surface, forming a complex that subsequently binds to RET (Fig. 14.5).[36,48–50] Binding of this complex results in receptor dimerization and autophosphorylation of tyrosine residues. This in turn initiates downstream signaling through the mitogen-activated protein kinase and other pathways.[34] Several other members of the GDNF ligand family have been shown to activate RET after binding to surface proteins. These include neurturin, artemin, and persephin.[36]

The RET receptor activates signaling pathways responsible for cell proliferation, survival, differentiation, motility, and chemotaxis.[34] RET is normally expressed by thyroid C cells and cells of the adrenal medulla, sympathetic ganglia, and kidneys. Populations of neural crest cells express RET during early embryogenesis and as they migrate to various regions of the body.[34] The normal development of the autonomic and enteric nervous systems and the excretory system is dependent on RET.[51]

Since the initial discovery of activating point mutations of RET as the primary cause of the hereditary forms of medullary carcinoma, a wide distribution of mutations have been identified in the extracellular cysteine-rich and the intracellular tyrosine kinase domains, as summarized in Figure 14.4 and Table 14.1.[33–36,41] Mutations of five cysteine-rich domain codons collectively account for about 95% of MEN2A and 85% of FMTC kindred.[35] Four are located on exon 10 (609, 611, 618, and 620) and one on exon 11 (634), and almost all mutations involve replacement of cysteine by another amino acid. Codon 634 is the most common site of mutations associated with MEN2A, being involved in 80% to 90% of cases. The most common mutation is substitution of arginine for cysteine (C634A), found in about 50% of MEN2A families.[34,35,41] The C634A mutation is also linked to parathyroid hyperplasia.[52] Most of the mutations associated with FMTC are found in extracellular cysteine-rich domain codons 618, 620, and 634 in a fairly even distribution.[35] FMTC also has been associated with mutations of the intracellular tyrosine kinase domain of *RET* including codons 768, 790, 791, 804, 848, 883, 891, and 904.[35,36,41]

About 95% of cases of MEN2B are associated with a point mutation in the tyrosine kinase domain codon 918 of exon 16, resulting in the replacement of a methionine by threonine (M918T).[34,41,53,54] A point mutation at codon 883 of exon 15 resulting in alanine replacement by phenylalanine accounts for almost all of the remaining small percentage of MEN2B cases.[34,36,55] A small number of MEN2B cases have been found to have double germline mutations involving codons 804+805, 804+806, and 804+904.[56–60] De novo mutations leading to MEN2B are more common compared with de novo mutations leading to MEN2A and FMTC.

Mutations in the cysteine-rich domain codons, which account for most cases of MEN2A and FMTC, activate the RET protein by constitutive dimerization (Fig. 14.5). The mutated forms of RET have unpaired cysteine residues that can form disulfide bonds with other RET monomers, and thus, dimerization occurs without the necessity of a ligand.[36,61,62] Mutation of the 918 codon, which is associated with MEN2B, affects the catalytic core region of the intracellular tyrosine kinase domain and causes constitutive

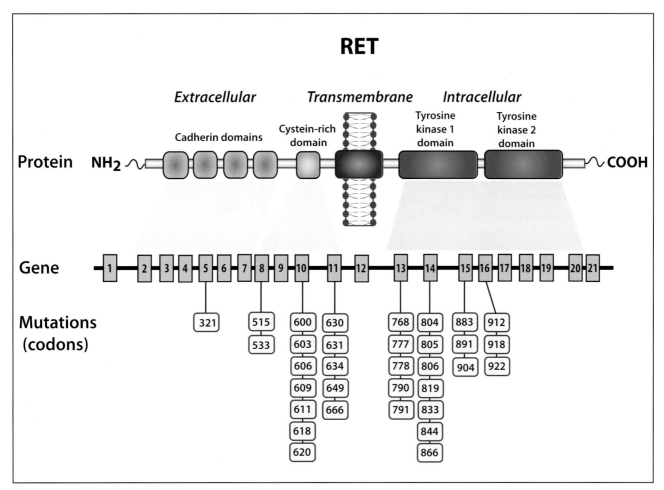

FIGURE 14.4. Schematic diagram of *RET* gene and associated RET protein. Codons reported to be sites of *RET* mutations resulting in hereditary medullary thyroid carcinoma are listed below their associated exon. The association between exons and the regions of the RET protein they encode is also shown.

activation of the monomeric form of RET.[36,54] A conformational change in the binding pocket of the tyrosine kinase domain leads to an altered substrate specificity. A small portion of FMTC cases have mutations involving the intracellular tyrosine kinase domain. The activation mechanisms associated with these mutations are not well defined at this time.

Somatic Mutations in Sporadic Medullary Thyroid Carcinoma

Somatic *RET* Mutations

Somatic *RET* mutations have been detected in 30% to 66% of sporadic medullary thyroid carcinomas.[34,63–65] The replacement of methionine by threonine at codon 918 (M918T) is most common, accounting for about 75% to 95% of somatic *RET* mutations.[34,46,63,64,66] This amino acid substitution at codon 918 is the same as that found in most MEN2B germline mutations. The remainder of somatic *RET* mutations have been reported at most of the other codons associated with hereditary carcinomas. Medullary carcinomas carrying a somatic *RET* mutation have been shown to have a higher frequency of metastasis involving regional lymph nodes and distant sites and to have a worse prognosis compared with those without *RET* mutation.[63] Of medullary carcinomas with somatic *RET* mutations, those with the codon 918 mutation appear to be more aggressive compared with those with other somatic *RET* mutations.[34,63]

Somatic RAS Mutations

RAS mutations have been recently found with substantial prevalence in sporadic medullary carcinomas. A study of 25 sporadic medullary carcinomas lacking a *RET* mutation identified *HRAS* (codons 12, 13, and 61) mutations in 14 cases (56%) and *KRAS* mutations (codon 61) in 3 cases (12%), whereas only 1 of 40 *RET* mutation-positive cases also had a *RAS* (*HRAS*) mutation.[67] No *NRAS* mutations were identified in any of the 65 medullary carcinomas. In contrast, the most common *RAS* mutation found in follicular and papillary thyroid carcinomas affects the *NRAS* gene (Chapters 10 and 11). Another study of 39 sporadic medullary carcinomas found two cases with an *HRAS* mutation and one with a *KRAS* mutation, and these cases were negative for *RET* mutations.[68] Although not all studies of sporadic medullary carcinoma found *RAS* mutations,[69] the available data and our experience Y. Nikiforov *personal communication, 2011* suggest that pathogenesis of sporadic medullary carcinomas is associated with nonoverlapping mutations involving the *RET* and *RAS* genes.

Other Genetic Abnormalities

Other genetic mutations and/or epigenetic events are likely to play a role in the development of sporadic and hereditary medullary carcinoma. The disease phenotype of hereditary tumors generally correlates with *RET* mutations of specific codons, but individuals with the same germline mutation still show some

A   **Normal RET Activation**

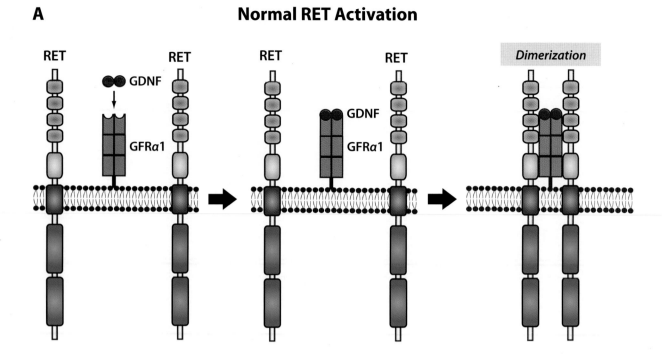

B   **Neoplastic RET Activation**

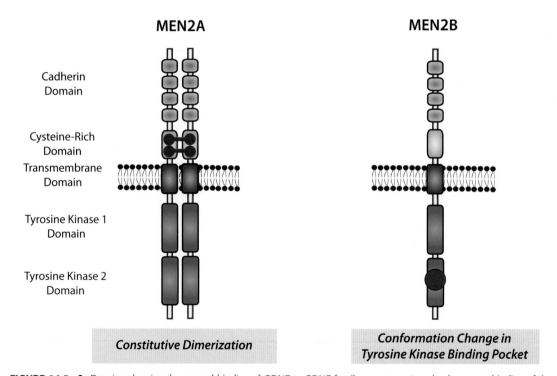

FIGURE 14.5. A: Drawing showing the normal binding of GDNF to GDNF family receptor α1 and subsequent binding of the complex with RET receptor and activation through dimerization. **B:** Drawings showing constitutive dimerization of *RET* in MEN2A and FTMC and monomeric activation in MEN2B due to change in tyrosine kinase binding pocket.

variation in regard to clinical manifestations of disease. Several potential oncoproteins and tumor suppressors are present in the signaling pathways utilized by the RET receptor, and mutations in genes encoding these proteins may play significant roles in the development of medullary carcinoma. Major signaling proteins activated downstream of RET are RAS and phosphatidylinositol 3-kinase. As discussed above, *RAS* mutations have been found in a significant number of sporadic medullary carcinomas. Loss

Table 14.1

Sites of *RET* Germline Mutations and Associated Forms of Hereditary Medullary Thyroid Carcinoma

Sites of Germline Mutations			Relative Risk of Aggressive Medullary Carcinoma (2001)[a]	ATA Risk Level (2009)[b]	Associated Form of Hereditary Medullary Carcinoma
Domain	Exon	Codon			
	8	533		A	FMTC
	10	609	1	B	MEN2A and FMTC
		611	2	B	MEN2A and FMTC
		618	2	B	MEN2A and FMTC
		620	2	B	MEN2A and FMTC
Extracellular cysteine-rich	11	630		B	MEN2A and FMTC
		634	2	C	MEN2A and FMTC
		649		A	FMTC
	13	768	1	A	MEN2A and FMTC
		790	1	A	MEN2A and FMTC
		791	1	A	MEN2A and FMTC
	13/14	804+778		B	MEN2A and FMTC
	14	804	1	A	MEN2A and FMTC
		804+805		D	MEN2B
Intracellular tyrosine kinase		804+806		D	MEN2B
	14/15	804+904		D	MEN2B
	15	883	3	D	MEN2B
		891	1	A	MEN2A and FMTC
	16	912		A	FMTC
		918	3	D	MEN2B

Note: The list of mutations in this table accounts for most cases of hereditary medullary thyroid carcinoma but is not all-inclusive. Additional, but relatively rare, sites of *RET* germline mutations include codons 321, 515,600, 603, 606, 631, 666, 777, 819, 833, 844, 866, 904, and 922. Most of these are associated with FMTC.
[a] Relative Risk Classification: 3, highest; 2, high; 1, least high. From 2001 Consensus Document of Seventh International Workshop on MEN; Brandi ML, Gagel RF, Angeli A, et al. Guidelines for diagnosis and therapy of MEN type 1 and type 2. *J Clin Endocrinol Metab.* 2001;86:5658–5671.
[b] ATA Risk Level: D, highest; C & B, intermediate, A, lowest. From Kloos RT, Eng C, Evans DB, et al. Medullary thyroid cancer: management guidelines of the American Thyroid Association. *Thyroid.* 2009;19:565–612.

of function of negative regulators of RET signaling such as the tyrosine phosphatases LAR, PTPRJ, or SHP-1 is another potential mechanism of tumorigenesis. Murine studies suggest that mutations of the tumor suppressor genes *RB1* and *TP53* may play a role in medullary carcinoma.

Loss of Heterozygosity

Analyses of both hereditary and sporadic cases of medullary carcinoma have shown loss of heterozygosity at one or more chromosomes other than 10q including 1p, 3p, 3q, 11p, 11q, 13q, 17p, 18p, 18q, 19p, 19q, and 22q.[70–72] About 25% of hereditary and 75% of sporadic cases show imbalances when analyzed by comparative genomic hybridization (CGH).[70] Medullary thyroid carcinomas with the somatic *RET* M918T mutation tend to have the highest number of chromosomal imbalances detected by CGH.[71] These chromosomal imbalances are due to both gains (amplification) and losses (deletions). The affected regions are known to be the location of tumor suppressor genes as well as the genes that code for proteins of the GDNF family of receptors and their ligands.[70] The developing picture of pathogenesis suggests that *RET* mutations cause C-cell hyperplasia, at least in familial cases, creating a favorable environment for the development of

medullary carcinoma and that additional somatic mutations lead to expansion of clones with more aggressive biologic properties.[70]

DNA Ploidy

Multiple studies have examined DNA ploidy of medullary carcinomas by flow cytometry.[73–78] Overall, about 30% of cases are aneuploid and the remaining 70% of cases diploid. Most studies found that DNA aneuploidy was an adverse prognostic indicator with univariate analysis but was not an independent prognostic factor when subjected to multivariate analysis.

C-CELL HYPERPLASIA AND RELATIONSHIP TO MEDULLARY CARCINOMA

Historical Comments

C cells, also known as parafollicular cells, are neuroendocrine cells of the thyroid that produce calcitonin and can give rise to medullary carcinoma. The first published descriptions of the

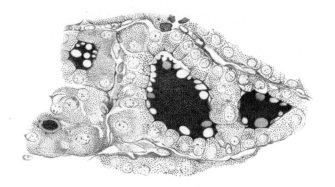

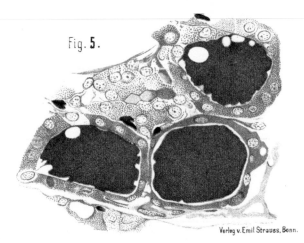

Fig. **5.**

Verlag v. Emil Strauss, Bonn.

FIGURE 14.6. Illustrations from Hürthle's 1894 article describing protoplasm-rich cells in the dog thyroid gland, which are now thought to represent C cells. The upper illustration shows the cells wedged between follicular cells, whereas the lower illustration shows them in a parafollicular location. (From Hürthle K. Beiträge zur Kenntniss des Secretionsvorgangs in der Schilddrüse. *Arch Gesammte Physiol.* 1894;56:1–44.)

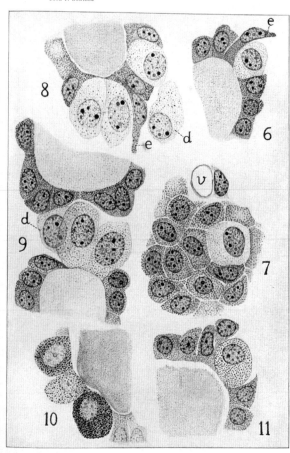

ORIGIN OF THE PARAFOLLICULAR CELL
JOSÉ F. NONIDEZ
PLATE 2

FIGURE 14.7. Illustration from Nonidez's 1932 article demonstrating argyrophilic granules within the cytoplasm of parafollicular cells of the dog thyroid gland. Parafollicular cells are designated "d" and elongated follicular cells "e." (From Nonidez JF. The origin of the "parafollicular" cell, a second epithelial component of the thyroid gland of the dog. *Am J Anat.* 1932;49:479–505.)

C cells are usually credited to E. Cresswell Baber[79,80] who in 1876 and 1878 described them within the dog thyroid. He noted their parafollicular location and different appearance from follicular cells, calling them parenchymatous cells. In 1894, Hürthle[81] provided additional description of what he thought were identical cells and applied the term *protoplasm-rich cells* (protoplasma-reichen Zellen) (Fig. 14.6). Although it appears that Hürthle described C cells, his name is often linked to metaplastic oncocytic follicular cells instead.

Nonidez[82] demonstrated in 1932 that the thyroid contained a population of cells with argyrophilic cytoplasmic granules and based on their location called them parafollicular cells (Fig. 14.7). Pearse[83] coined the term *C cell* in 1966 for cells he thought were comparable to those described by Baber, Hürthle, and Nonidez and that he postulated contained calcitonin. Bussolati and Pearse[84] confirmed the presence of calcitonin in C cells the following year.

Origin and Distribution of C Cells

The ultimobranchial bodies populate the thyroid with C cells after they fuse with the medial anlage during embryogenesis (see Chapter 2). After the ultimobranchial bodies are incorporated into the larger medial thyroid anlage, they begin a dissolution phase. Cells of the ultimobranchial bodies disperse into the lateral lobes and give rise to C cells. The ultimobranchial bodies usually fuse with

the middle to upper-middle region of the lateral lobes, and this is where the highest concentration of C cells is found in the normal thyroid gland.[85–87] Few, if any, C cells are found in the upper or lower poles or isthmus.

C cells are difficult, if not impossible, to recognize in routine histologic sections stained with hematoxylin and eosin (H&E). The prime exception is certain cases of C-cell hyperplasia as discussed below. Histologic clues for identifying C cells include cytoplasm that is clear or lightly staining and nuclei that are larger and more granular compared with adjacent follicular cells. Fortunately, immunohistochemical staining for calcitonin is readily available to most pathologists for the definitive identification of C cells.

C-Cell Hyperplasia

C-cell hyperplasia is recognized as the precursor of hereditary forms of medullary carcinoma.[88] The earliest reports of C-cell hyperplasia derived from studies of thyroids resected from individuals with MEN2A and MEN2B in which C-cell hyperplasia was a frequent finding. Thyroids removed prophylactically because of *RET* germline mutations may only show C-cell hyperplasia.[89]

Definition of C-Cell Hyperplasia

The criterion for C-cell hyperplasia used most commonly is >50 cells per low-power (100×) field (LPF).[30,90-93] In general, this is a reasonable and practical guideline for diagnostic histopathologists. There are, however, caveats for this criterion, and these are discussed later in this section.

Forms of C-Cell Hyperplasia

C-cell hyperplasia can exhibit focal, diffuse, and nodular growth patterns (Fig. 14.8 and Table 14.2). These patterns are not mutually exclusive, and more than one can be seen in a given case. The number of C cells and degree of aggregation can range in a continuum across the spectrum of hyperplasia. C-cell hyperplasia may be recognizable in H&E-stained sections, particularly in cases associated with hereditary forms of medullary carcinoma.

C-cell hyperplasia also has been observed in a number of other neoplastic and nonneoplastic conditions, although calcitonin immunostaining is generally necessary to identify the C cells. C-cell hyperplasia is one of the findings associated with PTEN-hamartoma tumor syndrome (PHTS).[94] PHTS is caused by a germline mutation of the *PTEN* tumor suppressor gene. Other associated lesions include multiple hyperplastic/adenomatous nodules, chronic lymphocytic thyroiditis, papillary carcinoma, follicular carcinoma, and/or follicular adenomas. C-cell hyperplasia has been observed

in chronic lymphocytic (Hashimoto) thyroiditis (Fig. 14.9), multinodular goiter, various forms of hypothyroidism, adjacent to follicular neoplasms and primary thyroid lymphoma, and following prior hemithyroidectomy.[95-99] From these observations, the concept has evolved that C-cell hyperplasia may be due to either an intrinsic genetic alteration or an external stimuli such as trophic hormones, hypercalcemia, hypergastrinemia, paracrine factors, or inflammation.[38,96] On this basis, C-cell hyperplasia can be separated into "neoplastic" and "reactive (or physiologic)" forms.[100]

Neoplastic C-cell hyperplasia is characterized by nodular and/or diffuse proliferation of relatively large cells with mild to moderate nuclear atypia that can be appreciated in H&E-stained sections (Fig. 14.10). These cells have more abundant cytoplasm that is clear or lighter staining relative to typical follicular cells in the section. It is of note that some consider C-cell hyperplasia a misnomer when it has "neoplastic" features and/or is associated with hereditary medullary carcinoma and instead prefer the term *medullary carcinoma in situ*.[95,101]

Calcitonin immunostaining is indicated whenever features suggestive of C-cell hyperplasia are seen in H&E-stained sections of thyroid. If C-cell hyperplasia is confirmed by calcitonin immunostaining, it is advisable that this finding be reported even if the thyroid was resected for reasons other than medullary carcinoma and/or *RET* germline mutation. Not every case in which C-cell hyperplasia is identifiable in H&E-stained sections will prove to be associated with a *RET* germline mutation, but consideration of

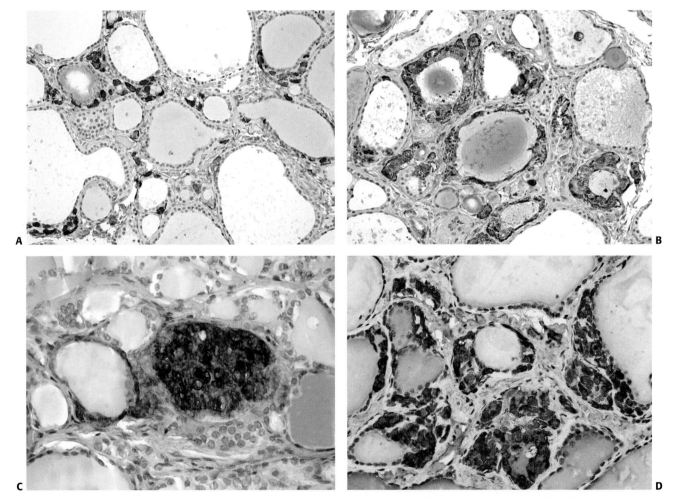

FIGURE 14.8. Growth patterns of C-cell hyperplasia. A: Focal hyperplasia with segmental proliferation. **B:** Focal and diffuse hyperplasia (encirclement of follicles). **C:** Nodular hyperplasia with obliteration of follicular lumen. **D:** Diffuse and nodular hyperplasia with central area suspicious for invasion beyond follicular basement membrane (early medullary carcinoma).

Table 14.2

C-Cell Hyperplasia—Definitions of Subtypes and Growth Patterns

Subtypes

"Neoplastic"	"Reactive"
• Detectable on H&E-stained sections	• Detectable only with calcitonin immunostain
• C cells enlarged	• C cells not enlarged
• Mild to moderate nuclear pleomorphism distinct from follicular cells	• No cytologic atypia
	• Usually unilateral
• More abundant cytoplasm, typically clear or lighter staining than follicular epithelium	• NCAM immunostain usually negative
	• Probably not associated with *RET* mutations
• Usually bilateral	
• NCAM immunostain usually positive	
• Associated with *RET* mutations	

Growth Patterns

Focal	Diffuse	Nodular
• Segmental proliferation within follicles	• Circumferential intrafollicular collar	• Obliteration of follicular lumen

NCAM, neural cell adhesion molecule.

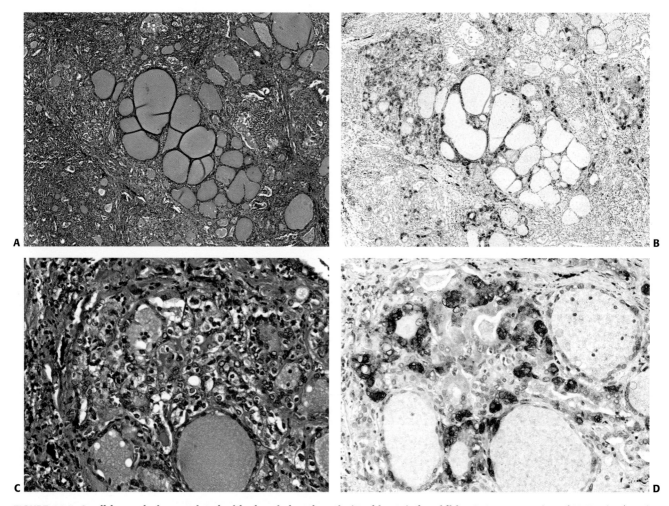

FIGURE 14.9. C-cell hyperplasia associated with chronic lymphocytic (Hashimoto) thyroiditis. A: Low-power view of H&E-stained section showing features of chronic lymphocytic thyroiditis. **B:** Calcitonin-stained section of same area as **(A)** showing numerous C cells. **C:** High-power view of H&E-stained section showing C cells with clear cytoplasm. **D:** High-power view of calcitonin-stained section showing encirclement of follicles by C cells.

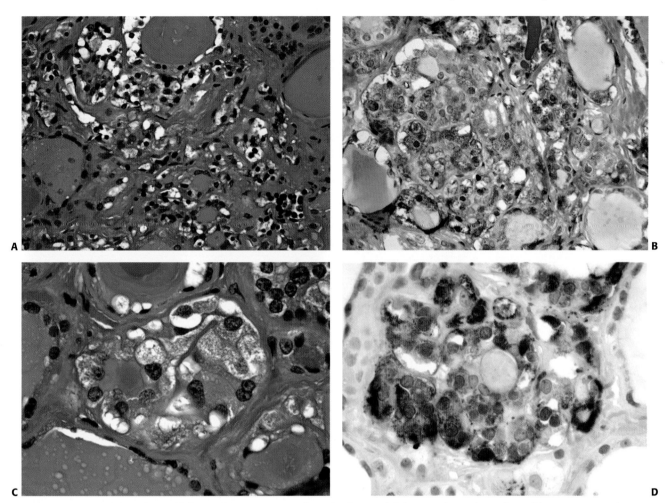

FIGURE 14.10. "Neoplastic" C-cell hyperplasia. Large C cells with clear or lightly stained cytoplasm detectable in H&E-stained sections **(A and C)**. Calcitonin-immunostained sections of same areas **(B and D)**.

genetic testing is advisable because of potential identification of a new hereditary kindred.

Reactive C-cell hyperplasia consists of an increase in C cells that meets the criterion for hyperplasia and requires calcitonin immunostaining for recognition. The C cells are not appreciably enlarged and lack cytologic atypia. Focal, diffuse, and nodular growth patterns are seen in the reactive subtype of C-cell hyperplasia with about the same relative frequency.[91,92,100]

Although the use of the terms *neoplastic and reactive C-cell hyperplasia* is common, these designations have not yet gained universal acceptance. Consistent differentiation of these two forms of C-cell hyperplasia on a histologic basis by pathologists may be problematic. Investigators have tried to identify other immunohistochemical markers that distinguish neoplastic from physiologic subtypes. Positive immunostaining for neural cell adhesion molecule (NCAM) favors neoplastic C-cell hyperplasia, but it is not 100% sensitive or specific.[93,102] Thus far, no immunostain has emerged that can serve as the criterion standard for distinguishing these putative subtypes. The lack of such a marker, however, has been offset by the development of molecular tests that identify specific *RET* germline mutations.

Differential Diagnosis of C-Cell Hyperplasia

The differential diagnosis of C-cell hyperplasia includes medullary microcarcinoma, spread of medullary carcinoma, solid cell nests, parathyroid tissue, focal squamous metaplasia, and palpation thyroiditis. Distinction of nodular C-cell hyperplasia from an early medullary microcarcinoma can be challenging. The criterion for medullary microcarcinoma is cells breaching the basement membrane of the follicle and extending into the adjacent stroma. Fibrosis around nests of tumor cells is a clue that invasion has occurred (Fig. 14.11). Immunostains for basement membrane components such as collagen IV may be helpful in some cases.[103] Tenascin C, an extracellular matrix glycoprotein, has been found to be expressed consistently in the stroma of both hereditary and sporadic medullary microcarcinomas and also in the stroma of concomitant and isolated foci of C-cell hyperplasia.[104] The significant overlapping of stromal expression in medullary microcarcinoma and C-cell hyperplasia limits the diagnostic utility of tenascin C, although the absence of stromal expression supports a diagnosis of C-cell hyperplasia.

Intrathyroidal spread of medullary carcinoma can have small foci similar in size to C-cell hyperplasia, but distinction between the two is generally not an issue with adequate sampling of the thyroid. Focal squamous metaplasia is typically associated with chronic lymphocytic (Hashimoto) thyroiditis. Squamous metaplasia associated with thyroiditis and palpation thyroiditis is discussed in Chapter 4. Solid cell nests are discussed in Chapter 1.

Controversial Aspects of C-Cell Hyperplasia

The definition of C-cell hyperplasia remains problematic. Although >50 cells per LPF (100× magnification: 10× objective

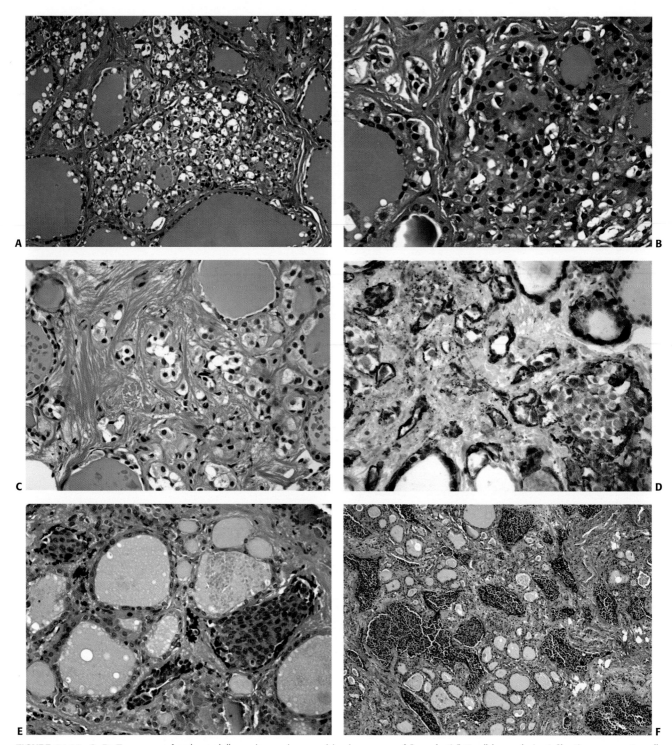

FIGURE 14.11. A–D: Two cases of early medullary microcarcinoma arising in an area of "neoplastic" C-cell hyperplasia. A fibrotic response to cells extending beyond the follicles is seen. **E and F:** Multifocal intrathyroidal spread of medullary carcinoma. Small isolated foci bear resemblance to nodular C-cell hyperplasia (**A–C, E,** and **F**, H&E; **D**, calcitonin immunostain).

combined with 10× eyepiece) is the most common criterion, even this has its variations as requirements range from this number of cells in just one field, to at least one field in each lobe, or to at least three fields in either or both lobes. Several other criteria have been used in the past.[105]

Distinct separation of C-cell hyperplasia from the upper limit of normal is difficult. Part of the problem is few studies have documented the concentration of C cells in the normal thyroid. Determining the normal concentration and distribution is difficult. C cells are relatively scant, comprising 0.1% or less of the thyroid cell population, and they are not equally distributed within the thyroid. Studies also indicate that C-cell concentration varies by age with a tendency of neonates and children to have more per unit region compared with adults. However, the ranges of concentration are broad with considerable overlap among the different age groups.[105] One autopsy study found >50 C cells in three or more LPFs in 33% of adults, whereas 62% had >50 C cells in at least one LPF.[106] Use of the term *hyperplasia* is problematic when a high percentage of the "normal" population meets the criterion.

Is C-cell hyperplasia, or at least the "neoplastic" form, specific for hereditary medullary carcinoma? The answer is not clear at this time. Hereditary medullary carcinoma is more likely to show foci of C-cell hyperplasia in thyroid tissue both adjacent to and more distant from the tumor.[107] Although C-cell hyperplasia is more frequently observed in thyroids of individuals with MEN2 and FMTC, it has also been observed in sporadic cases.[92,108,109] C-cell hyperplasia associated with sporadic cases has reportedly shown both neoplastic and physiologic features.[92,110] However, others have specifically linked neoplastic C-cell hyperplasia to germline mutations of *RET*.[93,96] A recent study of eight cases of sporadic medullary carcinoma with C-cell hyperplasia failed to detect a *RET* mutation in the hyperplastic foci, although three of the sporadic medullary carcinomas showed somatic M918T mutations.[93]

Thus, issues remain regarding the definition of C-cell hyperplasia and whether there are distinct subtypes. Fortunately, genetic analysis for *RET* germline mutations has relieved the pressure to differentiate hereditary from sporadic cases on the basis of C-cell hyperplasia. With future molecular-based studies, we will likely gain a more complete understanding of C-cell hyperplasia and greater insight into the neoplastic and reactive changes of C cells.

CLINICAL PRESENTATION AND IMAGING

The clinical presentation of sporadic medullary carcinoma is usually a painless solitary thyroid nodule. Most patients are in the fifth or sixth decade of life. About half of the patients have clinically detectable cervical lymph node metastasis.[23,24,111] Signs and symptoms of local mass effect such as hoarseness, stridor, or dysphagia occur in about 10% to 15% of cases.[23,111] Those with familial forms of medullary carcinoma usually present at an earlier age, typically in the third decade of life. Presentation in childhood or adolescence is possible, particularly for those affected by MEN2B. Many patients with hereditary medullary carcinoma are now detected and treated during childhood or adolescence before masses or symptoms are apparent.

Patients may experience various paraneoplastic syndromes because of the production of bioactive peptides and amines. Diarrhea is the most common, occurring in 10% to 30% of patients, and is usually attributed to elevated plasma calcitonin.[23,111] Rare cases of medullary carcinoma result in Cushing syndrome because of adrenocorticotropic hormone (ACTH) production.[112]

If medullary carcinoma is diagnosed by fine needle aspiration (FNA), the neck is usually examined by ultrasonography or CT scanning to evaluate lymph nodes. CT scanning or positron emission tomography–CT is used to detect distant metastasis.[113] Scintigraphic imaging studies of the thyroid with radioiodine reveal lack of uptake by the tumor.

GROSS FEATURES

Medullary carcinomas typically have well-defined borders but lack encapsulation (Fig. 14.12). However, rare cases may have a distinct fibrous capsule (Fig. 14.13).[114,115] Medullary carcinomas are usually firm in consistency and may feel gritty when sectioned owing to finely granular calcifications. However, some may have a soft consistency. Their color generally ranges from white to light gray or tan but may include shades of yellow or pink. Hemorrhage or necrosis is usually absent.

Medullary carcinomas can range in size from minute and barely discernible to 8 cm or more in diameter.[3] Larger tumors

may completely replace a lobe. Tumors <1 cm in diameter are called microcarcinomas, using the same nomenclature as with tumors derived from follicular epithelium. Pathologists seem to be encountering medullary microcarcinomas with increasing frequency because of screening programs that detect neoplastic lesions at an earlier stage. The thyroid capsule is usually intact, although it may be adherent to perithyroidal tissues without actual extrathyroid extension.

Medullary carcinomas are usually found in the middle regions of the lateral lobes. This region generally has the highest concentration of C cells, corresponding to the usual site of fusion of the ultimobranchial bodies with the medial thyroid analage. Involvement of the isthmus or poles of the lateral lobes is unusual unless the tumor is large. Tumor is limited to one lobe in most cases, but hereditary cases have about a 75% frequency of bilateral grossly identifiable masses, particularly if prophylactic resection is not performed early in life (Fig. 14.14).[21] Sporadic cases may have bilateral disease, with series reporting frequencies ranging from 0% to 22%.[116–119]

MICROSCOPIC FEATURES

Medullary carcinomas can exhibit a broad range of histologic features both in terms of growth patterns and cytologic features. The most common growth pattern is solid with sheets and nests of cells separated by fibrovascular stroma (Fig. 14.15). Tumor nests typically exhibit variable size and shape. Other common growth patterns include lobular and trabecular (Fig. 14.16). The lobular pattern, also known as organoid, nested, or insular, basically is the solid pattern with more definition of the tumor nests by the surrounding fibrovascular stroma. The trabecular pattern consists of curvilinear anatomosing bands of tumor.

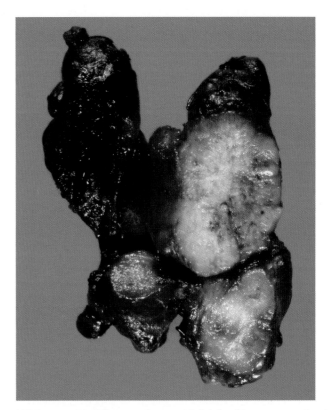

FIGURE 14.12. Medullary carcinoma. Well-defined but unencapsulated tumor in one lobe. Metastatic carcinoma is evident in the central lymph nodes inferior to the thyroid.

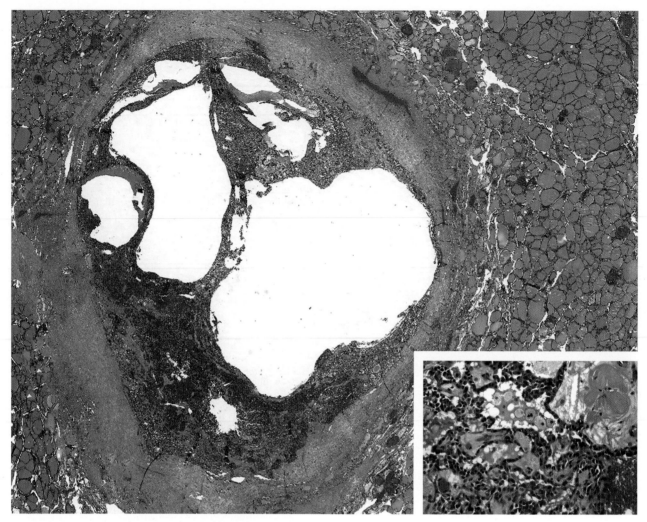

FIGURE 14.13. Encapsulated medullary carcinoma. Low-power photomicrograph showing fibrous capsule. The carcinoma has marked cystic change. The higher power inset shows discohesive cells.

These patterns may resemble carcinoid or islet cell tumors (Fig. 14.17). Intervening fibrovascular stroma ranges from thin and delicate to thick with abundant fibrous tissue. In many cases, the stroma has a hyalinized appearance because of amyloid deposition. Other, rare growth patterns define some tumor variants as described below.

Cells of medullary carcinoma are usually round to oval or polyhedral but frequently have an angulated or spindle shape (Fig. 14.18). Admixtures of these shapes are common in a single tumor. Cells usually range from 9 to 16 μm in greatest diameter.[3] Nuclei are round to oval and exhibit slight to moderate variation in size. The chromatin ranges from fine to moderately coarse and tends to have a uniform appearance within a particular tumor. The chromatin often gives nuclei a speckled or "salt and pepper" appearance, a feature common among neuroendocrine tumors. Binucleate cells are often present. Nucleoli are inconspicuous with the exception of the oncocytic variant (see Microscopic Variants section below). The nuclear:cytoplasmic ratio is generally low. Occasional large atypical nuclei may also be seen in tumors that are otherwise unremarkable. Nuclear pseudoinclusions similar to those seen in papillary thyroid carcinoma may be seen. Mitoses are sparse, usually ≤1 per 10 high-power fields (HPFs) and rarely >5 per HPF.[120]

The cytoplasm of most cells has a finely granular eosinophilic to amphophilic appearance with ill-defined cytoplasmic borders.

Neoplastic cells may exhibit a plasmacytoid appearance because of relatively abundant cytoplasm and an eccentrically placed nucleus. Some may exhibit clear cytoplasm, and clear mucin positive vacuoles are present occasionally. Mucin can be present within the cytoplasm or extracellularly, tends to be distributed focally, and its presence can be confirmed with histochemical stains.[121,122]

Several variants have been reported including tumors composed of a predominant, or at least significant, population of oncocytic, spindle, squamous, small, giant, mucinous, or melanotic cells (Table 14.3). Most of the variants represent extreme examples of features that can be seen to a limited extent in many more typical forms of medullary carcinoma. These variants are discussed further below.

Focal calcifications are common. Calcification is most commonly seen in the stroma, often in association with amyloid deposits (Fig. 14.19). Other calcific foci may be present among the neoplastic cells. Some calcifications resemble psammoma bodies but lack appreciable lamination. Occasionally, psammoma bodies with characteristic lamellae are seen. Necrosis and hemorrhage are uncommon and are generally limited to large tumors. Lymphocytic infiltrates are usually absent or light. Rare cases show significant infiltration by neutrophils. Tumor invasion of lymphatic and blood vessels may be evident in the surrounding thyroidal tissue.

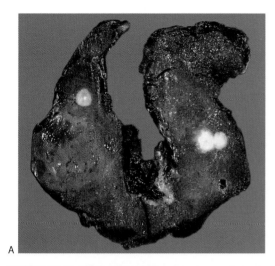
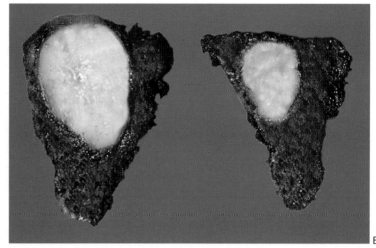

FIGURE 14.14. Bilateral medullary carcinoma is typically associated with familial forms of the disease. A: Bilateral microcarcinomas associated with MEN2A. **B:** Bilateral medullary carcinomas associated with MEN2B (mucosal neuromas shown in Fig. 14.3).

Amyloid stroma

Amyloid accumulation within the stroma is present in 70% to 80% or more of cases.[3,78,123] The amyloid may have a fairly diffuse distribution in the stroma or form small nodular deposits. The amyloid deposits are frequently associated with focal calcification, and multinucleated foreign body type giant cells are occasionally seen. The presence of amyloid can be confirmed with the Congo red stain and use of polarizing filters (Fig. 14.20).

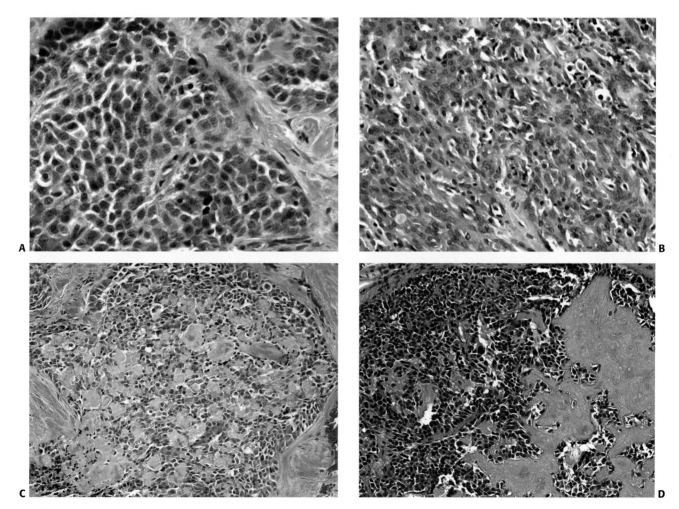

FIGURE 14.15. Medullary carcinoma showing solid growth patterns. Amyloid stroma is evident in images **(C)** and **(D)**.

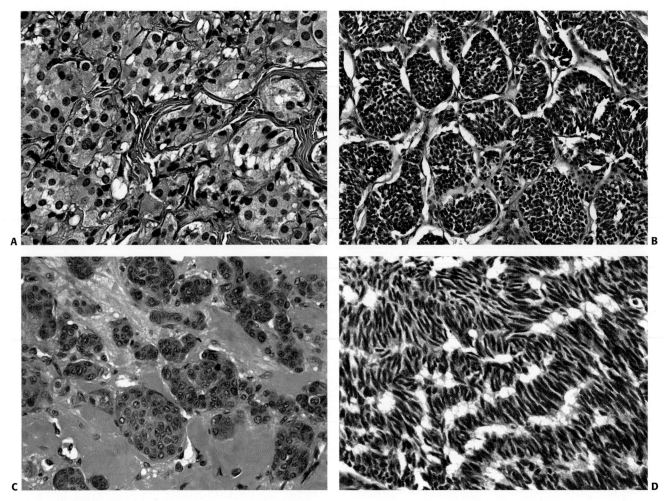

FIGURE 14.16. Medullary carcinoma. A–C: Nested or lobular architectural patterns. **D:** Trabecular growth pattern.

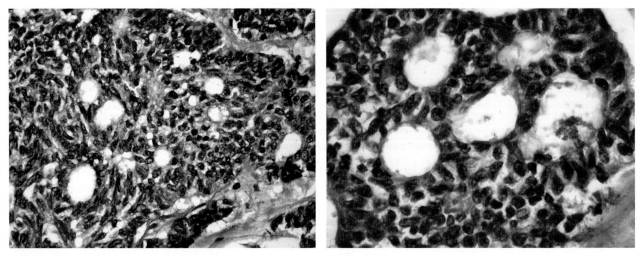

FIGURE 14.17. Medullary carcinoma with cribriform growth pattern resembling carcinoid tumor.

Amyloid appears to derive from calcitonin. An early study of medullary carcinoma and the subcellular distribution of calcitonin suggested an association with amyloid.[124] Subsequent ultrastructural studies using immunogold technique localized calcitonin immunoreactivity to amyloid fibers.[125,126] Recent

biophysical and structural analyses have shown that calcitonin monomers can indeed form amyloid fibrils under certain conditions.[127,128]

Some studies have found the absence of amyloid to be associated with an unfavorable prognosis.[74,118] However, this has not

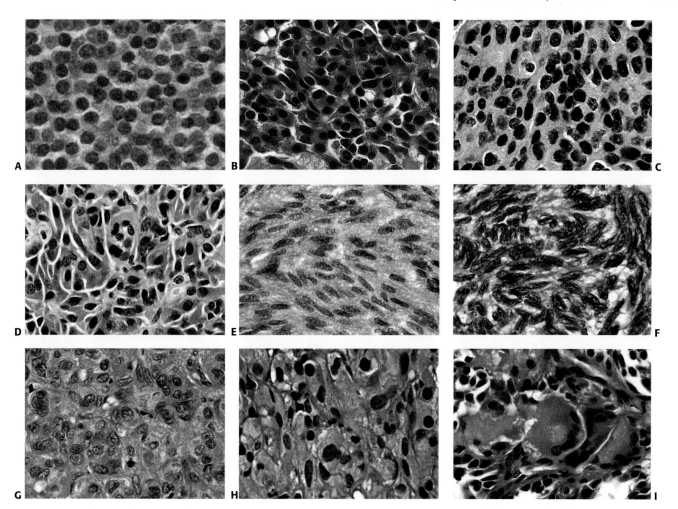

FIGURE 14.18. Broad range of cell types found in medullary carcinoma. A: Uniform round cells. **B:** Round to polygonal cells. **C:** Cells with round to oval hyperchromatic nuclei and mitotic activity. **D:** Polygonal to spindle cells. **E** and **F:** Spindle cells. **G** and **H:** Relatively large cells with pleomorphism and abundant cytoplasm. **I:** Multinucleated cells.

been a universal finding as other studies have found that absence of amyloid is not an independent prognostic factor when subjected to multivariate analysis.[73,77]

 ## SPREAD AND METASTASIS

Medullary thyroid carcinoma spreads by both lymphatic and hematogenous routes. At the time of diagnosis, about half will have cervical lymph node involvement that is clinical detectable.[23] Lymph nodes are the most common site of metastasis.[23,31,73,118,129] Pathologic examination of cervical lymph nodes may reveal metastatic disease undetected clinically, and some series report frequency of cervical lymph node involvement of 70% or higher.[73,118] The central paratracheal and/or superior mediastinal lymph nodes have a particularly high rate of involvement, not surprising given their proximity to the thyroid.[31]

The frequency of distant metastasis at the time of presentation and initial treatment is about 15%.[23,63,111,130,131] The lungs, liver, bone, adrenal glands, and brain are the most common sites of blood-borne metastases.[31,129] Patients who present with systemic symptoms of diarrhea, flushing, and/or bone pain almost always have distant metastasis.[111]

 ## MICROSCOPIC VARIANTS

Medullary Microcarcinoma

Medullary microcarcinoma is defined by size <1 cm in greatest dimension (Fig. 14.21). Microcarcinomas can exhibit one or more of the various cellular morphologies or architectural patterns associated with medullary carcinoma and may contain amyloid stroma. Microcarcinomas are particularly common in thyroids removed prophylactically because of a RET germline mutation. Microcarcinomas may be multifocal and bilateral, even in cases of sporadic medullary carcinoma.[109,117,132]

Very small microcarcinomas may be difficult to distinguish from nodular C-cell hyperplasia. Extension of C cells through the follicular basement membrane may be subtle and difficult to identify with certainty, even with the use of special stains to highlight the basement membrane. Isolated calcitonin-positive cells in a fibrotic stroma and/or the presence of amyloid support the diagnosis of medullary microcarcinoma (Fig. 14.22).

Medullary microcarcinomas tend to have a more favorable prognosis compared with larger tumors.[117] However, it is unclear whether the size <1 cm is an independent prognostic factor because of the lack of multivariate analysis. Medullary microcarcinomas still have the potential for adverse outcomes.

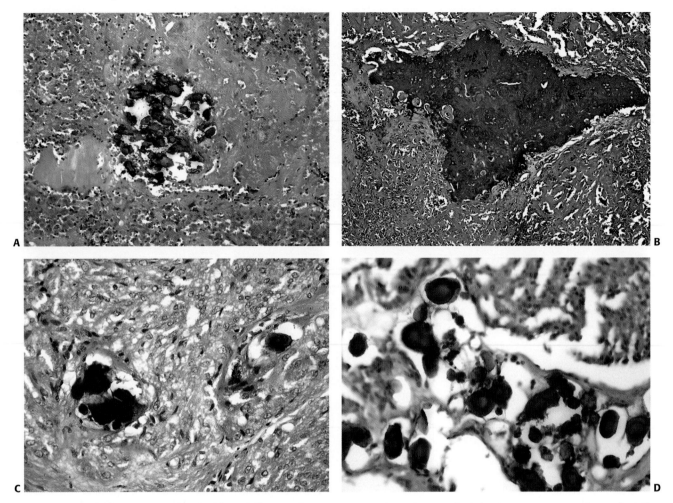

FIGURE 14.19. Calcifications associated with medullary carcinoma. A: Focus of granular stromal calcification. **B:** Larger area of stromal calcification with solid appearance. **C and D:** Calcifications resembling psammoma bodies.

Lymph node metastasis is associated with 10% to 30% of medullary microcarcinomas, including sporadic cases, and about 5% may have distant metastases and eventually die of disease.[109,117,132]

Spindle Cell Variant

Spindle cells are very common in medullary carcinoma and the dominant component in about 20% of cases (Fig. 14.23).[3] The

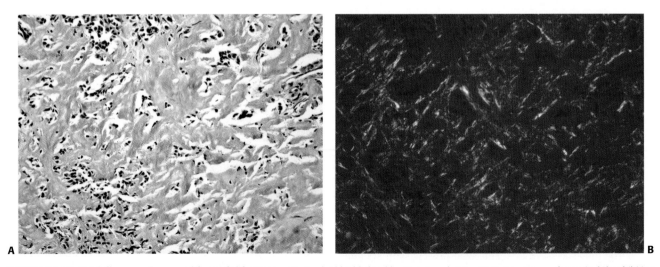

FIGURE 14.20. Medullary carcinoma with amyloid stroma. A: Amyloid highlighted by Congo red stain. **B:** Same area as shown in **(A)** exhibiting light green birefringence when viewed with polarizing filters.

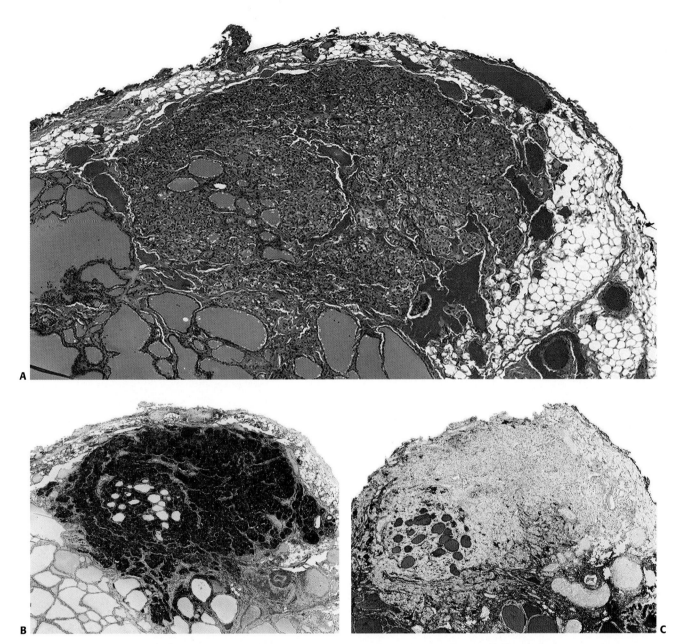

FIGURE 14.21. Medullary microcarcinoma measuring 0.2 cm. Tumor found in a thyroid removed prophylactically from an individual with a *RET* germline mutation. **B:** Neoplastic cells show strong positivity for calcitonin. **C:** Thyroglobulin immunostain highlights entrapped nonneoplastic follicles.

spindle cell variant is exclusively composed of spindle cells, or almost so. This variant can be confused with a sarcoma or other types of spindle cell neoplasms. Hyalinizing trabecular tumor, anaplastic carcinoma, and spindle cell tumor with thymus-like differentiation are other primary thyroid tumors that are included in the differential diagnosis of spindle cell lesions. Immunostains for cytokeratin and calcitonin are usually sufficient to resolve this differential diagnosis.

Papillary/Pseudopapillary Variant

Most medullary carcinomas exhibiting papillary architecture are actually pseudopapillary variants because of artifactual separation of neoplastic cells (Fig. 14.24). The cells of medullary carcinoma have a discohesive tendency; thus, they may adhere to the

fibrovascular stroma while detaching from adjacent neoplastic cells during histologic processing, resulting in a pseudopapillary appearance. Rare cases may show a true papillary growth pattern, at least in regions of the tumor.[133] The differential diagnosis includes mixed medullary and papillary carcinoma, and papillary carcinoma per se. Papillary variants of medullary carcinoma lack the spectrum of nuclear features characteristic of papillary carcinoma. Immunohistochemical stains for calcitonin and thyroglobulin should resolve most issues regarding the differential diagnosis.

Oncocytic/Oxyphilic Variant

Medullary carcinomas rarely may be composed predominately of oncocytic cells (Fig. 14.25).[120,134–136] Cells more typical of medullary

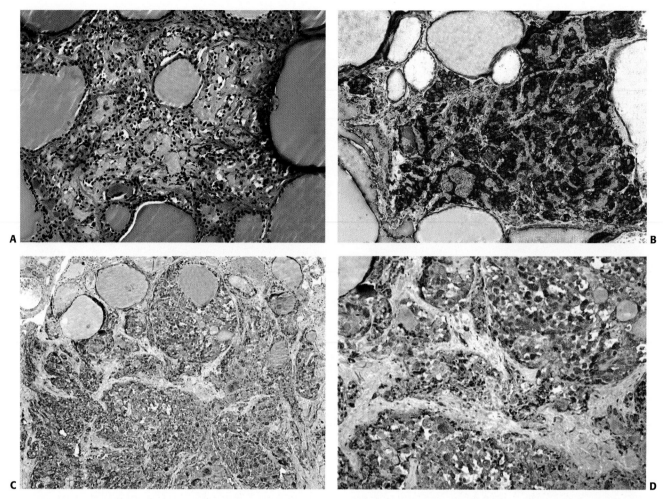

FIGURE 14.22. Two cases of early medullary microcarcinoma. The carcinoma in the first case **(A and B)** only measures 0.1 cm, but invasive growth is readily apparent, particularly in the calcitonin-stained section **(B)**. Amyloid stroma is also present **(A)**. The second case **(C and D)** is more subtle, but invasion of the perifollicular stroma is evident.

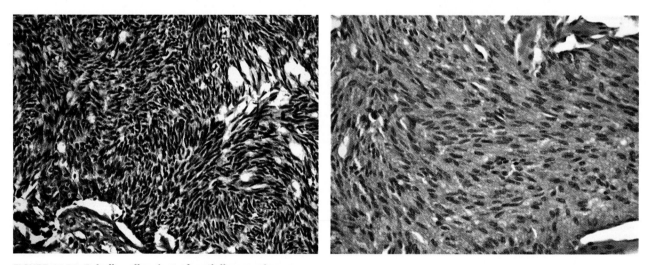

FIGURE 14.23. Spindle cell variant of medullary carcinoma.

carcinoma are seen in about half of the reported cases. Architecturally, oncocytic variants usually exhibit trabeculae, nests, and/or solid areas comparable with the common forms of medullary carcinoma. Some oncocytic variants exhibit follicle-like structures. More than half contain amyloid.

The neoplastic cells of almost all cases are immunoreactive for calcitonin and, if not, show argyrophilia with histochemical staining. Immunostains for thyroglobulin are negative. Ultrastructural examination of one case revealed abundant mitochondria as well as neurosecretory granules within the cytoplasm.[136]

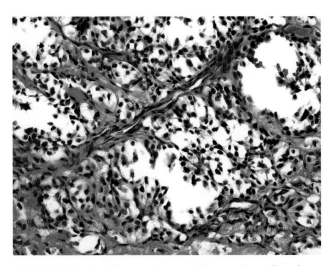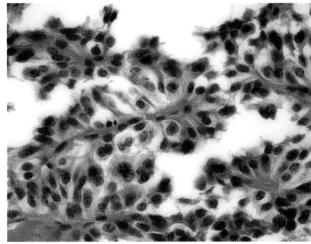

FIGURE 14.24. Medullary carcinoma with pseudopapillary features due to discohesive cells.

Clear-Cell Variant

Landon and Ordóñez[137] reported in 1985 a case of medullary carcinoma that appears to be composed almost entirely of clear cells. This carcinoma was composed of solid nests of polygonal and spindle cells that showed scattered immunostaining for calcitonin while having no immunoreactivity for thyroglobulin or parathyroid hormone. Electron microscopy revealed numerous neurosecretory granules within the cytoplasm. The explanation of the clear cytoplasm was unclear as staining for mucin was negative and significant amounts of glycogen were not found. The authors acknowledged that the clear cytoplasm could be a fixation artifact, but this seems unlikely given that similar features were seen in bone metastases sampled 6 years after thyroidectomy. Although occasional cases contain a minor population of clear cells, predominant or exclusive composition seems to be quite rare given the lack of other reported cases. The differential diagnosis includes clear-cell tumors derived from follicular epithelium and metastatic clear-cell tumors, particularly renal cell carcinoma. Clear-cell tumors of follicular derivation are typically immunoreactive for thyroglobulin in contrast to medullary thyroid carcinoma or metastatic renal cell carcinoma. Positive results for CD10 immunostaining support the diagnosis of metastatic renal cell carcinoma (see Chapter 18).

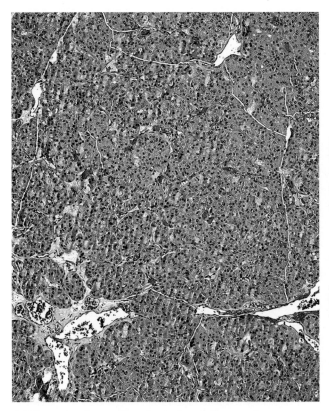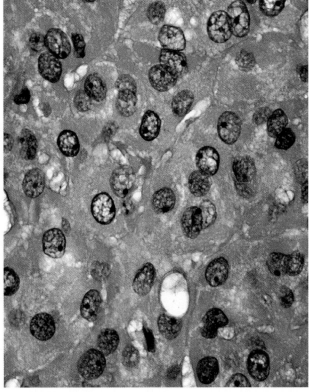

FIGURE 14.25. Oncocytic variant of medullary carcinoma.

Table 14.3

Variants of Medullary Thyroid Carcinoma

Microcarcinoma
Spindle cell
Papillary and pseudopapillary
Oncocytic/oxyphilic
Clear cell
Glandular/tubular/follicular
Amphicrine/composite calcitonin and mucin producing
Paraganglioma-like
Small cell
Giant cell
Angiosarcoma-like
Melanin producing/pigmented
Squamous cell (questionable)

Glandular/Tubular/Follicular Variant

This variant is characterized by glandular structures containing eosinophilic material resembling colloid (Fig. 14.26).[138,139] It is an extremely rare variant. These tumors can also exhibit solid and trabecular growth patterns in addition to the follicular structures. Immunohistochemical staining demonstrates calcitonin in the neoplastic cells and negative results for thyroglobulin. Ultrastructural examination has revealed that the cells forming follicular structures have cytoplasmic dense core secretory granules and microvilli that extend into the luminal spaces.[138] The composition and origin of the material within the lumina are unclear but may represent calcitonin or other proteins, although not thyroglobulin.[38] The differential diagnosis includes follicular thyroid carcinoma, entrapment of nonneoplastic thyroid follicles, and mixed medullary and follicular carcinoma.

Amphicrine/Composite Calcitonin and Mucin-Producing Variant

Medullary carcinoma may rarely show a significant population of signet-ring or goblet cells containing mucin.[140,141] These mucin-producing cells are admixed with more typical polygonal cells of medullary carcinoma, and both exhibit immunoreactivity for calcitonin. Ultrastructural examination shows both neurosecretory granules and glandular features in the neoplastic cells, and hence the application of the term *amphicrine*. Some have suggested that this variant supports the hypothesis that C cells may be of endodermal origin.

Paraganglioma-Like Variant

Encapsulated medullary carcinomas may show a nested or trabecular pattern in combination with a hyalinized stroma that resembles a paraganglioma.[114,142] Paragangliomas occur in the thyroid, albeit rarely, and differentiation from medullary carcinoma is important given the usually favorable prognosis of the former.[143,144] In addition to paraganglioma, the differential diagnosis includes hyalinizing trabecular tumor, atypical follicular and oncocytic thyroid neoplasms, and metastatic carcinoid tumor. Paragangliomas are negative for calcitonin, cytokeratin, and carcinoembryonic antigen (CEA). Hyalinizing trabecular tumors and follicular and oncocytic thyroid neoplasms are immunoreactive for thyroglobulin but not for calcitonin.

Small Cell Variant

The small cell medullary carcinoma is a rare variant histologically characterized by small cells with hyperchromatic nuclei and scant cytoplasm.[38,145] Stroma is usually scant, and growth patterns include sheets, small nodules, and trabeculae. A subset of the small cell variant may contain finely fibrillar perivascular material resembling that seen in neuroblastoma.[146] The mitotic rate is high, and necrotic foci may be present. Extensive sampling may reveal areas of more typical medullary carcinoma. The cells are positive for calcitonin, although the staining may be patchy.

Two cases of thyroid carcinoma with small cell features but without expression of calcitonin have been described.[147] The tumors exhibited positivity for chromogranin A and synaptophysin, but immunostains for calcitonin and thyroglobulin were negative. In addition, no calcitonin mRNA could be demonstrated with in situ hybridization. One tumor merged with an area of papillary carcinoma. The investigators concluded that thyroid tumors with small cell phenotype but no expression of calcitonin should be considered distinct from medullary carcinoma.

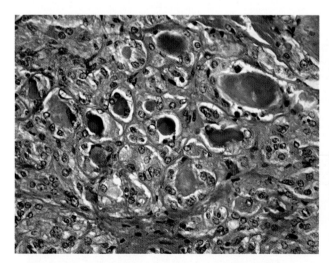 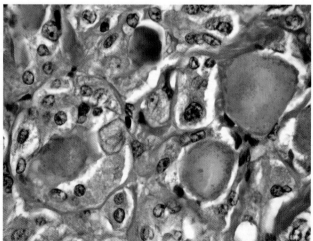

FIGURE 14.26. Glandular variant of medullary carcinoma with follicle-like structures. The neoplastic cells forming the follicle-like structures are comparable with the adjacent cells forming small, solid clusters. Immunostains revealed the expression of calcitonin but the absence of thyroglobulin.

The differential diagnosis includes lymphoma and metastatic small cell carcinoma. Identification of lymphoma is generally accomplished with a panel of lymphoid markers. Distinction from metastatic small cell carcinoma will likely depend on correlation with clinical information, imaging studies, and histologic examination of tissue from other sites.

Giant Cell Variant

The giant cell variant of medullary carcinoma is characterized by a predominant population of large pleomorphic cells with large, bizarre nuclei that may be multinucleated or multilobulated.[38,148] Areas of more typical medullary carcinoma may be present. An occasional giant cell can be seen in medullary carcinomas, and the giant cell variant probably represents a rare, extreme manifestation of this phenomenon. Metastatic lesions may contain a higher proportion of giant cells relative to the primary thyroid tumor. The giant cells are positive for calcitonin, although the staining may be variable.

The prime differential diagnosis is anaplastic thyroid carcinoma. This is an important distinction because of the significantly better prognosis of the giant cell variant of medullary carcinoma. Identification of areas of typical medullary carcinoma and demonstration of calcitonin immunoreactivity are keys to the correct diagnosis.

Angiosarcoma-Like Variant

Rare medullary carcinomas contain a prominent component of pseudovascular spaces resembling angiosarcoma.[149,150] The pseudovascular spaces appear as clefts among loosely cohesive spindle and polygonal neoplastic cells (Fig. 14.27). The neoplastic cells are positive for calcitonin, cytokeratin, and other markers characteristic of medullary carcinoma, whereas they are negative for vascular markers such as CD31 and CD34. Whether the angiosarcoma-like pattern is an artifact because of discohesive cells and/or histologic processing, FNA, or other manipulation is unclear.

Melanin-Producing/Pigmented Variant

Melanin production may be observed in medullary carcinomas. The amount of melanin ranges from microscopic foci to diffuse production and a grossly dark brown or black tumor.[142,151–154] In some cases, melanin and calcitonin are detectable within the same neoplastic cells, as are premelanosomes and dense core

granules ultrastructurally. In other cases, the melanin was found in dendritic cells interspersed among the round to polygonal tumor cells.[142,151] The dendritic cells have features comparable with sustentacular cells, having been shown immunoreactive for S-100 but not for HMB-45.[142] Melanin expression in medullary carcinoma is viewed as support for the neural crest origin of C cells. The main differential diagnosis is metastatic malignant melanoma. An immunohistochemical panel including calcitonin, cytokeratin, HMB-45, and Mart-1 (Melan-A) should allow distinction between the two entities.

Squamous Cell Variant

At the same time that Dominguez-Malagon et al.[136] reported an oncocytic variant in 1989, they also reported a case of medullary carcinoma with extensive squamous differentiation. Portions of the tumor had features of typical medullary carcinoma. The neoplastic cells were immunoreactive for chromogranin, neuron-specific enolase, and CEA but negative for calcitonin, so one could debate the appropriate diagnosis. If indeed a case of medullary carcinoma, this appears to be an extremely rare if not unique variant.

Other Proposed Variants

Other variants of medullary carcinoma have been proposed including carcinoid-like and encapsulated. At issue is where to draw the line between a distinct, rare variant and an unusual aspect in an otherwise typical medullary carcinoma. Harach and Bergholm[155] proposed recognition of a carcinoid-like subtype in 1993. They reported 15 cases that exhibited an appearance that raised the question of metastatic carcinoid tumor. Amyloid was absent or present in an isolated focus in about half of the cases, and two cases showed calcitonin immunostaining in 5% or less of the cells.

Medullary carcinomas may exhibit histologic patterns comparable with those of foregut, midgut, or hindgut carcinoids (Figs. 14.16D and 14.17). These include solid anastomosing nests characteristic of midgut carcinoids, a trabecular pattern typical of those originating in the hindgut, and any of the patterns seen in foregut carcinoids including trabecular, palisading, lobular, or glandular. Such patterns are often seen in medullary carcinomas, so it is debatable whether they should merit recognition as a variant. This may explain why carcinoid-like medullary carcinoma has not gained wide acceptance as a subtype. Cases with minimal expression of calcitonin may be difficult to distinguish from a rare

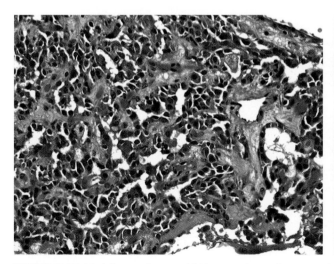
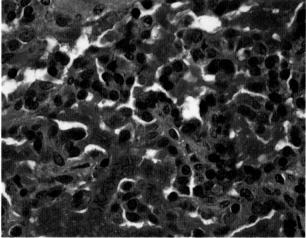

FIGURE 14.27. Medullary carcinoma exhibiting pseudovascular spaces due to discohesive cells and intratumoral hemorrhage.

case of metastatic carcinoid tumor on a histologic basis per se and require integration of clinical, imaging, and other ancillary information. However, carcinoid-like tumors with prominent immunostaining for calcitonin, CEA, and/or calcitonin gene–related peptide, however, should not pose a particular challenge for classification as medullary carcinoma.

Encapsulated medullary carcinomas are unusual and arguably warrant recognition as a variant (Fig. 14.13). Whether encapsulation of medullary carcinomas is a favorable prognostic indicator independent of other favorable indicators, such as tumor confined to the thyroid, is not clear at this time because of insufficient data. Some encapsulated tumors have been proffered as C-cell adenomas, but the concept of a benign C-cell neoplasm has not been embraced by experts in the field. The current general consensus is that all thyroid neoplasms exhibiting C-cell differentiation should be considered malignant, even if encapsulated, as the biologic behavior is unpredictable.[115]

C-cell adenoma is not recognized in the current World Health Organization (WHO) classification of thyroid tumors.[30] This is warranted given that evidence for C-cell adenoma is weak at best. A small number of putative cases of C-cell adenoma have been reported.[156,157] In one report, the tumors exhibiting C-cell differentiation reportedly were encapsulated, at least to some degree, lacked amyloid, and had a uniform population of spindle cells that were highlighted by an immunostain for calcitonin.[157] An earlier report describes 12 tumors containing "light" cells that exhibited histochemical enzyme reactions that the authors felt were demonstrative of C-cell differentiation.[158] Immunostaining for calcitonin was not performed. The accompanying photomicrographs consistently show follicular structures without features seen in most medullary carcinomas, and thus, their classification as C-cell neoplasms seems dubious.

 ## HISTOCHEMISTRY

Amyloid is demonstrable with the Congo red or crystal violet stain (Fig. 14.20).[120] Positive Congo red staining will show light green birefringence when viewed with polarizing filters. Amyloid shows purplish metachromatic staining with crystal violet. Most medullary carcinomas contain argyrophilic granules that are highlighted by the Grimelius stain but not by the Fontana-Masson stain.[120] A high percentage of medullary carcinomas show staining for extracellular and/or intracellular mucin with Alcian blue, PAS, and/or mucicarmine stains.[120–122]

 # IMMUNOHISTOCHEMISTRY

A wide variety of substances can be demonstrated immunohistochemically in medullary carcinoma, but a relatively small number have practical diagnostic or prognostic value (Table 14.4). The most useful diagnostic immunostains include calcitonin, CEA, chromogranin, synaptophysin, and calcitonin gene–related peptide. The ability to immunostain thyroid tumors for calcitonin has been of particular help in confirming the diagnosis of medullary carcinoma and appreciating its broad range of appearances.

Greater than 95% cases of tumors stain for calcitonin, although the degree of immunoreactivity is variable.[159] The percentage of calcitonin-positive cells can range from a minor fraction to >90%, and marked variation in staining intensity can occur within a given neoplasm.[160–165] However, most medullary carcinomas exhibit diffuse positivity (Fig. 14.28). The absence of immunostaining for calcitonin in a well-sampled tumor raises doubts about the diagnosis of medullary carcinoma. Alternative proof of C-cell differentiation can be achieved by demonstrating the immunoreactivity for calcitonin gene–releasing peptide (CGRP) or by detecting mRNA for calcitonin and/or CGRP by in situ hybridization.[159] CGRP is demonstrable immunohistochemically in most cases, but the extent of staining can vary and may be limited to small foci.[166–170]

Medullary carcinomas are usually positive for generic neuroendocrine markers such as chromogranin A, synaptophysin, and neuron-specific enolase.[120,159,163,165,166,170] Immunoreactivity for various peptides in addition to calcitonin and CGRP has been observed. These include somatostatin, gastrin-releasing peptide, ACTH, insulin, gastrin, and glucagon.[120,164,165,170] The bioactive amine serotonin is frequently detectable with immunostaining.[120,164,165]

CEA is demonstrable in most medullary carcinomas.[159,164,165,171] CEA immunostaining may be particularly helpful in cases of medullary carcinoma with little expression of calcitonin as CEA expression is usually retained. Medullary carcinomas typically express thyroid transcription factor 1 (TTF1), similar to follicular and papillary thyroid carcinomas.[159,172,173] Galectin-3 has been detected in the cytoplasm of 45% to 80% of medullary carcinomas.[171,174–177] The intensity and distribution of staining is variable, ranging from weak and focal to strong and more diffuse. This variability may explain some of the differences between studies. Most cases exhibit staining in the weak to moderate range.

Table 14.4		
Immunohistochemical Staining Characteristics of Medullary Thyroid Carcinoma		
Usually Positive (76%–100%)[a]	**Variably Positive (25%–75%)**	**Usually Negative (≤5%)**
Calcitonin	Galectin-3	Thyroglobulin
Calcitonin gene–related protein	Calretinin	Cytokeratin 20
CEA	Vimentin	
TTF1	S100[b]	
Synaptophysin	PAX8	
Chromogranin A		
Chromogranin B		
Neuron-specific enolase		
Pankeratin (AE1 + AE3)		
Cytokeratin 7		

[a]The division by percentage ranges reflects the frequency of positive staining of cases in most reports.
[b]May highlight occasional sustentacular-like cells.

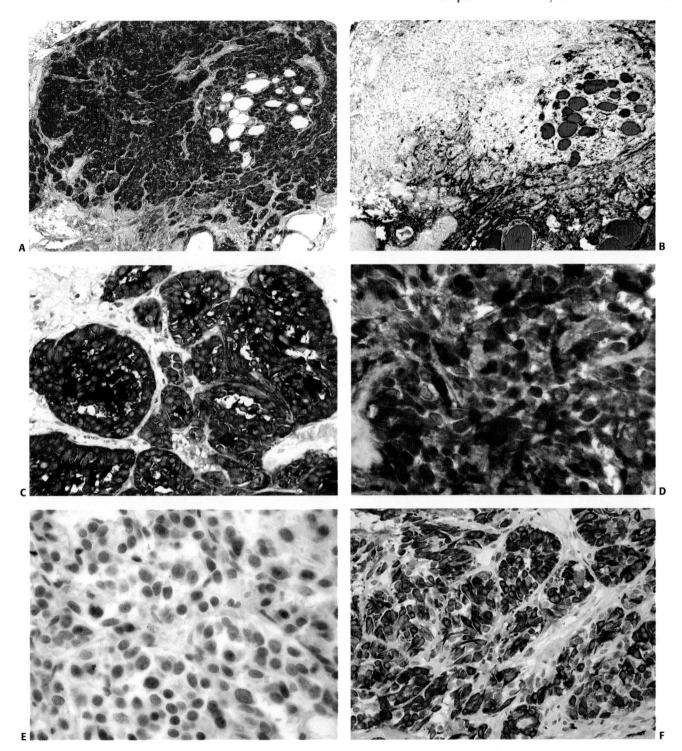

FIGURE 14.28. Immunohistochemical profile of medullary carcinoma. Expression of **(A)** calcitonin, **(C)** CEA, **(D)** chromogranin A, **(E)** TTF1, and **(F)** cytokeratin 7 (CK7). Immunostaining for thyroglobulin **(B)** highlights adjacent nonneoplastic thyroid tissue and entrapped follicles.

 MOLECULAR DIAGNOSTICS

Analysis of *RET* germline mutations is performed using peripheral blood to identify individuals with hereditary medullary thyroid carcinoma. Exons 10, 11, 13, 14, 15, and 16 of *RET* are typically analyzed by direct DNA sequencing. When the location of the mutation is known from the analysis of other family members, molecular testing can be performed targeting the specific region by restriction fragment length polymorphism assays, single-strand conformation polymorphism, hereroduplex techniques, or DNA sequencing (see Chapter 20).

Genetic screening for *RET* germline mutations is important for members of families known to be affected by hereditary medullary carcinoma and for first-degree relatives of individuals found to have medullary carcinoma and a *RET* germline mutation. Screening is also important in cases of apparent sporadic medullary carcinoma given that a significant number of cases will prove to be associated with a *RET* germline mutation.

Analysis of sporadic medullary carcinomas for somatic *RET* and *RAS* mutations is rarely performed in clinical practice. Finding a *RET* somatic mutation in the tumor would suggest medullary carcinoma, but testing is expensive and of limited sensitivity. In almost all cases of sporadic medullary carcinoma, the basic histologic examination combined with immunostains should be adequate for diagnosis.

 ## ULTRASTRUCTURAL FEATURES

Neurosecretory granules are the most distinct feature revealed by ultrastructural examination of medullary carcinoma (Fig. 14.29). These granules contain calcitonin and have been categorized as type I (mean diameter 270 to 280 nm) and the smaller type II

(mean diameter 130 to 135 nm).[125,178] The smaller type II granules are more electron dense than type I granules. However, not all ultrastructural studies have found such distinct segregation into two sizes.[126] The cytoplasm often contains abundant rough endoplasmic reticulum, polyribosomes, and Golgi apparatus. Within the extracellular space, amyloid is often seen and characterized by finely fibrillar material. Immunoelectron studies have demonstrated reactivity for calcitonin among the amyloid fibers.[126,179]

 ## CYTOLOGIC FEATURES

Aspirates can prove to be challenging specimens because of the broad range of cytologic features exhibited by medullary carcinomas.[180–184] The cytologic diagnosis of medullary carcinoma is

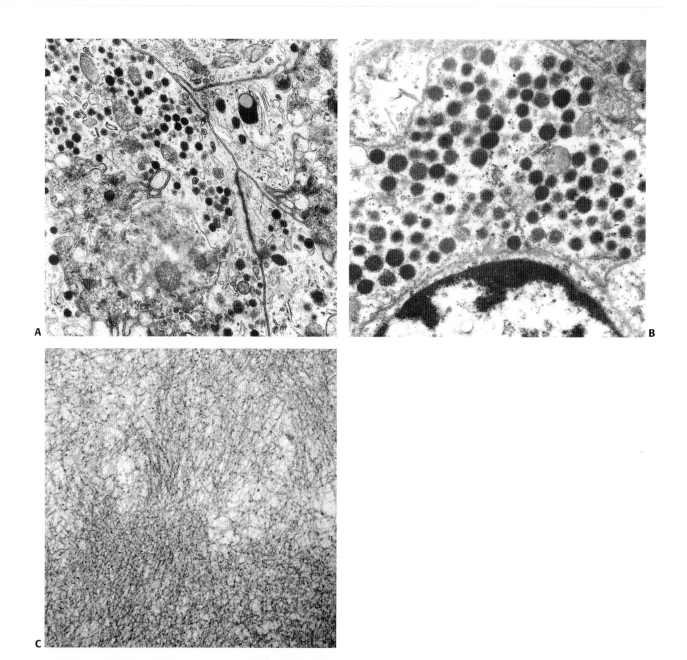

FIGURE 14.29. Electron photomicrographs of medullary carcinomas. Neurosecretory granules shown in Images **(A and B)** and amyloid fibrils in Image **(C)**. (Image **(A)** courtesy of Dr. JinRu Shia and Dr. Ronald Ghossein, Memorial Sloan-Kettering Cancer Center, New York, NY, and image **(B)** courtesy of Dr. Clara S. Heffess, Armed Forces Institute of Pathology, Washington, DC.)

often one of exclusion, and consideration of medullary carcinoma should be prompted whenever an aspirate does not show features of nodular hyperplasia or the more common well-differentiated follicular and papillary neoplasms. Immunostaining for calcitonin can prove to be a valuable adjunct but does require consideration of medullary carcinoma in the differential diagnosis.

Aspirates usually yield abundant cells, but the cellularity can vary, reflective of the variable amount of stromal fibrosis and amyloid accumulation within medullary carcinomas. Aspirated cells frequently show a lack of cohesiveness, so single and small groups of loosely attached cells are suspicious for medullary carcinoma. Cell clusters are usually solid, but microfollicular, rosette, and papillary-like arrangements can be seen. Cells may appear polygonal, round, oval, or spindle shaped, and mixed cell populations are seen in most cases (Fig. 14.30). Occasional cells may have a dendritic-like process.

Binucleate cells are commonly seen, as are cells with eccentric nuclei that bestow a plasmacytoid appearance. Nuclei usually have coarsely granular chromatin and lack prominent nucleoli. Scattered pleomorphic or multinucleated cells amidst a more uniform cell population are suggestive of medullary carcinoma. The degree of nuclear pleomorphism is variable and may be pronounced in some cases. Cells may exhibit intranuclear inclusions comparable with those seen in papillary thyroid carcinoma, but other characteristic nuclear features of papillary carcinoma are not typically found (Fig. 14.30C).

The cytoplasm in Diff-Quik (Dade Behring, Inc, Deerfield, Illinois) stained preparations is usually gray or reddish gray and often shows fine metachromatic cytoplasmic granules (Fig. 14.30G). Papanicolaou-stained preparations generally have pale cytoplasm with an amorphous or vaguely fibrillar appearance. Some cells may exhibit cytoplasmic vacuolization.

Fragments of amyloid are seen in about one-third of aspirates. It has a dark blue to violet color in Diff-Quik preparations. Amyloid tends to have a light greenish-blue appearance with the Papanicolaou stain but may be difficult to distinguish from colloid. Colloid is seen in a significant number of cases, deriving from follicles entrapped or immediately adjacent to the tumor.

 DIFFERENTIAL DIAGNOSIS

Medullary carcinomas are the chameleons of thyroid neoplasia. Owing to their protean manifestations, one should consider medullary carcinoma in the differential diagnosis of any thyroid neoplasm that is not a straightforward diagnosis. The differential diagnosis of medullary carcinomas includes primary thyroid tumors derived from follicular epithelium, other unusual primary thyroid neoplasms, intrathyroidal parathyroid tissue, and metastatic lesions (Table 14.5). Immunostaining for calcitonin plays a pivotal role in the histologic evaluation. Although staining for calcitonin may not differentiate all of these tumors, its sensitivity and specificity are sufficiently high to distinguish most medullary carcinomas from its mimics. Combining calcitonin with a panel of other immunostains can yield findings that approach 100% sensitivity and specificity. TTF1 is not useful in distinguishing medullary carcinoma from follicular and papillary carcinomas as all usually express this transcription factor in their nuclei.

Oncocytic follicular carcinoma, poorly differentiated thyroid carcinoma, follicular carcinoma with a trabecular pattern, solid variant of papillary carcinoma, anaplastic (undifferentiated) carcinoma, and hyalinizing trabecular tumor are the primary thyroid tumors of follicular derivation that are most likely to be confused with medullary carcinoma. All of these tumors are distinguished

Table 14.5									
Immunohistochemical Profiles of Tumors in Differential Diagnosis of Medullary Thyroid Carcinoma									
	Calcitonin	CEA	TTF1	Thyroglobulin	Cytokeratin 7	Parathyroid Hormone	Chromogranin	Synaptophysin	S100
Medullary thyroid carcinoma	+	+	+	−	+	−	+	+	− (+ sustentacular cells can be present)
Poorly differentiated thyroid carcinoma	−	−	+	±	+	−	−	−	−
Follicular carcinoma with trabecular pattern	−	−	+	+	+	−	−	−	−
Solid variant of papillary carcinoma	−	−	+	+	+	−	−	−	−
Hyalinizing trabecular tumor	−	−	+	+	+	−	−	−	−
Oncocytic follicular carcinoma	−	−	+	+	+	−	−	−	−
Intrathyroidal parathyroid tumor	−	−	−	−	+ (may be focal)	+	+	+	−
Paraganglioma	−	−	−	−	−	−	+	+	+ (sustentacular cells)
Metastatic neuroendocrine tumor	−	−	± (can vary by primary site)	−	±	−	+	+	±

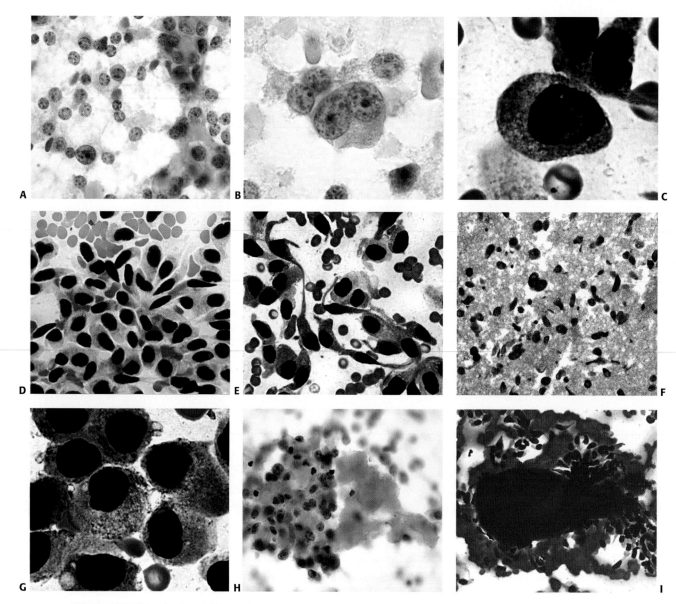

FIGURE 14.30. Cytologic fine needle aspirates of medullary carcinoma. A: Round cells with speckled chromatin seen singly and in aggregates. **B:** Binucleate cell. **C:** Intranuclear pseudoinclusion. **D:** Mixture of oval and spindle cells. **E:** Spindle cell with elongated, dendritic-like processes. **F:** Calcitonin immunostain highlighting neoplastic cells. **G:** Cytoplasmic granules highlighted by Diff-Quik stain. **H:** Amyloid in Papanicolaou-stained preparation. **I:** Amyloid in Diff-Quik–stained preparation (**A, B, and H**, Papanicolaou stain; **C–E, G,** and **I**, Diff-Quik stain).

from medullary carcinoma by their usual positivity for thyroglobulin and lack of calcitonin expression. Medullary carcinomas can have intranuclear pseudoinclusions, but they lack the spectrum of nuclear changes characteristic of papillary carcinoma and its variants. Medullary carcinomas may be mistaken for anaplastic thyroid carcinomas, particularly those with a relatively uniform spindle cell population. Immunoreactivity for calcitonin should distinguish medullary carcinoma. In addition, mitoses are infrequently seen in most medullary carcinomas, in contrast to the usual abundance in anaplastic carcinomas.

Intrathyroidal paragangliomas have been reported, and they exhibit S100 positive sustentacular cells while being negative for calcitonin and thyroglobulin.[171] Parathyroid tissue, either normal glands or neoplasms, may be found within the thyroid and raise the question of medullary carcinoma. The lack of staining for calcitonin and thyroglobulin combined with demonstration of parathyroid hormone should resolve this differential diagnosis.

The differential diagnosis of clear-cell tumors in the thyroid includes medullary thyroid carcinoma along with other primary thyroid tumor with clear-cell features, and metastatic clear-cell tumors, especially renal cell carcinoma. Immunostains for thyroglobulin and calcitonin are key to differentiation of clear-cell tumors of follicular derivation from medullary carcinoma. Immunoreactivity for CD10 supports the diagnosis of metastatic renal cell carcinoma. Metastatic malignant melanoma may enter the differential diagnosis, particularly if melanin is present. Immunostaining for melan-A, HMB-45, and/or tyrosinase will identify most malignant melanomas.

Metastatic neuroendocrine tumors are rare but a potential mimicker of medullary thyroid carcinoma.[185] These metastatic neoplasms can range from classic carcinoids to atypical carcinoids or high-grade neuroendocrine carcinomas and may consist of single or multiple lesions. Immunohistochemical studies can be very helpful as metastatic neuroendocrine tumors are typically negative for calcitonin and CEA.[185] However, medullary thyroid carcinomas and metastatic neuroendocrine tumors can have overlapping immunohistochemical staining patterns, and definitive diagnosis may require integration of clinical data, imaging studies, pathologic studies of tissue from other sites, and/or molecular analysis.

 TREATMENT AND PROGNOSIS

Patients with a clinically evident tumor, whether sporadic or hereditary, are usually treated with total thyroidectomy and resection of central neck lymph nodes.[21,186,187] A lateral neck dissection (levels IIA, III, IV, and V) is performed if metastasis is evident in lateral compartment lymph nodes with ultrasonic examination and there is no evidence of distant metastasis.[21] Less aggressive surgical therapy may be used if there is distant metastasis or advanced local disease because near-term preservation of speech, swallowing, and parathyroid function may outweigh any potential benefit from an attempt of locoregional control.[21]

Serum calcitonin concentration is usually determined before initial surgery to serve as a diagnostic aid, predictor of extent of metastatic disease, and as a baseline for future monitoring. Several other studies are usually performed, even for patients with apparent sporadic disease. Serum calcium is measured to screen for hyperparathyroidism, and blood is analyzed for the presence of a germline *RET* proto-oncogene mutation. Analysis of plasma or urine for metanephrines and normetanephrines or adrenal imaging studies are used to screen for pheochromocytoma.

Complete surgical resection of the primary tumor and regional lymph node metastasis is currently the only curative treatment of medullary carcinoma. Postoperative treatment is variable because the most appropriate single or combination modality is unclear. It is beyond the scope of this chapter to analyze the various treatment options, but they include external radiation therapy, ablation of residual thyroid with ^{131}I, additional surgery, conventional chemotherapy, somatostatin analogs, anti-CEA radioimmunotherapy, radiofrequency ablation, and targeted molecular therapy.[188] External radiation therapy is typically indicated for patients who have gross residual disease after surgical resection.[21] External radiation is also used for palliation of distant metastases. Radioimmunotherapy has shown increased survival in patients with advanced disease and may be appropriate particularly as part of a clinical trial.[21,189]

Increased understanding of the molecular biology of medullary carcinoma has yielded targeted therapy.[190] Clinical trials with tyrosine kinase inhibitors targeting RET kinase have shown encouraging results in terms of remissions and reduction in size of metastatic disease.[32,191,192] As our understanding of the RET protein and its downstream signaling pathways progresses, new generations of therapeutic inhibitors can be anticipated in the future.

Prophylatic Thyroidectomy and Specimen Processing

Prophylactic thyroidectomy is recommended for individuals with germline *RET* mutations. The recommended time of surgery varies according to the *RET* genotype, and the ATA stratifies the risk at four levels, A to D (Table 14.6).[21] Individuals with MEN2B due to germline mutations at codons 918 and 883 have the highest level of risk (level D) and are advised to undergo thyroidectomy as soon as possible within the first year of life. Those with *RET* germline mutations at the most frequent codon site, 634, have an intermediate level of risk (level C), and thyroidectomy before age 5 is recommended. Those with lower levels of risk (A and B) may delay surgery past age 5 if their family has a history of less aggressive MTC and they lack clinical evidence of neoplasia. Individuals with lower risk tend to be members of FMTC kindred.

Prophylactic thyroidectomies performed on patients with a *RET* germline mutation may yield thyroid specimens without gross lesions. Careful examination for C-cell hyperplasia and medullary microcarcinoma is advisable. The lobes should be serially sectioned transversely, and the sections submitted sequentially from superior to inferior (see Chapter 19). Submission of tissue blocks in this manner allows one to know the relative spatial location of a given section, which is important as the highest concentration of C cells is usually found in the mid to upper regions of the lateral lobes. Immunostains for calcitonin and CEA may be necessary to identify the C cells and fully assess the degree of hyperplasia and microcarcinoma.

Prognosis

Numerous studies have examined clinical and pathologic features of medullary carcinoma for prognostic factors. The most consistent prognostic indicator is tumor stage or specific features that determine stage such as extrathyroidal extension or metastasis (see Chapter 7 for staging criteria of medullary carcinoma).[23,24,63,73,111,118,193,194] This is particularly true when

Table 14.6
ATA Management Guidelines for Hereditary Medullary Thyroid Carcinoma

ATA Risk Level	RET Genotype (Codon Site of Mutation)	Recommended Age of *RET* Testing	Recommended Time of Prophylactic Thyroidectomy
D	883, 918, V804M+E805K, V804M+Y806C, V804M+S904C	As soon as possible and within the 1st year of life	As soon as possible and within the 1st year of life
C	634	<3–5 years	Before 5 years of age
B	609, 611, 618, 620, 630, V804M+V778I	<3–5 years	Consider before age 5; may delay if criteria met[a]
A	533, 649, 768, 790, 791, 804, 891, 912	<3–5 years	May delay after age 5 if criteria met[a]

[a]Criteria: Normal calcitonin, normal neck ultrasound examination, less aggressive family history, and family preference.
Table based on Kloos RT, Eng C, Evans DB, et al. Medullary thyroid cancer: management guidelines of the American Thyroid Association. *Thyroid*. 2009;19:565–612.

multivariate analysis is performed to identify independent predictors of survival.

The current Cancer Staging Manual (Seventh Edition) of the American Joint Commission on Cancer lists the following 5-year *observed* and *relative* survival rates for medullary carcinoma during 1985 to 1991 as follows: Stage I, 100% and 100%; Stage II, 88% and 98%; Stage III, 74% and 81%; Stage IV, 25% and 28%.[195] About one half of patients with medullary carcinoma will have metastasis at the time of diagnosis, particularly when one does not include those having prophylactic thyroidectomies because of *RET* germline mutations. Combining the data from four studies published during the past 11 years, each with at least 100 cases (679 total), reveals the following distribution by stage: Stage I, 19%; Stage II, 33%; Stage III, 32%; and Stage IV, 14%.[63,111,130,131] These studies and others reveal that Stage I disease, or medullary microcarcinomas, has almost 100% survival at 5 and 10 years. Stage III disease with metastasis involving central neck (level VI) lymph nodes has a 10-year survival in the range of 65% to 85%, whereas Stage IV disease (extrathyroidal extension and/or metastasis to lateral cervical lymph nodes or beyond) has 10-year survival in the range of 20% to 50%. Even with metastatic disease, however, survival may extend for more than two decades.[111,131,193]

Age is frequently found to be a prognostic factor, and one that often remains an independent factor in multivariate analyses.[23,24,73,111,118,123,193] Younger individuals tend to have better outcomes. The dividing line between younger and older varies between 40 and 60 years of age, with most studies reporting 45 years as the watershed mark. Male gender has been identified as an adverse prognostic factor in multiple studies.[23,24,118,196]

However, gender does not always prove significant in multivariate analyses, and thus, it is probably a minor risk factor.

Several other adverse prognostic factors have been identified, but these usually have not been consistently confirmed or examined in multiple studies or proven to be independent prognostic factors when subjected to multivariate analysis. This seems to be the case regarding the prognostic significance of the sporadic versus MEN2A versus MEN2B versus FMTC forms of medullary carcinoma. MEN2B has been reported to have a higher mortality rate relative to sporadic and other hereditary forms in some studies. However, whether medullary carcinoma is sporadic or one of the hereditary forms does not appear to be an independent prognostic factor when controlled for stage or considered in a multivariate analysis.[24,111]

 ## MIXED MEDULLARY AND FOLLICULAR CARCINOMA

Mixed medullary and follicular carcinoma is defined as having features of both medullary carcinoma with immunoreactive calcitonin and follicular carcinoma with immunoreactive thyroglobulin (Fig. 14.31). The follicular component may also exhibit oncocytic features (Fig. 14.32). A small but substantial number of cases have been reported, and they are a recognized entity in the 2004 WHO classification of thyroid tumors.[30,197–208]

The presence of both types of tumor in a metastatic lesion (in addition to the thyroid primary site) is generally regarded as sufficient proof of the diagnosis.[30] For those without mixed

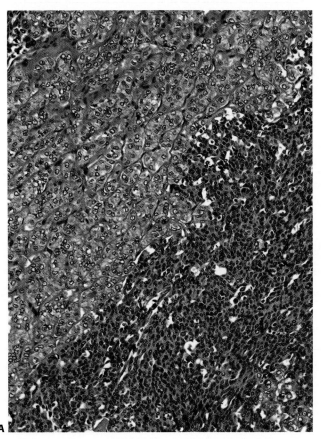
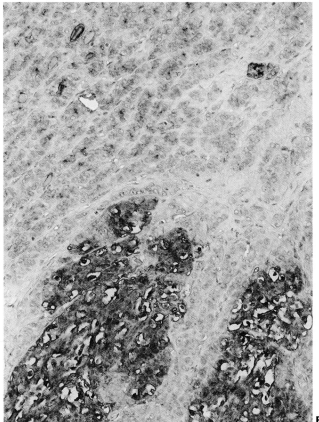

FIGURE 14.31. Mixed medullary and follicular carcinoma. Composite photomicrographs of **(A)** H&E and **(B)** immunostained sections. The follicular component has a solid growth pattern (**upper left**), and the medullary carcinoma component has a spindle cell pattern and small regular dark nuclei (**bottom right**). **B:** Double immunohistochemical staining (calcitonin red, thyroglobulin brown). (Images courtesy of Dr. Marco Volante and Dr. Mauro Papotti, University of Turin, Turin, Italy.)

metastatic lesions, the follicular component should be deep within the tumor, stain positive for thyroglobulin, and be composed of relatively large follicular cells with hyperchromatic nuclei before the diagnosis is considered.[30] Given the protean manifestations of medullary carcinoma, it may be very difficult, if not impossible, to make a definitive diagnosis based on histologic examination of the primary tumor alone.

This form of thyroid carcinoma poses a number of challenges in terms of histogenesis and diagnosis. Putative cases may represent nonneoplastic thyroid follicles entrapped within an expanding medullary carcinoma. If the follicular component is indeed neoplastic, histogenetic possibilities include (1) origin from stem cells capable of both follicular and C-cell differentiation, (2) follicular differentiation, or at least production of thyroglobulin, by a subpopulation of a medullary carcinoma owing to additional molecular alterations, (3) development of both populations from remnants of the ultimobranchial body, (4) coincidental development of medullary and follicular carcinomas ("collision" tumors), or (5) the "hostage" theory in which normal follicles are entrapped within medullary carcinoma and then undergo hyperplasia and eventual neoplastic transformation.[209–211] Studies suggest that mixed medullary and follicular carcinomas are a heterogeneous group of tumors with different pathogenic mechanisms. Most of the mixed tumors studied thus far contain mixtures of neoplastic cells that express either medullary or follicular features but usually not both.[209,212] However, a minority of cases contain cells in which mRNA for both calcitonin and thyroglobulin has been detected.[212,213]

MIXED MEDULLARY AND PAPILLARY CARCINOMA

Medullary and papillary carcinomas may either occur as separate, coincidental tumors or occur as an intimate admixture of the two.[214–216] The term *mixed medullary and papillary carcinoma* is reserved for those exhibiting the latter (Fig. 14.33). These true mixed tumors are exceedingly rare, although separate occult papillary microcarcinomas can be found coexisting with medullary carcinomas relatively often. Four different series of medullary carcinomas reported incidental papillary microcarcinomas in 4% to 19% of cases.[111,216–218] Spatially distinct carcinomas with exclusive medullary or papillary features or those in proximity but with no appreciable intermingling should be reported as separate medullary and papillary carcinomas.

The histogenetic possibilities for mixed medullary and papillary carcinoma are similar to those noted in the above section on mixed medullary and follicular carcinoma. Molecular analysis of most cases has not revealed common genetic abnormalities of the medullary and papillary components.[216,217] The possibility exists that some cases derive from a common cell, but clarification of the pathogenic options awaits further molecular studies.

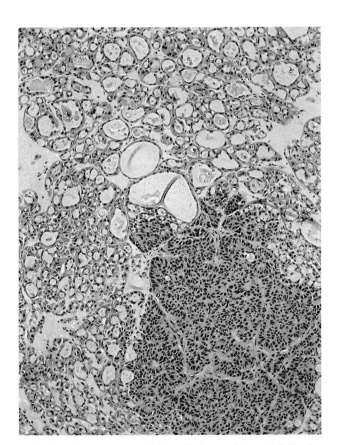

FIGURE 14.32. Mixed medullary (lower right) and follicular (oncocytic type) carcinoma. The follicular component exhibits distinct follicular growth pattern and oncocytic cytologic features **(top and left)** and the medullary carcinoma component has a solid growth pattern and small irregular dark nuclei **(bottom, right)**. (Image courtesy of Dr. Marco Volante and Dr. Mauro Papotti, University of Turin, Turin, Italy.)

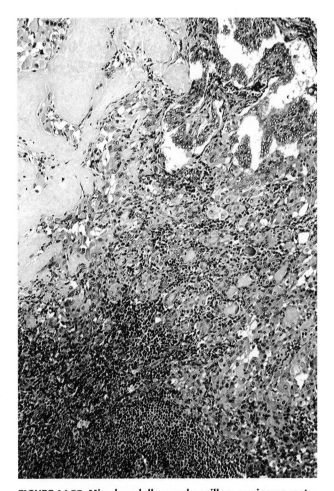

FIGURE 14.33. Mixed medullary and papillary carcinoma metastatic to a lymph node. Medullary carcinoma constitutes the majority of metastatic tumor. Papillary carcinoma is evident in the upper right region. Amyloid stroma is seen in the upper left region. (Image courtesy of Dr. Marco Volante and Dr. Mauro Papotti, University of Turin, Turin, Italy.)

REFERENCES

1. Hazard JB, Crile G Jr, Dinsmore RS, et al. Neoplasms of the thyroid: classification, morphology, and treatment. *AMA Arch Pathol.* 1955;59:502–513.
2. Hazard JB, Hawk WA, Crile G Jr. Medullary (solid) carcinoma of the thyroid; a clinicopathologic entity. *J Clin Endocrinol Metab.* 1959;19:152–161.
3. Hazard JB. The C cells (parafollicular cells) of the thyroid gland and medullary thyroid carcinoma. A review. *Am J Pathol.* 1977;88:213–250.
4. Jacquet J. Ein Fall von metastasierenden amyloidtumoren (lymphosarkom). *Virchows Arch Pathol Anat.* 1906;185:251–268.
5. Stoffel E. Lokales amyloid der Schilddrüse. *Virchows Arch Pathol Anat.* 1910;201:245–252.
6. Horn RC Jr. Carcinoma of the thyroid: description of a distinctive morphological variant and report of seven cases. *Cancer.* 1951;4:697–707.
7. Williams ED. Histogenesis of medullary carcinoma of the thyroid. *J Clin Pathol.* 1966;19:114–118.
8. Meyer JS, Abdel-Bari W. Granules and thyrocalcitonin-like activity in medullary carcinoma of the thyroid gland. *N Engl J Med.* 1968;278:523–529.
9. Bussolati G, Foster GV, Clark MB, et al. Immunofluorescent localisation of calcitonin in medullary C-cell thyroid carcinoma, using antibody to the pure porcine hormone. *Virchows Arch B Cell Pathol.* 1969;2:234–238.
10. Sipple JH. The association of pheochromocytoma with carcinoma of the thyroid gland. *Am J Med.* 1961;31:163–166.
11. Schimke RN, Hartmann WH. Familial amyloid-producing medullary thyroid carcinoma and pheochromocytoma. A distinct genetic entity. *Ann Intern Med.* 1965;63:1027–1039.
12. Steiner AL, Goodman AD, Powers SR. Study of a kindred with pheochromocytoma, medullary thyroid carcinoma, hyperparathyroidism and Cushing's disease: multiple endocrine neoplasia, type 2. *Medicine (Baltimore).* 1968;47:371–409.
13. Williams ED, Pollock DJ. Multiple mucosal neuromata with endocrine tumours: a syndrome allied to von Recklinghausen's disease. *J Pathol Bacteriol.* 1966;91:71–80.
14. Schimke RN, Hartmann WH, Prout TE, et al. Syndrome of bilateral pheochromocytoma, medullary thyroid carcinoma and multiple neuromas. A possible regulatory defect in the differentiation of chromaffin tissue. *N Engl J Med.* 1968;279:1–7.
15. Gorlin RJ, Sedano HO, Vickers RA, et al. Multiple mucosal neuromas, pheochromocytoma and medullary carcinoma of the thyroid—a syndrome. *Cancer.* 1968;22:293–299.
16. Wagenmann A. Multiple neurome des auges und der Zunge. *Ber Dtsch Ophthalmol Ges.* 1922;43:282–285.
17. Froboese C. Das aus markhaltigen nervenfasern bestehende gangliezenllenlose echte neurom in rankenformzugleich ein beitrag zu den nervosen Geschwulsten der zunge und des augenlides. *Virchows Arch Pathol Anat.* 1923;240:312–327.
18. Farndon JR, Leight GS, Dilley WG, et al. Familial medullary thyroid carcinoma without associated endocrinopathies: a distinct clinical entity. *Br J Surg.* 1986;73:278–281.
19. Hundahl SA, Fleming ID, Fremgen AM, et al. A National Cancer Data Base report on 53,856 cases of thyroid carcinoma treated in the U.S., 1985–1995 [see comments]. *Cancer.* 1998;83:2638–2648.
20. Howlader N, Noone AM, Krapcho M, et al. SEER cancer statistics review, 1975–2008. National Cancer Institute. SEER web site. http://seer.cancer.gov/csr/1975_2008/. Accessed July, 2011.
21. Kloos RT, Eng C, Evans DB, et al. Medullary thyroid cancer: management guidelines of the American Thyroid Association. *Thyroid.* 2009;19:565–612.
22. Cramer JD, Fu P, Harth KC, et al. Analysis of the rising incidence of thyroid cancer using the Surveillance, Epidemiology and End Results national cancer data registry. *Surgery.* 2010;148:1147–1152; discussion 1152–1143.
23. Saad MF, Ordonez NG, Rashid RK, et al. Medullary carcinoma of the thyroid. A study of the clinical features and prognostic factors in 161 patients. *Medicine (Baltimore).* 1984;63:319–342.
24. Raue F, Kotzerke J, Reinwein D, et al. Prognostic factors in medullary thyroid carcinoma: evaluation of 741 patients from the German Medullary Thyroid Carcinoma Register. *Clin Investig.* 1993;71:7–12.
25. Kilfoy BA, Zheng T, Holford TR, et al. International patterns and trends in thyroid cancer incidence, 1973–2002. *Cancer Causes Control.* 2009;20:525–531.
26. Ahmed SR, Ball DW. Incidentally discovered medullary thyroid cancer: diagnostic strategies and treatment. *J Clin Endocrinol Metab.* 2011;96:1237–1245.
27. Valle LA, Kloos RT. The prevalence of occult medullary thyroid carcinoma at autopsy. *J Clin Endocrinol Metab.* 2011;96:E109–E113.
28. Komorowski RA, Hanson GA. Occult thyroid pathology in the young adult: an autopsy study of 138 patients without clinical thyroid disease. *Hum Pathol.* 1988;19:689–696.
29. Martinez-Tello FJ, Martinez-Cabruja R, Fernandez-Martin J, et al. Occult carcinoma of the thyroid. A systematic autopsy study from Spain of two series performed with two different methods. *Cancer.* 1993;71:4022–4029.
30. DeLellis RA, Lloyd RV, Heitz PU, et al, eds. *Pathology and Genetic of Tumours of Endocrine Organs.* World Health Organization Classification of Tumours. Lyon, France: IARC Press; 2004.
31. Clark JR, Fridman TR, Odell MJ, et al. Prognostic variables and calcitonin in medullary thyroid cancer. *Laryngoscope.* 2005;115:1445–1450.
32. Lakhani VT, You YN, Wells SA. The multiple endocrine neoplasia syndromes. *Annu Rev Med.* 2007;58:253–265.
33. Brandi ML, Gagel RF, Angeli A, et al. Guidelines for diagnosis and therapy of MEN type 1 and type 2. *J Clin Endocrinol Metab.* 2001;86:5658–5671.
34. de Groot JW, Links TP, Plukker JT, et al. RET as a diagnostic and therapeutic target in sporadic and hereditary endocrine tumors. *Endocr Rev.* 2006;27:535–560.
35. Eng C, Mulligan LM. Mutations of the *RET* proto-oncogene in the multiple endocrine neoplasia type 2 syndromes, related sporadic tumours, and Hirschsprung disease. *Hum Mutat.* 1997;9:97–109.
36. Asai N, Jijiwa M, Enomoto A, et al. RET receptor signaling: dysfunction in thyroid cancer and Hirschsprung's disease. *Pathol Int.* 2006;56:164–172.
37. Morrison PJ, Nevin NC. Multiple endocrine neoplasia type 2B (mucosal neuroma syndrome, Wagenmann-Froboese syndrome). *J Med Genet.* 1996;33:779–782.
38. Rosai J, Carcangiu ML, DeLellis RA. *Tumors of the Thyroid Gland.* Washington, DC: Armed Forces Institute of Pathology; 1992.
39. Wiench M, Wygoda Z, Gubala E, et al. Estimation of risk of inherited medullary thyroid carcinoma in apparent sporadic patients. *J Clin Oncol.* 2001;19:1374–1380.
40. Bugalho MJ, Domingues R, Santos JR, et al. Mutation analysis of the *RET* proto-oncogene and early thyroidectomy: results of a Portuguese cancer centre. *Surgery.* 2007;141:90–95.
41. Elisei R, Romei C, Cosci B, et al. *RET* genetic screening in patients with medullary thyroid cancer and their relatives: experience with 807 individuals at one center. *J Clin Endocrinol Metab.* 2007;92:4725–4729.
42. Takahashi M, Ritz J, Cooper GM. Activation of a novel human transforming gene, ret, by DNA rearrangement. *Cell.* 1985;42:581–588.
43. Mathew CG, Chin KS, Easton DF, et al. A linked genetic marker for multiple endocrine neoplasia type 2A on chromosome 10. *Nature.* 1987;328:527–528.
44. Mulligan LM, Kwok JB, Healey CS, et al. Germline mutations of the *RET* proto-oncogene in multiple endocrine neoplasia type 2A. *Nature.* 1993;363:458–460.
45. Donis-Keller H, Dou S, Chi D, et al. Mutations in the *RET* proto-oncogene are associated with MEN 2A and FMTC. *Hum Mol Genet.* 1993;2:851–856.
46. Eng C, Smith DP, Mulligan LM, et al. Point mutation within the tyrosine kinase domain of the *RET* proto-oncogene in multiple endocrine neoplasia type 2B and related sporadic tumours. *Hum Mol Genet.* 1994;3:237–241.
47. Pasini B, Hofstra RM, Yin L, et al. The physical map of the human *RET* proto-oncogene. *Oncogene.* 1995;11:1737–1743.
48. Durbec P, Marcos Gutierrez CV, Kilkenny C, et al. GDNF signalling through the Ret receptor tyrosine kinase. *Nature.* 1996;381:789–793.
49. Jing S, Wen D, Yu Y, et al. GDNF-induced activation of the ret protein tyrosine kinase is mediated by GDNFR-alpha, a novel receptor for GDNF. *Cell.* 1996;85:1113–1124.
50. Treanor JJ, Goodman L, de Sauvage F, et al. Characterization of a multicomponent receptor for GDNF. *Nature.* 1996;382:80–83.
51. Schuchardt A, D'Agati V, Larsson-Blomberg L, et al. Defects in the kidney and enteric nervous system of mice lacking the tyrosine kinase receptor Ret. *Nature.* 1994;367:380–383.
52. Mulligan LM, Eng C, Healey CS, et al. Specific mutations of the *RET* proto-oncogene are related to disease phenotype in MEN 2A and FMTC. *Nat Genet.* 1994;6:70–74.
53. Eng C. Seminars in medicine of the Beth Israel Hospital, Boston. The *RET* proto-oncogene in multiple endocrine neoplasia type 2 and Hirschsprung's disease. *N Engl J Med.* 1996;335:943–951.
54. Carlson KM, Dou S, Chi D, et al. Single missense mutation in the tyrosine kinase catalytic domain of the *RET* protooncogene is associated with multiple endocrine neoplasia type 2B. *Proc Natl Acad Sci U S A.* 1994;91:1579–1583.
55. Gimm O, Marsh DJ, Andrew SD, et al. Germline dinucleotide mutation in codon 883 of the *RET* proto-oncogene in multiple endocrine neoplasia type 2B without codon 918 mutation. *J Clin Endocrinol Metab.* 1997;82:3902–3904.
56. Cranston AN, Carniti C, Oakhill K, et al. *RET* is constitutively activated by novel tandem mutations that alter the active site resulting in multiple endocrine neoplasia type 2B. *Cancer Res.* 2006;66:10179–10187.
57. Miyauchi A, Futami H, Hai N, et al. Two germline missense mutations at codons 804 and 806 of the *RET* proto-oncogene in the same allele in a patient with multiple endocrine neoplasia type 2B without codon 918 mutation. *Jpn J Cancer Res.* 1999;90:1–5.
58. Kameyama K, Okinaga H, Takami H. *RET* oncogene mutations in 75 cases of familial medullary thyroid carcinoma in Japan. *Biomed Pharmacother.* 2004;58:345–347.
59. Iwashita T, Murakami H, Kurokawa K, et al. A two-hit model for development of multiple endocrine neoplasia type 2B by *RET* mutations. *Biochem Biophys Res Commun.* 2000;268:804–808.
60. Menko FH, van der Luijt RB, de Valk IA, et al. Atypical MEN type 2B associated with two germline *RET* mutations on the same allele not involving codon 918. *J Clin Endocrinol Metab.* 2002;87:393–397.
61. Santoro M, Carlomagno F, Romano A, et al. Activation of *RET* as a dominant transforming gene by germline mutations of MEN2A and MEN2B. *Science.* 1995;267:381–383.
62. Borrello MG, Smith DP, Pasini B, et al. *RET* activation by germline MEN2A and MEN2B mutations. *Oncogene.* 1995;11:2419–2427.
63. Elisei R, Cosci B, Romei C, et al. Prognostic significance of somatic *RET* oncogene mutations in sporadic medullary thyroid cancer: a 10-year follow-up study. *J Clin Endocrinol Metab.* 2008;93:682–687.
64. Marsh DJ, Learoyd DL, Andrew SD, et al. Somatic mutations in the *RET* proto-oncogene in sporadic medullary thyroid carcinoma. *Clin Endocrinol (Oxf).* 1996;44:249–257.
65. Dvorakova S, Vaclavikova E, Sykorova V, et al. Somatic mutations in the *RET* proto-oncogene in sporadic medullary thyroid carcinomas. *Mol Cell Endocrinol.* 2008;284:21–27.
66. Zedenius J, Wallin G, Hamberger B, et al. Somatic and MEN 2A de novo mutations identified in the *RET* proto-oncogene by screening of sporadic MTC:s. *Hum Mol Genet.* 1994;3:1259–1262.
67. Moura MM, Cavaco BM, Pinto AE, et al. High prevalence of *RAS* mutations in RET-negative sporadic medullary thyroid carcinomas. *J Clin Endocrinol Metab.* 2011;96:E863–E868.

68. Schlumberger MJ, Elisei R, Bastholt L, et al. Phase II study of safety and efficacy of motesanib in patients with progressive or symptomatic, advanced or metastatic medullary thyroid cancer. *J Clin Oncol.* 2009;27:3794–3801.

69. Bockhorn M, Frilling A, Kalinin V, et al. Absence of *H*- and *K-ras* oncogene mutations in sporadic medullary thyroid carcinoma. *Exp Clin Endocrinol Diabetes.* 2000;108:49–53.

70. Marsh DJ, Theodosopoulos G, Martin-Schulte K, et al. Genome-wide copy number imbalances identified in familial and sporadic medullary thyroid carcinoma. *J Clin Endocrinol Metab.* 2003;88:1866–1872.

71. Frisk T, Zedenius J, Lundberg J, et al. CGH alterations in medullary thyroid carcinomas in relation to the *RET* M918T mutation and clinical outcome. *Int J Oncol.* 2001;18:1219–1225.

72. Hemmer S, Wasenius VM, Knuutila S, et al. DNA copy number changes in thyroid carcinomas. *Am J Pathol.* 1999;154:1539–1547.

73. Schröder S, Böcker W, Baisch H, et al. Prognostic factors in medullary thyroid carcinomas. Survival in relation to age, sex, stage, histology, immunocytochemistry, and DNA content. *Cancer.* 1988;61:806–816.

74. Bergholm U, Adami HO, Auer G, et al. Histopathologic characteristics and nuclear DNA content as prognostic factors in medullary thyroid carcinoma. A nationwide study in Sweden. The Swedish MTC Study Group. *Cancer.* 1989;64:135–142.

75. Galera-Davidson H, González-Cámpora R, Mora-Marín JA, et al. Cytophotometric DNA measurements in medullary thyroid carcinoma. *Cancer.* 1990;65:2255–2260.

76. Hay ID, Ryan JJ, Grant CS, et al. Prognostic significance of nondiploid DNA determined by flow cytometry in sporadic and familial medullary thyroid carcinoma. *Surgery.* 1990;108:972–979; discussion 979–980.

77. el-Naggar AK, Ordonez NG, McLemore D, et al. Clinicopathologic and flow cytometric DNA study of medullary thyroid carcinoma. *Surgery.* 1990;108:981–985.

78. Pyke CM, Hay ID, Goellner JR, et al. Prognostic significance of calcitonin immunoreactivity, amyloid staining, and flow cytometric DNA measurements in medullary thyroid carcinoma. *Surgery.* 1991;110:964–970; discussion 970–961.

79. Baber EC. Contributions to the minute anatomy of the thyroid gland of the dog. *Proc R Soc Lond.* 1876;24:240–241.

80. Baber EC. Further researches on the minute structure of the thyroid gland. *Proc R Soc Lond.* 1878;27:56–60.

81. Hürthle K. Beiträge zur Kenntniss des Secretionsvorgangs in der Schilddrüse. *Arch Gesammte Physiol.* 1894;56:1–44.

82. Nonidez JF. The orignin of the "parafollicular" cell, a second epithelial component of the thyroid gland of the dog. *Am J Anat.* 1932;49:479–505.

83. Pearse AG. The cytochemistry of the thyroid C cells and their relationship to calcitonin. *Proc R Soc Lond B Biol Sci.* 1966;164:478–487.

84. Bussolati G, Pearse AG. Immunofluorescent localization of calcitonin in the "C" cells of pig and dog thyroid. *J Endocrinol.* 1967;37:205–209.

85. Wolfe HJ, Voelkel EF, Tashjian AH Jr. Distribution of calcitonin-containing cells in the normal adult human thyroid gland: a correlation of morphology with peptide content. *J Clin Endocrinol Metab.* 1974;38:688–694.

86. McMillan PJ, Hooker WM, Deptos LJ. Distribution of calcitonin-containing cells in the human thyroid. *Am J Anat.* 1974;140:73–79.

87. Harach HR. Solid cell nests of the thyroid. *J Pathol.* 1988;155:191–200.

88. Wolfe HJ, Melvin KE, Cervi-Skinner SJ, et al. C-cell hyperplasia preceding medullary thyroid carcinoma. *N Engl J Med.* 1973;289:437–441.

89. Etit D, Faquin WC, Gaz R, et al. Histopathologic and clinical features of medullary microcarcinoma and C-cell hyperplasia in prophylactic thyroidectomies for medullary carcinoma: a study of 42 cases. *Arch Pathol Lab Med.* 2008;132:1767–1773.

90. Albores-Saavedra J, Monforte H, Nadji M, et al. C-cell hyperplasia in thyroid tissue adjacent to follicular cell tumors. *Hum Pathol.* 1988;19:795–799.

91. Kaserer K, Scheuba C, Neuhold N, et al. C-cell hyperplasia and medullary thyroid carcinoma in patients routinely screened for serum calcitonin. *Am J Surg Pathol.* 1998;22:722–728.

92. Guyetant S, Josselin N, Savagner F, et al. C-cell hyperplasia and medullary thyroid carcinoma: clinicopathological and genetic correlations in 66 consecutive patients. *Mod Pathol.* 2003;16:756–763.

93. Saggiorato E, Rapa I, Garino F, et al. Absence of *RET* gene point mutations in sporadic thyroid C-cell hyperplasia. *J Mol Diagn.* 2007;9:214–219.

94. Nosé V. Familial thyroid cancer: a review. *Mod Pathol.* 2011;24(suppl 2): S19–S33.

95. Albores-Saavedra JA, Krueger JE. C-cell hyperplasia and medullary thyroid microcarcinoma. *Endocr Pathol.* 2001;12:365–377.

96. Guyetant S, Blechet C, Saint-Andre JP. C-cell hyperplasia. *Ann Endocrinol (Paris).* 2006;67:190–197.

97. Biddinger PW, Brennan MF, Rosen PP. Symptomatic C-cell hyperplasia associated with chronic lymphocytic thyroiditis. *Am J Surg Pathol.* 1991;15: 599–604.

98. Matias-Guiu X, DeLellis R, Moley JF, et al. Medullary thyroid carcinoma. In: DeLellis R, Lloyd R, Heitz P, Eng C, eds. *Pathology and Genetics of Tumours of Endocrine Organs.* Lyon: IARC Press; 2004:86–91.

99. Scheuba C, Kaserer K, Kotzmann H, et al. Prevalence of C-cell hyperplasia in patients with normal basal and pentagastrin-stimulated calcitonin. *Thyroid.* 2000;10:413–416.

100. Perry A, Molberg K, Albores-Saavedra J. Physiologic versus neoplastic C-cell hyperplasia of the thyroid: separation of distinct histologic and biologic entities. *Cancer.* 1996;77:750–756.

101. LiVolsi VA. C cell hyperplasia/neoplasia. *J Clin Endocrinol Metab.* 1997;82:39–41.

102. Komminoth P, Roth J, Saremaslani P, et al. Polysialic acid of the neural cell adhesion molecule in the human thyroid: a marker for medullary thyroid carcinoma and primary C-cell hyperplasia. An immunohistochemical study on 79 thyroid lesions. *Am J Surg Pathol.* 1994;18:399–411.

103. McDermott MB, Swanson PE, Wick MR. Immunostains for collagen type IV discriminate between C-cell hyperplasia and microscopic medullary carcinoma in multiple endocrine neoplasia, type 2a. *Hum Pathol.* 1995;26:1308–1312.

104. Koperek O, Prinz A, Scheuba C, et al. Tenascin C in medullary thyroid microcarcinoma and C-cell hyperplasia. *Virchows Arch.* 2009;455:43–48.

105. Biddinger PW, Ray M. Distribution of C cells in the normal and diseased thyroid gland. *Pathol Annu.* 1993;28:205–229.

106. Guyetant S, Rousselet MC, Durigon M, et al. Sex-related C cell hyperplasia in the normal human thyroid: a quantitative autopsy study. *J Clin Endocrinol Metab.* 1997;82:42–47.

107. Block MA, Jackson CE, Greenawald KA, et al. Clinical characteristics distinguishing hereditary from sporadic medullary thyroid carcinoma. Treatment implications. *Arch Surg.* 1980;115:142–148.

108. Ekblom M, Valimaki M, Pelkonen R, et al. Familial and sporadic medullary thyroid carcinoma: clinical and immunohistological findings. *Q J Med.* 1987;65:899–910.

109. Kaserer K, Scheuba C, Neuhold N, et al. Sporadic versus familial medullary thyroid microcarcinoma: a histopathologic study of 50 consecutive patients. *Am J Surg Pathol.* 2001;25:1245–1251.

110. Hinze R, Gimm O, Brauckhoff M, et al. ["Physiological" and "neoplastic" C-cell hyperplasia of the thyroid. Morphologically and biologically distinct entities?]. *Pathologe.* 2001;22:259–265.

111. Kebebew E, Ituarte PH, Siperstein AE, et al. Medullary thyroid carcinoma: clinical characteristics, treatment, prognostic factors, and a comparison of staging systems. *Cancer.* 2000;88:1139–1148.

112. Barbosa SL, Rodien P, Lebouleux S, et al. Ectopic adrenocorticotropic hormone-syndrome in medullary carcinoma of the thyroid: a retrospective analysis and review of the literature. *Thyroid.* 2005;15:618–623.

113. Oudoux A, Salaun PY, Bournaud C, et al. Sensitivity and prognostic value of positron emission tomography with F-18-fluorodeoxyglucose and sensitivity of immunoscintigraphy in patients with medullary thyroid carcinoma treated with anticarcinoembryonic antigen-targeted radioimmunotherapy. *J Clin Endocrinol Metab.* 2007;92:4590–4597.

114. Huss LJ, Mendelsohn G. Medullary carcinoma of the thyroid gland: an encapsulated variant resembling the hyalinizing trabecular (paraganglioma-like) adenoma of thyroid. *Mod Pathol.* 1990;3:581–585.

115. Driman D, Murray D, Kovacs K, et al. Encapsulated medullary carcinoma of the thyroid. A morphologic study including immunocytochemistry, electron microscopy, flow cytometry, and in situ hybridization. *Am J Surg Pathol.* 1991;15:1089–1095.

116. Miyauchi A, Matsuzuka F, Hirai K, et al. Prospective trial of unilateral surgery for nonhereditary medullary thyroid carcinoma in patients without germline *RET* mutations. *World J Surg.* 2002;26:1023–1028.

117. Beressi N, Campos JM, Beressi JP, et al. Sporadic medullary microcarcinoma of the thyroid: a retrospective analysis of eighty cases. *Thyroid.* 1998;8:1039–1044.

118. Scopsi L, Sampietro G, Boracchi P, et al. Multivariate analysis of prognostic factors in sporadic medullary carcinoma of the thyroid. A retrospective study of 109 consecutive patients. *Cancer.* 1996;78:2173–2183.

119. Scollo C, Baudin E, Travagli JP, et al. Rationale for central and bilateral lymph node dissection in sporadic and hereditary medullary thyroid cancer. *J Clin Endocrinol Metab.* 2003;88:2070–2075.

120. Uribe M, Fenoglio-Preiser CM, Grimes M, et al. Medullary carcinoma of the thyroid gland. Clinical, pathological, and immunohistochemical features with review of the literature. *Am J Surg Pathol.* 1985;9:577–594.

121. Zaatari GS, Saigo PE, Huvos AG. Mucin production in medullary carcinoma of the thyroid. *Arch Pathol Lab Med.* 1983;107:70–74.

122. Martin-Lacave I, Gonzalez-Campora R, Moreno Fernandez A, et al. Mucosubstances in medullary carcinoma of the thyroid. *Histopathology.* 1988;13:55–66.

123. Franc B, Rosenberg-Bourgin M, Caillou B, et al. Medullary thyroid carcinoma: search for histological predictors of survival (109 proband cases analysis). *Hum Pathol.* 1998;29:1078–1084.

124. Meyer JS, Hutton WE, Kenny AD. Medullary carcinoma of thyroid gland. Subcellular distribution of calcitonin and relationship between granules and amyloid. *Cancer.* 1973;31:433–441.

125. Dämmrich J, Ormanns W, Schäffer R. Electron microscopic demonstration of calcitonin in human medullary carcinoma of thyroid by the immuno gold staining method. *Histochemistry.* 1984;81:369–372.

126. Silver MM, Hearn SA, Lines LD, et al. Calcitonin and chromogranin A localization in medullary carcinoma of the thyroid by immunoelectron microscopy. *J Histochem Cytochem.* 1988;36:1031–1036.

127. Reches M, Porat Y, Gazit E. Amyloid fibril formation by pentapeptide and tetrapeptide fragments of human calcitonin. *J Biol Chem.* 2002;277:35475–35480.

128. Avidan-Shpalter C, Gazit E. The early stages of amyloid formation: biophysical and structural characterization of human calcitonin pre-fibrillar assemblies. *Amyloid.* 2006;13:216–225.

129. Williams ED, Brown CL, Doniach I. Pathological and clinical findings in a series of 67 cases of medullary carcinoma of the thyroid. *J Clin Pathol.* 1966;19:103–113.

130. Greene FL, Page DL, Fleming ID, et al, eds. *AJCC Cancer Staging Manual.* 6th ed. New York, NY: Springer-Verlag; 2002.

131. Pelizzo MR, Boschin IM, Bernante P, et al. Natural history, diagnosis, treatment and outcome of medullary thyroid cancer: 37 years experience on 157 patients. *Eur J Surg Oncol.* 2007;33:493–497.

132. Guyetant S, Dupre F, Bigorgne JC, et al. Medullary thyroid microcarcinoma: a clinicopathologic retrospective study of 38 patients with no prior familial disease. *Hum Pathol.* 1999;30:957–963.

133. Kakudo K, Miyauchi A, Takai S, et al. C cell carcinoma of the thyroid—papillary type. *Acta Pathol Jpn.* 1979;29:653–659.

134. Gordon PR, Huvos AG, Strong EW. Medullary carcinoma of the thyroid gland. A clinicopathologic study of 40 cases. *Cancer*. 1973;31:915–924.

135. Harach HR, Bergholm U. Medullary (C cell) carcinoma of the thyroid with features of follicular oxyphilic cell tumours. *Histopathology*. 1988;13:645–656.

136. Dominguez-Malagon H, Delgado-Chavez R, Torres-Najera M, et al. Oxyphil and squamous variants of medullary thyroid carcinoma. *Cancer*. 1989;63:1183–1188.

137. Landon G, Ordóñez NG. Clear cell variant of medullary carcinoma of the thyroid. *Hum Pathol*. 1985;16:844–847.

138. Lertprasertsuke N, Kakudo K, Nakamura A, et al. C cell carcinoma of the thyroid. Follicular variant. *Acta Pathol Jpn*. 1989;39:393–399.

139. Cakir M, Altunbas H, Balci MK, et al. Medullary thyroid carcinoma, follicular variant. *Endocr Pathol*. 2002;13:75–79.

140. Golouh R, Us-Krasovec M, Auersperg M, et al. Amphicrine—composite calcitonin and mucin-producing—carcinoma of the thyroid. *Ultrastruct Pathol*. 1985;8:197–206.

141. Dominguez-Malagon H, Macias-Martinez V, Molina-Cardenas H, et al. Amphicrine medullary carcinoma of the thyroid with luminal differentiation: report of an immunohistochemical and ultrastructural study. *Ultrastruct Pathol*. 1997;21:569–574.

142. Ikeda T, Satoh M, Azuma K, et al. Medullary thyroid carcinoma with a paraganglioma-like pattern and melanin production: a case report with ultrastructural and immunohistochemical studies. *Arch Pathol Lab Med*. 1998;122:555–558.

143. Mitsudo SM, Grajower MM, Balbi H, et al. Malignant paraganglioma of the thyroid gland. *Arch Pathol Lab Med*. 1987;111:378–380.

144. LaGuette J, Matias-Guiu X, Rosai J. Thyroid paraganglioma: a clinicopathologic and immunohistochemical study of three cases. *Am J Surg Pathol*. 1997;21:748–753.

145. Mendelsohn G, Baylin SB, Bigner SH, et al. Anaplastic variants of medullary thyroid carcinoma: a light-microscopic and immunohistochemical study. *Am J Surg Pathol*. 1980;4:333–341.

146. Harach HR, Bergholm U. Small cell variant of medullary carcinoma of the thyroid with neuroblastoma-like features. *Histopathology*. 1992;21:378–380.

147. Eusebi V, Damiani S, Riva C, et al. Calcitonin free oat-cell carcinoma of the thyroid gland. *Virchows Arch A Pathol Anat Histopathol*. 1990;417:267–271.

148. Kakudo K, Miyauchi A, Ogihara T, et al. Medullary carcinoma of the thyroid. Giant cell type. *Arch Pathol Lab Med*. 1978;102:445–447.

149. Papotti M, Sapino A, Abbona G, et al. Pseudoangiosarcomatous features in medullary carcinomas of the thyroid. Report of two cases. *Int J Surg Pathol*. 1995;3:29–34.

150. Laforga JB, Aranda FI. Pseudoangiosarcomatous features in medullary thyroid carcinoma spindle-cell variant. Report of a case studied by FNA and immunohistochemistry. *Diagn Cytopathol*. 2007;35:424–428.

151. Marcus JN, Dise CA, LiVolsi VA. Melanin production in a medullary thyroid carcinoma. *Cancer*. 1982;49:2518–2526.

152. Eng HL, Chen WJ. Melanin-producing medullary carcinoma of the thyroid gland. *Arch Pathol Lab Med*. 1989;113:377–380.

153. Beerman H, Rigaud C, Bogomoletz WV, et al. Melanin production in black medullary thyroid carcinoma (MTC). *Histopathology*. 1990;16:227–233.

154. Singh K, Sharma MC, Jain D, et al. Melanotic medullary carcinoma of thyroid—report of a rare case with brief review of literature. *Diagn Pathol*. 2008;3:2.

155. Harach HR, Bergholm U. Medullary carcinoma of the thyroid with carcinoid-like features. *J Clin Pathol*. 1993;46:113–117.

156. Beskid M. C cell adenoma of the human thyroid gland. *Oncology*. 1979;36:19–22.

157. Kodama T, Okamoto T, Fujimoto Y, et al. C cell adenoma of the thyroid: a rare but distinct clinical entity. *Surgery*. 1988;104:997–1003.

158. Beskid M, Lorenc R, Rosciszewska A. C-cell thyroid adenoma in man. *J Pathol*. 1971;103:1–4.

159. Erickson LA, Lloyd RV. Practical markers used in the diagnosis of endocrine tumors. *Adv Anat Pathol*. 2004;11:175–189.

160. Lippman SM, Mendelsohn G, Trump DL, et al. The prognostic and biological significance of cellular heterogeneity in medullary thyroid carcinoma: a study of calcitonin, L-dopa decarboxylase, and histaminase. *J Clin Endocrinol Metab*. 1982;54:233–240.

161. Mendelsohn G, Wells SA Jr, Baylin SB. Relationship of tissue carcinoembryonic antigen and calcitonin to tumor virulence in medullary thyroid carcinoma. An immunohistochemical study in early, localized, and virulent disseminated stages of disease. *Cancer*. 1984;54:657–662.

162. Saad MF, Ordonez NG, Guido JJ, et al. The prognostic value of calcitonin immunostaining in medullary carcinoma of the thyroid. *J Clin Endocrinol Metab*. 1984;59:850–856.

163. Viale G, Roncalli M, Grimelius L, et al. Prognostic value of *bcl-2* immunoreactivity in medullary thyroid carcinoma. *Hum Pathol*. 1995;26:945–950.

164. Krisch K, Krisch I, Horvat G, et al. The value of immunohistochemistry in medullary thyroid carcinoma: a systematic study of 30 cases. *Histopathology*. 1985;9:1077–1089.

165. Holm R, Sobrinho-Simoes M, Nesland JM, et al. Medullary carcinoma of the thyroid gland: an immunocytochemical study. *Ultrastruct Pathol*. 1985;8:25–41.

166. Schmid KW, Kirchmair R, Ladurner D, et al. Immunohistochemical comparison of chromogranins A and B and secretogranin II with calcitonin and calcitonin gene-related peptide expression in normal, hyperplastic and neoplastic C-cells of the human thyroid. *Histopathology*. 1992;21:225–232.

167. Mansson B, Ahren B, Nobin A, et al. Calcitonin, calcitonin gene-related peptide, and gastrin-releasing peptide in familial thyroid medullary carcinoma. *Surgery*. 1990;107:182–186.

168. Pacini F, Fugazzola L, Basolo F, et al. Expression of calcitonin gene-related peptide in medullary thyroid cancer. *J Endocrinol Invest*. 1992;15:539–542.

169. Schifter S, Williams ED, Craig RK, et al. Calcitonin gene-related peptide and calcitonin in medullary thyroid carcinoma. *Clin Endocrinol (Oxf)*. 1986;25:703–710.

170. Sikri KL, Varndell IM, Hamid QA, et al. Medullary carcinoma of the thyroid. An immunocytochemical and histochemical study of 25 cases using eight separate markers. *Cancer*. 1985;56:2481–2491.

171. Fischer S, Asa SL. Application of immunohistochemistry to thyroid neoplasms. *Arch Pathol Lab Med*. 2008;132:359–372.

172. Bejarano PA, Nikiforov YE, Swenson ES, et al. Thyroid transcription factor-1, thyroglobulin, cytokeratin 7, and cytokeratin 20 in thyroid neoplasms. *Appl Immunohistochem Mol Morphol*. 2000;8:189–194.

173. Katoh R, Miyagi E, Nakamura N, et al. Expression of thyroid transcription factor-1 (TTF-1) in human C cells and medullary thyroid carcinomas. *Hum Pathol*. 2000;31:386–393.

174. Fernandez PL, Merino MJ, Gomez M, et al. Galectin-3 and laminin expression in neoplastic and non-neoplastic thyroid tissue. *J Pathol*. 1997;181:80–86.

175. Cvejic D, Savin S, Golubovic S, et al. Galectin-3 and carcinoembryonic antigen expression in medullary thyroid carcinoma: possible relation to tumour progression. *Histopathology*. 2000;37:530–535.

176. Faggiano A, Talbot M, Lacroix L, et al. Differential expression of galectin-3 in medullary thyroid carcinoma and C-cell hyperplasia. *Clin Endocrinol (Oxf)*. 2002;57:813–819.

177. Kovacs RB, Foldes J, Winkler G, et al. The investigation of galectin-3 in diseases of the thyroid gland. *Eur J Endocrinol*. 2003;149:449–453.

178. DeLellis RA, May L, Tashjian AH Jr, et al. C-cell granule heterogeneity in man. An ultrastructural immunocytochemical study. *Lab Invest*. 1978;38:263–269.

179. Berger G, Berger N, Guillaud MH, et al. Calcitonin-like immunoreactivity of amyloid fibrils in medullary thyroid carcinomas. An immunoelectron microscope study. *Virchows Arch A Pathol Anat Histopathol*. 1988;412:543–551.

180. Kini SR, Miller JM, Hamburger JI, et al. Cytopathologic features of medullary carcinoma of the thyroid. *Arch Pathol Lab Med*. 1984;108:156–159.

181. Zeppa P, Vetrani A, Marino M, et al. Fine needle aspiration cytology of medullary thyroid carcinoma: a review of 18 cases. *Cytopathology*. 1990;1:35–44.

182. Mendonca ME, Ramos S, Soares J. Medullary carcinoma of thyroid: a re-evaluation of the cytological criteria of diagnosis. *Cytopathology*. 1991;2:93–102.

183. Papaparaskeva K, Nagel H, Droese M. Cytologic diagnosis of medullary carcinoma of the thyroid gland. *Diagn Cytopathol*. 2000;22:351–358.

184. Kaushal S, Iyer VK, Mathur SR, et al. Fine needle aspiration cytology of medullary carcinoma of the thyroid with a focus on rare variants: a review of 78 cases. *Cytopathology*. 2010;22:95-105.

185. Matias-Guiu X, LaGuette J, Puras-Gil AM, et al. Metastatic neuroendocrine tumors to the thyroid gland mimicking medullary carcinoma: a pathologic and immunohistochemical study of six cases. *Am J Surg Pathol*. 1997;21:754–762.

186. Fleming JB, Lee JE, Bouvet M, et al. Surgical strategy for the treatment of medullary thyroid carcinoma. *Ann Surg*. 1999;230:697–707.

187. Kebebew E, Clark OH. Medullary thyroid cancer. *Curr Treat Options Oncol*. 2000;1:359–367.

188. Schlumberger M, Carlomagno F, Baudin E, et al. New therapeutic approaches to treat medullary thyroid carcinoma. *Nat Clin Pract Endocrinol Metab*. 2008;4:22–32.

189. Chatal JF, Campion L, Kraeber-Bodere F, et al. Survival improvement in patients with medullary thyroid carcinoma who undergo pretargeted anti-carcinoembryonic-antigen radioimmunotherapy: a collaborative study with the French Endocrine Tumor Group. *J Clin Oncol*. 2006;24:1705–1711.

190. Cerrato A, De Falco V, Santoro M. Molecular genetics of medullary thyroid carcinoma: the quest for novel therapeutic targets. *J Mol Endocrinol*. 2009;43:143–155.

191. Ye L, Santarpia L, Gagel RF. The evolving field of tyrosine kinase inhibitors in the treatment of endocrine tumors. *Endocr Rev*. 2010;31:578–599.

192. Sherman SI. Targeted therapy of thyroid cancer. *Biochem Pharmacol*. 2010;80:592–601.

193. Girelli ME, Nacamulli D, Pelizzo MR, et al. Medullary thyroid carcinoma: clinical features and long-term follow-up of seventy-eight patients treated between 1969 and 1986. *Thyroid*. 1998;8:517–523.

194. Miccoli P, Minuto MN, Ugolini C, et al. Clinically unpredictable prognostic factors in the outcome of medullary thyroid cancer. *Endocr Relat Cancer*. 2007;14:1099–1105.

195. Edge SB, Byrd DR, Compton CC, et al, eds. *AJCC Cancer Staging Manual*. 7th ed. New York, NY: Springer; 2010.

196. Roncalli M, Viale G, Grimelius L, et al. Prognostic value of N-myc immunoreactivity in medullary thyroid carcinoma. *Cancer*. 1994;74:134–141.

197. Hales M, Rosenau W, Okerlund MD, et al. Carcinoma of the thyroid with a mixed medullary and follicular pattern: morphologic, immunohistochemical, and clinical laboratory studies. *Cancer*. 1982;50:1352–1359.

198. Pfaltz M, Hedinger CE, Muhlethaler JP. Mixed medullary and follicular carcinoma of the thyroid. *Virchows Arch A Pathol Anat Histopathol*. 1983;400:53–59.

199. Ljungberg O, Bondeson L, Bondeson AG. Differentiated thyroid carcinoma, intermediate type: a new tumor entity with features of follicular and parafollicular cell carcinoma. *Hum Pathol*. 1984;15:218–228.

200. Polliack A, Freund U. Mixed papillary and follicular carcinoma of the thyroid gland with stromal amyloid. *Am J Clin Pathol*. 1970;53:592–595.

201. Perrone T. Mixed medullary-follicular thyroid carcinoma. *Am J Surg Pathol*. 1986;10:362–363.

202. Ogawa H, Kino I, Arai T. Mixed medullary-follicular carcinoma of the thyroid. Immunohistochemical and electron microscopic studies. *Acta Pathol Jpn*. 1989;39:67–72.

203. Mizukami Y, Michigishi T, Nonomura A, et al. Mixed medullary-follicular carcinoma of the thyroid occurring in familial form. *Histopathology*. 1993;22:284–287.
204. Kashima K, Yokoyama S, Inoue S, et al. Mixed medullary and follicular carcinoma of the thyroid: report of two cases with an immunohistochemical study. *Acta Pathol Jpn*. 1993;43:428–433.
205. Sobrinho-Simoes M. Mixed medullary and follicular carcinoma of the thyroid. *Histopathology*. 1993;23:287–289.
206. Mizukami Y, Nonomura A, Michigishi T, et al. Mixed medullary-follicular carcinoma of the thyroid gland: a clinicopathologic variant of medullary thyroid carcinoma. *Mod Pathol*. 1996;9:631–635.
207. Shiroko T, Yokoo N, Okamoto K, et al. Mixed medullary-papillary carcinoma of the thyroid with lymph node metastases: report of a case. *Surg Today*. 2001;31:317–321.
208. Hanna AN, Michael CW, Jing X. Mixed medullary-follicular carcinoma of the thyroid: diagnostic dilemmas in fine-needle aspiration cytology. *Diagn Cytopathol*. 2010.
209. Volante M, Papotti M, Roth J, et al. Mixed medullary-follicular thyroid carcinoma. Molecular evidence for a dual origin of tumor components. *Am J Pathol*. 1999;155:1499–1509.
210. Matias-Guiu X. Mixed medullary and follicular carcinoma of the thyroid. On the search for its histogenesis. *Am J Pathol*. 1999;155:1413–1418.
211. Sadow PM, Hunt JL. Mixed medullary-follicular-derived carcinomas of the thyroid gland. *Adv Anat Pathol*. 2010;17:282–285.
212. Papotti M, Negro F, Carney JA, et al. Mixed medullary-follicular carcinoma of the thyroid. A morphological, immunohistochemical and in situ hybridization analysis of 11 cases. *Virchows Arch*. 1997;430:397–405.
213. Noel M, Delehaye MC, Segond N, et al. Study of calcitonin and thyroglobulin gene expression in human mixed follicular and medullary thyroid carcinoma. *Thyroid*. 1991;1:249–256.
214. Albores-Saavedra J, Gorraez de la Mora T, de la Torre-Rendon F, et al. Mixed medullary-papillary carcinoma of the thyroid: a previously unrecognized variant of thyroid carcinoma. *Hum Pathol*. 1990;21:1151–1155.
215. Lax SF, Beham A, Kronberger-Schonecker D, et al. Coexistence of papillary and medullary carcinoma of the thyroid gland-mixed or collision tumour? Clinicopathological analysis of three cases. *Virchows Arch*. 1994;424:441–447.
216. Rossi S, Fugazzola L, De Pasquale L, et al. Medullary and papillary carcinoma of the thyroid gland occurring as a collision tumour: report of three cases with molecular analysis and review of the literature. *Endocr Relat Cancer*. 2005;12:281–289.
217. Biscolla RP, Ugolini C, Sculli M, et al. Medullary and papillary tumors are frequently associated in the same thyroid gland without evidence of reciprocal influence in their biologic behavior. *Thyroid*. 2004;14:946–952.
218. Kim WG, Gong G, Kim EY, et al. Concurrent occurrence of medullary thyroid carcinoma and papillary thyroid carcinoma in the same thyroid should be considered as coincidental. *Clin Endocrinol (Oxf)*. 2010;72:256–263.

Rare Primary Thyroid Epithelial Tumors

 ## MUCOEPIDERMOID CARCINOMA

Mucoepidermoid carcinoma (MEC) is a malignant epithelial neoplasm. By definition, an MEC contains a combination of mucinous and epidermoid components.[1] There are two histologic variants of MEC: mucoepidermoid carcinoma and sclerosing mucoepidermoid carcinoma with eosinophilia. The sclerosing variant with eosinophilia will be described in the next section.

Etiology

Although a well-developed etiology has not been elucidated, radiation exposure during childhood may be a factor.[2–4]

Histogenesis and Molecular Genetics

The hypothesis that MEC derives from follicular epithelial cells or from the ultimobranchial body remains unconfirmed.[4–7] The detection of squamous metaplasia within papillary thyroid carcinoma and in MEC suggests a follicular derivation. Furthermore, a transition from follicular epithelium is supported by the neoplastic cells reacting with thyroglobulin, thyroid transcription factor 1 (TTF1), TTF2, paired box gene 8 (PAX8), and specific keratin reactions in MEC.[8,9] Lymphocytic thyroiditis with squamous metaplasia is present in the background of most cases of MEC, another finding that supports a thyroid follicular epithelial derivation.[4] Some authors believe that MEC may in fact be a variant of papillary carcinoma, or at the least very closely related.[3,6,10–13] In contrast to the cells in MEC, solid cell nests (SCNs) typically lack intercellular bridges and are thought to be remnants of the ultimobranchial body, the structure that gives rise to C-cells rather than follicular cells (see Chapter 1). In addition, there is no calcitonin or chromogranin immunoreactivity in MEC. SCNs have mucin-positive debris in their centers and rounded apical portions of cells. Finally, MECs may arise in the isthmus and pyramidal lobes, locations in which SCNs are not found.[4,7]

BRAF mutations, characteristic of thyroid papillary carcinomas, have not been found in these tumors.[14] The *CRTC1/MAML2* fusion corresponding to the cytogenetically detectable translocation t(11;19), which is common in MEC of salivary glands, has been detected in one of three thyroid MECs.[15]

Clinical Presentation

MEC accounts for <0.5% of all thyroid gland malignancies. Women are affected more frequently than men (2:1). There is a bimodal age distribution at 20 to 40 years and 60 to 80 years. Patients are euthyroid and present clinically with a firm, painless mass in the thyroid gland. Recurrent laryngeal nerve compression is not common.[1,4,10,16]

Pathology

Gross Presentation

Extrathyroidal extension is noted in up to 20% of patients.[4,13,17] The tumors can be as large as 10 cm in their greatest dimension, and they feature a firm cut surface with a tan-brown to yellow-white mass. Although they are well demarcated, they are seldom encapsulated (Fig. 15.1). Cystic degeneration, sometimes with a myxoid–mucoid appearance, and necrosis are sometimes identified.[1,4]

Microscopic Description

The tumor is infiltrative, demonstrating intertwined cords and nests of epidermoid cells and mucocytes in a stroma of fibrous connective tissue (Fig. 15.2). The epidermoid component may appear as sheets of atypical cells, sometimes with keratinization (Fig. 15.3). Keratin pearl formation is noted. Cystic spaces may be present; when they are, they frequently contain keratinaceous and mucinous debris with inflammatory cells (Fig. 15.3). The goblet-like cells may be seen within the cystic spaces, lining the cords of epidermoid cells, or within gland-like lumina (Fig. 15.4). The cytoplasm of the mucocyte may be clear to foamy or vacuolated. Mucin can be intra- and/or extracellular (Fig. 15.5). Ciliated cells may be seen.[1,4] Hyaline bodies (positive with periodic acid–Schiff [PAS] staining) resembling colloid may be seen in the cytoplasm of mucocytes.[12] The cells are intermediate in size. Their nuclei have pale nuclear chromatin similar to papillary thyroid carcinoma. Nuclear grooves and intranuclear cytoplasmic inclusions can be seen.[1] Psammoma bodies are occasionally present.[9,12] Lymphocytic thyroiditis is usually present in the surrounding thyroid parenchyma, and although germinal center formation is common, oncocytic metaplasia of the follicular epithelium is not.[1,4,10,12,16] Squamous metaplasia is seen in lymphocytic thyroiditis (Hashimoto thyroiditis) and is present in papillary thyroid carcinoma. Areas of transition between MEC and papillary thyroid carcinoma can be seen.[1,6,8,18,19] Concurrent papillary carcinoma has been identified in up to 50% of cases (Fig. 15.6).[4,10,12,19] In rare cases, anaplastic (undifferentiated) carcinoma may develop, a finding that often alters the prognosis.[10–12,20]

Immunohistochemistry and Molecular Diagnostics

The mucinous material is highlighted with PAS (Fig. 15.4), mucicarmine, and Alcian blue pH 2.5.[12] The tumor cells are positive with keratins (high and low molecular weight), with polyclonal carcinoembryonic antigen (CEA) (mucocytes only), and focally with thyroglobulin and TTF1 (Fig. 15.7).[1,4,9,16,19,20] p63 and CK5/6 may be of value in highlighting the epidermoid epithelium (Fig. 15.7). P-cadherin neoexpression and E-cadherin abnormalities are seen in the epidermoid tumor cells.[21] Calcitonin is negative.[4,16,19] Expression of thyroid-specific genes (*TTF1, TTF2, PAX8,* and thyroid peroxidase) detected by RT-PCR supports a follicular epithelial derivation,[9] although *BRAF* (V600E) mutation is not detected.[14,22] The *CRTC1/MAML2* fusion is detected in about one-third of cases.[15]

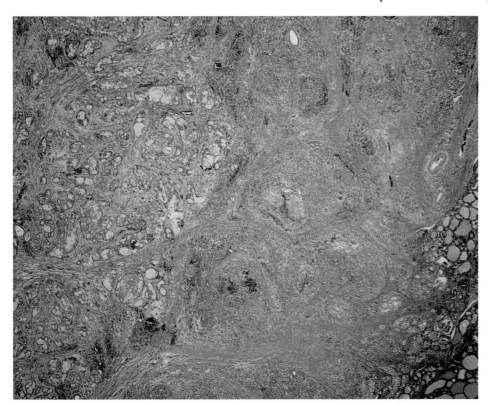

FIGURE 15.1. Mucoepidermoid carcinoma. A low-power magnification demonstrates poor circumscription with heavy fibrosis and a background of lymphocytic thyroiditis.

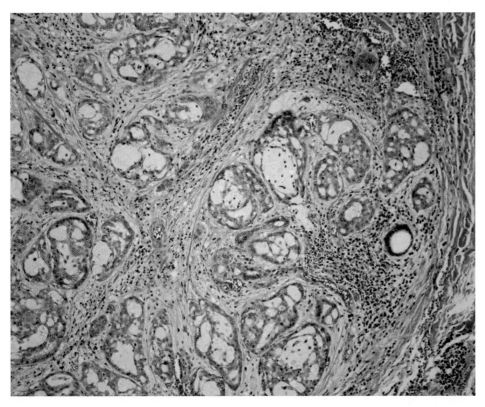

FIGURE 15.2. Mucoepidermoid carcinoma. There are intertwined cords, nests, and glands of neoplastic cells set in a background of lymphocytic thyroiditis.

FIGURE 15.3. Mucoepidermoid carcinoma. A: Sheets of atypical squamous cells showing keratin pearl formation. Inflammatory cells, including eosinophils, are present. **B:** Sheets of atypical squamous epithelium are arranged within cystic spaces. Keratin pearl formation is noted. Keratinaceous debris is present within the cysts.

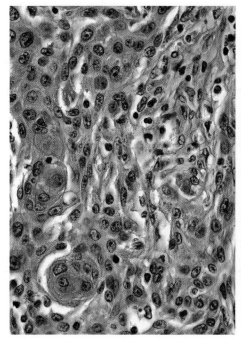
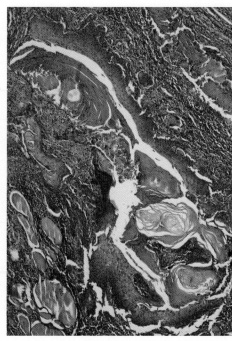

Cytopathology

Smears are cellular, with cohesive monolayered and syncytial sheets of cells within a background of amorphous debris and necrotic and mucinous material. A dual cell population of mucocytes (vacuolated to foamy cytoplasm compressing the nucleus) and epidermoid cells (polygonal cells with distinct cell borders and round nuclei, vesicular nuclear chromatin, prominent nucleoli, and opaque, homogeneous eosinophilic cytoplasm) are intermingled.[1,3,20,23,24] In rare cases, anaplastic cells may also be present.[11,20]

Differential Diagnosis

Prominent squamous metaplasia can be seen in lymphocytic thyroiditis, but a tumor mass is not identified. Prominent SCNs may also have mucocytes and mucinous detritus present in the cystic lumina. But SCNs usually appear as isolated microscopic foci rather than as a clinical

FIGURE 15.4. Mucoepidermoid carcinoma. Goblet cells containing basophilic mucin line a cystic space and are arranged within glandular spaces. The inset demonstrates a PAS with diastase-positive intracytoplasmic mucin droplet.

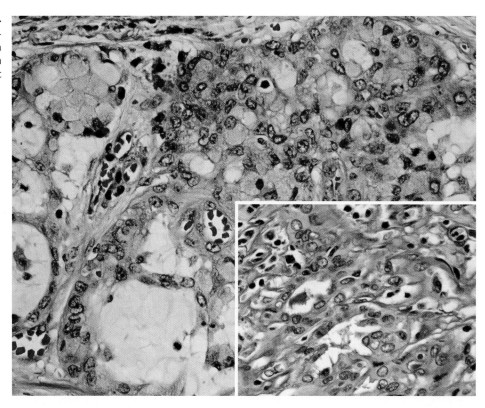

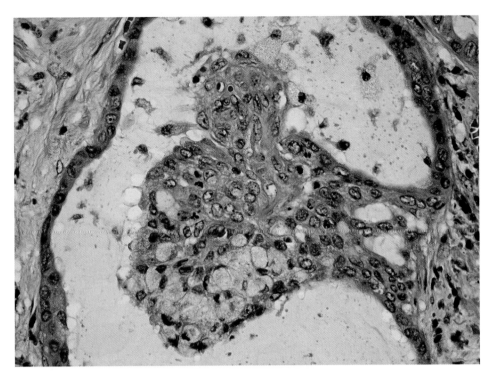

FIGURE 15.5. Mucoepidermoid carcinoma. Intra- and extracellular mucin is present. Note the signet-ring appearance with nuclear compression.

mass. Squamous cell carcinoma (SCC) is characterized by marked cytologic atypia, but it lacks mucocytes and extracellular mucin.[25] Furthermore, there is usually no associated papillary carcinoma. Squamous metaplasia can be seen in papillary carcinoma, but mucocytes and areas of transitional type epithelium are not seen in papillary carcinoma.

Treatment and Prognosis

Surgery is the treatment of choice, but if there is extensive local invasion, external beam radiation or radioablation can be employed.[8] Many consider MEC of the thyroid gland to be an indolent tumor with a good long-term prognosis (similar to that of papillary thyroid carcinoma).[1,4,10] Although death from tumor may occur in older patients, it is usually limited to those cases in which an anaplastic or undifferentiated component has been identified histologically.[10–12,20,26] Lymph node metastasis, which has been seen in up to 40% of patients,[1,4,9,12,13,20] is much more common than distant metastasis, although lung, bone, and pleural metastases have been reported.[3,23]

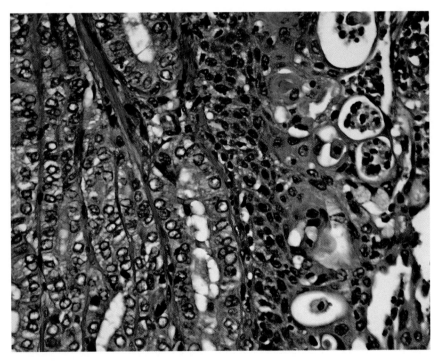

FIGURE 15.6. Mucoepidermoid carcinoma. There is a concurrent papillary carcinoma (left). Notice the mucocytes (right).

FIGURE 15.7. Mucoepidermoid carcinoma. **Left:** Thyroglobulin shows focal
positive staining in the glandular profiles.
Right: A p63 highlights the epidermoid
component.

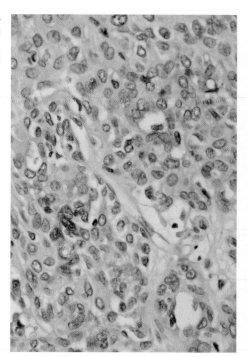
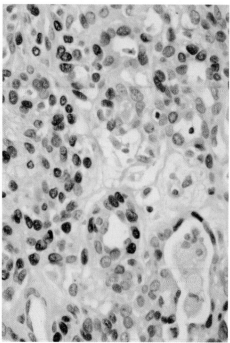

SCLEROSING MUCOEPIDERMOID CARCINOMA WITH EOSINOPHILIA

Sclerosing mucoepidermoid carcinoma with eosinophilia (SMECE) is an extremely rare primary thyroid gland neoplasm. It exhibits epidermoid and glandular differentiation set in a prominently sclerotic background with a rich investment of eosinophils and lymphocytes.[27,28] It is distinct from MEC, although eosinophils can be seen in both types of tumor.

Etiology

There is no known etiologic agent, although nearly all cases are associated with lymphocytic thyroiditis—specifically, the fibrosing Hashimoto thyroiditis.[27,29]

Histogenesis and Molecular Genetics

The tumor is presumed to arise from squamous metaplasia of the thyroid follicular epithelium, usually in the setting of lymphocytic thyroiditis (Hashimoto thyroiditis).[27,29] Origin from the ultimobranchial body is a possibility,[30] but immunohistochemistry results are equivocal because p63 immunoreactivity is seen in squamous metaplasia and in ultimobranchial body remnants (SCNs).[31]

Clinical Presentation

Fewer than 50 cases of SMECE have been reported. The vast majority of these occurred in women. Patients generally present with a slowly growing, painless neck mass.[10,27,32-36] The nonfunctional tumor rarely presents with rapid enlargement, hoarseness, or vocal fold paralysis.[28,29,37]

Pathology

Gross Presentation

Tumor size ranges from 1 to 13 cm. Tumors usually appear as ill-defined, white to yellow, firm, solid masses.[27,34] Cystic change may occur, but this is uncommon.[28]

Microscopic Description

Anastomosing cords, strands, and nests of tumor cells are identified in a stroma of very sclerotic fibrohyaline connective tissue (Fig. 15.8). Innumerable eosinophils are seen throughout (Fig. 15.9). The neoplastic cells are biphasic, with cohesive nests of epidermoid, polygonal cells with well-developed cell borders. Intercellular bridges are noted, with opacified, *thick* eosinophilic cytoplasm. Keratin pearls and keratin debris can be identified (Figs. 15.9 and 15.10) There is only mild to moderate pleomorphism. Nucleoli are prominent. Occasionally, clear cells are present.[29] Mucocytes with squashed nuclei are intermingled in the epidermoid sheets, highlighted with mucicarmine stain or PAS with diastase (Fig. 15.10). Mucus pools are uncommon.[27] In rare cases, the tumor cells may grow in a pseudoangiomatous pattern. Extrathyroidal extension is seen in as many as one-half of all cases, with lymph node metastasis in about one-third.[10,27,28,36,37] Perineural and vascular invasion is common. Lymphoid infiltration (lymphocytes and plasma cells), including a finding of lymphocytic thyroiditis (Hashimoto thyroiditis), is seen in the adjacent thyroid parenchyma in nearly all cases. Squamous metaplasia is also seen in the areas of lymphocytic thyroiditis.[10,27,33,35] Papillary carcinoma is identified in a few cases, although transition between the two is less common than it is in MEC.

Immunohistochemistry and Molecular Diagnostics

Cytokeratins are positive in the tumor cells (Fig. 15.11); TTF1 is identified less often. CEA is sometimes expressed in the mucocytes but not in the areas of squamous differentiation. Calcitonin and thyroglobulin immunoreactive is not present.[10,27-29] p63 strongly stains the epidermoid tumor cells (Fig. 15.11),[30] a finding that is also seen in the basaloid cells of squamous metaplasia.[31] TP53 staining is occasionally seen in the epidermoid cells. *BRAF* mutations are not identified.[22]

Cytopathology

In general, a definitive diagnosis by fine needle aspiration cytology is difficult because of the nonspecific nature of the findings. There tends to be a combination of malignant epithelial cells set

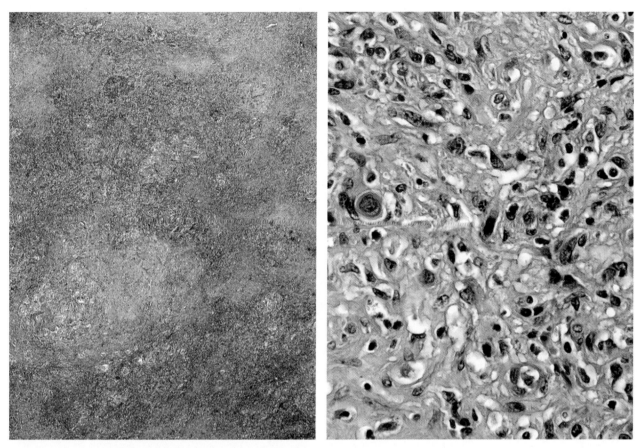

FIGURE 15.8. Sclerosing mucoepidermoid carcinoma with eosinophilia. Left: A well-developed lymphocytic thyroiditis is identified in association with sclerotic fibrous connective tissue. Neoplastic cells are embedded in this background. **Right:** The sclerotic background is sometimes quite heavy, almost concealing the isolated and infiltrating epidermoid cells. Eosinophils are present.

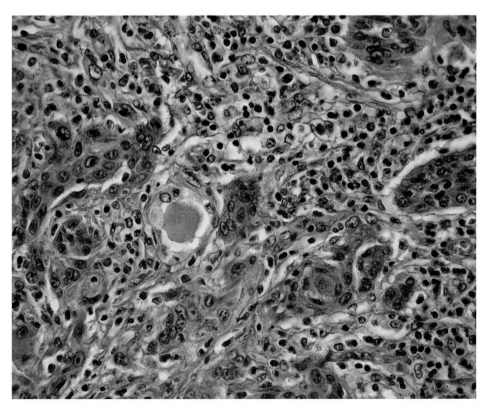

FIGURE 15.9. Sclerosing mucoepidermoid carcinoma with eosinophilia. Countless eosinophils are present in the background. The epidermoid component demonstrates keratin pearl formation and well-developed intercellular borders.

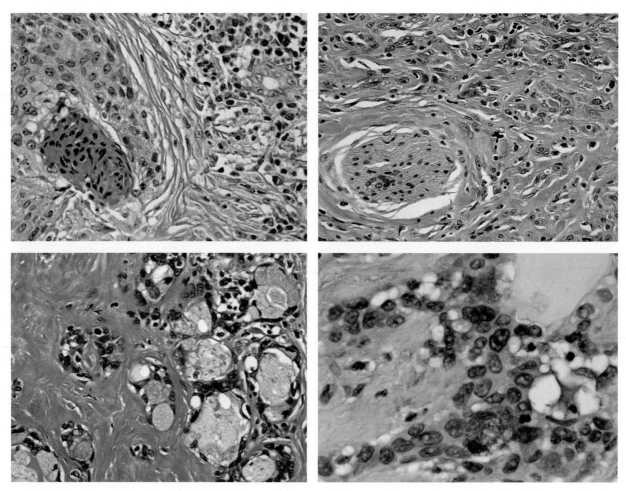

FIGURE 15.10. Sclerosing mucoepidermoid carcinoma with eosinophilia. A: Cohesive epidermoid cells with well-defined cell borders. Opacified cytoplasm is noted with keratin debris. **B:** Perineural invasion is present along with a background hyalinization. **C:** Mucocytes with squashed nuclei are present. **D:** Mucicarmine highlights the mucocytes.

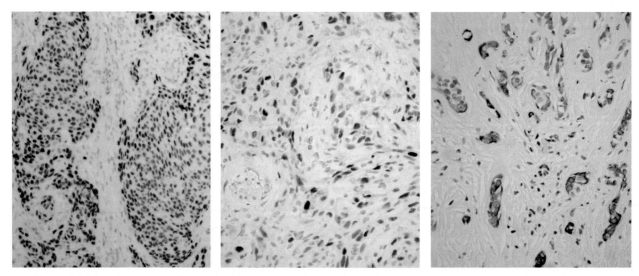

FIGURE 15.11. Sclerosing mucoepidermoid carcinoma with eosinophilia. Left: The epidermoid cells are strongly and diffusely immunoreactive with p63. **Center:** TP53 immunoreactivity in the epidermoid component. **Right:** CK7 highlights the glandular component.

in a mucinous and debris-filled background with eosinophils. Cohesive clusters of cells with either epidermoid or glandular differentiation are present. These findings suggest malignancy, but they may also raise the possibility of metastatic tumor or Hashimoto thyroiditis.[35,38]

Differential Diagnosis

Anaplastic (undifferentiated) thyroid carcinoma, SCC, carcinoma showing thymus-like differentiation (CASTLE), Hodgkin lymphoma, direct extension of adjacent organ tumors, and florid squamous metaplasia enter the differential diagnosis.[27] Undifferentiated carcinoma has more pleomorphism, sheetlike growth, increased mitotic activity, and necrosis, and it lacks mucocytes and significant eosinophils. Pure SCC has significantly greater pleomorphism, sheetlike growth, and necrosis, and it lacks mucocytes and mucin pools.[25] CASTLE can have mucinous material, but it is spindled, tends not to have lymphoid infiltrate, and has a unique immunohistochemical profile. Hodgkin lymphoma may have a rich eosinophilic infiltrate and contains lymphocytes and plasma cells, but it also has Reed–Sternberg cells, which are not present in SMECE.[39] Primary carcinomas of the larynx and esophagus can invade the thyroid gland, but in general, the clinical and/or radiographic findings will help make this distinction. Florid squamous metaplasia tends not to form a mass, is present in lymphocytic thyroiditis, and does not have mucocytes or eosinophils.[31,40]

Treatment and Prognosis

Total thyroidectomy is the treatment of choice, especially since extrathyroidal extension is common. Selected cervical lymph node sampling is recommended for patients with clinically apparent lymph node enlargement—up to 30% of cases at presentation.[10,29,34–37] Lung, liver, and bone metastases are uncommon.[35–37] The tumor is usually indolent, and the long-term clinical prognosis is intermediate.[10,28,33] Specific prognostic factors are unknown.

 # SQUAMOUS CELL CARCINOMA

A primary SCC in the thyroid gland is composed entirely of cells with squamous differentiation, without mucocytes, and without direct invasion from an adjacent organ (larynx, trachea, or esophagus).[41] Therefore, endoscopic evaluation (laryngoscopy, esophagoscopy, bronchoscopy) and radiographic studies are often required to establish a definitive diagnosis.[42–45]

Histogenesis and Molecular Genetics

SCC is thought to arise from thyroid follicular epithelium, either directly or through squamous metaplasia, which then undergoes additional alterations to yield a malignant tumor. The squamous epithelium may represent a persistence of thyroglossal duct or branchial pouch remnants. Association with Hashimoto thyroiditis may also be seen.[41,44,46–49] Previous radiation has been reported as an etiologic factor in a few cases.[45,50]

Clinical Presentation

SCC accounts for <0.5% of all malignant thyroid tumors, with fewer than 100 reported cases.[51] Its clinical presentation is similar to that of undifferentiated carcinoma. In both cases, there is a rapidly enlarging neck mass that is very often associated with recurrent laryngeal nerve compression and pressure symptoms, including airway obstruction and dyspnea (Fig. 15.12). Cervical lymph node enlargement is common.[52] Most affected patients are in the sixth or seventh decade of life, and the

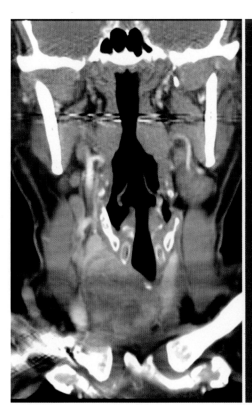
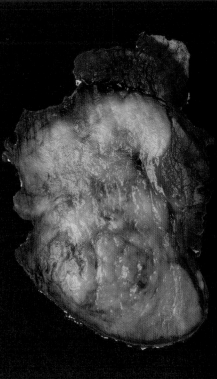

FIGURE 15.12. Squamous cell carcinoma. Left: A CT scan demonstrates a large destructive mass, pushing aside the trachea and expanding into the lower neck soft tissues. **Right:** The cut surface shows near complete replacement of the thyroid gland by a necrotic tumor mass.

female-to-male ratio is 2:1.[25,43–45,48,49,52–59] Hashimoto thyroiditis is concurrently identified in a few patients.[25] The paraneoplastic syndrome of *hypercalcemia, fever,* and *leukocytosis* is rare and probably develops as a result of tumor-derived humoral mediators.[60–62]

Pathology

Gross Presentation

Like undifferentiated carcinomas, SCCs are usually large (up to 8 cm), firm, tan-white masses, often involving one or both lobes of the thyroid gland. Additional nodules of tumor are frequently identified, and extrathyroidal extension is frequent. Necrosis is common (Fig. 15.12).[41,52,56,57]

Microscopic Description

Before making a diagnosis of a primary thyroid SCC, direct extension from the larynx or esophagus (clinically, radiographically, or operatively) must be excluded. A primary SCC is an invasive neoplasm with extensive destruction, composed entirely of squamous cells (Fig. 15.13).[63] Vascular and perineural invasion, as well as extensive local extension, is common. The cells are cohesive and arranged in sheets, ribbons, and nests (Fig. 15.14) of pleomorphic cells with a variable nucleus-to-cytoplasm ratio (Fig. 15.15). Tumor cell spindling can be seen. Keratinization is frequently present, with keratin pearl formation (Fig. 15.15). Mitotic figures are common, including atypical forms. Tumors are graded as *well differentiated, moderately differentiated,* and *poorly differentiated.* They are also classified as *keratinizing* or *nonkeratinizing*; most thyroid tumors are *poorly differentiated.* An inflammatory infiltrate and stromal fibroplasia are frequently present (Fig. 15.16), sometimes in association with mucin production.[41,44,46,49,52,56,58] It is important to note that papillary carcinoma and undifferentiated carcinoma can both exhibit areas of squamous differentiation,[47,56,59,64–70] and these are much more common

than in primary thyroid SCC. Fine needle aspiration may induce squamous metaplasia in the tumor.[67] Therefore, although rare cases of SCC associated with follicular neoplasms have been reported,[44,64,71] by definition and convention, a primary SCC of the thyroid gland must be a pure tumor without any other type of differentiation. If other differentiation is present, the primary tumor is diagnosed and coupled with a statement about squamous differentiation—for example, *anaplastic carcinoma with squamous differentiation.* Collision tumors (from different lobes) have been reported.[72]

Immunohistochemistry and Molecular Diagnostics

Pankeratin, CK19, and p63 are strongly positive within the neoplastic cells. CK7 and CK18 are focally immunoreactive, whereas epithelial membrane antigen (EMA) is occasionally reactive.[25,53,57,70,73] CK1, CK4, CK6, CK10/13, CK20, and CD5 are nonreactive.[57,73,74] S-100A9 is highlighted in a diffuse, laminated reaction that is different from the reaction seen with thymus-derived tumors.[75] Diffusion artifacts may cause a false-positive thyroglobulin reaction, but TTF1 immunoreactivity has been reported.[53] The tumor cells usually demonstrate a high proliferation index with MIB-1 antibodies.[25,41,53,56] Although only a few cases have been studied, abnormal p53 expression and loss of p21 expression have been reported.[25,53,56,57] *TP53* expression becomes greater as the neoplasm exhibits less squamous differentiation.[57] Epidermal growth factor receptor (EGFR) may be overexpressed in these tumors (which showed gene polysomy), possibly providing a therapeutic alterative for these tumors.[54,76]

Cytopathology

Fine needle aspiration cytology easily establishes the diagnosis, although it does not always correctly identify the source (thyroid, larynx, lymph node, esophagus, metastasis, thyroglossal duct

FIGURE 15.13. Squamous cell carcinoma. A widely invasive carcinoma invades between the thyroid gland follicles and extends into the perithyroidal soft tissues.

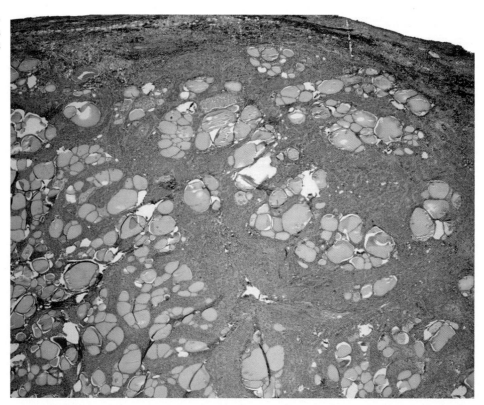

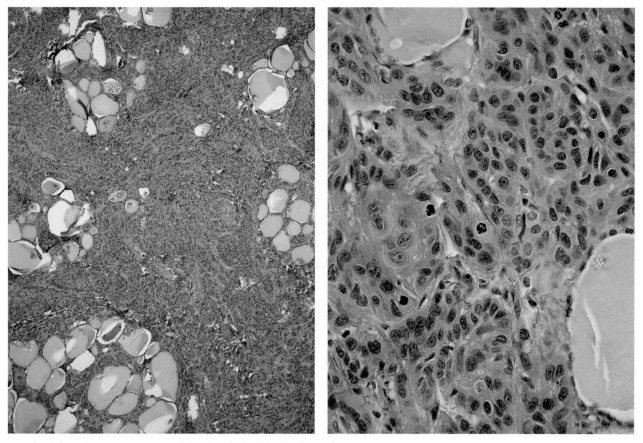

FIGURE 15.14. Squamous cell carcinoma. Cohesive sheets and ribbons of squamous cell destroy the thyroid gland parenchyma.

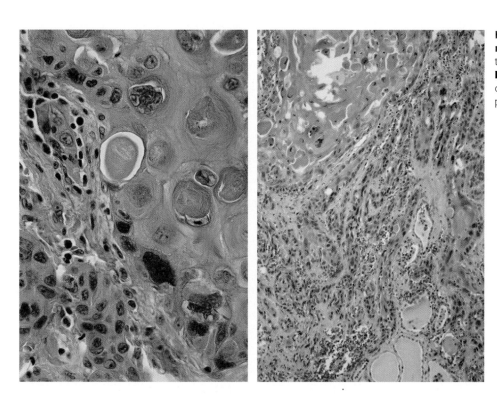

FIGURE 15.15. Squamous cell carcinoma. Left: Profound pleomorphism is identified. Dyskeratosis is present in many cells. **Right:** Keratinization is easily identified in this carcinoma with dyskeratosis and squamous pearl formation.

FIGURE 15.16. Squamous cell carcinoma. Left: A desmoplastic stromal fibroplasia is noted in this invasive carcinoma. **Right:** A poorly differentiated SCC with associated desmoplastic stroma.

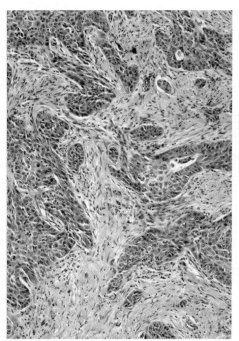 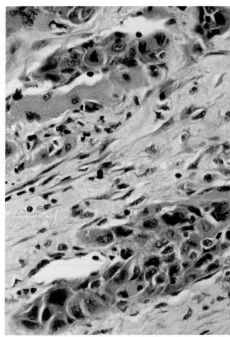

cyst). Cellular smears contain cohesive clusters and isolated cells set in a necrotic and granular, eosinophilic keratin-debris–filled background. Irregular shapes (tadpole cells), nuclear hyperchromasia, and cytoplasmic orangophilia and dyskeratosis are noted in the neoplastic cells. Distinguishing a metastatic SCC from a direct extension is impossible on cytology alone.[77–80]

Differential Diagnosis

Primary thyroid gland SCC frequently invades into the surrounding tissues, including the larynx, esophagus, and trachea, sometimes causing confusion about the primary site of origin. The larynx, esophagus, and trachea may all be sources of a primary tumor. In cases of tumor in the thyroid gland and an adjacent location, radiographic studies or clinical symptoms may help determine the center point of the bulk of the tumor mass. It is important to make this distinction because patients with primary thyroid SCC have a worse prognosis than do those with an extension from an adjacent tumor.[48,51,53,56,63,81] SCC metastasis to the thyroid gland is possible, but it is rare; when it does occur, the patient usually has a known clinical history of an SCC in a different location. Metastases to the thyroid gland generally develop within 3 years of identification of the primary site.[51,77,82] An SCC may develop within a thyroglossal duct cyst, a developmental anomaly that is intimately associated with the thyroid gland in many cases.[78]

Cytopathology squamous differentiation in an undifferentiated carcinoma is usually focal and is not the dominant histologic finding. Papillary carcinoma (particularly of diffuse sclerosing variant) can exhibit areas of squamous differentiation, but the papillary carcinoma tends to predominate. Squamous metaplasia within lymphocytic thyroiditis does not present as a mass lesion, lacks infiltrative growth and cytologic atypia, and is not associated with necrosis.[31]

Cytopathology CASTLE usually manifests a greater degree of tumor spindling, may contain Hassall corpuscles, demonstrates more keloid-like collagen deposition, has inflammatory cells, and immunophenotypically, the cells are positive with thymic markers (CD5, scattered S-100A9 cells).[73–75,83]

Treatment and Prognosis

Early total resection along with radical dose radiotherapy is the treatment of choice for SCC. The tumor is usually unaltered by radioiodine or chemotherapy. Radiation alone can be used for patients with unresectable tumors and for those who are poor surgical candidates.[41,45,48,52,53,58,69,84] Thyroid hormone suppression may help, since thyroid-stimulating hormone could be a growth factor.[60] Pharmaceutical targeting of EGFR may show promise in the future.[76] Local invasion and lymph node metastasis are common; distant metastasis (lung) is less common, occurring in fewer than 30% of cases.[41,52,58] Airway compromise is the usual cause of death. The overall prognosis is poor; mean survival is <12 months, and 5-year survival is <10%.[41,44,49,52,53,57,58,69,84] However, patients who have only localized disease and who are managed with combination surgery and radiation may survive longer.[52,58,84] By convention, SCC is placed in the same staging category as undifferentiated carcinoma.[85,86]

MUCINOUS CARCINOMA

Mucinous carcinoma of the thyroid is an exceeding rare tumor characterized by nests of neoplastic cells floating in pools of extracellular mucin.[87]

Histogenesis and Molecular Genetics

The ultimobranchial body and its remnant, SCNs, may be the cells of origin. SCNs demonstrate *mixed thyroid follicles* by having follicular epithelium and epidermoid-like cells. Histochemically, SCNs demonstrate intraluminal acid mucins and immunoreactivity for CEA and cytokeratins.[88,89]

Clinical Presentation

Clinical presentation is nonspecific as patients can present with either a slowly growing or a rapidly growing nodule.[89–92] Lymph

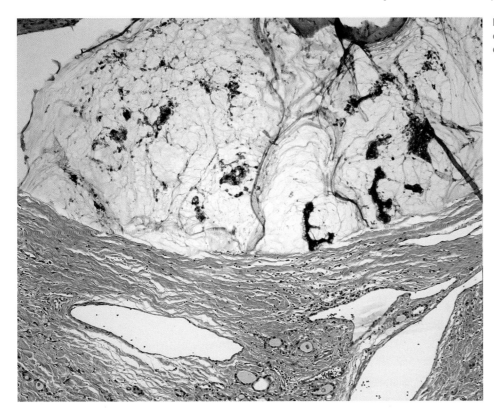

FIGURE 15.17. Mucinous carcinoma. Mucinous pools contain small nests of glandular epithelium.

node metastasis may occur.[93] The results of thyroid function studies are normal.[89]

Pathology

Gross Presentation

Tumors are intermediate in size (2.5 cm). Their cut surface is gelatinous, glistening, and white-gray, and their borders can be either well or ill defined.[89,93]

Microscopic Description

The neoplasm is contained in a capsule that separates it from the surrounding thyroid gland parenchyma. Necrosis, mitotic figures, and invasion (capsule or vessel) are seen in some tumors. By definition, mucinous carcinoma contains pools of abundant mucoid material surrounding collections of epithelial neoplastic cells (Fig. 15.17). The tumor cells can be arranged in a glandular, microfollicular, trabecular, or spindled pattern.[89,93–95] The cells are cuboidal to columnar; they contain intracytoplasmic mucin vacuoles with a bland histology, although the nuclei are large with prominent nucleoli (Fig. 15.18).[89] Focal areas of squamous differentiation have been reported.[89,90,92]

Immunohistochemistry and Molecular Diagnostics

The mucin is sulfated acid mucin, positive with mucicarmine, Alcian blue, and PAS (with and without diastase).[89,93,95] Ultrastructural studies have shown the cells to be follicular, with colloid secretion and intracytoplasmic mucin droplets in the same cells. The nuclei have irregular contours and prominent nucleoli. A well-developed basal lamina is present, and desmosomes are easily identified. The luminal aspects of the cells have microvilli and a glycocalyx, but they lack rootlets. Neuroendocrine granules are not present.[89,90,96]

The cells are immunoreactive with low molecular weight cytokeratins, vimentin, TTF1, MUC2, and CEA, and focally with thyroglobulin. The cells are negative with calcitonin, chromogranin, and Sw100 protein.[89,93–95] It is important to note that simple mucin-type antigens (T, Tn, and sialyl Tn) are identified in thyroid gland neoplasms, and MUC1 and MUC2 are seen in papillary and follicular carcinoma.[97–99] Therefore, the presence of mucin-type antigens alone does not specifically identify this tumor type. *TP53* has been detected in isolated cases.[93]

Differential Diagnosis

The differential diagnosis includes primary MEC, metastatic mucin-producing tumors (colon, lung, breast, salivary gland),[89,91,100] mucinous parathyroid carcinoma,[101] and primary thyroid gland tumors with mucin production. The latter include follicular adenoma, follicular carcinoma, papillary carcinoma, and medullary carcinoma with extracellular mucin production or signet-ring morphology. It is important to remember that the extracellular mucin-producing or signet-ring thyroid tumors preserve a characteristic growth pattern, such as encapsulated microfollicular pattern of follicular adenoma or carcinoma, contain much more abundant tumor epithelium, and exhibit characteristic nuclear features of the specific tumor type, such as nuclear features of papillary carcinoma or speckled chromatin of medullary carcinoma. These features have to be lost before a diagnosis of mucinous carcinoma can be established, and focal mucinous differentiation in other thyroid gland tumors does not change the diagnosis. Metastatic carcinomas can be ruled out based on the positive staining for thyroglobulin, PAX8, and TTF1.

Treatment and Prognosis

Because the literature contains only a few isolated case reports, any purportedly definitive comment about treatment and prognosis would be unreliable. Lung, liver, and bone metastases have been reported. Overall, patients appear to die from their disease after a period of months to years.[90,92,93,102]

FIGURE 15.18. Mucinous carcinoma. The cuboidal to columnar cells have intracytoplasmic mucin vacuoles. Lakes of mucin are noted in the background.

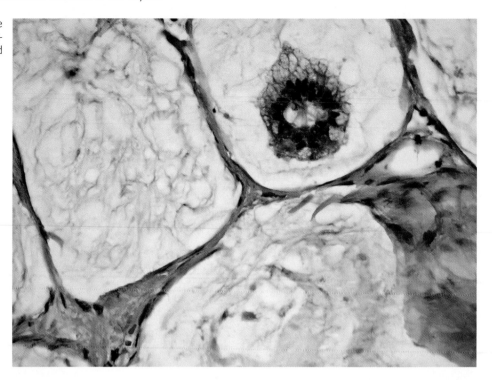

SPINDLE CELL TUMOR WITH THYMUS-LIKE DIFFERENTIATION

Spindle cell tumor with thymus-like differentiation (SETTLE) is a very rare thyroid gland malignancy. It is characterized by a peripheral lobulation and the biphasic appearance of spindle-shaped epithelial cells that blend almost imperceptibly with glandular structures.[103] As a distinct thyroid gland primary that is histologically similar to fetal thymus (thymoblastoma), SETTLE must be topographically separate from the thymus gland. Sometimes this is difficult to document, since the thyroid gland and thymus development overlap embryologically. The diagnostic use of the terms *malignant teratoma* and *thyroid thymoma of childhood* should be discouraged because they are inaccurate. SETTLE is one of two malignant tumors on the morphologic spectrum of thymic gland–related lesions; the other is CASTLE.[104]

Histogenesis and Molecular Genetics

In view of the rare nature of these tumors, it is difficult to make a definitive comment about pathogenesis. However, it has been proposed that SETTLE arises either from intrathyroidal ectopic thymic tissue or from other remnants of the branchial pouches that have retained the ability to differentiate into a tumor of thymic type.[104–106]

Clinical Presentation

SETTLE generally affects the young as most patients present in the second decade of life. However, the tumor has been reported in a broad range of ages (2 to 59 years). There is a male predominance (2:1).[103–120] Patients experience a thyroid or neck mass, sometimes painful, over a period of anywhere from a few weeks to a decade.[108–110,113,116–118,121] In rare cases, a rapidly enlarging neck mass with compression symptoms is identified.[105,116] Local tenderness sometimes mimics

thyroiditis,[103,114] but the results of thyroid function studies are normal.[109] Radiographic studies reveal a mixed solid and cystic mass.[103]

Pathology

Gross Presentation

The macroscopic appearance is variable, although a vaguely lobular appearance is usually noted (Fig. 15.19). The mass may be encapsulated, partially circumscribed, or infiltrative. Sometimes the tumor extends into the soft tissues (skeletal

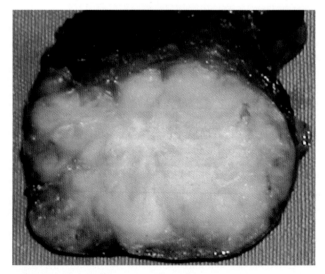

FIGURE 15.19. SETTLE. The macroscopic appearance is lobular, tan-white, with a predominantly solid appearance, focally showing small cysts. (Courtesy of Dr. A. Nihan Haberal, Baskent University, School of Medicine, Ankara, Turkey.)

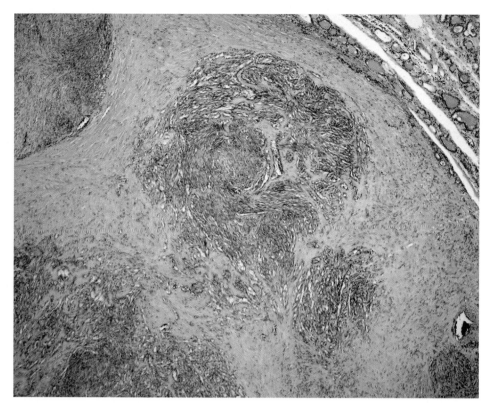

FIGURE 15.20. SETTLE. Lobules of tumor invade the thyroid gland. Sclerotic fibrous connective tissue separates the tumor into vague nodules which have a biphasic appearance.

muscle) of the neck. The tumors are usually intermediate in size (mean: 3.6 cm; range: 1 to 12 cm). Tumors are predominantly unilateral.[116,121] The cut surface is firm to hard, gray-white to tan, and predominantly solid; occasionally, small cysts and a gritty appearance is noted. Yellow areas suggest necrosis.[103,105,106,109,111–113,116–118,120–122]

Microscopic Description

SETTLE is a highly cellular tumor with primitive thymus-like histology. The tumor contains lobules of cells separated by acellular, sclerotic fibrous septa (Fig. 15.20). Vascular invasion may be noted at the periphery. The tumors are most

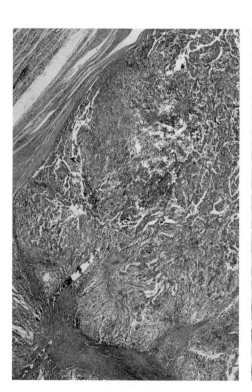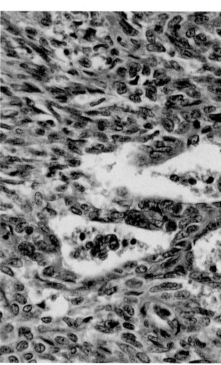

FIGURE 15.21. SETTLE. Left: The biphasic tumor contains spindle cell fascicles and gland-papillary groups. The thyroid gland parenchyma is present in the upper left. **Right:** An abrupt transition between spindle and glandular cells is common.

FIGURE 15.22. SETTLE. A predominantly spindled cell population arranged in short, interlacing fascicles. There is a syncytial architecture. The thyroid follicular epithelium is noted at the top of the photograph.

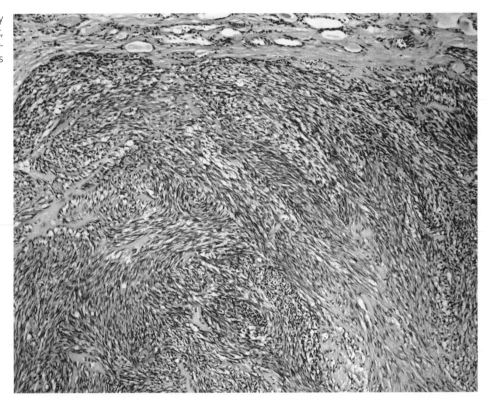

frequently biphasic, composed of short, reticulated, interlacing, and streaming fascicles of long, spindled tumor cells that blend almost imperceptibly with glandular and tubulopapillary structures (Fig. 15.21).[103–106,110,111,113,116–118,120,122] In rare cases, only one component or the other (spindle cells or glandular cells) is present; such a tumor is called the *monophasic variant*.[107,109,112,119]

The spindle cells have scant cytoplasm surrounding elongated nuclei with fine, delicate nuclear chromatin distribution (Fig. 15.22). The cells are often syncytial without distinct cell borders (Fig. 15.23). Nucleoli are small. Isolated foci of nuclear pleomorphism are occasionally present.[103,105,109] Mitotic figures are scant, although a high mitotic index is seen along with necrosis

FIGURE 15.23. SETTLE. Left: A syncytial arrangement in short, streaming fascicles of spindle cells with focal myxoid change. **Right:** Remarkably atypical nuclei can occasionally be present.

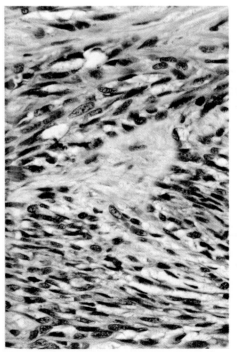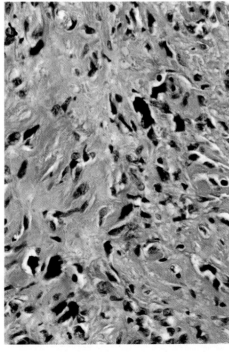

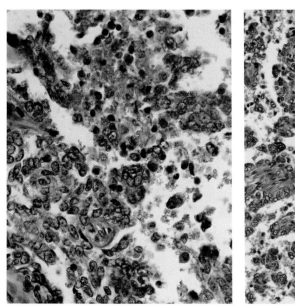 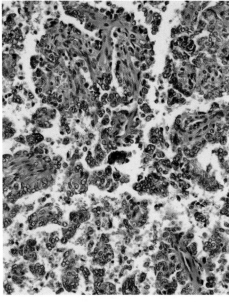

FIGURE 15.24. SETTLE. Left: Tumor necrosis is present within the glandular proliferation. **Right:** A calcification within the tubulopapillary structures.

in a few cases (Fig. 15.24).[113] The appearance of the glandular structures ranges from large cystic spaces lined with respiratory epithelium to mucinous glands, cords, nests, or tubules of pale-staining cuboidal to columnar cells arranged around cystic spaces (Fig. 15.25). The cells may be goblet-like or ciliated (Fig. 15.26).[118] The nuclei tend to be more round than the spindle cells, but the chromatin distribution is similar to that of the spindled cells.[104,113,116,117,122] Intercellular fluid and mucin may be seen. Squamous metaplasia or keratin pearls are exceptional.[107,109,113,118,120] A sprinkling of lymphocytes may be noted,

usually toward the periphery. Calcifications can be seen, but they are not common (Fig. 15.24).[109]

Immunohistochemistry and Molecular Diagnostics

Both the spindle and glandular cells express AE1/AE3 (Fig. 15.26), CAM5.2, and vimentin.[106,107,109,111–113,113,116–120] A limited expression with low–molecular weight keratins and EMA can

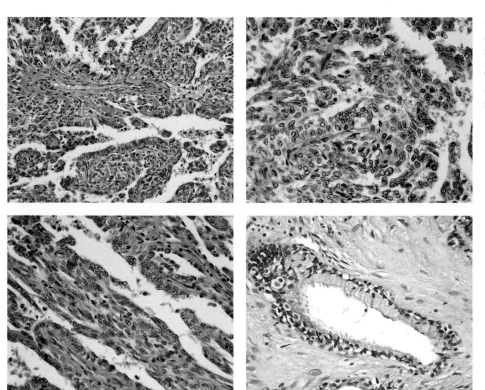

FIGURE 15.25. SETTLE. This quartet of images demonstrates the various patterns of the glandular component, arranged around cystic spaces, in papillary projections and in tubules. The nuclei are round to oval with irregular contours. Stratification and ciliated cells can be seen. Goblet cells are present.

FIGURE 15.26. SETTLE. Left: The biphasic appearance is illustrated here. There are cilia on the glandular cells. Goblet-type cells are noted in the upper center. **Right:** The neoplastic cells are strongly and diffusely keratin (AE1/AE3) immunoreactive.

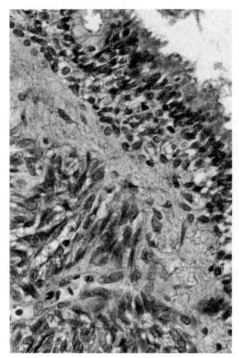 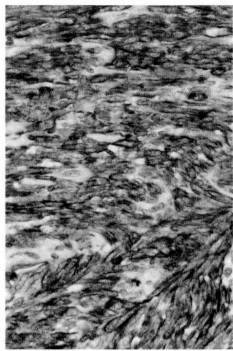

be seen.[106] CK7 shows cytoplasmic reactivity, whereas CK20 is negative.[106] In rare cases, the spindle cells demonstrate myoepithelial differentiation (smooth muscle actin, muscle-specific actin) and may react with bcl-2 and CD99 (MIC-2).[106,113,116–118,120] Reactivity with CD117 (75%), INI-1 (100%), and TLE1 (20%) has also been reported.[106] The tumor cells are negative for thyroglobulin, TTF1, calcitonin, CEA, CD5, S100 protein, neuron-specific enolase, synaptophysin, chromogranin, and deoxynucleotidyl transferase (TdT).[103,107,112,113,117–119,122] On electron microscopy, the spindle cells demonstrate numerous desmosomes, bundles of cytoplasmic tonofilaments, dense bodies, and basal lamina, findings that support the presence of an epithelial type cell.[111–113,118,122] Flow cytometry has a diploid DNA content.[112] There are only single case reports of the molecular findings; in these reports, a *KRAS* gene mutation was noted at codons 13 and 15 on the same allele.[120]

Cytopathology

Fine needle aspiration smears are cellular, showing cohesive and single dissociated spindle cells in a background of red metachromatic extracellular material arranged in fine, dust-like granules or irregular clumps (air-dried Romanowsky stains).[119] Epithelioid cells are occasionally seen. The spindle cells have scant fibrillar cytoplasm and bland uniform nuclei without conspicuous nucleoli. Columnar cells can be seen as well as background mucinous material.[118] Mitotic figures, necrosis, and pleomorphism are not seen. Immunohistochemistry studies can yield a correct preoperative diagnosis.[113,114,118]

Differential Diagnosis

SETTLE must be distinguished from undifferentiated thyroid carcinoma, ectopic thymoma, synovial sarcoma, and spindle cell medullary carcinoma. Undifferentiated carcinoma does not involve the very young, is not usually well circumscribed, and demonstrates marked nuclear pleomorphism and extensive necrosis. The neoplastic cells rarely show strong immunoreactivity with keratins. An ectopic thymoma has more

a jigsaw-puzzle–like lobulation and a very rich, immature TdT-positive T-cell population. Synovial sarcoma develops in young patients. It may develop in the neck, and it is often a biphasic tumor with a spindle cell population. SETTLE may be positive with INI-1 and TLE1, which is when the characteristic molecular alteration t(X;18) *SYT-SSX* gene fusion (detected by RT-PCR or fluorescence in situ hybridization) confirms the diagnosis of synovial carcinoma.[106,109,119] The spindle cell variant of medullary carcinoma may contain amyloid in the stroma, focal necrosis, and a more coarse nuclear chromatin distribution; calcitonin, CEA, chromogranin, and synaptophysin are positive.

Treatment and Prognosis

Surgery is the treatment of choice for the primary tumor, and it can also yield a good result in patients with metastatic disease, which is seen in up to 70% of cases. Metastatic disease tends to develop later in the course of this indolent tumor (as many as 22 years later); the most common sites of metastasis, in order of frequency, are the lung, lymph nodes, kidney, and soft tissues.[105–107,110,116,123] As there is often a protracted clinical course, aggressive resection of metastases, when they develop, can help to achieve a longer survival.[103] Although uncommon, regional lymph node metastases at presentation have been identified.[107,116,122] Combination chemotherapy and radiation therapy may treat metastatic disease.[110,116] The 5-year survival rate is approximately 90%, but this belies the indolent nature of the tumor, which can cause metastatic disease many years after the primary tumor's initial presentation.

 CARCINOMA SHOWING THYMUS-LIKE DIFFERENTIATION

Carcinoma showing thymus-like differentiation (CASTLE) is a primary thyroid gland malignancy that is architecturally and cytologically similar to thymic epithelial tumors.[83,104] CASTLE accounts for <0.1% of all thyroid gland malignancies.

Histogenesis and Molecular Genetics

It has been proposed that CASTLE arises from thymic rests adjacent to or within the thyroid gland (1) as a persistence of cervical thymic tissue left behind during its embryologic descent into the anterior mediastinum or (2) from remnants of the branchial pouches that can differentiate along the thymic line (such as SCNs).[104] Expression of CD5 by CASTLE cells provides support for this theory.[73,124]

Clinical Presentation

Generally, middle-aged adults (5th decade) present with a painless mass in the thyroid gland. Women are affected slightly more often than men (1.3:1). Tracheal compression and hoarseness are seen.[104,124–128] Patients are euthyroid. The mass appears as a cold nodule on scintigraphy, as a solid noncalcified soft-tissue density on CT, as an isointense mass on T1-weighted MRI, as a hyperintense mass on T2-weighted MR imaging, and as a hypoechoic and heterogeneous mass on ultrasonography.[129] Enlarged neck lymph nodes are seen in up to 30% of patients as a result of metastatic disease.[127] It is interesting that the frequent clinical associations with thymoma (myasthenia gravis, hypogammaglobulinemia, red cell aplasia/hypoplasia, and dermatomyositis) are not yet documented in patients with CASTLE.

Pathology

Gross Presentation

Involvement of the thyroid gland is requisite for the diagnosis, although sometimes a perithyroidal soft-tissue primary may obscure the point of origin. The tumor develops most often in the lower poles of the thyroid. The tumors are well circumscribed, slightly lobulated, and easily demarcated. Their cut surfaces are firm to fleshy, and their color is a mixture of yellow, gray, and tan.[124,125,127,130]

Microscopic Description

CASTLE is similar to thymic carcinoma (synonyms include *intrathyroidal epithelial thymoma* and *primary thyroid thymoma*[124,125]). The tumor is arranged in broad, pushing, smooth-bordered islands abutted against a desmoplastic cellular stroma (Fig. 15.27). Extrathyroidal extension is common (Fig. 15.28). As a result, sometimes separation from a perithyroidal origin is difficult.[126] The lobules of tumor are associated with delicate vessels that are frequently surrounded by lymphocytes and plasma cells, which spill into the tumor nests.[104,124,125,127,131] Mitotic figures are present, but they are not numerous (<3/10 high-power fields). The tumor cells are squamoid and syncytial to spindled, with pale to eosinophilic cytoplasm (Fig. 15.29). Well-defined cell borders, intercellular bridges, and frank keratinization are uncommon (Fig. 15.30).[131] The nuclei have only mild to moderate pleomorphism, and they are generally oval with a fine pale to vesicular chromatin distribution. Nucleoli are usually small, but they are easy to identify. Hassall corpuscles within lymphoid stroma may be seen at the periphery of the tumor, suggesting thymic remnants.[131] Granulomas are usually not identified. Electron microscopy demonstrates elongated epithelial cells with prominent desmosomes, bundles of cytoplasmic tonofilaments, and a lack of secretory granules and amyloid fibers.[125]

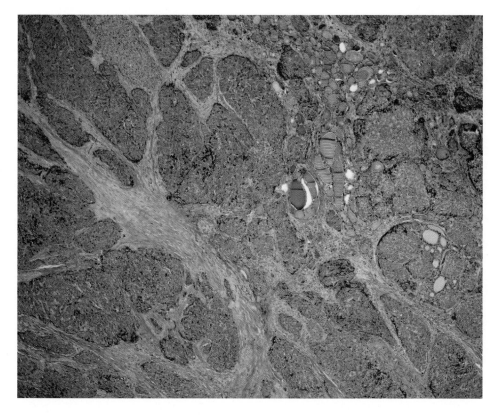

FIGURE 15.27. CASTLE. Broad, anastomosing islands of tumor cells are surrounded by desmoplastic stroma. Thyroid parenchyma is destroyed and overtaken by the neoplasm.

FIGURE 15.28. CASTLE. Tumor islands invade into an adjacent parathyroid gland.

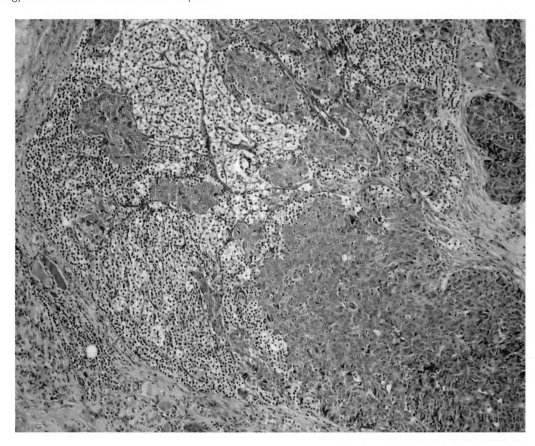

FIGURE 15.29. CASTLE. Left: A syncytium of cells with mild pleomorphism. The nuclear chromatin is vesicular with small but easily identified nucleoli. **Right:** Vague tumor spindling is noted in the center, along with areas of squamoid differentiation.

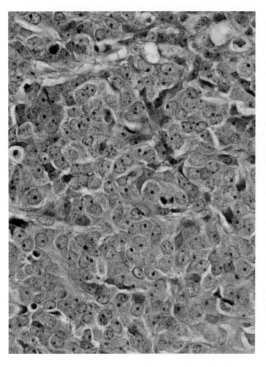 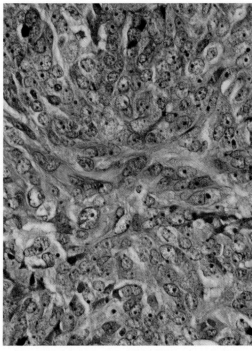

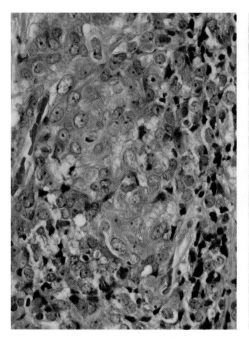 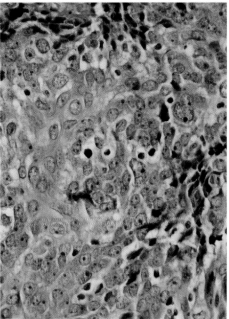

FIGURE 15.30. CASTLE. Both of these tumors show areas of squamous differentiation. Intercellular bridges and cytoplasmic keratinization is better developed in the tumor in the left panel. Note the lymphocytes at the periphery and scattered within the tumor nests.

Immunohistochemistry and Molecular Diagnostics

The neoplastic cells are strongly immunoreactive with pancytokeratin, CD5 (Fig. 15.31), p63, and CEA, whereas the lymphoid cells are *negative* for *immature* T-cell markers (TdT+/CD1a+).[73,124,127,130,132] The tumor cells exhibit a scattered pattern of S100A9–positive cells, similar to that of thymoma.[75] Synaptophysin and chromogranin-A reactivity has been reported.[130] The neoplastic cells are nonreactive with TTF1, thyroglobulin, chromogranin, calcitonin, and Epstein–Barr virus–encoded RNA (EBER).[57,125,133] CASTLE is also immunoreactive with *bcl-1* and *mcl-1* (antiapoptosis proto-oncogenes), which are also expressed by most thymic carcinomas but only rarely by thymomas.[124]

Cytopathology

Cellular smears display atypical epithelial cells arranged in sheets and single cells. The cells have easily identified nucleoli within nuclei that have delicate and vesicular nuclear chromatin. A background of lymphoid elements is present. Definitive separation from metastatic tumors (such as nonkeratinizing nasopharyngeal carcinoma) is difficult.[128,134]

Differential Diagnosis

The major differential diagnostic considerations include undifferentiated thyroid carcinoma, primary thyroid gland SCC, medullary carcinoma, follicular dendritic cell sarcoma, direct extension from a thymic tumor, and metastatic lymphoepithelial carcinoma (a previously used term for CASTLE). Separation is important because many of the tumors in the differential diagnosis are associated with a significantly worse prognosis.[127] Undifferentiated thyroid carcinoma generally has significant invasion, remarkable pleomorphism, atypical mitotic figures, and tumor necrosis.[75] SCC tends to display more keratinization, is invasive, and is nonreactive with CD5.[57,73,131] Medullary carcinoma may have spindle cell morphology, contains amyloid, and is immunoreactive with calcitonin, chromogranin, and CEA.[125] Follicular dendritic cell sarcoma may have a lobulated growth with extensive vascular space invasion, but it is negative with keratin and CD5.[135] Radiographs should help define any direct extension or continuity from a thymic tumor—specifically, from the cervical thymus, although CD5 will be positive in both tumors. Lymphoepithelial carcinoma is strongly associated with Epstein–Barr virus (EBV), the latter supported by a strong in situ hybridization with EBER (Fig. 15.32), whereas CASTLE is negative for EBER.[133]

Treatment and Prognosis

Thyroidectomy and selected lymph node dissection with adjuvant therapy (usually radiotherapy) is the treatment of choice. Local recurrences and local lymph node metastases are seen in as many as 30% of patients, findings associated with a worse prognosis.[126,127,136] Patients managed with radiation tend not

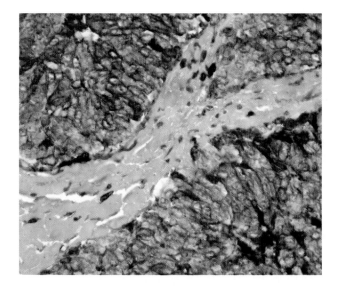

FIGURE 15.31. CASTLE. The tumor cells have cell membrane CD5 immunostaining. T cells within the tumor and in the stroma serve as an internal positive control.

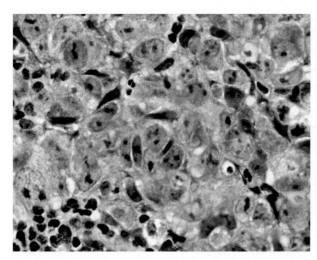 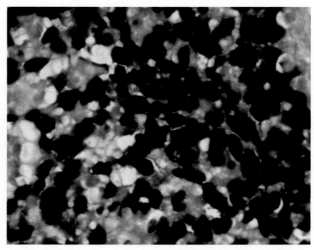

FIGURE 15.32. **Lymphoepithelial carcinoma.** The syncytial architecture with prominent nucleoli can mimic CASTLE **(left)**; however, the strong and diffuse in situ hybridization with EBER confirms the diagnosis **(right)**.

to develop locoregional recurrence.[127,136] Adjuvant chemotherapy may shrink the tumor to prevent airway compromise and thereby allow for definitive surgery.[126,136] Because only a limited number of cases have been reported, any definitive comment about prognosis would be unreliable. Even so, most patients survive many years (10-year cause-specific survival: 82%); only occasionally do patients experience a rapidly fatal course.[126,127,131,132,136,137]

 # ECTOPIC THYMOMA

An epithelial tumor of thymic derivation, ectopic thymoma of the thyroid is distinctly different from ectopic hamartomatous thymoma, which is a branchial cleft anlage tumor, and CASTLE and SETTLE, the latter two with evidence of thymic differentiation.[104,138]

Histogenesis and Molecular Genetics

During embryologic development, the thyroid primordia come into direct contact with the third and fourth branchial pouches, structures that give rise to the parathyroid glands and the thymus (see Chapter 2). It has been postulated that ectopic, trapped, or residual thymic tissue retains the potential to give rise to this neoplasm.[104,138-140]

Clinical Presentation

An exceedingly rare tumor, ectopic thymoma affects middle-aged patients, with an almost exclusive presentation in women. A nodular mass lesion is identified in the thyroid that has often been present for years. Compressive symptoms (dyspnea, hoarseness) may be noted.[104,138-148] Myasthenia gravis has not been reported in the thyroid gland tumors. Radiographic studies are nondiscriminating, but they may demonstrate attachment to the thymus.[144,146,149,150] The results of thyroid function studies are normal.

Pathology

Gross Presentation

Almost all reported cases of ectopic thymoma in the thyroid have been noninvasive. The cut surfaces show lobulated yellow-tan tumor interspersed with whitish fibrous septa.[104,138,140]

Microscopic Description

The tumor is well circumscribed and encapsulated, although it is often nodular to bosselated at the periphery; compressed or atrophic thymic tissue may also be identified at the periphery.[104,138,140,143] The tumors are separated into nodules by fibrous septa. The epithelial cells are interspersed with lymphocytes, often arranged in a jumbled fashion (Fig. 15.33). The epithelial cells are polygonal to spindled, occasionally appearing epidermoid (Fig. 15.34). Mitotic figures may be seen. The histologic appearance of this tumor in the thyroid is identical to that of the subtypes described by the World Health Organization (type A, B, or AB) in the thymus.[104,138,140]

Immunohistochemistry and Molecular Diagnostics

The epithelial cells are reactive with keratins, whereas the lymphoid component has T-cell antigens and terminal TdT. A high proliferation index can be highlighted with Ki-67. EBV is negative.[138,143,148]

Cytopathology

The smears are variably cellular, with tissue fragments, isolated spindled to polygonal cells, and a background of blood and lymphoid cells. The epithelial nuclei are round to elongated with delicate to finely granular chromatin and inconspicuous nucleoli. The lymphoid population may sometimes demonstrate atypia. The smears may mimic lymphocytic thyroiditis or a lymphoma if the lymphoid component dominates. Necrosis, mitotic figures, and pleomorphism are not identified.[141,142,146,147] Flow cytometry may be gated for a thymoma.[147]

Differential Diagnosis

The main differential diagnosis depends on the type of thymoma: epithelium-rich tumors are to be distinguished from undifferentiated thyroid carcinoma, SCC, and ectopic hamartomatous thymoma, whereas lymphocyte-rich neoplasms are to be differentiated from lymphoma.[148] Undifferentiated carcinoma has significantly more pleomorphism, is widely invasive, and may have thyroid follicular differentiation immunohistochemically.[138] *Ectopic hamartomatous thymoma*, which is actually a misnomer (no thymic differentiation), presents as a benign lesion of the low-anterior neck (sternoclavicular region) predominantly in men; it features plump, spindled cells arranged in fascicles, solid and

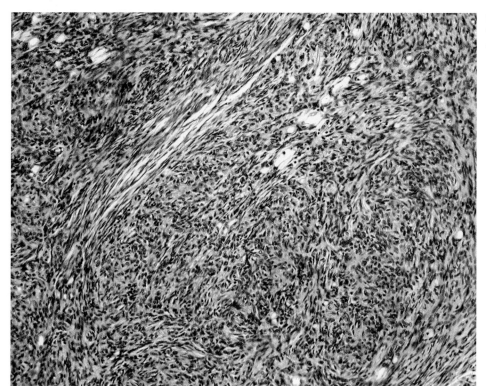

FIGURE 15.33. Ectopic thymoma. An intersection of spindled and epithelioid cells comprises this thymoma.

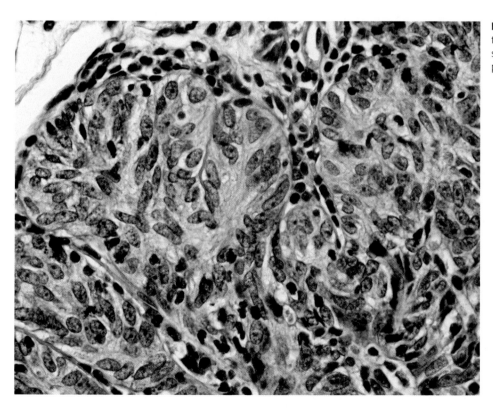

FIGURE 15.34. Ectopic thymoma. The epithelioid cells have elongated nuclei. Note the scattered lymphocytes within the tumor at the periphery.

FIGURE 15.35. Ectopic hamartomatous thymoma. Fascicles of plump spindled cells interspersed with solid and cystic squamous epithelium and fat.

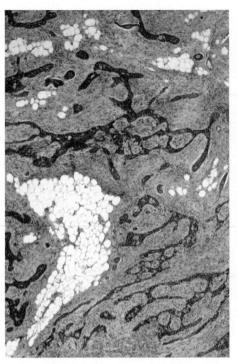
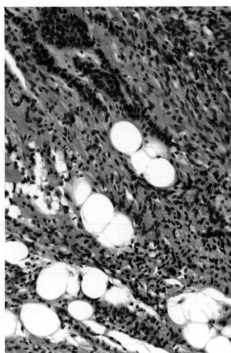

cystic squamous epithelium, glandular areas, and fat (Fig. 15.35). The cells have a mixed epithelial and myoepithelial phenotype (keratin 5/6, smooth muscle actin, CD10, calponin).[151]

Treatment and Prognosis

Ectopic thymomas are benign tumors, although isolated cases of lymph node metastasis have been reported. Surgical excision is the treatment of choice.[104,138,143,144]

REFERENCES

1. Cameselle-Teijeiro J, Wenig BM, Sobrinho-Simões M, et al. Mucoepidermoid carcinoma. In: DeLellis RA, Lloyd RV, Heitz PU, Eng C, eds. *Pathology and Genetics of Tumours of Endocrine Organs.* Lyon, France: IARC Press; 2004:82–83.
2. Bakri K, Shimaoka K, Rao U, et al. Adenosquamous carcinoma of the thyroid after radiotherapy for Hodgkin's disease. A case report and review. *Cancer.* 1983;52:465–470.
3. Bondeson L, Bondeson AG, Thompson NW. Papillary carcinoma of the thyroid with mucoepidermoid features. *Am J Clin Pathol.* 1991;95:175–179.
4. Wenig BM, Adair CF, Heffess CS. Primary mucoepidermoid carcinoma of the thyroid gland: a report of six cases and a review of the literature of a follicular epithelial-derived tumor. *Hum Pathol.* 1995;26:1099–1108.
5. Ando M, Nakanishi Y, Asai M, et al. Mucoepidermoid carcinoma of the thyroid gland showing marked ciliation suggestive of its pathogenesis. *Pathol Int.* 2008;58:741–744.
6. Cameselle-Teijeiro J. Mucoepidermoid carcinoma and solid cell nests of the thyroid. *Hum Pathol.* 1996;27:861–863.
7. Harach HR. A study on the relationship between solid cell nests and mucoepidermoid carcinoma of the thyroid. *Histopathology.* 1985;9:195–207.
8. Arezzo A, Patetta R, Ceppa P, et al. Mucoepidermoid carcinoma of the thyroid gland arising from a papillary epithelial neoplasm. *Am Surg.* 1998;64:307–311.
9. Minagawa A, Iitaka M, Suzuki M, et al. A case of primary mucoepidermoid carcinoma of the thyroid: molecular evidence of its origin. *Clin Endocrinol.* 2002;57:551–556.
10. Baloch ZW, Solomon AC, Li V, V. Primary mucoepidermoid carcinoma and sclerosing mucoepidermoid carcinoma with eosinophilia of the thyroid gland: a report of nine cases. *Mod Pathol.* 2000;13:802–807.
11. Cameselle-Teijeiro J, Febles-Perez C, Sobrinho-Simoes M. Cytologic features of fine needle aspirates of papillary and mucoepidermoid carcinoma of the thyroid with anaplastic transformation. A case report. *Acta Cytol.* 1997;41:1356–1360.
12. Franssila KO, Harach HR, Wasenius VM. Mucoepidermoid carcinoma of the thyroid. *Histopathology.* 1984;8:847–860.
13. Miranda RN, Myint MA, Gnepp DR. Composite follicular variant of papillary carcinoma and mucoepidermoid carcinoma of the thyroid. Report of a case and review of the literature. *Am J Surg Pathol.* 1995;19:1209–1215.
14. Trovisco V, Vieira de Castro I, Soares P, et al. *BRAF* mutations are associated with some histological types of papillary thyroid carcinoma. *J Pathol.* 2004;202:247–251.
15. Tirado Y, Williams MD, Hanna EY, et al. *CRTC1/MAML2* fusion transcript in high grade mucoepidermoid carcinomas of salivary and thyroid glands and Warthin's tumors: implications for histogenesis and biologic behavior. *Genes Chromosomes Cancer.* 2007;46:708–715.
16. Katoh R, Sugai T, Ono S, et al. Mucoepidermoid carcinoma of the thyroid gland. *Cancer.* 1990;65:2020–2027.
17. Bhandarkar ND, Chan J, Strome M. A rare case of mucoepidermoid carcinoma of the thyroid. *Am J Otolaryngol.* 2005;26:138–141.
18. Monroe MM, Sauer DA, Samuels MH, et al. Pathology quiz case 1. Coexistent conventional mucoepidermoid carcinoma of the thyroid (MECT) and papillary thyroid carcinoma. *Arch Otolaryngol Head Neck Surg.* 2009;135:720, 722.
19. Viciana MJ, Galera-Davidson H, Martin-Lacave I, et al. Papillary carcinoma of the thyroid with mucoepidermoid differentiation. *Arch Pathol Lab Med.* 1996;120:397–398.
20. Vazquez Ramirez F, Otal Salaverri C, Argueta Manzano O, et al. Fine needle aspiration cytology of high grade mucoepidermoid carcinoma of the thyroid. A case report. *Acta Cytol.* 2000;44:259–264.
21. Rocha AS, Soares P, Machado JC, et al. Mucoepidermoid carcinoma of the thyroid: a tumour histotype characterised by P-cadherin neoexpression and marked abnormalities of E-cadherin/catenins complex. *Virchows Arch.* 2002;440:498–504.
22. Hunt JL. Unusual thyroid tumors: a review of pathologic and molecular diagnosis. *Expert Rev Mol Diagn.* 2005;5:725–734.
23. Larson RS, Wick MR. Primary mucoepidermoid carcinoma of the thyroid: diagnosis by fine-needle aspiration biopsy. *Diagn Cytopathol.* 1993;9:438–443.
24. Cameselle-Teijeiro J, Sobrinho-Simoes M. Cytomorphologic features of mucoepidermoid carcinoma of the thyroid. *Am J Clin Pathol.* 1999;111:134–136.
25. Sanchez-Sosa S, Rios-Luna NP, Tamayo BR, et al. Primary squamous cell carcinoma of the thyroid arising in Hashimoto's thyroiditis in an adolescent. *Pediatr Dev Pathol.* 2006;9:496–500.
26. Franca SR, Caldas D, Alcebiades V, et al. [Mucoepidermoid carcinoma of the thyroid: a case report and literature review]. *Arq Bras Endocrinol Metabol.* 2006;50:968–976.
27. Chan JK, bores-Saavedra J, Battifora H, et al. Sclerosing mucoepidermoid thyroid carcinoma with eosinophilia. A distinctive low-grade malignancy arising from the metaplastic follicles of Hashimoto's thyroiditis. *Am J Surg Pathol.* 1991;15:438–448.
28. Chan JKC, LiVolsi V, Bondeson L, et al. Sclerosing mucoepidermoid carcinoma with eosinophilia. In: DeLellis RA, Lloyd RV, Heitz PU, Eng C, eds. *Pathology and Genetics of Tumours of Endocrine Organs.* Lyon, France: IARC Press; 2004:84.

29. Albores-Saavedra J, Gu X, Luna MA. Clear cells and thyroid transcription factor I reactivity in sclerosing mucoepidermoid carcinoma of the thyroid gland. *Ann Diagn Pathol.* 2003;7:348–353.
30. Hunt JL, LiVolsi VA, Barnes EL. p63 expression in sclerosing mucoepidermoid carcinomas with eosinophilia arising in the thyroid. *Mod Pathol.* 2004;17:526–529.
31. Ryska A, Ludvikova M, Rydlova M, et al. Massive squamous metaplasia of the thyroid gland—report of three cases. *Pathol Res Pract.* 2006;202:99–106.
32. Calo PG, Maxia S, Lai ML, et al. Sclerosing mucoepidermoid thyroid carcinoma requiring cervical reconstruction: a case report and review of the literature. *Am Surg.* 2010;76:918–919.
33. Cavazza A, Toschi E, Valcavi R, et al. [Sclerosing mucoepidermoid carcinoma with eosinophilia of the thyroid: description of a case]. *Pathologica.* 1999;91:31–35.
34. Chung J, Lee SK, Gong G, et al. Sclerosing mucoepidermoid carcinoma with eosinophilia of the thyroid glands: a case report with clinical manifestation of recurrent neck mass. *J Korean Med Sci (Korea).* 1999;14:338–341.
35. Geisinger KR, Steffee CH, McGee RS, et al. The cytomorphologic features of sclerosing mucoepidermoid carcinoma of the thyroid gland with eosinophilia. *Am J Clin Pathol.* 1998;109:294–301.
36. Sim SJ, Ro JY, Ordonez NG, et al. Sclerosing mucoepidermoid carcinoma with eosinophilia of the thyroid: report of two patients, one with distant metastasis, and review of the literature. *Hum Pathol.* 1997;28:1091–1096.
37. Shehadeh NJ, Vernick J, Lonardo F, et al. Sclerosing mucoepidermoid carcinoma with eosinophilia of the thyroid: a case report and review of the literature. *Am J Otolaryngol.* 2004;25:48–53.
38. Bondeson L, Bondeson AG. Cytologic features in fine-needle aspirates from a sclerosing mucoepidermoid thyroid carcinoma with eosinophilia. *Diagn Cytopathol.* 1996;15:301–305.
39. Solomon AC, Baloch ZW, Salhany KE, et al. Thyroid sclerosing mucoepidermoid carcinoma with eosinophilia: mimic of Hodgkin disease in nodal metastases. *Arch Pathol Lab Med.* 2000;124:446–449.
40. Musso-Lassalle S, Butori C, Bailleux S, et al. A diagnostic pitfall: nodular tumor-like squamous metaplasia with Hashimoto's thyroiditis mimicking a sclerosing mucoepidermoid carcinoma with eosinophilia. *Pathol Res Pract.* 2006;202:379–383.
41. Lam KY, Sakamoto A. Squamous cell carcinoma. In: DeLellis RA, Lloyd RV, Heitz PU, Eng C, eds. *Pathology and Genetics of Tumours of Endocrine Organs.* Lyon, France: IARC Press; 2004:81.
42. Chen CY, Tseng HS, Lee CH, et al. Primary squamous cell carcinoma of the thyroid gland with eggshell calcification: sonographic and computed tomographic findings. *J Ultrasound Med.* 2010;29:1667–1670.
43. Korovin GS, Kuriloff DB, Cho HT, et al. Squamous cell carcinoma of the thyroid: a diagnostic dilemma. *Ann Otol Rhinol Laryngol.* 1989;98:59–65.
44. Sahoo M, Bal CS, Bhatnagar D. Primary squamous-cell carcinoma of the thyroid gland: new evidence in support of follicular epithelial cell origin. *Diagn Cytopathol.* 2002;27:227–231.
45. Yucel H, Schaper NC, van BM, et al. Primary squamous cell carcinoma of the thyroid years after radioactive iodine treatment. *Neth J Med.* 2010;68:224–226.
46. Chaudhary RK, Barnes EL, Myers EN. Squamous cell carcinoma arising in Hashimoto's thyroiditis. *Head Neck.* 1994;16:582–585.
47. Harada T, Shimaoka K, Yakumaru K, et al. Squamous cell carcinoma of the thyroid gland—transition from adenocarcinoma. *J Surg Oncol.* 1982;19:36–43.
48. Kampsen EB, Jager N, Max MH. Squamous cell carcinoma of the thyroid: a report of two cases. *J Surg Oncol.* 1977;9:567–578.
49. Tsuchiya A, Suzuki S, Nomizu T, et al. Squamous cell carcinoma of the thyroid—a report of three cases. *Jpn J Surg.* 1990;20:341–345.
50. Onai T, Maruta S, Yamada M, et al. [Primary squamous cell carcinoma of the thyroid gland possibly transformed from papillary adenocarcinoma after irradiation]. *Nippon Naika Gakkai Zasshi.* 1989;78:1775–1776.
51. Syed MI, Stewart M, Syed S, et al. Squamous cell carcinoma of the thyroid gland: primary or secondary disease? *J Laryngol Otol.* 2011;125:3–9.
52. Cook AM, Vini L, Harmer C. Squamous cell carcinoma of the thyroid: outcome of treatment in 16 patients. *Eur J Surg Oncol.* 1999;25:606–609.
53. Booya F, Sebo TJ, Kasperbauer JL, et al. Primary squamous cell carcinoma of the thyroid: report of ten cases. *Thyroid.* 2006;16:89–93.
54. Cameselle-Teijeiro J. Uncommon tumors of the thyroid gland. *Int J Surg Pathol.* 2010;18:205S–208S.
55. Ezaki H, Ebihara S, Fujimoto Y, et al. Analysis of thyroid carcinoma based on material registered in Japan during 1977–1986 with special reference to predominance of papillary type. *Cancer.* 1992;70:808–814.
56. Kleer CG, Giordano TJ, Merino MJ. Squamous cell carcinoma of the thyroid: an aggressive tumor associated with tall cell variant of papillary thyroid carcinoma. *Mod Pathol.* 2000;13:742–746.
57. Lam KY, Lo CY, Liu MC. Primary squamous cell carcinoma of the thyroid gland: an entity with aggressive clinical behaviour and distinctive cytokeratin expression profiles. *Histopathology.* 2001;39:279–286.
58. Simpson WJ, Carruthers J. Squamous cell carcinoma of the thyroid gland. *Am J Surg.* 1988;156:44–46.
59. Kasantikul V, Maneesri S, Panichabhong V, et al. Adenosquamous carcinoma of the thyroid: a case report and review of the literature. *J Med Assoc Thai.* 1995;78:197–203.
60. Burman KD, Ringel MD, Wartofsky L. Unusual types of thyroid neoplasms. *Endocrinol Metab Clin North Am.* 1996;25:49–68.
61. Riddle PE, Dincsoy HP. Primary squamous cell carcinoma of the thyroid associated with leukocytosis and hypercalcemia. *Arch Pathol Lab Med.* 1987;111:373–374.
62. Saito K, Kuratomi Y, Yamamoto K, et al. Primary squamous cell carcinoma of the thyroid associated with marked leukocytosis and hypercalcemia. *Cancer.* 1981;48:2080–2083.
63. Nakhjavani M, Gharib H, Goellner JR, et al. Direct extension of malignant lesions to the thyroid gland from adjacent organs: report of 17 cases. *Endocr Pract.* 1999;5:69–71.
64. Ashraf MJ, Azarpira N, Khademi B, et al. Squamous cell carcinoma associated with tall cell variant of papillary carcinoma of the thyroid. *Indian J Pathol Microbiol.* 2010;53:548–550.
65. Harada T, Shimaoka K, Katagiri M, et al. Rarity of squamous cell carcinoma of the thyroid: autopsy review. *World J Surg.* 1994;18:542–546.
66. Katoh R, Sakamoto A, Kasai N, et al. Squamous differentiation in thyroid carcinoma. With special reference to histogenesis of squamous cell carcinoma of the thyroid. *Acta Pathol Jpn.* 1989;39:306–312.
67. Noh SJ, Cha EJ, Choi KH, et al. Papillary carcinoma of the thyroid with massive squamous metaplasia after fine needle aspiration: a potential diagnostic pitfall. *Acta Cytol.* 2009;53:605–607.
68. Thompson LD, Wieneke JA, Heffess CS. Diffuse sclerosing variant of papillary thyroid carcinoma: a clinicopathologic and immunophenotypic analysis of 22 cases. *Endocr Pathol.* 2005;16:331–348.
69. Sarda AK, Bal S, Arunabh Singh MK, et al. Squamous cell carcinoma of the thyroid. *J Surg Oncol.* 1988;39:175–178.
70. Sutak J, Armstrong JS, Rusby JE. Squamous cell carcinoma arising in a tall cell papillary carcinoma of the thyroid. *J Clin Pathol.* 2005;58:662–664.
71. Jung TS, Oh YL, Min YK, et al. A patient with primary squamous cell carcinoma of the thyroid intermingled with follicular thyroid carcinoma that remains alive more than 8 years after diagnosis. *Korean J Intern Med.* 2006;21:73–78.
72. Motoyama T, Watanabe H. Simultaneous squamous cell carcinoma and papillary adenocarcinoma of the thyroid gland. *Hum Pathol.* 1983;14:1009–1010.
73. Reimann JD, Dorfman DM, Nose V. Carcinoma showing thymus-like differentiation of the thyroid (CASTLE): a comparative study: evidence of thymic differentiation and solid cell nest origin. *Am J Surg Pathol.* 2006;30:994–1001.
74. Dorfman DM, Shahsafaei A, Miyauchi A. Intrathyroidal epithelial thymoma (ITET)/carcinoma showing thymus-like differentiation (CASTLE) exhibits CD5 immunoreactivity: new evidence for thymic differentiation. *Histopathology.* 1998;32:104–109.
75. Ito Y, Miyauchi A, Arai K, et al. Usefulness of S100A9 for diagnosis of intrathyroid epithelial thymoma (ITET)/carcinoma showing thymus-like differentiation (CASTLE). *Pathology.* 2006;38:541–544.
76. Bonetti LR, Lupi M, Trani M, et al. EGFR polysomy in squamous cell carcinoma of the thyroid. Report of two cases and review of the literature. *Tumori.* 2010;96:503–507.
77. Dequanter D, Lothaire P, Larsimont D, et al. [Intrathyroid metastasis: 11 cases]. *Ann Endocrinol (Paris).* 2004;65:205–208.
78. Hanna E. Squamous cell carcinoma in a thyroglossal duct cyst (TGDC): clinical presentation, diagnosis, and management. *Am J Otolaryngol.* 1996;17:353–357.
79. Kumar PV, Malekhusseini SA, Talei AR. Primary squamous cell carcinoma of the thyroid diagnosed by fine needle aspiration cytology. A report of two cases. *Acta Cytol.* 1999;43:659–662.
80. Mai KT, Yazdi HM, MacDonald L. Fine needle aspiration biopsy of primary squamous cell carcinoma of the thyroid. *Acta Cytol.* 1999;43:1194–1196.
81. Jacobson AS, Wenig BM, Urken ML. Collision tumor of the thyroid and larynx: a patient with papillary thyroid carcinoma colliding with laryngeal squamous cell carcinoma. *Thyroid.* 2008;18:1325–1328.
82. Chen H, Nicol TL, Udelsman R. Clinically significant, isolated metastatic disease to the thyroid gland. *World J Surg.* 1999;23:177–180.
83. Cheuk W, Chan JKC, Dorfman DM, et al. Carcinoma showing thymus-like differentiation. In: DeLellis RA, Lloyd RV, Heitz PU, Eng C, eds. *Pathology and Genetics of Tumours of Endocrine Organs.* Lyon, France: IARC Press; 2004:96–97.
84. Zhou XH. Primary squamous cell carcinoma of the thyroid. *Eur J Surg Oncol.* 2002;28:42–45.
85. *AJCC Cancer Staging Manual.* 7th ed. New York, NY: Springer; 2010.
86. *International Union against Cancer (UICC): TNM Classification of Malignant Tumours.* 6th ed. New York, NY: Wiley, John & Sons; 2002.
87. Sobrinho-Simões M, Cameselle-Teijeiro J, Harach HR. Mucinous carcinoma. In: DeLellis RA, Lloyd RV, Heitz PU, Eng C, eds. *Pathology and Genetics of Tumours of Endocrine Organs.* Lyon, France: IARC Press; 2004:85.
88. Cameselle-Teijeiro J, Varela-Duran J, Sambade C, et al. Solid cell nests of the thyroid: light microscopy and immunohistochemical profile. *Hum Pathol.* 1994;25:684–693.
89. Sobrinho-Simoes MA, Nesland JM, Johannessen JV. A mucin-producing tumor in the thyroid gland. *Ultrastruct Pathol.* 1985;9:277–281.
90. Deligdisch L, Subhani Z, Gordon RE. Primary mucinous carcinoma of the thyroid gland: report of a case and ultrastructural study. *Cancer.* 1980;45:2564–2567.
91. Diaz-Perez R, Quiroz H, Nishiyama RH. Primary mucinous adenocarcinoma of thyroid gland. *Cancer.* 1976;38:1323–1325.
92. Harada T, Shimaoka K, Hiratsuka M, et al. Mucin-producing carcinoma of the thyroid gland—a case report and review of the literature. *Jpn J Clin Oncol.* 1984;14:417–424.
93. Kondo T, Kato Y, Nakazawa T, et al. Mucinous carcinoma (poorly differentiated carcinoma with extensive extracellular mucin deposition) of the thyroid: a case report with immunohistochemical studies. *Hum Pathol.* 2005;36:698–701.
94. Mizukami Y, Nakajima H, Annen Y, et al. Mucin-producing poorly differentiated adenocarcinoma of the thyroid. A case report. *Pathol Res Pract.* 1993;189:608–612.

95. Sobrinho-Simoes M, Stenwig AE, Nesland JM, et al. A mucinous carcinoma of the thyroid. *Pathol Res Pract.* 1986;181:464–471.
96. Rigaud C, Peltier F, Bogomoletz WV. Mucin producing microfollicular adenoma of the thyroid. *J Clin Pathol.* 1985;38:277–280.
97. Fonseca E, Castanhas S, Sobrinho-Simoes M. Expression of simple mucin type antigens and Lewis type 1 and type 2 chain antigens in the thyroid gland: an immunohistochemical study of normal thyroid tissues, benign lesions, and malignant tumors. *Endocr Pathol.* 1996;7:291–301.
98. Alves P, Soares P, Fonseca E, et al. Papillary thyroid carcinoma overexpresses fully and underglycosylated mucins together with native and sialylated simple mucin antigens and histo-blood group antigens. *Endocr Pathol.* 1999;10:315–324.
99. Patel KN, Maghami E, Wreesmann VB, et al. MUC1 plays a role in tumor maintenance in aggressive thyroid carcinomas. *Surgery.* 2005;138:994–1001.
100. Haraguchi S, Hioki M, Yamashita K, et al. Metastasis to the thyroid from lung adenocarcinoma mimicking thyroid carcinoma. *Jpn J Thorac Cardiovasc Surg.* 2004;52:353–356.
101. Edelson GW, Kleerekoper M, Talpos GB, et al. Mucin-producing parathyroid carcinoma. *Bone.* 1992;13:7–10.
102. Uccella S, La RS, Finzi G, et al. Mixed mucus-secreting and oncocytic carcinoma of the thyroid: pathologic, histochemical, immunohistochemical, and ultrastructural study of a case. *Arch Pathol Lab Med.* 2000;124:1547–1552.
103. Cheuk W, Chan JKC, Dorfman DM, et al. Spindle cell tumour with thymus-like differentiation. In: DeLellis RA, Lloyd RV, Heitz PU, Eng C, eds. *Pathology and Genetics of Tumours of Endocrine Organs.* Lyon, France: IARC Press; 2004:94–95.
104. Chan JK, Rosai J. Tumors of the neck showing thymic or related branchial pouch differentiation: a unifying concept. *Hum Pathol.* 1991;22:349–367.
105. Cheuk W, Jacobson AA, Chan JK. Spindle epithelial tumor with thymus-like differentiation (SETTLE): a distinctive malignant thyroid neoplasm with significant metastatic potential. *Mod Pathol.* 2000;13:1150–1155.
106. Folpe AL, Lloyd RV, Bacchi CE, et al. Spindle epithelial tumor with thymus-like differentiation: a morphologic, immunohistochemical, and molecular genetic study of 11 cases. *Am J Surg Pathol.* 2009;33:1179–1186.
107. Abrosimov AY, LiVolsi VA. Spindle epithelial tumor with thymus-like differentiation (SETTLE) of the thyroid with neck lymph node metastasis: a case report. *Endocr Pathol.* 2005;16:139–143.
108. Casco F, Illanes MM, Gonzalez CR, et al. Spindle epithelial tumor with thymus-like differentiation in a 2-year-old boy: a case report. *Anal Quant Cytol Histol.* 2010;32:53–57.
109. Chetty R, Goetsch S, Nayler S, et al. Spindle epithelial tumour with thymus-like element (SETTLE): the predominantly monophasic variant. *Histopathology.* 1998;33:71–74.
110. Grushka JR, Ryckman J, Mueller C, et al. Spindle epithelial tumor with thymus-like differentiation of the thyroid: a multi-institutional case series and review of the literature. *J Pediatr Surg.* 2009;44:944–948.
111. Hofman P, Mainguene C, Michiels JF, et al. Thyroid spindle epithelial tumor with thymus-like differentiation (the "SETTLE" tumor). An immunohistochemical and electron microscopic study. *Eur Arch Otorhinolaryngol.* 1995;252:316–320.
112. Iwasa K, Imai MA, Noguchi M, et al. Spindle epithelial tumor with thymus-like differentiation of the thyroid. *Head Neck.* 2002;24:888–893.
113. Kirby PA, Ellison WA, Thomas PA. Spindle epithelial tumor with thymus-like differentiation (SETTLE) of the thyroid with prominent mitotic activity and focal necrosis. *Am J Surg Pathol.* 1999;23:712–716.
114. Kloboves-Prevodnik V, Jazbec J, Us-Krasovec M, et al. Thyroid spindle epithelial tumor with thymus-like differentiation (SETTLE): is cytopathological diagnosis possible? *Diagn Cytopathol.* 2002;26:314–319.
115. Nisa A, Barakzai A, Minhas K, et al. Spindle epithelial tumor with thymus-like differentiation of thyroid gland: report of two cases with follow-up. *Indian J Pathol Microbiol.* 2010;53:781–784.
116. Raffel A, Cupisti K, Rees M, et al. Spindle epithelial tumour with thymus-like differentiation (SETTLE) of the thyroid gland with widespread metastases in a 13-year-old girl. *Clin Oncol (R Coll Radiol).* 2003;15:490–495.
117. Satoh S, Toda S, Narikawa K, et al. Spindle epithelial tumor with thymus-like differentiation (SETTLE): youngest reported patient. *Pathol Int.* 2006;56:563–567.
118. Su L, Beals T, Bernacki EG, et al. Spindle epithelial tumor with thymus-like differentiation: a case report with cytologic, histologic, immunohistologic, and ultrastructural findings. *Mod Pathol.* 1997;10:510–514.
119. Tong GX, Hamele-Bena D, Wei XJ, et al. Fine-needle aspiration biopsy of monophasic variant of spindle epithelial tumor with thymus-like differentiation of the thyroid: report of one case and review of the literature. *Diagn Cytopathol.* 2007;35:113–119.
120. Xu B, Hirokawa M, Yoshimoto K, et al. Spindle epithelial tumor with thymus-like differentiation of the thyroid: a case report with pathological and molecular genetics study. *Hum Pathol.* 2003;34:190–193.
121. Haberal AN, Aydin H, Turan E, et al. Unusual spindle cell tumor of thyroid (SETTLE). *Thyroid.* 2008;18:85–87.
122. Erickson ML, Tapia B, Moreno ER, et al. Early metastasizing spindle epithelial tumor with thymus-like differentiation (SETTLE) of the thyroid. *Pediatr Dev Pathol.* 2005;8:599–606.
123. Kingsley DPE, Elton A, Bennett MH. Malignant teratomas of the thyroid. Case report and a review of the literature. *Br J Cancer.* 1968;22:7–11.
124. Dorfman DM, Shahsafaei A, Miyauchi A. Immunohistochemical staining for *bcl-2* and *mcl-1* in intrathyroidal epithelial thymoma (ITET)/carcinoma showing thymus-like differentiation (CASTLE) and cervical thymic carcinoma. *Mod Pathol.* 1998;11:989–994.
125. Asa SL, Dardick I, Van Nostrand AW, et al. Primary thyroid thymoma: a distinct clinicopathologic entity. *Hum Pathol.* 1988;19:1463–1467.
126. Chow SM, Chan JK, Tse LL, et al. Carcinoma showing thymus-like element (CASTLE) of thyroid: combined modality treatment in 3 patients with locally advanced disease. *Eur J Surg Oncol.* 2007;33:83–85.
127. Ito Y, Miyauchi A, Nakamura Y, et al. Clinicopathologic significance of intrathyroidal epithelial thymoma/carcinoma showing thymus-like differentiation: a collaborative study with Member Institutes of The Japanese Society of Thyroid Surgery. *Am J Clin Pathol.* 2007;127:230–236.
128. Youens KE, Bean SM, Dodd LG, et al. Thyroid carcinoma showing thymus-like differentiation (CASTLE): case report with cytomorphology and review of the literature. *Diagn Cytopathol.* 2011;39:204–209.
129. Musella M, De Franciscis S, Amorosi A, et al. CASTLE tumour of the thyroid. Value of multiplanar imaging acquisition. *Ann Ital Chir.* 2006;77:509–512.
130. Yamazaki M, Fujii S, Daiko H, et al. Carcinoma showing thymus-like differentiation (CASTLE) with neuroendocrine differentiation. *Pathol Int.* 2008;58:775–779.
131. Da J, Shi H, Lu J. [Thyroid squamous-cell carcinoma showing thymus-like element (CASTLE): a report of eight cases]. *Zhonghua Zhong Liu Za Zhi.* 1999;21:303–304.
132. Chan LP, Chiang FY, Lee KW, et al. Carcinoma showing thymus-like differentiation (CASTLE) of thyroid: a case report and literature review. *Kaohsiung J Med Sci.* 2008;24:591–597.
133. Shek TW, Luk IS, Ng IO, et al. Lymphoepithelioma-like carcinoma of the thyroid gland: lack of evidence of association with Epstein-Barr virus. *Hum Pathol.* 1996;27:851–853.
134. Ng WK, Collins RJ, Shek WH, et al. Cytologic diagnosis of "CASTLE" of thyroid gland: report of a case with histologic correlation. *Diagn Cytopathol.* 1996;15:224–227.
135. Moz U, Pignatelli U, Forner P, et al. Follicular dendritic cell tumour of the cervical lymph node: case report and brief review of literature. *Acta Otorhinolaryngol Ital.* 2004;24:223–225.
136. Roka S, Kornek G, Schuller J, et al. Carcinoma showing thymic-like elements—a rare malignancy of the thyroid gland. *Br J Surg.* 2004;91:142–145.
137. Cappelli C, Tironi A, Marchetti GP, et al. Aggressive thyroid carcinoma showing thymic-like differentiation (CASTLE): case report and review of the literature. *Endocr J.* 2008;55:685–690.
138. Chan JKC, Cheuk W, Dorfman DM, et al. Ectopic thymoma. In: DeLellis RA, Lloyd RV, Heitz PU, Eng C, eds. *Pathology and Genetics of Tumours of Endocrine Organs.* Lyon, France: IARC Press; 2004:112.
139. Chang ST, Chuang SS. Ectopic cervical thymoma: a mimic of T-lymphoblastic lymphoma. *Pathol Res Pract.* 2003;199:633–635.
140. Yamashita H, Murakami N, Noguchi S, et al. Cervical thymoma and incidence of cervical thymus. *Acta Pathol Jpn.* 1983;33:189–194.
141. Cohen JB, Troxell M, Kong CS, et al. Ectopic intrathyroidal thymoma: a case report and review. *Thyroid.* 2003;13:305–308.
142. Gerhard R, Kanashiro EH, Kliemann CM, et al. Fine-needle aspiration biopsy of ectopic cervical spindle-cell thymoma: a case report. *Diagn Cytopathol.* 2005;32:358–362.
143. Kwon Y, Koo H, Cho K, et al. Clinicopathological and immunohistochemical studies in three ectopic cervical thymomas (ECT) and one carcinoma showing thymus-like differentiation (CASTLE). *Korean J Pathol.* 2002;36:S133.
144. Miller WT Jr, Gefter WB, Miller WT. Thymoma mimicking a thyroid mass. *Radiology.* 1992;184:75–76.
145. Mourra N, Duron F, Parc R, et al. Cervical ectopic thymoma: a diagnostic pitfall on frozen section. *Histopathology.* 2005;46:583–585.
146. Oh YL, Ko YH, Ree HJ. Aspiration cytology of ectopic cervical thymoma mimicking a thyroid mass. A case report. *Acta Cytol.* 1998;42:1167–1171.
147. Ponder TB, Collins BT, Bee CS, et al. Diagnosis of cervical thymoma by fine needle aspiration biopsy with flow cytometry. A case report. *Acta Cytol.* 2002;46:1129–1132.
148. Vengrove MA, Schimmel M, Atkinson BF, et al. Invasive cervical thymoma masquerading as a solitary thyroid nodule. Report of a case studied by fine needle aspiration. *Acta Cytol.* 1991;35:431–433.
149. Kaplan IL, Swayne LC, Widmann WD, et al. CT demonstration of "ectopic" thymoma. *J Comput Assist Tomogr.* 1988;12:1037–1038.
150. Nagasawa K, Takahashi K, Hayashi T, et al. Ectopic cervical thymoma: MRI findings. *AJR Am J Roentgenol.* 2004;182:262–263.
151. Fetsch JF, Laskin WB, Michal M, et al. Ectopic hamartomatous thymoma: a clinicopathologic and immunohistochemical analysis of 21 cases with data supporting reclassification as a branchial anlage mixed tumor. *Am J Surg Pathol.* 2004;28:1360–1370.

Rare Primary Thyroid Nonepithelial Tumors and Tumor-like Conditions

 ## PRIMARY ANGIOSARCOMA

Primary thyroid gland angiosarcoma is a malignant tumor of endothelial cell differentiation. This generally rare thyroid tumor is more common in the Alpine countries of central Europe where there is iodine deficiency.[1] Although a pseudoangiomatous pattern can be seen in undifferentiated carcinoma, angiosarcoma is a distinct clinical, histologic, and immunophenotypic entity.

Etiology

Although the cause of thyroid angiosarcoma is considered to be multifactorial, its incidence is higher in countries where there is a dietary iodine deficiency—particularly the Alpine countries of central Europe.[2,3] Interestingly, iodized salt prophylaxis in the mountain areas of Austria where there was previously iodine deficiency resulted in a decrease in the prevalence of angiosarcoma from 3% of all thyroid gland cancers[4] in 1957–1975 to 0.7% in 1986–1995. Even so, these tumors are also reported in many countries where the intake of dietary iodine is adequate.[1,5–8] Significant occupational exposure to industrial vinyl chloride and other polymeric materials may also be contributory.[3]

Histogenesis and Molecular Genetics

An endothelial origin seems to have been confirmed, although the possibility of an undifferentiated stem cell with both epithelial and endothelial differentiation has not been entirely ruled out.[2,9]

Clinical Presentation

Thyroid angiosarcomas account for <2% of all thyroid gland malignancies, although there is geographic variability, as discussed above. Women are affected much more frequently than men (4:1). Most cases arise in the seventh decade of life. Patients present with a painless mass that has often developed in the setting of long-standing goiter; other symptoms include dyspnea, asthenia, and weight loss.[2,5,7,8,10–17] Occasionally, a rapidly growing mass is noted with pressure symptoms.[1,6,11,12] Hyperthyroidism is rare, with some authors suggesting that the angiosarcoma has a trophic effect on the follicular epithelium.[18] Scintigraphic studies usually show a "cold" nodule,[2] although ultrasound and CT studies can also be used to evaluate the nodule, showing a vascular tumor with irregular Doppler flow.[12]

Pathology

Gross Presentation

Macroscopically, the tumors may appear circumscribed, although in many cases it presents as an ill-defined mass infiltrating the thyroid parenchyma (Fig. 16.1). Tumors are usually large, measuring up to 10 cm. The cut surface is variegated, extensively hemorrhagic, with solid and cystic areas. Necrosis is common and extensive. Invasion of the surrounding soft tissues may be grossly identifiable.[1,2,7,8,13,19]

Microscopic Description

The periphery of the tumor is irregular. Freely anastomosing vascular channels infiltrate the adjacent parenchyma and soft tissues (Fig. 16.2). Tumor necrosis and hemorrhage are seen throughout. Various patterns can be seen, from solid, spindled, and papillary to pseudoglandular. Irregular, cleft-like to patulous, gaping vascular channels are common (Fig. 16.3A,B). The neoplastic large cells that line the vascular channels or are present in the solid areas are epithelioid (Fig. 16.3C,D). The cells have abundant eosinophilic cytoplasm surrounding round nuclei with vesicular nuclear chromatin (Fig. 16.4). The nuclei contain prominent, basophilic nucleoli, occasionally attached to the nuclear membrane by chromatin strands.[1,5,8,11,13,20] The cells simulate undifferentiated carcinoma.[2,5,20] Neolumen formation with erythrocytes within the newly formed channels is occasionally noted, although sometimes just vacuoles within the solid nests are present (Fig. 16.5).[7,8,13,19] Mitotic figures, including atypical forms, are frequent. Multinucleated tumor giant cells are rare, although binucleated forms are occasionally present. Hemosiderin-laden macrophages are common. Single membrane-bound, rod-shaped cytoplasmic structures (Weibel–Palade bodies) can be identified only by electron microscopy (Fig. 16.5); a pericellular basal lamina, tight junctions, and subplasmalemmal pinocytotic vesicles are also noted.[7,8,10,13,14,21]

Immunohistochemistry and Molecular Diagnostics

The neoplastic cells are strongly and diffusely immunoreactive with vimentin and various vascular endothelial markers, including factor VIII–related antigen (FVIII-RA), CD34, CD31, and *Ulex europaeus* I lectin.[1,2,5–8,10–14,17,20,22] It is important to identify cytoplasmic immunoreactivity and not just diffusion artifact or nonspecific uptake from the surrounding serum or from phagocytosis by cells in contact with the blood elements.[23] The FVIII-RA staining is quite granular and seen in all tumor cells, not just in the luminal cells. Keratins are variably positive, ranging from a few isolated cells to diffuse immunoreactive of all tumor cells (Fig. 16.5). The variability of immunoreactivity may depend on the specific keratin used (AE1/AE3, CAM5.2, or CK7), although AE1/AE3 seems to be the most frequently positive.[2,6,22] Thyroglobulin and thyroid transcription factor-1 (TTF1) are negative. Smooth muscle actin and type IV collagen react around the endothelial cells, the former highlighting smooth muscle.[1,2,6–8,13,19,20,22,24] TP53 nuclear immunoreactivity is rarely seen.[8]

Cytopathology

The interpretation of smears from a thyroid angiosarcoma is difficult, as the background is composed of necrotic material and

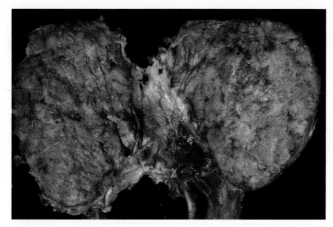 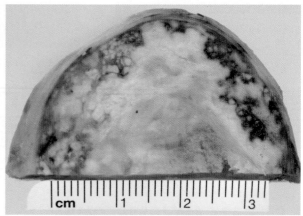

FIGURE 16.1. Primary thyroid angiosarcoma. Left: The tumor does not form a discrete nodule and shows complete effacement of thyroid parenchyma. **Right:** Another case of angiosarcoma showing a mass with extensive necrosis and focal hemorrhage. (Courtesy of Dr. A. Ryška, Department of Pathology, Charles University Medical Faculty Hospital, Hradec Kralove, Czech Republic.)

blood.[11,15,25] Isolated large, neoplastic "epithelioid" cells are identified. They usually contain abundant eosinophilic to vacuolated cytoplasm with central, round nuclei that contain prominent nucleoli. Clusters of oval to round neoplastic cells are also noted. Cell borders are indistinct.[6] Occasional intracytoplasmic lumina or vacuoles may be seen.[11] It is important to not misinterpret these findings as a metastatic tumor or as an undifferentiated carcinoma.

Differential Diagnosis

An angiomatous pattern can be seen in undifferentiated carcinoma,[2,9,15,21,23,26] but there is often a greater degree of pleomorphism and significantly more giant tumor cells. Immunostains for endothelial markers confirm the diagnosis. Adenomatoid nodules with degenerative or retrogressive changes may contain areas of

vascular proliferation. Organization of clot within a nodule can yield a mass lesion.[15] In the post–fine-needle aspiration (FNA) setting, a Masson papillary endothelial hyperplasia type of reaction may be seen; sometimes, it is quite florid. However, a well-defined area of involvement, a finding of involvement within a vessel or nodule, a lack of cytologic atypia, and a lack of freely anastomosing vessels help make the distinction.[15,27] Metastatic tumors (renal cell carcinoma and angiosarcoma[25]) and direct invasion into the thyroid gland from a soft-tissue primary should be separable based on clinical, radiographic, and histologic findings and immunophenotypic studies.[28]

Treatment and Prognosis

Combination adjuvant therapy (particularly rapid radiation) and surgical eradication may not alter the prognosis, as most patients

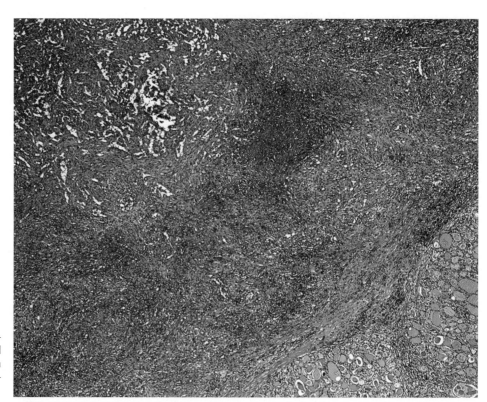

FIGURE 16.2. Angiosarcoma. Freely anastomosing vascular channels and a spindle-cell population admixed with blood are seen destroying the adjacent thyroid gland parenchyma (lower right).

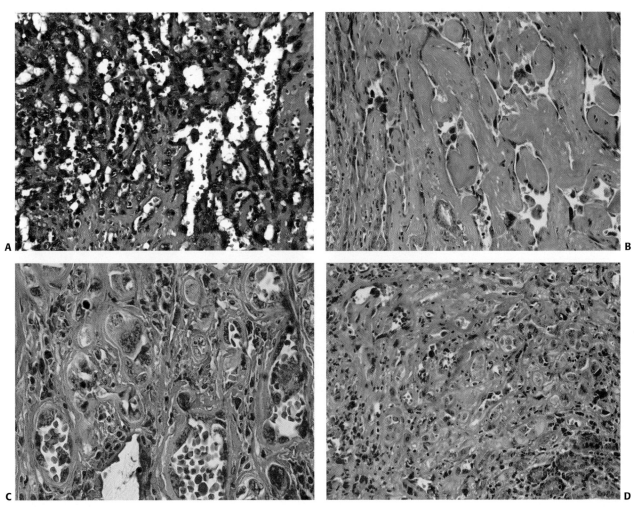

FIGURE 16.3. Angiosarcoma. A, B: Irregular, freely anastomosing to cleft-like and gaping vascular channels are seen. Large, highly atypical epithelioid cells line the vascular channels **(C)** or the gland-like profiles **(D)**.

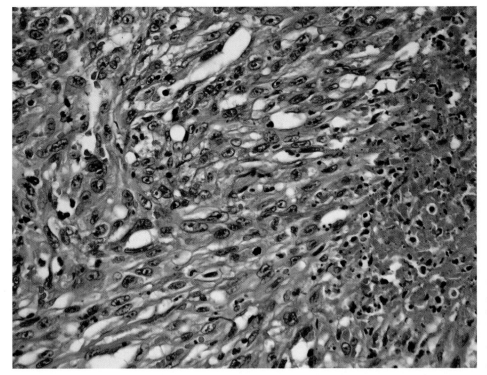

FIGURE 16.4. Angiosarcoma. The spindled-epithelioid cells have abundant eosinophilic cytoplasm surrounding nuclei with vesicular nuclear chromatin and prominent nucleoli. Note the tumor necrosis in the right field. This angiosarcoma appearance simulates an anaplastic carcinoma.

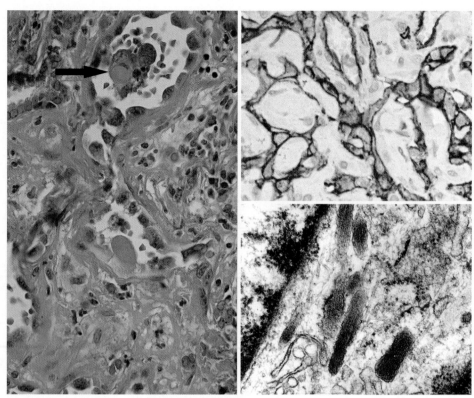

FIGURE 16.5. Angiosarcoma. Left: Neolumen formation contains erythrocytes within the cytoplasm of neoplastic endothelial cells *(arrow)*. **Right upper:** The neoplastic cells can show strong and diffuse keratin immunoreactivity in the endothelial cells. **Right lower:** Electron microscopy of Weibel–Palade bodies, a single membrane-bound, rod-shaped cytoplasmic structure characteristic of endothelium. (EM courtesy of Dr. S. Bhuta.)

die of their tumors in <6 months, frequently from massive hemorrhage.[2,3,5,7,11,12,14,18,20] Razoxane may benefit patients as a radiation sensitizer.[3,8,16] In rare cases, a patient will survive beyond 5 years. Tumors confined to the thyroid gland seem to behave less aggressively than do tumors that spread extrathyroidally.[3,7,8,16] Distant metastases (lung, gastrointestinal tract [Fig. 16.6], and bone) may cause fatal bleeding.[1–3,20,24,28,29] Fibrinogen, factor VIII, and FVIII-RA in the serum may be used as surrogate markers during follow-up.[16]

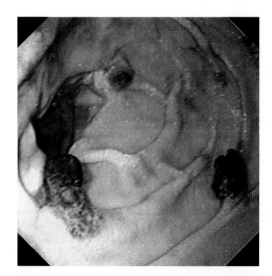

FIGURE 16.6. Primary thyroid angiosarcoma metastatic to the small bowel. An endoscopic view of mucosal deposits of metastatic angiosarcoma. (Courtesy of Dr. A. Ryška, Department of Pathology, Charles University Medical Faculty Hospital, Hradec Kralove, Czech Republic.)

TERATOMA

Tumors of the cervical region are regarded as thyroid teratomas if (1) the tumor occupies a portion of the thyroid gland, (2) there is direct continuity or a close anatomic relationship between the tumor and the thyroid gland, and/or (3) a cervical teratoma is accompanied by a complete absence of the thyroid gland.[30,31] The latter circumstance has been explained by two postulates: (1) total replacement of the gland by the tumor or (2) a thyroid anlage that failed to develop into a mature thyroid gland. In a given case, it may be difficult to rule out the possibility that the thyroid tissue found adjacent to a teratoma represents either normal thyroid gland secondarily replaced by a primary teratoma or just another component of the teratoma.[30] Histologically, by definition, teratoma displays mature or immature tissues from *all three* embryonic germ cell layers: ectoderm, endoderm, and mesoderm.[30,32] The interrelationship of these constituents and the percentage of each element that is present are used to classify the tumors into one of three types: *mature, immature,* or *malignant.* The terms *teratoma, choristoma, hamartoma, heterotopia, epignathus,* and *dermoid* are sometimes used interchangeably, but *teratoma* should be used only to describe a tumor with trilineage differentiation.

Histogenesis and Molecular Genetics

Teratomas include tissues from all three primordial layers (ectoderm, mesoderm, and endoderm). They are believed to arise from misplaced embryonic germ cells (rests) in the thyroid gland that continue to develop in the new location.[30]

Clinical Presentation

Teratomas represent <0.1% of all primary thyroid gland neoplasms. The age range of affected patients at the initial presentation extends from newborns to 85 years, but the average age is <10 years. This average is skewed by the number of older patients with malignant teratomas; the median age at presentation is <1 month.[30,31,33–37] When neonates and infants are considered apart from children and adults, two distinct biologic groups appear: >90% of the tumors in the neonatal group are benign and >50% of tumors in the older group are malignant. There is no predilection for either sex.[30] All patients present with a neck mass that often reaches a significant size. In addition, patients experience dyspnea, difficulty breathing, and/or stridor. Other congenital anomalies may be present in neonatal patients. Ultrasonographic images (in utero, at the time of birth, or later) provide the best information and are easiest to obtain. The most common finding is a multicystic mass lesion of the thyroid gland. CT demonstrates an inhomogeneous mass arising in the thyroid gland and compressing the upper airway for both benign and malignant teratomas (Fig. 16.7).[30,38–42]

Pathology

Gross Presentation

Teratomas range in size up to 13 cm in their greatest dimension (mean size 6 cm). Tumors associated with compression symptoms (stridor, hoarseness, and difficulty breathing) are on average larger than those not associated with these symptoms.[30,31,33,36,37] The outer tumor surface varies from smooth to bosselated or lobulated. The tumor periphery is well circumscribed to widely infiltrative into the surrounding thyroid parenchyma. The tumor is firm to soft and cystic, the cut surface is multiloculated, and the cystic spaces contain white-tan creamy material, mucoid glairy material, or dark brown hemorrhagic fluid admixed with necrotic debris (Fig. 16.8). Material resembling brain tissue along with gritty bone or cartilage is frequently noted during gross examination.[30,31,33,34,36,37]

Microscopic Description

In order for a tumor to qualify as a thyroid teratoma, thyroid parenchyma should be identified somewhere within the mass

(Fig. 16.9); even so, residual thyroid follicles are frequently scarce or absent in malignant teratomas. Teratomas display a wide array of tissue types and growth patterns within a single lesion (Fig. 16.10). Small cystic spaces to solid nests contain various different epithelia: squamous epithelium (simple and stratified), pseudostratified ciliated columnar epithelium (respiratory), cuboidal epithelium (with and without goblet cells) glandular epithelium (Fig. 16.11), and transitional epithelium. Pilosebaceous and other adnexal structures are seen (Fig. 16.11). True *organ* differentiation (pancreas, liver, or lung) can be found. Neural tissue (ectodermal derivation) is the most common element; it is composed variously of mature glial tissue (Figs. 16.10 and 16.12), choroid plexus, pigmented retinal anlage (Fig. 16.13), and/or immature neuroblastemal elements. The latter are composed of small-to-medium-sized cells with a high nucleus-to-cytoplasm ratio, arranged in sheets or rosette-like structures (Homer Wright or Flexner–Wintersteiner types; Fig. 16.13). The nuclear chromatin is hyperchromatic. There are frequent mitoses. The maturation of the neural-type tissue determines the grade: *completely mature* (grade 0), *predominantly mature* (grade 1 or 2), and *exclusively immature* (grade 3 or malignant). Cartilage, bone, striated skeletal muscle, smooth muscle, adipose tissue, and loose myxoid to fibrous embryonic mesenchymal connective tissue are intermixed with the other components.[30,38–41,43–46]

The grading criteria for gonadal and sacrococcygeal teratomas[47–49] have been modified for thyroid teratomas. *Benign, immature,* and *malignant* teratomas are classified as such on the basis of the relative proportions of immature neuroectodermal tissues (see Table 16.1). Benign mature teratomas are classified as grade 0; benign immature teratomas are classified as grade 1 or 2; and malignant teratomas are classified as grade 3.[30] The presence of embryonal carcinoma or yolk sac tumor would place a teratoma into the malignant category (grade 3).

Immunohistochemistry and Molecular Diagnostics

Malignant teratomas may require immunohistochemical evaluation. The immature glial components are immunoreactive with S100

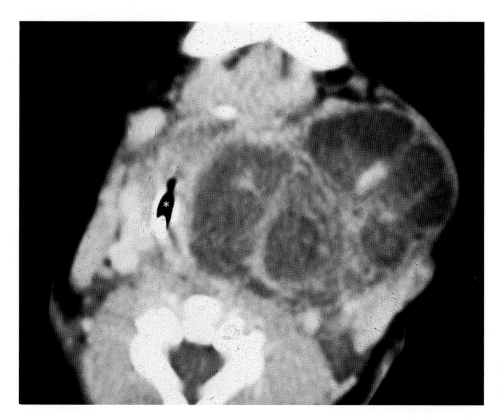

FIGURE 16.7. Teratoma. A CT scan demonstrates a large multicystic neoplasm in the anterior neck, completely replacing the thyroid gland. *marks the laryngeal lumen.

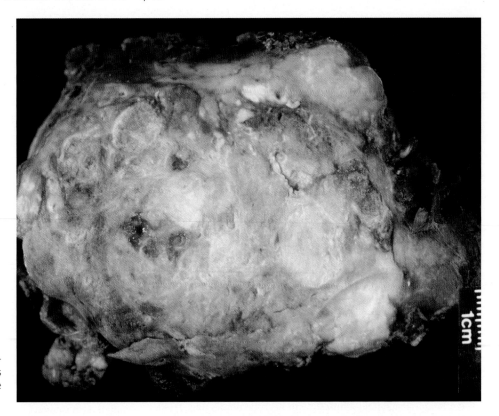

FIGURE 16.8. Teratoma. Tumors are multinodular with a white-tan appearance. Cysts are noted in this tumor that replaces the thyroid gland.

protein, glial fibrillary acidic protein (GFAP) (Fig. 16.14), neuron-specific enolase, and neural filament protein. Early skeletal muscle differentiation can be highlighted with myo-D1, myogenin (Fig. 16.14) or myoglobulin.[30,36,39,46] Immature areas produce an increased proliferation fraction (MIB-1) that is often >10% in malignant cases.

Cytopathology

Smears from an FNA sample demonstrate various cellular components that are often misinterpreted as *contamination* or *a missed* lesion (i.e., the *tumor* was not sampled). The smears from malignant teratomas have a *neuroepithelial* small, round, blue cell appearance when taken from the immature neural elements. These cells result in a *positive* or *malignant* interpretation, rather than the pathologist making a specific diagnosis of malignant teratoma.[30,38,39,41,50]

Differential Diagnosis

The clinical differential diagnosis, especially in neonates, includes lymphangioma, thyroglossal duct cyst, and branchial cleft cyst.

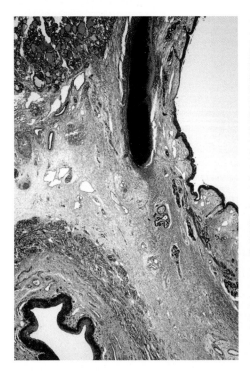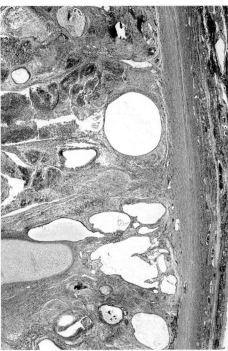

FIGURE 16.9. Teratoma. Thyroid parenchyma is noted at the periphery of each of these teratomas. Note the presence of a trachea and esophagus (**left**) in this benign mature teratoma. **Right:** There is a haphazard arrangement of components in this benign immature teratoma (thyroid parenchyma on far right).

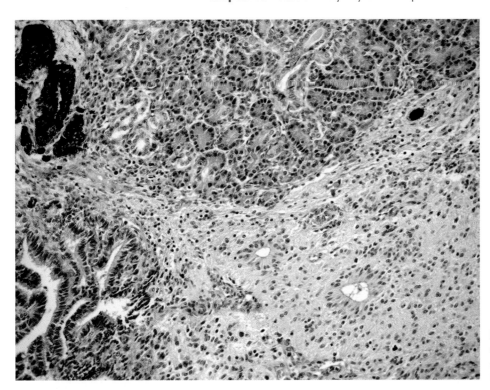

FIGURE 16.10. Teratoma. Mature glial tissue, pigmented retinal anlage, salivary gland, and glandular epithelium are haphazardly arranged in benign mature teratoma.

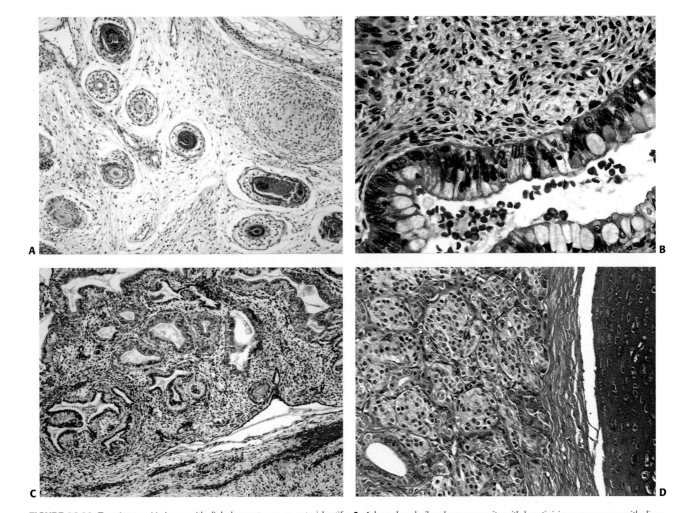

FIGURE 16.11. Teratoma. Various epithelial elements are easy to identify. **A:** Adnexal and pilosebaceous units with keratinizing squamous epithelium. **B:** Goblet cells are present in this cuboidal epithelium. **C:** Immature salivary gland tissue with ducts. **D:** Pancreatic tissue juxtaposed to mature cartilage.

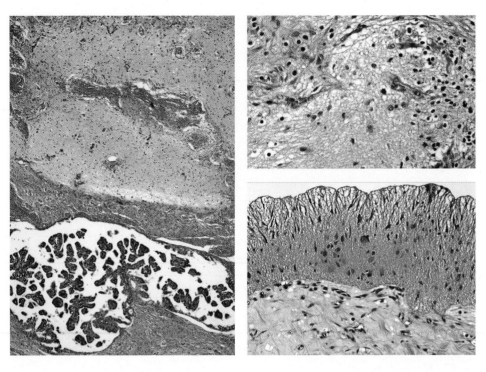

FIGURE 16.12. Teratoma. This composite demonstrates mature glial tissue with choroid plexus (**left**), and axons (**right upper**) or ganglia (**right lower**) in a benign mature teratoma.

Histologically, teratomas should be separated from dermoids (which only contain skin elements), extraskeletal Ewing sarcoma, rhabdomyosarcoma, small-cell carcinoma, lymphoma, and melanoma.[51] The diagnosis of teratoma under these circumstances is largely dependent on the identification of other tissue elements and a confirmatory immunohistochemical panel.[30,31,41,45,51]

Treatment and Prognosis

The outcome for patients with thyroid teratomas depends on the patient's age, the size of the tumor at the time of presentation,

and the presence and proportion of immaturity. The age at presentation and tumor histology are strongly correlated. In neonates and infants, there is a preponderance of immature teratomas (grade 1 or 2 immaturity) and a near-absence of malignant tumors. Conversely, among children and adults, there is a preponderance of malignant teratomas (grade 3 immaturity). No patient with a grade 0, 1, or 2 tumor (*benign mature* or *benign immature*) dies *of* disease, although some die *with* disease; when death does occur in such cases, it is generally a direct result of significant morbidity secondary to tracheal compression or a lack of development of vital structures in the neck during

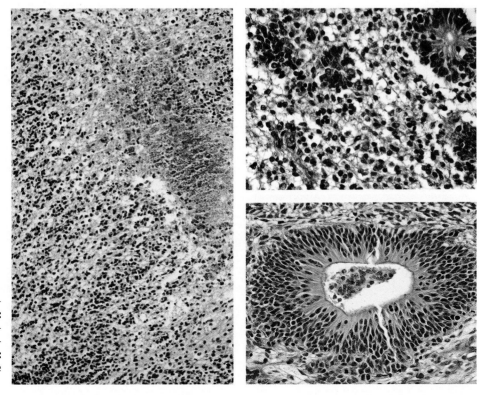

FIGURE 16.13. Teratoma. Immature neuroblastemal elements comprise this teratoma. **Left:** Necrosis is present in malignant (Grade 3) teratoma. **Right upper:** Rosettes are noted in a background of immature neural tissue. **Right lower:** A well-formed Flexner–Wintersteiner rosette shows a gland-like lumen.

Table 16.1

Thyroid Gland Teratoma Histologic Grading

Grade	Tumor Type	Histologic Appearance
0	Benign mature	Only mature elements present
1	Benign immature	Embryonal-type tissue in only 1 low-power field
2	Benign immature	>1 but <4 low-power fields of immature foci
3	Malignant	>4 low-power fields of immature tissue, pleomorphism, and increased mitotic figures

Low-power magnification field = 4 × objective with a 10 × ocular.[30]

fetal growth. Therefore, surgery for benign thyroid teratomas should be instituted without delay because preoperative morbidity (mass effect) and mortality are significant.[30,48] Malignant teratomas exhibit a clinically malignant behavior, thus emphasizing the importance of identifying their morphology and distinguishing them from the benign mature and benign immature types of teratoma.[30,52] Malignant teratomas may invade by direct extension into the esophagus, trachea, salivary glands, and/or the soft tissues of the neck. Recurrence and dissemination (usually in the lungs) are known to occur in about one-third of these patients; most of these cases are fatal. These patients are managed with radiation and chemotherapy, although treatment is palliative.[30,31,35,38–41,43–46] Staging does not apply to malignant teratomas.

SMOOTH MUSCLE TUMORS

Smooth muscle tumors primary to the thyroid gland are defined by criteria similar to those used to define leiomyomas and leiomyosarcomas in other noncutaneous and nonuterine sites. These neoplasms are composed of cells with distinct smooth muscle differentiation histologically; the diagnosis is confirmed by immunohistochemical techniques.[53]

Etiology

There is no known etiology for smooth muscle tumors of the thyroid gland, specifically including radiation exposure.[54] A single case of an EBV-associated thyroid smooth muscle tumor has been reported in a child with a congenital immunodeficiency disease.[55] No specific thyroid topographic location is seen in smooth muscle tumors, although association with smooth muscle–walled vessels at the periphery of the gland (thyroid gland capsule) has been shown (Fig. 16.15).[54]

Histogenesis and Molecular Genetics

Although not experimentally proven, the histogenesis of thyroid smooth muscle tumors occurs in the thyroid vessels—that is, the smooth muscle in the vascular walls (Fig. 16.15). Smooth muscle tumors are classified into cutaneous and subcutaneous, deep soft tissue, and vascular origins; the latter is the favored histogenesis for thyroid gland primaries.[53,54,56]

Clinical Presentation

Primary smooth muscle tumors of the thyroid gland are exceedingly rare, representing <0.02% of all thyroid gland tumors.[54–66] According to reports, no patient with a leiomyoma has died of disease, but almost all patients with a leiomyosarcoma in whom follow-up was available did die from their disease.[56,60,61,63–68]

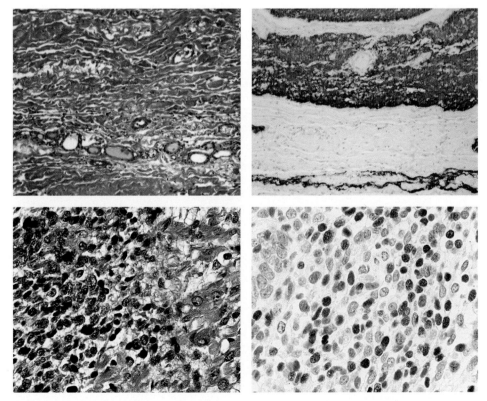

FIGURE 16.14. Teratoma. Top: What appears to be dense collagenized tissue in this teratoma with thyroid epithelium, is mature glial tissue with gliosis (GFAP immunohistochemistry, **right upper**). **Bottom:** Immature round to spindle cells react strongly with myogenin (**right bottom**).

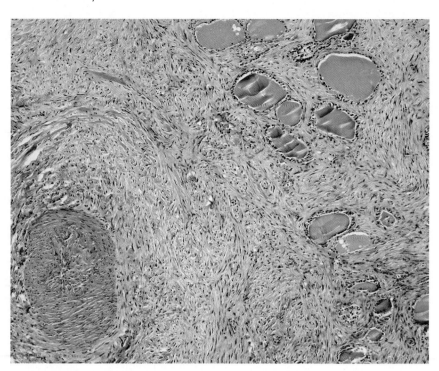

FIGURE 16.15. Smooth muscle tumor. Origin from a perithyroidal vessel wall can be seen as the neoplastic cells scroll off the muscle wall in this leiomyosarcoma.

Unlike their benign counterparts, primary thyroid leiomyosarcomas tend to occur in older patients. In view of the limited number of cases, no predilection for either sex has been established.

Patients present with nonspecific signs and symptoms. A thyroid mass, usually increasing in size (leiomyosarcoma cases), is associated with dyspnea, difficulty breathing, and/or stridor. The duration of symptoms ranges from days to years, depending on the extent of the tumor. Thyroid scans with radioactive isotopes demonstrate a cold nodule. CT reveals an inhomogeneous low-density mass in the thyroid gland; the signal intensity is similar to that of the surrounding soft tissue. Compression of the upper airway, infiltration into the soft tissues or destruction of the thyroid gland, and necrosis suggest a malignant process, but these signs are not specific for a leiomyosarcoma. In general, lymphadenopathy is absent. Ultrasonographic examination does not yield a specific diagnosis, although an ill-defined hypoechoic mass without halo has been reported.[54,65]

Pathology

Gross Presentation

Tumors range in size up to 12 cm in their greatest dimension; on average, leiomyosarcomas tend to be larger than leiomyomas (6 cm vs. 2 cm). Macroscopically, the outer tumor surface is smooth to nodular, depending on the diagnosis. The tumor periphery is well circumscribed to widely infiltrative into the surrounding soft tissue.[54–57,59–66]

Microscopic Description

Tumor cells are arranged in bundles or fascicles of smooth muscle fibers that intersect in an orderly fashion. The cells are spindled, and blunt-ended, cigar-shaped, slightly hyperchromatic nuclei occupy a central location within the cell. Perinuclear cytoplasmic vacuoles can be seen (Fig. 16.16). In many malignant cases,

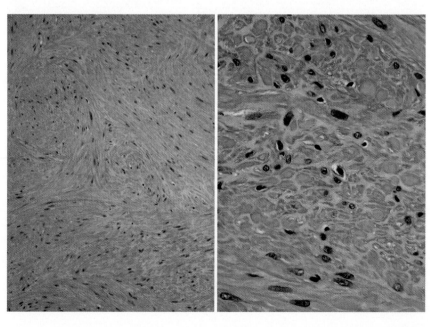

FIGURE 16.16. Smooth muscle tumor. The spindled cells are fascicular, with perinucleolar halos in these leiomyomas.

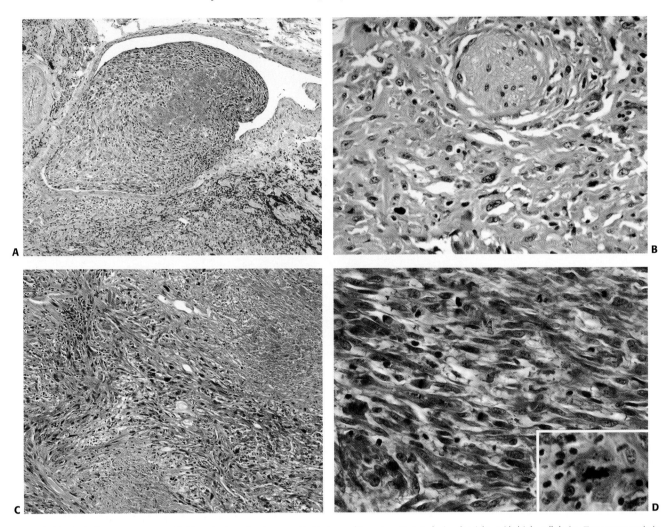

FIGURE 16.17. Leiomyosarcoma. A: Vascular invasion is seen. **B:** Perineural invasion. **C:** Interlacing fascicles with high cellularity. Tumor necrosis is prominent. **D:** Note the increased number of mitotic figures, including atypical forms (inset).

capsular invasion, vascular invasion, and perineural invasion (Fig. 16.17) are present. Entrapment of normal thyroid follicles can be seen. Leiomyosarcomas feature the morphologic characteristics of malignant smooth muscle tumors—that is, high cellularity, disordered fascicular growth pattern, and tumor necrosis (Fig. 16.17). Nuclei are markedly atypical and pleomorphic, and there is an increased number of mitotic figures (>5/10 high power fields [HPF]). Atypical mitotic figures are usually easily identified (Fig. 16.17).[54–66] Electron microscopic examination of the spindle cells reveals microfilament bundles with dense patches and a discontinuous basal lamina. Grading of primary thyroid gland leiomyosarcomas has not been proposed, but doubtless would include nuclear anaplasia, increased mitotic figures, and the presence of tumor necrosis.

Immunohistochemistry and Molecular Diagnostics

Trichrome will reveal smooth muscle and the background collagen, although rarely performed for diagnostic purposes (Fig. 16.18). Both leiomyomas and leiomyosarcomas show myogenic immunoreactivity with smooth muscle actin (Fig. 16.18), muscle-specific actin, and desmin; vimentin is always present. Myo-D1, myogenin, and CD117 may show focal reactivity.[54,61] Thyroglobulin, cytokeratin, S100 protein, chromogranin, and calcitonin are negative.[54,56,60,63,68] Ki-67 fractions are increased in

leiomyosarcoma, but they have not been correlated with patient survival.

Cytology

Only single case reports of leiomyosarcoma have been published. The FNA smears are cellular with individual cells to small clusters of spindled cells (Fig. 16.19). Nuclear pleomorphism is noted, and mitotic figures are identified.[58,68,69]

Differential Diagnosis

It is difficult to distinguish leiomyosarcoma from anaplastic (undifferentiated) thyroid carcinoma with a spindle-cell pattern (Table 16.2). A primary thyroid leiomyosarcoma should be diagnosed only when there is a complete lack of all epithelial differentiation and there is definite evidence (histologic, immunophenotypic, or ultrastructural) of specific sarcomatous differentiation.[53,54] Anaplastic thyroid carcinoma usually occurs in older patients who have a longstanding history of a preexisting thyroid lesion that has rapidly enlarged. Marked nuclear atypia also favor anaplastic carcinoma. The presence of residual well-differentiated thyroid carcinoma is virtually diagnostic for anaplastic carcinoma in this setting. Anaplastic carcinoma may lose its epithelial phenotype, but it does not express desmin or actins. The other major considerations are direct extension from neoplasms in the neck[70]

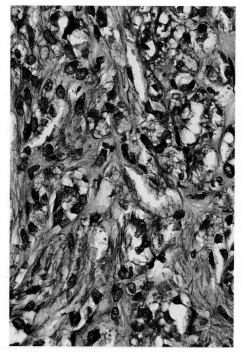 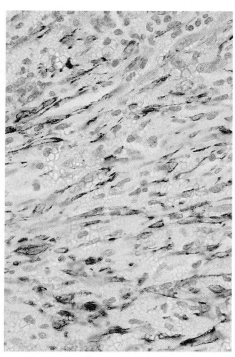

FIGURE 16.18. Smooth muscle tumor. Left: A trichrome stain highlights the muscle (*red*) and the surrounding supporting fibrous connective tissue (*blue*). **Right:** The neoplastic spindle cells are desmin immunoreactive.

and metastatic leiomyosarcoma in the thyroid gland.[71–74] Before a primary diagnosis can be established, a primary tumor elsewhere (uterine, gastrointestinal tract, or soft tissue) should be excluded, even though sarcomas rarely metastasize to the thyroid gland. Primary leiomyosarcoma is solitary, although metastatic disease tends to be multifocal in the thyroid and is frequently identified in other organs also. Clinical and radiographic evaluations may be useful in making the distinction.[54,56,74–78]

Treatment and Prognosis

Leiomyomas are excised without sequelae. By contrast, the diagnosis of primary leiomyosarcoma of the thyroid is associated with a poor clinical outcome irrespective of clinical features, size, grade, or stage of the tumor. Staging is not usually applied because the local effect is more prognostically significant than other features.

PERIPHERAL NERVE SHEATH TUMORS

The criteria for defining primary peripheral nerve sheath tumors (PNSTs) of the thyroid gland are similar to those used for schwannoma and malignant PNSTs (MPNSTs) at other sites. To be called a thyroid gland primary, the tumor must arise within

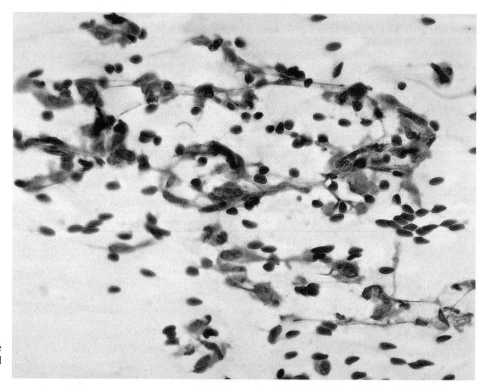

FIGURE 16.19. Smooth muscle tumor. The atypical spindle cells in a bloody background are present in an FNA of a leiomyosarcoma.

Table 16.2

Differential Diagnosis of Nonepithelial Spindle Cell Tumors of the Thyroid Gland

Feature	Leiomyosarcoma	MPNST	Solitary Fibrous Tumor	SETTLE	Anaplastic Carcinoma
Histogenesis	Vessels of thyroid capsule	Nerve plexus around thyroid	Mesenchymal cells with myofibroblastic differentiation	Ectopic thymus or solid cell nests (branchial pouch)	Follicular cell origin
Clinical presentation	Age usually > 60 years; F = M; Thyroid gland mass; Dyspnea, difficulty breath and stridor occasionally	Any age, but syndrome associated tend to be young; F = M; Mass increasing in size; May be associated with von Recklinghausen disease	Middle age (mean, 48 years); F > M; Asymptomatic enlarging mass; Hoarseness rare; Tumor may be present for years	Young age, second decade peak; M > F (2:1); Often long-standing thyroid mass; Local tenderness or pain is infrequent	Age > 60 years usually; F > M (2:1); Rapidly enlarging mass in patient with long history of thyroid disease; Hoarseness; Vocal cord paralysis
Macroscopic features	Mean size 6 cm; Nodular external surface; Infiltrative	Effaced thyroid; Preferentially at gland periphery; Tan-white, glistening	Mean size 4.5 cm; Well-delineated mass; Firm, solid, white-grey-tan; Can be perithyroidal	Mean size 3.6 cm; Lobular; Circumscribed to infiltrative; Hard, grey-white cut surface; Small cysts may be present	Large, fleshy mass; Extensively invasive; Hemorrhage and necrosis ubiquitous
Microscopic features	Infiltrative, with vascular and perineural invasion; Fascicular growth; Spindle, blunt-ended, cigar-shaped cells; Perinuclear cytoplasmic vacuoles; Central nuclei; Tumor necrosis; Increased mitotic figures	Infiltrative tumors; Highly cellular; Herringbone pattern; Fusiform cells with tapered, elongated nuclei; Pleomorphism; Tumor necrosis; Increased mitotic figures	Syncytial architecture; Variably cellular spindle-cell proliferation entrapping thyroid follicles; Keloid-like collagen deposition; Open, patulous vessels; Bland, monotonous cell population; Slender nuclei with delicate chromatin	Highly cellular, biphasic; Lobules separated by fibrous septa; Short, interlacing fascicles; Long spindled cells blend with glandular–papillary structures; Vascular invasion; Lymphocytes may be seen	Infiltrative; Highly pleomorphic spindled and epithelioid cells, tumor giant cells; Increased and atypical mitotic figures; Inflammatory infiltrate; Frequent coexistent papillary or follicular carcinoma
Immunohistochemistry	Positive: SMA, MSA, desmin, myogenin, MYOD1, vimentin; Negative: S100 protein, TTF1, thyroglobulin, calcitonin	Positive: S100, vimentin, TP53; Negative: Thyroglobulin, SMA, MSA, desmin	Positive: Vimentin, CD34, CD99, bcl-2; Negative: TTF1, thyroglobulin, GFAP, HMB-45, CD117, keratin, FVIII-Rag	Positive: Keratins, CAM5.2, vimentin; Negative: TTF1, thyroglobulin, CD5, neuroendocrine markers	Positive: Keratin, but focal or isolated (>50% cases positive), PAX8, TP53; Negative: TTF1, thyroglobulin
Molecular	None reported	None reported	None reported	KRAS mutation	TP53, β-catenin, NRAS, HRAS, BRAF mutations
Pitfalls	Must separate from other tumors, as outcome may be different	S100 protein may be diminished in MPNST; Anaplastic carcinoma may not have epithelial markers	Rare tumor requiring inclusion in differential of other spindle-cell lesions	Spindle-cell component may be dominant (monophasic variant); Metastatic spindle-cell lesions can mimic; Medullary carcinoma also occurs in young patients	Metastatic disease should be excluded; Squamous differentiation can be present

F, Female; M, Male.

the thyroid parenchyma or be contained within the capsule of the thyroid gland. These neoplasms are composed of cells with evidence of distinct peripheral nerve sheath differentiation histologically; the diagnosis is confirmed using immunohistochemical techniques.[79] PNSTs include schwannoma and neurofibroma; the designation MPNST is used to describe the malignant counterpart of these neoplasms.

Histogenesis and Molecular Genetics

The histogenesis of thyroid gland PNST includes the sympathetic and parasympathetic innervation (cervical plexus) or possibly the sensory nerves—that is, any of the nerves in or around the thyroid gland.[80,81] In general, the prevalence of PNSTs is higher among kindred with von Recklinghausen disease and neurofibromatosis, although this association has been documented only in patients with isolated thyroid gland primary PNST.[79,81-83]

Clinical Presentation

PNSTs and MPNSTs of the thyroid are exceedingly rare, representing <0.02% of all thyroid gland tumors.[57,80-90] Neurogenic tumors of the thyroid occur in patients of all ages, but patients with syndrome-associated tumors tend to develop tumors at a younger age at presentation.[79,82,83] No predilection for either sex has been determined. The presenting signs and symptoms are nonspecific; they include a thyroid mass that has usually increased in size. In malignant cases, there may be associated dyspnea, difficulty breathing, and weight loss. Ultrasound usually shows a circumscribed hypoechoic mass, whereas CT demonstrates an inhomogeneous low-density mass in the thyroid; the signal density is similar to that of the surrounding soft tissue. Compression of the upper airway, infiltration into the soft tissues or destruction of the thyroid gland, and necrosis suggest a malignant process, but these signs are not specific for MPNST. In general, lymphadenopathy

is absent. Thyroid radionuclide scans (^{99m}Tc) demonstrate a cold nodule, but they are nonspecific.[81,84,90-92]

Pathology

Gross Presentation

Tumors grow as large as 7 cm in their greatest dimension. Given the small number of reported cases, no specific difference in the size of benign and malignant PNSTs can be inferred. Macroscopically, the outer tumor surface is smooth and encapsulated (PNSTs). The cut surface may focally appear cystic with yellow fluid. Effacement of the thyroid parenchyma and invasion beyond the tumor capsule is seen in MPNSTs, although soft-tissue invasion is not usually identified. These tumors are tan to white and glistening.[57,80-90] No specific thyroid topographic location is seen in PNSTs, although an association with medium to large nerves at the periphery of the gland (thyroid gland capsule) has been shown.[81]

Microscopic Description

Schwannomas are variably cellular, with either densely packed spindle-cell areas (Antoni A) or loosely arranged hypocellular degenerated myxoid areas (Antoni B). The slender spindle cells are arranged in interlacing fascicles in a variably hyalinized matrix. Palisading of the nuclei (Verocay bodies) is seen (Fig. 16.20). The cells are fusiform with elongated cytoplasmic extensions, presenting a wavy to spindled appearance. The nuclei are elongated, and they reveal little pleomorphism. They have a coarse nuclear chromatin distribution and inconspicuous nucleoli. Rare mitotic figures are present, but atypical forms are not encountered. Small-to-medium-sized blood vessels may have hyalinized walls. Axons are not identified within the tumors.[57,79-81,85-88,90] MPNSTs invade into the surrounding thyroid gland parenchyma, entrapping and destroying the follicles (Fig. 16.21). MPNSTs have increased cellularity with fusiform

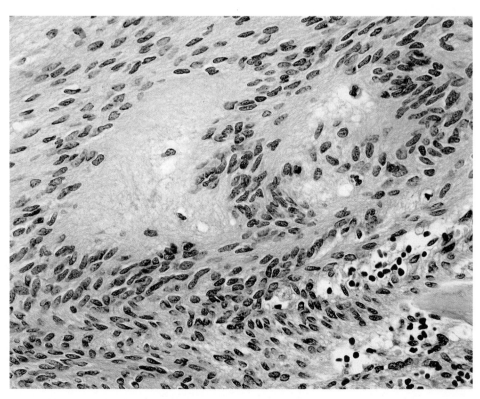

FIGURE 16.20. Peripheral nerve sheath tumor. A schwannoma has wavy cells arranged in a palisade (Verocay body).

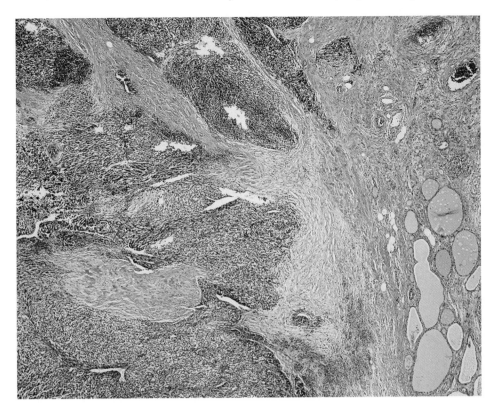

FIGURE 16.21. Malignant peripheral nerve sheath tumor. This tumor is widely invasive, showing a small amount of residual thyroid parenchyma at the periphery.

cells arranged in tightly packed fascicles that are woven into a vague herringbone pattern (Fig. 16.22). Antoni B areas can also be seen; they are composed of wavy cells with fibrillar cytoplasmic extensions arranged in a loose background. Cellular pleomorphism, increased mitotic figures (including atypical forms), necrosis (Fig. 16.23), hemorrhage, and vascular invasion are features typical of MPNSTs.[81,84,89,93] Ultrastructural features of Schwann cell derivation include cells with narrow to broad, entangled cell processes covered by a discrete basement membrane substance. Collagen fibers are banded together and inserted into the basal lamina. Intermediate filaments are contained within the cytoplasm. Primitive junctions are identified

between tumor cells. The so-called *fibrous long-spacing collagen*, with its distinct periodicity, is demonstrated.[81,94,95] Whereas grading of MPNST of the thyroid gland has not been specifically proposed, it would include nuclear anaplasia, increased mitotic figures, tumor necrosis, and vascular invasion.[81,84,89,93]

Immunohistochemistry and Molecular Diagnostics

Schwann cell-derived tumors of the thyroid gland are diffusely and strongly immunoreactive with S100 protein (Fig. 16.23),

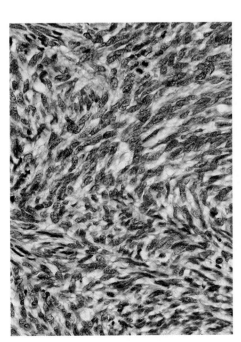
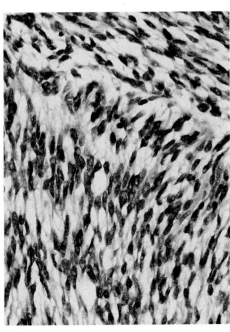

FIGURE 16.22. Malignant peripheral nerve sheath tumor. A herringbone pattern (**left**) or palisade (**right**) can be seen in this MPNST of the thyroid gland. Note the mitotic figures.

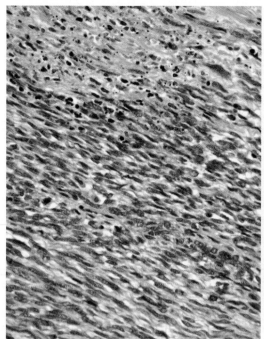
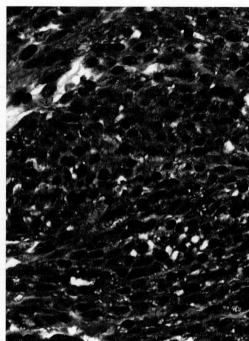

FIGURE 16.23. Malignant peripheral nerve sheath tumor. Left: Tumor necrosis is present in this MPNST. Note the wavy nuclei with elongated, pointed nuclei. **Right:** A strong and diffuse S100 protein reaction is identified in the nucleus and cytoplasm of the cells in this MPNST.

vimentin, and TP53 (nuclear overexpression) and nonreactive with thyroglobulin, chromogranin, smooth muscle actin, muscle-specific actin, and desmin.[57,80,81,84,88,90] S100 protein is often less intense in MPNSTs. In rare instances, keratin reactivity has been reported.[89] Clonal chromosome aberrations can be seen in both benign and malignant PNSTs; they include a loss of 22q, monosomy 17, and trisomy 7. Triploid or tetraploid clones are associated with high-grade tumors.[96]

Cytopathology

FNA may be attempted. The cytologic features are similar to those of schwannoma elsewhere: spindled tumor cells with elongated, slender, and wavy nuclei. A fibrillary metachromatic stroma (on air-dried Romanovsky-stained slides) may be present. There is a lack of colloid and thyroid follicular epithelial cells. MPNSTs may contain highly atypical spindled or epithelioid cells that have no specific features. Immunohistochemistry (S100 protein) may help establish a definitive diagnosis of a neural tumor. However, distinction between primary and metastatic soft-tissue tumors is impossible on cytology alone.[81,85,88,91,97]

Differential Diagnosis

Benign PNSTs are usually sufficiently well developed to be accurately diagnosed on hematoxylin- and eosin-stained slides alone. Sometimes, a mass of the soft tissues of the neck may masquerade as a thyroid gland mass, but surgical observation or radiographic studies may lead to a correct identification.[98] It may be difficult to distinguish an MPNST from an anaplastic thyroid carcinoma with a spindle cell pattern (Table 16.2). A primary MPNST of the thyroid should be diagnosed only when there is a complete absence of all epithelial and thyroid differentiation and there is definite evidence of specific Schwann cell derivation histologically, immunophenotypically, and/or ultrastructurally.[79,81] MPNSTs occur as isolated masses that are not associated with any preexisting thyroid lesion. They are uniformly negative with thyroglobulin, keratin, TTF1,

chromogranin, and calcitonin; this, in concert with the aforementioned findings, virtually negates the possibility of epithelial or neuroendocrine derivation from follicular epithelial cells or C cells, respectively.[81,84,88,90,97,99] Isolated reports of malignant triton tumors (malignant schwannoma with rhabdomyoblastic differentiation) in the thyroid gland may be included in the differential diagnosis of MPNST.[100,101] Other sarcomas (fibrosarcoma, leiomyosarcoma, rhabdomyosarcoma, malignant fibrous histiocytoma, or angiosarcoma) either by direction extension or by metastatic disease, can usually be eliminated by growth pattern and immunohistochemical differences.[10,54,72,78,97,98,102-105] A metastatic melanoma can mimic a PNST, especially when it is spindled and if only an S100 protein immunostain is obtained.[81,106,107] However, HMB-45, melan-A, and tyrosinase can usually distinguish these lesions.

Treatment and Prognosis

Schwannoma can be removed without clinical consequence or further management. Primary MPNST of the thyroid gland is associated with a poor clinical outcome irrespective of clinical features, size, grade, or stage of the tumor.[79,81,84] Radiotherapy may be of palliative value in malignant cases.[89] Staging is not usually applied. Whereas no patient with a *benign* PNST died of disease, all patients with a *malignant* PNST for whom follow-up was available did die of their disease.[81,84]

 # PARAGANGLIOMA

Extra-adrenal gland paraganglia are derived from the primitive neural crest. They are functionally separated into two types: *sympathetic* and *parasympathetic*. Most parasympathetic tumors occur in the head and neck region. Although they produce catecholamines immunohistochemically, thyroid gland primaries may be functionally silent. Thyroid gland primary paragangliomas (PGLs) are intrathyroidal neuroendocrine tumors of paraganglionic origin.[108]

Etiology

Primary thyroid gland tumors appear sporadically, although familial tumors are possible. Chronic hypoxia is not an identified cause, as it is in vagal PGL.[108,109]

Histogenesis and Molecular Genetics

Thyroid PGLs probably arise from the inferior laryngeal paraganglia, which may rarely be found within the thyroid gland instead of adjacent to the larynx.[109] Genetic studies have identified genes implicated in the pathogenesis of hereditary PGLs. Familial PGL1 syndrome is caused by mutation in the succinate dehydrogenase subunit D (*SDHD*) gene on chromosome 11q23; PGL3 is caused by mutation in the *SDHC* gene (1q21); and PGL4 by mutation in the *SDHB* gene (1p36). These genes encode mitochondrial respiratory chain proteins. Genetic testing may help identify syndrome-associated patients.[108] In sporadic PGLs, somatic mutations in these genes are rarely found, whereas deletions on chromosome 11q and other involved regions are common.[110]

Clinical Presentation

Thyroid PGLs are exceedingly rare.[109,111–119] Females are almost exclusively affected. The range of ages at initial presentation varies widely, but most patients are in the fifth decade of life. Patients usually present with an asymptomatic neck mass; extension into the soft tissues has been reported.[118,120] Multifocal tumors may be identified, which raises the possibility of syndrome association.[114] Octreotide or Sestamibi scintigraphy may highlight the tumor.

Pathology

Gross Presentation

These tumors are typically circumscribed, grey-brown, and about 3 cm in their greatest dimension.

Microscopic Description

PGLs are usually well-circumscribed and encapsulated intrathyroidal tumors (Fig. 16.24), although extension into the perithyroidal soft tissues is present occasionally.[120] The tumors are highly vascular. The chief cells and supporting sustentacular cells are arranged in an alveolar, lobular, or zellballen pattern (Fig. 16.25). In rare instances, anastomosing cords or sheets are noted. The fibrovascular septa are delicate and discontinuous. The chief cells are polygonal with abundant granular amphophilic cytoplasm, occasionally containing vacuoles. The nuclei are round to oval, and they feature a coarse nuclear chromatin distribution and small nucleoli. Isolated pleomorphic nuclei may be appreciated (Fig. 16.26). The spindled sustentacular cells are histologically inconspicuous, found at the periphery of the lobules. Necrosis and mitotic figures are absent. Melanin pigment and globules have not been described in the thyroid gland.[108,109,111–113,115,117–119] Ultrastructurally, the chief cells are associated with neurosecretory granules; they are not present in the sustentacular supporting cells.[113]

Immunohistochemistry and Molecular Diagnostics

The chief cells are typically positive for synaptophysin, chromogranin, neuron-specific enolase, tyrosine hydroxylase,

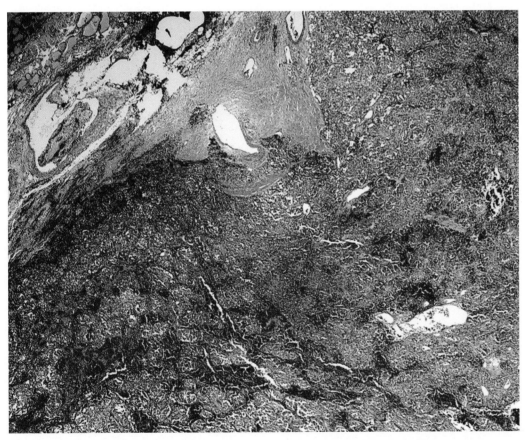

FIGURE 16.24. Paraganglioma. A fibrous connective tissue capsule surrounds this paraganglioma. Thyroid parenchyma is noted in the upper left corner.

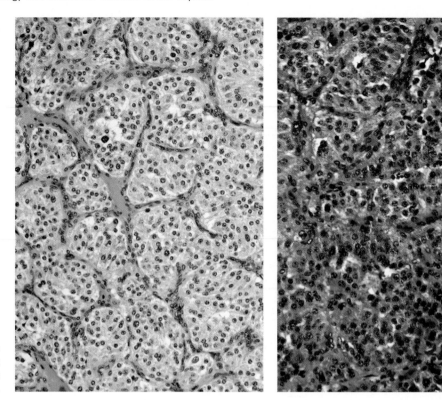

FIGURE 16.25. Paraganglioma. The characteristic zellballen pattern (**left**) may sometimes be more lobular or trabecular (**right**).

and CD56; S100 protein and glial fibrillary acidic protein highlight the wisps of cytoplasm that confirm they are sustentacular cells (Fig. 16.27). Cytokeratins, EMA, thyroglobulin, TTF1, calcitonin, serotonin, and vimentin are negative.[112,115,116,119]

Cytopathology

The cytopathologic features of a single case of thyroid PGL have been reported.[121] Aspirates have single cells and loose clusters of large cells with ovoid nuclei, focally discrete nucleoli, and moderate anisocytosis and anisonucleosis. A few

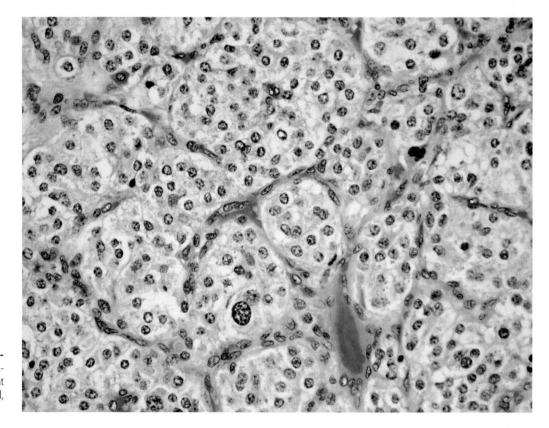

FIGURE 16.26. Paraganglioma. The chief cells have a syncytial architecture with abundant cytoplasm. Note the isolated, pleomorphic cell.

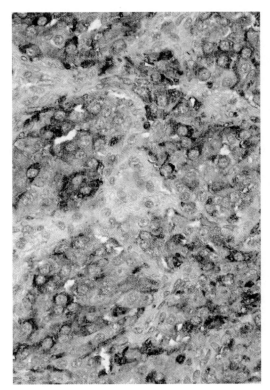
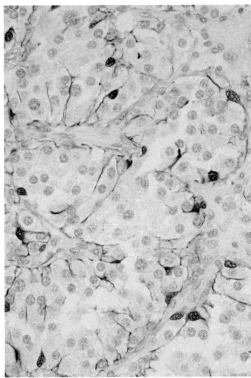

FIGURE 16.27. Paraganglioma. The chief cells are chromogranin immunoreactive (**left**), while the supporting sustentacular cells are highlighted with S100 protein (**right**).

cells with irregular nuclei and coarse chromatin were also present.[115,121]

Differential Diagnosis

Hyalinizing trabecular tumor, medullary thyroid carcinoma, papillary carcinoma, and metastatic carcinoid are the main tumors to consider in the differential diagnosis. Hyalinizing trabecular tumor (a previous name was *paraganglioma-like tumor*) features a well-developed intratumoral fibrosis, trabecular architecture, perinucleolar halos (vacuoles), intranuclear cytoplasmic inclusions, and yellow bodies. The neoplastic cells react with TTF1 and thyroglobulin and have a characteristic MIB-1 membrane immunohistochemistry. Medullary thyroid carcinoma is invasive, demonstrates fibrosis, produces amyloid, and possesses cytokeratin, calcitonin, and CEA immunoreactivity. Papillary carcinoma exhibits characteristic nuclear features not seen in PGL. Metastatic carcinoid tends to be multifocal, exhibits more cytologic atypia, may contain more spindled tumor cells, and is keratin-immunoreactive.[111,112,114,115,119,122,123]

Treatment and Prognosis

Nearly all thyroid gland PGLs are benign, although invasive growth into the trachea or larynx may be seen.[109,115,118] Surgical excision is the treatment of choice; clinical follow-up is recommended, especially if multifocal tumors are identified.[108,109,114–116]

 SOLITARY FIBROUS TUMOR

Solitary fibrous tumor is a mesenchymal tumor composed of collagen-producing spindle cells arranged in a characteristic vascular pattern. This tumor is identical to pleural tumors of a similar nature (i.e., not mesothelioma). However, there is significant debate about the taxonomy of this tumor, thought to lie within the morphologic spectrum of solitary fibrous tumor—hemangiopericytoma as a tumor group.[124–126]

Histogenesis and Molecular Genetics

Solitary fibrous tumor is thought to arise from a primitive mesenchymal cell that is capable of myofibroblastic and/or fibroblastic differentiation in which a vascular component (hemangiopericytoma) can be identified.[124]

Clinical Presentation

This exceedingly rare thyroid neoplasm (<25 cases reported[125–138]) tends to affect middle-aged patients (mean age 48 years). There is a female preponderance. Most patients present clinically with an asymptomatic enlarging mass in the neck; in some cases, hoarseness is noted. The tumor is slowly growing and may have been present for years before patients seek medical attention. The tumor presents as a solid or hyperechoic nodule on ultrasonography.[132]

Pathology

Gross Presentation

These tumors may involve the thyroid gland proper or may be identified in the immediately adjacent soft tissues. They are well-circumscribed and frequently encapsulated masses with a firm, solid, white-grey-tan cut appearance. The masses are large (mean: approximately 4.5 cm). Cystic change is occasionally observed, but necrosis and calcification are not.[125,126,137]

Microscopic Description

A solitary fibrous tumor may lie anywhere along the spectrum of benign to malignant disease. These tumors have various architectural and cytologic features within the spectrum

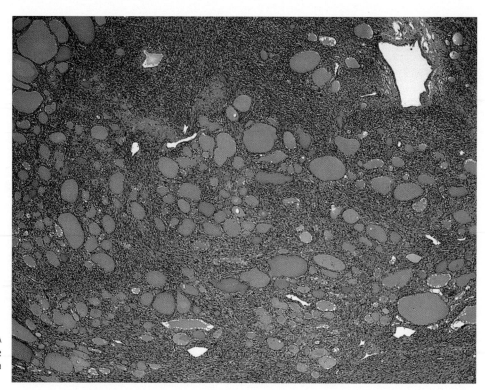

FIGURE 16.28. Solitary fibrous tumor. A spindle-cell proliferation infiltrates between the thyroid follicular epithelium without forming a well-defined nodule.

between solitary fibrous tumor and hemangiopericytoma. They typically have a well-defined border or capsule, although an infiltrative growth pattern can also be seen with extension of the spindle–cell proliferation into the surrounding thyroid gland parenchyma, trapping the thyroid follicles (Fig. 16.28). The neoplasm is composed of a variegated, cellular,

mesenchymal proliferation of bland, monotonous, spindle-shaped cells without any specific growth pattern, although storiform, fascicular, or herringbone patterns are noted (Fig. 16.29). The cells are separated by bundles of keloid-like collagen and delicate, open to patulous vascular spaces. The vascular spaces tend not to be dominant, but they give the

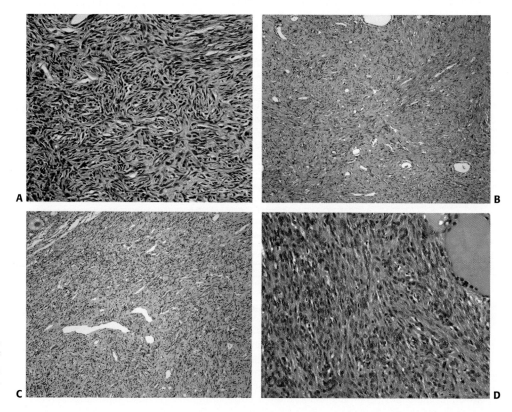

FIGURE 16.29. Solitary fibrous tumor. A number of different patterns of growth can be seen, including storiform **(A)**, fascicular **(B)**, hemangiopericytoma-like **(C)**, and fascicular **(D)**.

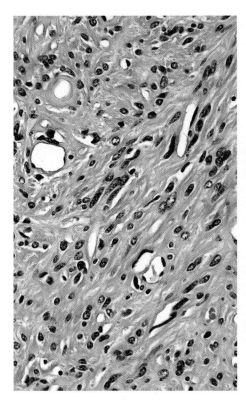
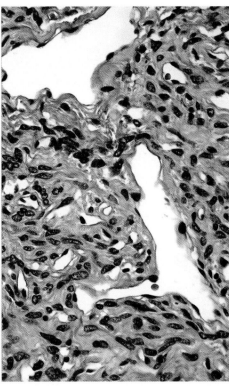

FIGURE 16.30. Solitary fibrous tumor. **Left:** The neoplastic cells are spindled with elongated, slender nuclei. There is a syncytial architecture. The nuclear chromatin is even and delicate. **Right:** Patulous vessels are noted in this solitary fibrous tumor.

appearance of a hemangiopericytoma-like pattern (Fig. 16.30). Some of the vessels may have thick walls. Cysts can be seen, but they are not common; myxoid change is noted. Hypocellular areas alternate with hypercellular areas (Fig. 16.31). Extravasated erythrocytes and inflammatory cells, specifically mast cells, are common. Mitotic figures are rare, and necrosis is not appreciated. The neoplastic cells are spindled with elongated, slender nuclei surrounded by scant cytoplasm. The cells are often considered to be syncytial with indistinct cell borders. The nuclear chromatin is delicate and fine to vesicular (Fig. 16.30).[125–138] A lipomatous variant (adipocytic variant) has been reported.[130,137] On electron microscopy, the cells are nonspecific; the cytoplasm contains few organelles, a poorly developed rough endoplasmic reticulum, scant mitochondria, and intercellular junctions. Filaments are identified, and collagen is noted in the background.[126,129,137]

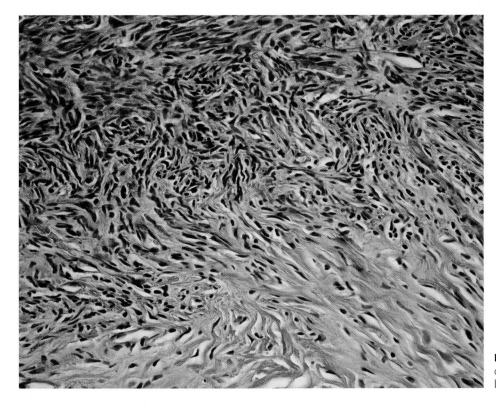

FIGURE 16.31. Solitary fibrous tumor. A cellular area blends into an area of hypocellularity with increased collagen deposition.

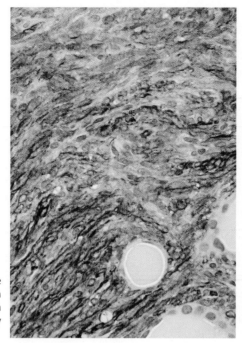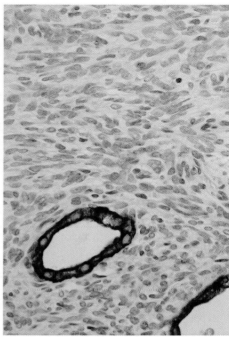

FIGURE 16.32. Solitary fibrous tumor. The neoplastic cells are immunoreactive with CD34 (**left**) while non-reactive with keratin (**right**). Note the mirror image-type reactivity of the thyroid follicular epithelial cells.

Immunohistochemistry and Molecular Diagnostics

As is the case with solitary fibrous tumors in other anatomic sites, the neoplastic cells in thyroid tumors are immunoreactive with vimentin, CD34 (Fig. 16.32), CD99, and bcl-2, whereas S100 protein may highlight the occasional fatty-cell infiltrate. There are reports of actin immunoreactivity.[126] The neoplastic cells are negative with TTF1, thyroglobulin, FVIII-RAg, glial fibrillary acidic protein, HMB-45, EMA, ALK-1, desmin, CD117, and keratins.[126–129,132,135,136,138] Trisomy 21 has not been identified.[132]

Cytopathology

FNA smears are paucicellular. A dyscohesive, slender, spindle-shaped cell population is interspersed with fragments of collagenized stromal tissue.[126,127,135,139]

Differential Diagnosis

Solitary fibrous tumor is considered to be on the opposite end of the morphologic spectrum from hemangiopericytoma. In the thyroid gland, discrimination from smooth muscle tumors, PNSTs, spindle-cell follicular adenoma, anaplastic carcinoma, medullary carcinoma, and post-FNA nodules is usually augmented by a pertinent immunohistochemistry panel applied to the tumors within the differential diagnosis (Table 16.2). Medullary carcinoma cells can be spindled, but they are immunoreactive to keratin and calcitonin. A post-FNA nodule is a localized phenomenon in a nodule that has the characteristic histology of the underlying tumor. CD34 immunoreactivity can be seen in PNSTs, but the other histologic features help make the correct diagnosis. Spindle-cell follicular adenoma does not have collagen deposition, still has colloid production, and is immunoreactive with keratin, TTF1, and thyroglobulin. Carcinomas are usually high grade and epithelial, and they are easily distinguished from solitary fibrous tumors. The paucicellular variant of anaplastic carcinoma has remarkable pleomorphism in isolated cells and lacks CD34 immunoreactivity.[140]

Treatment and Prognosis

Excision is thought to be the treatment of choice for solitary fibrous tumors, although too few cases have been reported to yield definitive treatment recommendations. These tumors are benign by definition, but if increased cellularity, a high-mitotic index, pleomorphism, necrosis, and/or invasive growth with perineural or vascular invasion are noted, a malignant transformation would need to be excluded.[126,128] Recurrence and metastasis have not been reported.[126,131,137,138]

 # FOLLICULAR DENDRITIC CELL TUMOR

A follicular dendritic cell tumor is a primary thyroid gland neoplasm composed of follicular dendritic cells. The term *reticulum-cell sarcoma* is no longer used.[141]

Etiology

There is no known etiologic association for tumors arising in the thyroid gland, although in extrathyroidal locations, this tumor has been associated with exposure to Epstein–Barr virus or Castleman disease of the hyaline-vascular type.[141,142]

Histogenesis and Molecular Genetics

Follicular dendritic cells are the antigen-presenting cells found within the primary and secondary germinal centers of lymph nodes, and these cells are the putative cells of origin for follicular dendritic-cell tumor.[143] Extranodal tumors are uncommon, but when they do occur, they are derived from the same cell type.

Clinical Presentation

These tumors are exceedingly rare in the thyroid gland. Affected adults of both sexes present with a slowly growing painless mass.

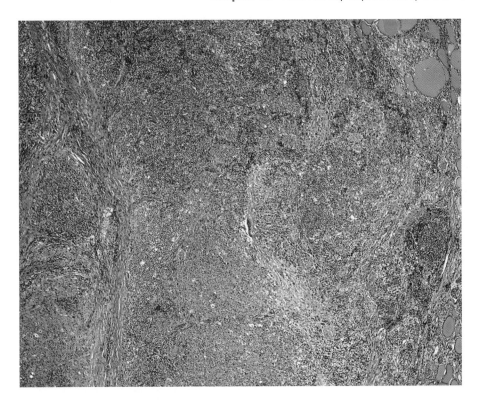

FIGURE 16.33. Follicular dendritic cell tumor. The spindled neoplasm blends with the thyroid parenchyma. Note the lymphocytic thyroiditis. Heavy bands of fibrosis are present.

In up to 20% of cases, cervical lymph nodes express alterations of the hyaline-vascular type of Castleman disease.[141,144]

Pathology

Gross Presentation

These neoplasms are well circumscribed, solid, and tan-gray. Foci of necrosis and blood may be present, especially in large tumors.[144,145]

Microscopic Description

The masses are not encapsulated histologically, but they blend with the thyroid gland parenchyma (Fig 16.33). Lymphatic and blood vessel invasion is common (Fig. 16.34). Tumors are cellular, and they feature a syncytial arrangement of spindled to epithelioid cells arranged in diffuse, fascicular, and whorled patterns (Fig. 16.35). Ample eosinophilic cytoplasm surrounds round to spindled nuclei. The nuclear chromatin is open (vesicular), and

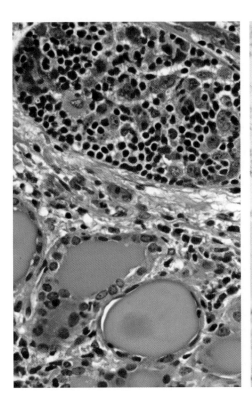
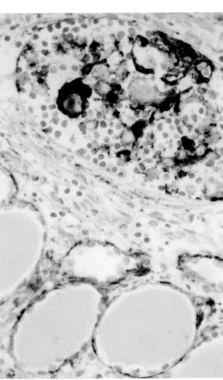

FIGURE 16.34. Follicular dendritic cell tumor. Left: An aggregate of tumor cells is present within a vessel. **Right:** The neoplastic cells within the vessel are CD21 immunoreactive.

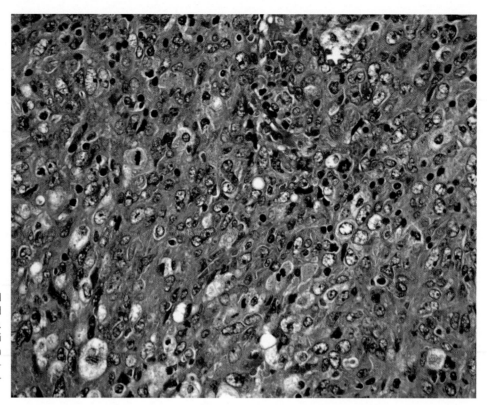

FIGURE 16.35. Follicular dendritic cell tumor. A syncytial arrangement of epithelioid and spindled cells in a diffuse architecture. Eosinophilic cytoplasm surrounds large nuclei with vesicular-open nuclear chromatin with prominent nucleoli. There are numerous mitotic figures, including atypical forms. Lymphocytes are intermingled.

the nucleus contains small, well-defined nucleoli. The mitotic index is quite variable; a high rate is seen in some cases. Grape-like clusters of nuclei occasionally create giant cells that resemble Warthin-Finkeldey cells histologically. Lymphocytes are invariably present, both as part of the neoplasm and in the surrounding thyroid parenchyma (lymphocytic thyroiditis). Perivascular lymphoid cuffing may be seen.[141,144]

Immunohistochemistry and Molecular Diagnostics

The lesional cells are strongly immunoreactive with CD21 (Fig. 16.34), CD35, CD23 (Fig. 16.36), fascin, clusterin, KiM4p, and vimentin and variably immunoreactive with EMA, S100 protein, CD45RB, CD15, and CD68.[146] The cells are nonreactive with keratins (AE1/AE3, CAM5.2) and EBV latent membrane

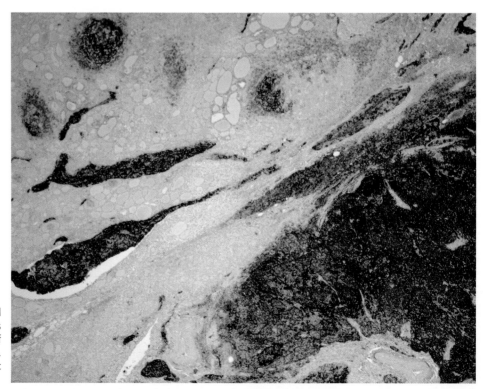

FIGURE 16.36. Follicular dendritic cell tumor. CD23 strongly and diffusely stains the neoplastic cells. Note the many areas of vascular invasion highlighted by the CD23. Lymphoid follicles, part of the lymphocytic thyroiditis, serve as an internal control.

protein-1. Isolated cells react with CD45RB and CD20. The reactive lymphocytes and plasma cells include a mixed T- and B-cell phenotype.[141,144,147]

Differential Diagnosis

The spindled nature of this rare tumor includes it in the differential diagnosis with mesenchymal tumors, medullary carcinoma, spindle cell tumor with thymus-like differentiation (SETTLE), and anaplastic carcinoma. The tumor has a unique cytologic and immunohistochemical profile that allows for separation from other thyroid gland neoplasm, but a high index of suspicion is necessary to make a diagnosis of this rare neoplasm.

Treatment and Prognosis

With only isolated case reports available, it is not possible to issue a definitive statement about prognosis or management. Cervical lymph node metastases may develop; if so, they require complete surgical excision and adjuvant chemotherapy and/or radiation. Secondary thyroid involvement may also be seen.[141,144,145]

LANGERHANS CELL HISTIOCYTOSIS

Langerhans cell histiocytosis (LCH) is a complex entity. It is made up of three distinct clinical syndromes that share identical histologic features. These syndromes are eosinophilic granuloma, which is predominantly osseous or pulmonary; Hand–Schüller–Christian disease, which involves multiple organ systems, most typically the skull base; and Letterer–Siwe disease, the most severe manifestation, which typically involves the abdominal viscera. All of these interrelated diseases are manifestations of an increase in the number of Langerhans cells, unique histiocytic cells that contain Birbeck granules on electron microscopy. The presence of Langerhans cells within the thyroid gland may be either an isolated phenomenon or part of a more widespread disease. Special studies are required to confirm the diagnosis; findings include the characteristic binding of peanut lectin or a positive stain for ATPase, CD207 (Langerin), CD1a, S100 protein, or α-D-mannosidase; or identifying Birbeck granules ultrastructurally.[148,149]

Etiology

Although the etiology of LCH is unknown, possible causes include a neoplastic process,[150] a viral agent,[151–153] or an abnormal proliferative process with varying degrees of cellular differentiation.[149]

Histogenesis and Molecular Genetics

The Langerhans histiocyte is the putative cell of origin. This cell is believed to be a modified histiocyte derived from the dendritic system.[154]

Clinical Presentation

LCH isolated to the thyroid gland is exceptionally rare. It has been reported to occur with greater frequency when it is a part of systemic disease. Affected patients range in age from a few months to old age; a young age at initial presentation (<20 years) is more common with systemic disease, and an older age is more common with isolated thyroid gland involvement.[155–166] Distribution of cases by sex is equal. In most cases, a thyroid gland nodule,

usually unilateral, is identified. Patients also exhibit associated nonspecific symptoms, including sore throat, upper respiratory tract infection, skin rash, pulmonary distress, gastrointestinal symptoms, and lymph node enlargement. These symptoms are usually noted in patients with systemic involvement (bone, skin, liver, lymph nodes, lungs, CNS, spleen, and gastrointestinal tract).[165,167,168] The duration of symptoms ranges from days to years, depending on whether the patient has isolated (longer duration) or systemic disease.[155–160,162–165]

Radiographic findings are not specific. A thyroid scan demonstrates a cold nodule; its size depends on the extent of disease. Ultrasonography demonstrates a mixed-density mass lesion.[156,163–165]

Pathology

Gross Presentation

The nodules of LCH are macroscopically indistinguishable from other thyroid nodules. Lesions can be as small as 2 mm, or they can be very large and almost completely replace the thyroid parenchyma.[165]

Microscopic Description

Thyroid gland involvement by LCH can be either diffuse or focal (Fig. 16.37); there is no specific anatomic predilection, although a subcapsular and septal location appears to be more common. The Langerhans cell histiocytes are characterized by the presence of enlarged cells that contain delicate pale or eosinophilic cytoplasm surrounding vesicular nuclei. The nuclei have an indented, notched, lobulated, folded, grooved, or coffee-bean–shaped appearance, with one or two nucleoli (Fig. 16.38). The cytoplasm is often finely vacuolated, with phagocytized cellular debris. The cellular infiltrate pushes or destroys the thyroid parenchyma, effacing the thyroid follicular architecture. The histiocytic cells may extend beyond the confines of the thyroid capsule, causing the thyroid gland to adhere to the surrounding soft tissue or skeletal muscle. An increased number of eosinophils can be seen intermingled with the Langerhans cells, concentrated in collections around areas of necrosis (Fig. 16.38). Lymphocytic thyroiditis appears to be a common background disorder (Fig. 16.37), while hyperplastic (adenomatoid) nodules, diffuse hyperplasia, and papillary thyroid carcinoma topographically distant from the foci of LCH are occasionally noted.[159,164,165,169–172]

On ultrastructural studies, Langerhans cells have folded, convoluted, and lobulated nuclei with cytoplasmic filopodial extensions that exhibit an uneven cell contour. The cells contain a variable number of invaginations of the cell membrane; these are called *Birbeck granules* or *Langerhans granules*. Outwardly, these granules are disk-shaped, but when they are cross-sectioned, they are rod-shaped. The granules are pentalaminar, with cross-striations, often with the characteristic vesicular expansions imparting a *tennis-racquet* appearance.[158,160,164,173]

Immunohistochemistry and Molecular Diagnostics

The immunohistochemical antigenic profile of Langerhans cells includes diffuse cytoplasmic and nuclear reactivity with S100 protein and cytoplasmic reactivity with CD1a, Langerin (CD207), CD68 (KP-1), lysozyme, (sialated) Leu-M1, Ki-1, CD2, CD3, placental alkaline phosphatase, peanut agglutinin, CD4, CD11c, Cdw32, ATPase or T-6 antigenic determinants, α-1-antichymotrypsin, and anti-Mac. Specifically, Langerin is localized in the Birbeck granules and is a transmembrane cell surface receptor

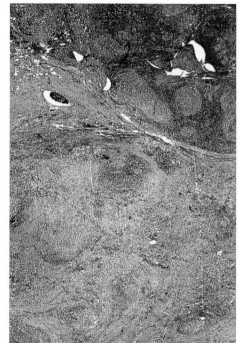
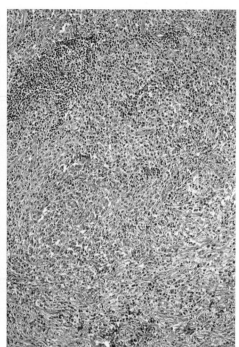

FIGURE 16.37. Langerhans cell histiocytosis. Left: A focus of Langerhans cells is immediately adjacent to an area of lymphocytic thyroiditis. **Right:** Eosinophils are easily identified, even at an intermediate power.

encoded by the *CD207* gene.[174,175] The macrophage antigens generally demonstrate a concentration in the perinuclear space and Golgi region. The cells react with proliferating cell nuclear antigen and Ki-67, but this just confirms local proliferation. The cells are nonreactive with cytokeratin, thyroglobulin, and TTF1.[154,158,160,163–165,175] Practically, a positive reaction with S100, CD1a, CD207 (Langerin) and/or CD68 should yield a diagnosis of LCH.

Cytopathology

FNA cytology reveals scant colloid in a hemorrhagic background with high cellularity. Thyroid follicular epithelial cells are sparse. There are collections of eosinophils, lymphocytes, and isolated discrete, large mononucleated or multinucleated Langerhans cells with prominent nuclear folds (grooves) and abundant foamy, granular cytoplasm. Mitotic figures are common.[157–160,163,164,166,175] The Langerhans cells may mimic papillary thyroid carcinoma cells.

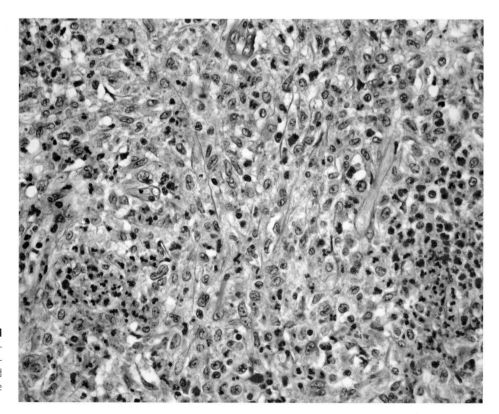

FIGURE 16.38. Langerhans cell histiocytosis. The Langerhans cell histiocytes are large, with abundant, foamy cytoplasm surrounding elongated, grooved, and folded nuclei with grooves. Eosinophils are scattered throughout.

Differential Diagnosis

The main differential diagnoses are other histiocytic disorders, papillary carcinoma, and anaplastic thyroid carcinoma. Massive lymphadenopathy with sinus histiocytosis (Rosai–Dorfman disease) exhibits a characteristic emperipolesis (phagocytized nuclear debris in the cytoplasm of the histiocyte), but the cells have also S100 protein immunoreactivity.[176] The inflammatory infiltrate of lymphocytic thyroiditis may obscure the histiocytes and the eosinophils of LCH, potentially leading one to overlook its presence. Papillary thyroid carcinoma demonstrates cohesive clusters of epithelial cells with nuclear enlargement, nuclear chromatin clearing, nuclear grooves, and intranuclear cytoplasmic inclusions. Anaplastic carcinoma exhibits a much greater degree of pleomorphism and extensive necrosis, tends to lack inflammatory infiltrate, and has a different immunohistochemistry profile.[158,164,165,170]

Treatment and Prognosis

The treatment of LCH differs according to whether it is localized or systemic. For LCH localized to the thyroid, resection is the only treatment necessary. For systemic disease that includes thyroid involvement, combination chemotherapy is the treatment of choice.[158,161,177] Recognition of this lesion should prompt exclusion of systemic disease. The prognosis for LCH is closely related to localized (excellent) versus systemic disease (aggressive, with a poor prognosis).[155–160,162–165] Curiously, when localized thyroid disease is documented, patients tend not to develop subsequent systemic disease.[165,167,168]

 # ROSAI–DORFMAN DISEASE

Rosai–Dorfman disease, also known as *sinus histiocytosis with massive lymphadenopathy*, may primarily affects the thyroid gland. Although some cases of isolated thyroid involvement have been reported, most cases appear to involve the thyroid as part of systemic disease.[178,179]

Histogenesis and Molecular Genetics

Rosai–Dorfman disease is thought to be derived from a functionally activated macrophage, possibly from circulating monocytes.[179]

Clinical Presentation

Extranodal involvement of the thyroid gland is limited to single case reports,[176,180–182] although involvement as part of systemic disease may be seen.[176,183] Painless cervical adenopathy may be present. The only reported cases of isolated thyroid gland involvement have all occurred in women, most of whom were between 20 and 40 years old. This condition is usually discovered incidentally, but the thyroid enlargement may masquerade as anaplastic thyroid carcinoma clinically.[180,181] Leukocytosis, an elevated erythrocyte sedimentation rate, and hypergammaglobulinemia may also be present.[183] Radiographic findings (nodularity) are not specific.[176,184]

Pathology

Microscopic Description

Lymphoid aggregates with plasma cells alternate with pale-appearing areas of histiocytes and lymphocytes in what appear to be dilated vascular spaces (Fig. 16.39). The overall architecture of the lesion simulates a germinal center surrounded by sinuses, such as those seen in a lymph node. Mature lymphocytes, plasma cells, and histiocytes make up the lymphoid aggregates without truly forming a germinal center. The histiocytes can appear in clusters or nests. The histiocytes are the characteristic cells of this lesion. The cells are large with a uniform overall appearance; they contain round to oval,

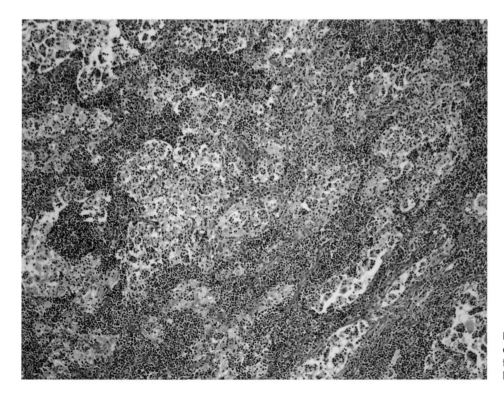

FIGURE 16.39. Rosai-Dorfman disease. Dilated vascular spaces (sinuses) are filled with pale histiocytes. A background of lymphoid aggregates is noted.

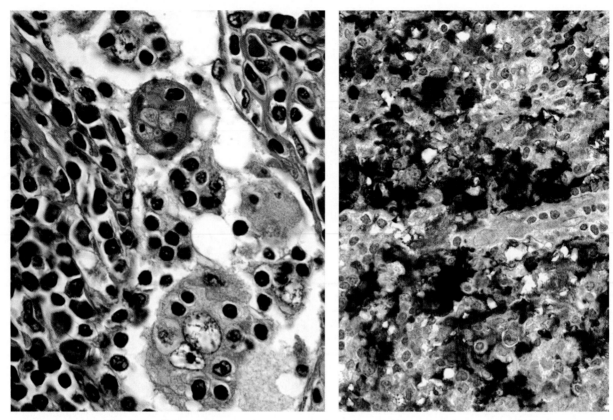

FIGURE 16.40. Rosai-Dorfman disease. Left: Large histiocytes are filled with emperipolesed lymphocytes. Note the "perinuclear" halo surrounding the engulfed nucleus within the cytoplasm of the histiocyte. **Right:** The histiocytes stain strongly and diffusely with S100 protein.

vesicular to hyperchromatic nuclei surrounded by abundant foamy, vacuolated, or clear cytoplasm (Fig. 16.40). There are no nuclear grooves or indentations in the nuclei. Emperipolesis (cytophagocytosis) of lymphocytes (lymphophagocytosis), plasma cells, neutrophils, or erythrocytes within the histiocyte cell cytoplasm is characteristic (Fig. 16.40). A perinuclear halo separates the engulfed nucleus/cell from the cytoplasm of the histiocyte.[176,178,180,181]

Immunohistochemistry and Molecular Diagnostics

The histiocytic cells are diffusely immunoreactive with S100 protein (Fig. 16.40) and CD68 and negative with CD1a. The histiocytes may also be positive with Leu-M3, lysozyme, α-1-antichymotrypsin, α-1-antitrypsin, Leu-M1, and Ki-1.[185,186] The plasma cells in the background are polyclonal, and they exhibit both kappa and lambda light-chain cytoplasmic reactivity.[178]

Differential Diagnosis

The differential diagnosis includes several histiocytic disorders, as well as papillary and anaplastic thyroid carcinoma.[184] The inflammatory infiltrate of lymphocytic thyroiditis may overshadow the histiocytes, potentially leading one to overlook their presence. LCH has grooved nuclei and xanthomatous cytoplasm, lacks emperipolesis, usually has many eosinophils, and the lesional cells are immunoreactive with CD1a.[154] Sarcoidosis reveals epithelioid histiocytes and giant cells in tightly clustered nodules, while also lacking emperipolesis. Hodgkin lymphoma is exceedingly uncommon in the thyroid gland, but sometimes

the Reed–Sternberg variants can simulate the histiocytes of Rosai–Dorfman disease. However, the Reed–Sternberg variants contain prominent nucleoli, tend to be binucleated or multinucleated, and are negative with S100 protein and positive with CD15 and CD30.

Treatment and Prognosis

Steroid therapy may result in regression of the disease, but disease isolated to the thyroid gland generally must be managed by surgery.[176,178,180,181,183]

 # GRANULAR CELL TUMOR

Primary granular cell tumor of the thyroid gland is exceedingly uncommon, with only isolated case reports.[187–195]

Histogenesis and Molecular Genetics

Although only anecdotal, a neural crest origin is suggested for this tumor type derived from nerve sheath.[194]

Clinical Presentation

The patients present with a nonspecific mass in the neck, not associated with thyroid gland dysfunction. The tumor may be identified incidentally. There seems to be a preponderance of female to male patients (6:1). Although any age can be affected, patients seem to be young at initial presentation (mean, 21 years). An FNA may be used to identify the tumor.[194]

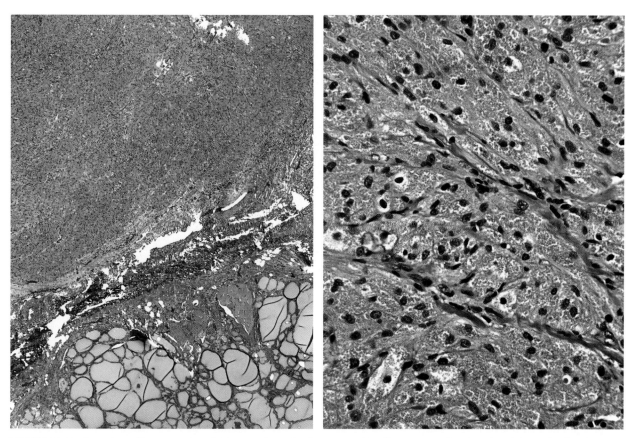

FIGURE 16.41. Granular cell tumor. Note the large, polygonal cells, separated by fibrous connective tissue bands immediately adjacent to thyroid gland parenchyma. There is abundant granular, eosinophilic cytoplasm.

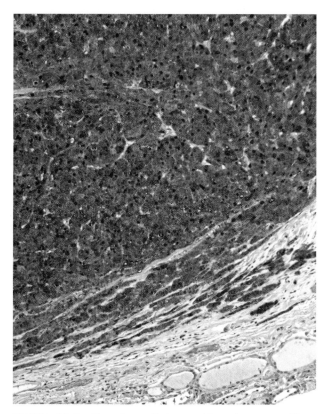

FIGURE 16.42. Granular cell tumor. There is strong, diffuse, nuclear, and cytoplasmic immunoreactivity with S100 protein.

Pathology

Microscopic Description

The tumor may appear macroscopically as a circumscribed tumor nodule. The cells are separated into nests by fibrous septa, which mingle with the surrounding thyroid follicular epithelium. The cells are large, epithelioid to polygonal, with abundant granular, eosinophilic cytoplasm (Fig. 16.41). The cell borders may be inconspicuous. The nuclei are round and regular with coarse to uniform nuclear chromatin distribution and inconspicuous nucleoli. Mitoses are inconspicuous. Although malignancy is not well defined in this location, tumor cell spindling, necrosis, prominent nucleoli, increased nuclear to cytoplasmic ratio, nuclear pleomorphism, and increased mitoses are known to be associated with malignant clinical behavior in soft tissue locations.[196]

Cytology, Immunohistochemistry, and Molecular Diagnostics

Smears show single cells, pseudofollicles or syncytial clusters of large cells. The large cells have small round to oval or spindled nuclei, small nucleoli, and abundant grayish, granular fragile cytoplasm. Owing to the cytoplasmic fragility, there are many naked nuclei and granular debris in the background.[188,192] The cytologic features of atypical tumors include focal spindle–cell morphology, increased nuclear to cytoplasmic ratio, and prominent nucleoli.[187,190] The immunohistochemistry results are similar for their soft tissue counterparts, with strong nuclear and cytoplasmic reactivity with S100 protein (Fig. 16.42) and calretinin, cytoplasmic reactivity with vimentin, NSE, PGP9.5, myelin basic protein, and CD68, whereas negative for keratin, TTF1, thyroglobulin, calcitonin, and chromogranin.[191]

Differential Diagnosis

The tumor most closely resembles any primary oncocytic neoplasms (adenoma, papillary or follicular carcinoma, and medullary carcinoma) or may look like a PGL. However, the unique immunohistochemistry profile helps with separation.

Treatment and Prognosis

Surgery (lobectomy) seems to yield a cure, although there are only limited case reports.

REFERENCES

1. Eusebi V. Angiosarcoma. In: DeLellis RA, Lloyd RV, Heitz PU, et al., eds. *Pathology and Genetics of Tumours of Endocrine Organs*. Lyon, France: IARC Press; 2004:113–114.
2. Eusebi V, Carcangiu ML, Dina R, et al. Keratin-positive epithelioid angiosarcoma of thyroid. A report of four cases. *Am J Surg Pathol*. 1990;14:737–747.
3. Rhomberg W, Gruber-Mosenbacher U, Eiter H, et al. Prognosis and epidemiology of malignant hemangioendotheliomas of the thyroid gland. *Schweiz Med Wochenschr*. 1993;123:1640–1644.
4. Bacher-Stier C, Riccabona G, Totsch M, et al. Incidence and clinical characteristics of thyroid carcinoma after iodine prophylaxis in an endemic goiter country. *Thyroid*. 1997;7:733–741.
5. Goh SG, Chuah KL, Goh HK, et al. Two cases of epithelioid angiosarcoma involving the thyroid and a brief review of non-Alpine epithelioid angiosarcoma of the thyroid. *Arch Pathol Lab Med*. 2003;127:E70–E73.
6. Lin O, Gerhard R, Coelho Siqueira SA, et al. Cytologic findings of epithelioid angiosarcoma of the thyroid. A case report. *Acta Cytol*. 2002;46:767–771.
7. Maiorana A, Collina G, Cesinaro AM, et al. Epithelioid angiosarcoma of the thyroid. Clinicopathological analysis of seven cases from non-Alpine areas. *Virchows Arch*. 1996;429:131–137.
8. Ryska A, Ludvikova M, Szepe P, et al. Epithelioid haemangiosarcoma of the thyroid gland. Report of six cases from a non-Alpine region. *Histopathology*. 2004;44:40–46.
9. Ritter JH, Mills SE, Nappi O, et al. Angiosarcoma-like neoplasms of epithelial organs: true endothelial tumors or variants of carcinoma? *Semin Diagn Pathol*. 1995;12:270–282.
10. Chan YF, Ma L, Boey JH, et al. Angiosarcoma of the thyroid. An immunohistochemical and ultrastructural study of a case in a Chinese patient. *Cancer*. 1986;57:2381–2388.
11. Isa NM, James DT, Saw TH, et al. Primary angiosarcoma of the thyroid gland with recurrence diagnosed by fine needle aspiration: a case report. *Diagn Cytopathol*. 2009;37:427–432.
12. Kalitova P, Plzak J, Kodet R, et al. Angiosarcoma of the thyroid. *Eur Arch Otorhinolaryngol*. 2009;266:903–905.
13. Lamovec J, Zidar A, Zidanik B. Epithelioid angiosarcoma of the thyroid gland. Report of two cases. *Arch Pathol Lab Med*. 1994;118:642–646.
14. Liu M, Ba E, Zhao P, et al. A clinicopathological study of fifteen epithelioid angiosarcoma. *Zhonghua Bing Li Xue Za Zhi*. 2002;31:407–410.
15. Papotti M, Arrondini M, Tavaglione V, et al. Diagnostic controversies in vascular proliferations of the thyroid gland. *Endocr Pathol*. 2008;19:175–183.
16. Rhomberg W, Boehler F, Eiter H, et al. Treatment options for malignant hemangioendotheliomas of the thyroid. *Int J Radiat Oncol Biol Phys*. 2004;60:401–405.
17. Totsch M, Dobler G, Feichtinger H, et al. Malignant hemangioendothelioma of the thyroid. Its immunohistochemical discrimination from undifferentiated thyroid carcinoma. *Am J Surg Pathol*. 1990;14:69–74.
18. Proces S, Schroeyers P, Delos M, et al. Angiosarcoma of the thyroid and concurrent hyperthyroidism. *J Endocrinol Invest*. 1998;21:67–69.
19. Papotti M, Volante M, Negro F, et al. Thyroglobulin mRNA expression helps to distinguish anaplastic carcinoma from angiosarcoma of the thyroid. *Virchows Arch*. 2000;437:635–642.
20. Mills SE, Gaffey MJ, Watts JC, et al. Angiomatoid carcinoma and 'angiosarcoma' of the thyroid gland. A spectrum of endothelial differentiation. *Am J Clin Pathol*. 1994;102:322–330.
21. Bisceglia M, Vairo M, Tardio G, et al. Primary angiosarcoma of the thyroid. Presentation of a case (epithelioid type) and nosological problems. *Pathologica*. 1995;87:154–161.
22. Kim NR, Ko YH, Sung CO. A case of coexistent angiosarcoma and follicular carcinoma of the thyroid. *J Korean Med Sci*. 2003;18:908–913.
23. Mills SE, Stallings RG, Austin MB. Angiomatoid carcinoma of the thyroid gland. Anaplastic carcinoma with follicular and medullary features mimicking angiosarcoma. *Am J Clin Pathol*. 1986;86:674–678.
24. Bandorski D, Arps H, Jaspersen D, et al. Severe intestinal bleeding caused by intestinal metastases of a primary angiosarcome of the thyroid gland. *Z Gastroenterol*. 2002;40:811–814.
25. Eng SP, Goh CH, Khoo JB, et al. Metastatic angiosarcoma to the thyroid. *Rev Laryngol Otol Rhinol*. 2005;126:111–114.
26. Njim L, Moussa A, Hadhri R, et al. Angiomatoid tumor of the thyroid gland: primitive angiosarcoma or variant of anaplastic carcinoma?. *Ann Pathol*. 2008;28:221–224.
27. Aulicino MR, Kaneko M, Unger PD. Excessive endothelial cell proliferation occurring in an organizing thyroid hematoma: report of a case and review of the literature. *Endocr Pathol*. 1995;6:153–158.
28. Yu J, Steiner FA, Muench JP, et al. Juxtathyroidal neck soft tissue angiosarcoma presenting as an undifferentiated thyroid carcinoma. *Thyroid*. 2002;12:427–432.
29. Yilmazlar T, Kirdak T, Adim S, et al. A case of hemangiosarcoma in thyroid with severe anemia due to bone marrow metastasis. *Endocr J*. 2005;52:57–59.
30. Thompson LDR, Rosai J, Heffess CS. Primary thyroid teratomas: a clinicopathologic study of 30 cases. *Cancer*. 2000;88:1149–1158.
31. Thompson LDR, Craver RD. Teratoma. In: DeLellis RA, Lloyd RV, Heitz PU, et al., eds. *Pathology and Genetics of Tumours of Endocrine Organs*. Lyon, France: IARC Press; 2004:106–108.
32. Rosai J, Carcangiu ML, DeLellis RA. *Tumors of the Thyroid Gland*. Vol. 5. 3rd ed. Washington, DC: Armed Forces Institute of Pathology; 1992:280–282.
33. Jordan RB, Gauderer MWL. Cervical teratomas: an analysis, literature review and proposed classification. *J Pediatr Surg*. 1988;23:583–591.
34. Lack EE. Extragonadal germ cell tumors of the head and neck region: review of 16 cases. *Hum Pathol*. 1985;16:56–64.
35. Perez-Mies B, Regojo Zapata RM, Garcia-Fernandez E, et al. Malignant teratoma of the thyroid in a pregnant woman. *Ann Diagn Pathol*. 2010;14:264–267.
36. Vujanic GM, Harach HR, Minic P, et al. Thyroid/cervical teratomas in children: immunohistochemical studies for specific thyroid epithelial cell markers. *Pediatr Pathol*. 1994;14:369–375.
37. Zerella JT, Finberg FJ. Obstruction of the neonatal airway from teratomas. *Surg Gynecol Obstet*. 1990;170:126–131.
38. Buckley NJ, Burch WM, Leight GS. Malignant teratoma in the thyroid gland of an adult: a case report and a review of the literature. *Surgery*. 1986;100:932–937.
39. Jayaram G, Cheah PL, Yip CH. Malignant teratoma of the thyroid with predominantly neuroepithelial differentiation. Fine needle aspiration cytologic, histologic and immunocytochemical features of a case. *Acta Cytol*. 2000;44:375–379.
40. Kier R, Silverman PM, Korobkin M, et al. Malignant teratoma of the thyroid in an adult: CT appearance. *J Comput Assist Tomogr*. 1985;9:174–176.
41. Ueno NT, Amato RJ, Ro JJ, et al. Primary malignant teratoma of the thyroid gland: report and discussion of two cases. *Head Neck*. 1998;20:649–653.
42. Zhang YZ, Li WH, Zhu MJ, et al. An unusual mature thyroid teratoma on CT and 99Tcm scintigraphy imaging in a child. *Pediatr Radiol*. 2010;40:1831–1833.
43. Bowker CM, Whittaker RS. Malignant teratoma of the thyroid: case report and literature review of thyroid teratoma in adults. *Histopathology*. 1992;21:81–83.
44. Chen JS, Lai GM, Hsueh S. Malignant thyroid teratoma of an adult: a long-term survival after chemotherapy. *Am J Clin Oncol*. 1998;21:212–214.
45. Craver RD, Lipscomb JT, Suskind D, et al. Malignant teratoma of the thyroid with primitive neuroepithelial and mesenchymal sarcomatous components. *Ann Diagn Pathol*. 2001;5:285–292.
46. Lecomte-Houcke M, Parent M, Carnaille B, et al. Teratomes malins primitifs de la thyroide. Deux observations avec etudes immunohistochimique et ultrastructurale. *Ann Pathol*. 1992;12:12–19.
47. Valdiserri RO, Yunis EJ. Sacrococcygeal teratomas: a review of 68 cases. *Cancer*. 1981;48:217–221.
48. Kooijman CD. Immature teratomas in children. *Histopathology*. 1988;12:491–502.
49. Norris HJ, Zirkin HJ, Benson WL. Immature (malignant) teratoma of the ovary, a clinical and pathological study of 58 cases. *Cancer*. 1976;37:2359–2372.
50. Kahle M, Filler RD. Das maligne Teratom der Schilddruse. *Dtsch Med Wochenschr*. 1990;115:784–786.
51. Akoojee SB. A case of cervical teratoma arising in the thyroid gland and causing obstructive respiratory symptoms in a neonate is described. *S Afr Med J*. 1980;57:93–94.
52. Kemp DR. Teratoma of the neck in the adult. Report of a case and review of the literature. *Aust NZ J Surg*. 1967;36:323–327.
53. Thompson LDR. Smooth muscle tumours. In: DeLellis RA, Lloyd RV, Heitz PU, et al., eds. *Pathology and Genetics of Tumours of Endocrine Organs*. Lyon, France: IARC Press, 2004:115.
54. Thompson LDR, Wenig BM, Adair CF, et al. Primary smooth muscle tumors of the thyroid gland. *Cancer*. 1997;79:579–587.
55. Tulbah A, Al Dayel F, Fawaz I, et al. Epstein-Barr virus-associated leiomyosarcoma of the thyroid in a child with congenital immunodeficiency: a case report. *Am J Surg Pathol*. 1999;23:473–476.
56. Kawahara E, Nakanishi I, Terahata S, et al. Leiomyosarcoma of the thyroid gland. A case report with a comparative study of five cases of anaplastic carcinoma. *Cancer*. 1988;62:2558–2563.
57. Andrion A, Bellis D, Delsedime L, et al. Leiomyoma and neurilemoma: report of two unusual non-epithelial tumours of the thyroid gland. *Virchows Arch A Pathol Anat Histopathol*. 1988;413:367–372.
58. Bertelli AA, Massarollo LC, Volpi EM, et al. Thyroid gland primary leiomyosarcoma. *Arq Bras Endocrinol Metabol*. 2010;54:326–330.
59. Biankin SA, Cachia AR. Leiomyoma of the thyroid gland. *Pathology*. 1999;31:64–66.
60. Chetty R, Clark SP, Dowling JP. Leiomyosarcoma of the thyroid: immunohistochemical and ultrastructural study. *Pathology*. 1993;25:203–205.
61. Day AS, Lou PJ, Lin WC, et al. Over-expression of c-kit in a primary leiomyosarcoma of the thyroid gland. *Eur Arch Otorhinolaryngol*. 2007;264:705–708.
62. Erkilic S, Erkilic A, Bayazit YA. Primary leiomyoma of the thyroid gland. *J Laryngol Otol*. 2003;117:832–834.

63. Iida Y, Katoh R, Yoshioka M, et al. Primary leiomyosarcoma of the thyroid gland. *Acta Pathol Jpn.* 1993;43:71–75.

64. Ozaki O, Sugino K, Mimura T, et al. Primary leiomyosarcoma of the thyroid gland. *Surg Today.* 1997;27:177–180.

65. Takayama F, Takashima S, Matsuba H, et al. MR imaging of primary leiomyosarcoma of the thyroid gland. *Eur J Radiol.* 2001;37:36–41.

66. Tsugawa K, Koyanagi N, Nakanishi K, et al. Leiomyosarcoma of the thyroid gland with rapid growth and tracheal obstruction: a partial thyroidectomy and tracheostomy using an ultrasonically activated scalpel can be safely performed with less bleeding. *Eur J Med Res.* 1999;4:483–487.

67. Adachi M, Wellmann KF, Garcia R. Metastatic leiomyosarcoma in brain and heart. *J Pathol.* 1969;98:294–296.

68. Kaur A, Jayaram G. Thyroid tumors: cytomorphology of medullary, clinically anaplastic, and miscellaneous thyroid neoplasms. *Diagn Cytopathol.* 1990;6:383–389.

69. Nemenqani D, Yaqoob N, Khoja H. Leiomyosarcoma metastatic to the thyroid diagnosed by fine needle aspiration cytology. *J Pak Med Assoc.* 2010;60:307–309.

70. Marioni G, Bertino G, Mariuzzi L, et al. Laryngeal leiomyosarcoma. *J Laryngol Otol.* 2000;114:398–401.

71. Ivy HK. Cancer metastatic to the thyroid: a diagnostic problem. *Mayo Clin Proc.* 1984;59:856–859.

72. Chen H, Nicol TL, Udelsman R. Clinically significant, isolated metastatic disease to the thyroid gland. *World J Surg.* 1999;23:177–180.

73. Deng XR, Wang G, Kuang CJ, et al. Metastasis of leiomyosarcoma to the thyroid. *Chin Med J(Engl.)* 2005;118:174–176.

74. Leath CA, III, Huh WK, Straughn JM Jr., et al. Uterine leiomyosarcoma metastatic to the thyroid. *Obstet Gynecol.* 2002;100:1122–1124.

75. Akata D, Aralasmak A, Ozmen MN, et al. US and CT findings of multicentric leiomyosarcomatosis. *Eur Radiol.* 1999;9:711–714.

76. Bode-Lesniewska B, Schroder S, Gemsenjager E, et al. Leiomyosarcoma in the thyroid gland—primary tumor or metastasis? *Pathologe.* 1994;15:303–307.

77. Cruickshank JC. Leiomyosarcoma metastatic to the thyroid gland. *Ear Nose Throat J.* 1988;67:899–904.

78. Wang TY, Lee CH, Yang AH, et al. Metastatic leiomyosarcoma of the thyroid: a case report. *Zhonghua Yi Xue Za Zhi. Taipei* 1998;61:353–357.

79. Thompson LDR. Peripheral nerve sheath tumours. In: DeLellis RA, Lloyd RV, Heitz PU, et al., eds. *Pathology and Genetics of Tumours of Endocrine Organs.* Lyon, France: IARC Press; 2004:116.

80. Goldstein J, Tovi F, Sidi J. Primary Schwannoma of the thyroid gland. *Int Surg.* 1982;67:433–434.

81. Thompson LDR, Wenig BM, Adair CF, et al. Peripheral nerve sheath tumors of the thyroid gland: a series of four cases and a review of the literature. *Endocr Pathol.* 1996;7:309–318.

82. Anagnostouli M, Piperingos G, Yapijakis C, et al. Thyroid gland neurofibroma in a NF1 patient. *Acta Neurol Scand.* 2002;106:58–61.

83. Leslie MD, Cheung KY. Malignant transformation of neurofibromas at multiple sites in a case of neurofibromatosis. *Postgrad Med J.* 1987;63:131–133.

84. Al Ghamdi S, Fageeh N, Dewan M. Malignant schwannoma of the thyroid gland. *Otolaryngol Head Neck Surg.* 2000;122:143–144.

85. Andrion A, Mazzucco G, Torchio B. FNA cytology of thyroid neurilemmoma (schwannoma). *Diagn Cytopathol.* 1992;8:311–312.

86. Aoki T, Kumeda S, Iwasa T, et al. Primary neurilemoma of the thyroid gland: report of a case. *Surg Today.* 1993;23:265–268.

87. Gustafson LM, Liu JH, Rutter MJ, et al. Primary neurilemoma of the thyroid gland: a case report. *Am J Otolaryngol.* 2001;22:84–86.

88. Jayaram G. Neurilemmoma (schwannoma) of the thyroid diagnosed by fine needle aspiration cytology. *Acta Cytol.* 1999;43:743–744.

89. Pallares J, Perez-Ruiz L, Ros S, et al. Malignant peripheral nerve sheath tumor of the thyroid: a clinicopathological and ultrastructural study of one case. *Endocr Pathol.* 2004;15:167–174.

90. Sugita R, Nomura T, Yuda F. Primary schwannoma of the thyroid gland: CT findings. *AJR Am J Roentgenol.* 1998;171:528–529.

91. An J, Oh YL, Shin JH, et al. Primary schwannoma of the thyroid gland: a case report. *Acta Cytol.* 2010;54:857–862.

92. Uri O, Baron E, Lefel O, et al. Primary schwannoma of the thyroid gland presenting as an asymptomatic cold nodule. *Am J Otolaryngol.* 2009;30:427–429.

93. Vege DS, Chinoy RF, Ganesth B, et al. Malignant peripheral nerve sheath tumors of the head and neck: a clinicopathological study. *J Surg Oncol.* 1994;55:100–103.

94. Dickersin GR. The electron microscopic spectrum of nerve sheath tumors. *Ultrastruct Pathol.* 1987;11:103–146.

95. Hirose T, Scheithauer BW, Sano T. Perineurial malignant peripheral nerve sheath tumor (MPNST): a clinicopathologic, immunohistochemical, and ultrastructural study of seven cases. *Am J Surg Pathol.* 1998;22:1368–1378.

96. Mertens F, Dal Cin P, De Wever I, et al. Cytogenetic characterization of peripheral nerve sheath tumours: a report of the CHAMP study group. *J Pathol.* 2000;190:31–38.

97. Wojcik EM. Fine needle aspiration of metastatic malignant schwannoma to the thyroid gland. *Diagn Cytopathol.* 1997;16:94–95.

98. Badawi RA, Scott-Coombes D. Ancient schwannoma masquerading as a thyroid mass. *Eur J Surg Oncol.* 2002;28:88–90.

99. Aldinger KA, Samaan NA, Ibanez M, et al. Anaplastic carcinoma of the thyroid: a review of 84 cases of spindle and giant cell carcinoma of the thyroid. *Cancer.* 1978;41:2267–2275.

100. Boos S, Meyer E, Wimmer B, et al. Malignant triton tumor of the thyroid gland. *Radiat Med.* 1991;9:159–161.

101. Naruse T, Koike A, Suzumura K, et al. Malignant "triton" tumor in the thyroid—a case report. *Jpn J Surg.* 1991;21:466–70.

102. Gattuso P, Castelli MJ, Reyes CV. Fine needle aspiration cytology of metastatic sarcoma involving the thyroid. *South Med J.* 1989;82:1158–1160.

103. Ferrozzi F, Bova D, Campodonico F, et al. US and CT findings of secondary neoplasms of the thyroid—a pictorial essay. *Clin Imaging.* 1998;22:157–161.

104. McCabe DP, Farrar WB, Petkov TM, et al. Clinical and pathologic correlations in disease metastatic to the thyroid gland. *Am J Surg.* 1985;150:519–523.

105. Michelow PM, Leiman G. Metastases to the thyroid gland: diagnosis by aspiration cytology. *Diagn Cytopathol.* 1995;13:209–213.

106. King R, Busam K, Rosai J. Metastatic malignant melanoma resembling malignant peripheral nerve sheath tumor: report of 16 cases. *Am J Surg Pathol.* 1999;23:1499–1505.

107. Chung SY, Kim EK, Kim JH, et al. Sonographic findings of metastatic disease to the thyroid. *Yonsei Med J.* 2001;42:411–417.

108. DeLellis RA. Paraganglioma. In: DeLellis RA, Lloyd RV, Heitz PU, et al., eds. *Pathology and Genetics of Tumours of Endocrine Organs.* Lyon, France: IARC Press; 2004:117.

109. Brownlee RE, Shockley WW. Thyroid paraganglioma. *Ann Otol Rhinol Laryngol.* 1992;101:293–299.

110. Bikhazi PH, Messina L, Mhatre AN, et al. Molecular pathogenesis in sporadic head and neck paraganglioma. *Laryngoscope.* 2000;110:1346–1348.

111. Baloch ZW, LiVolsi VA. Neuroendocrine tumors of the thyroid gland. *Am J Clin Pathol.* 2001;115(suppl):S56–S67.

112. Bizollon MH, Darreye G, Berger N. Thyroid paraganglioma: report of a case. *Ann Pathol.* 1997;17:416–418.

113. Buss DH, Marshall RB, Baird FG, et al. Paraganglioma of the thyroid gland. *Am J Surg Pathol.* 1980;4:589–593.

114. Cayot F, Bastien H, Justrabo E, et al. Multiple paragangliomas of the neck localized in the thyroid region. Papillary thyroid cancer associated with parathyroid adenoma. *Sem Hop.* 1982;58:2004–2007.

115. Corrado S, Montanini V, De GC, et al. Primary paraganglioma of the thyroid gland. *J Endocrinol Invest* 2004;27:788–792.

116. Ferri E, Manconi R, Armato E, et al. Primary paraganglioma of thyroid gland: a clinicopathologic and immunohistochemical study with review of the literature. *Acta Otorhinolaryngol Ital.* 2009;29:97–102.

117. Kay S, Montague JW, Dodd RW. Nonchromaffin paraganglioma (chemodectoma) of thyroid region. *Cancer.* 1975;36:582–855.

118. Mitsudo SM, Grajower MM, Balbi H, et al. Malignant paraganglioma of the thyroid gland. *Arch Pathol Lab Med.* 1987;111:378–380.

119. Napolitano L, Francomano F, Angelucci D, et al. Thyroid paraganglioma: report of a case and review of the literature. *Ann Ital Chir.* 2000;71:511–513.

120. Tytor M, Olofsson J. Thyroid tumors invading the larynx and trachea. *J Otolaryngol.* 1986;15:74–79.

121. Vodovnik A. Fine needle aspiration cytology of primary thyroid paraganglioma. Report of a case with cytologic, histologic and immunohistochemical features and differential diagnostic considerations. *Acta Cytol.* 2002;46:1133–1137.

122. Carney JA, Ryan J, Goellner JR. Hyalinizing trabecular adenoma of the thyroid gland. *Am J Surg Pathol.* 1987;11:583–591.

123. Ikeda T, Satoh M, Azuma K, et al. Medullary thyroid carcinoma with a paraganglioma-like pattern and melanin production: a case report with ultrastructural and immunohistochemical studies. *Arch Pathol Lab Med.* 1998;122:555–558.

124. Sobrinho-Simões M, Cameselle-Teijeiro J. Solitary fibrous tumour. In: DeLellis RA, Lloyd RV, Heitz PU, et al., eds. *Pathology and Genetics of Tumours of Endocrine Organs.* Lyon, France: IARC Press; 2004:118–119.

125. Papi G, Corrado S, Uberti ED, et al. Solitary fibrous tumor of the thyroid gland. *Thyroid.* 2007;17:119–126.

126. Rodriguez I, Ayala E, Caballero C, et al. Solitary fibrous tumor of the thyroid gland: report of seven cases. *Am J Surg Pathol.* 2001;25:1424–1428.

127. Babouk NL. Solitary fibrous tumor of the thyroid gland. *Saudi Med J.* 2004;25:805–807.

128. Bohorquez CL, Gonzalez-Campora R, Loscertales MC, et al. Solitary fibrous tumor of the thyroid with capsular invasion. *Pathol Res Pract.* 2003;199:687–690.

129. Cameselle-Teijeiro J, Varela-Duran J, Fonseca E, et al. Solitary fibrous tumor of the thyroid. *Am J Clin Pathol.* 1994;101:535–538.

130. Cameselle-Teijeiro J, Manuel LJ, Villanueva JP, et al. Lipomatous haemangiopericytoma (adipocytic variant of solitary fibrous tumour) of the thyroid. *Histopathology.* 2003;43:406–408.

131. Deshmukh NS, Mangham DC, Warfield AT, et al. Solitary fibrous tumour of the thyroid gland. *J Laryngol Otol.* 2001;115:940–942.

132. Larsen SR, Godballe C, Krogdahl A. Solitary fibrous tumor arising in an intrathoracic goiter. *Thyroid.* 2010;20:435–437.

133. Kie JH, Kim JY, Park YN, et al. Solitary fibrous tumour of the thyroid. *Histopathology.* 1997;30:365–368.

134. Papi G, Corrado S, Ruggiero C, et al. Solitary fibrous tumor of the thyroid gland associated with papillary thyroid carcinoma. *Thyroid.* 2006;16:319–320.

135. Parwani AV, Galindo R, Steinberg DM, et al. Solitary fibrous tumor of the thyroid: cytopathologic findings and differential diagnosis. *Diagn Cytopathol.* 2003;28:213–216.

136. Santeusanio G, Schiaroli S, Ortenzi A, et al. Solitary fibrous tumour of thyroid: report of two cases with immunohistochemical features and literature review. *Head Neck Pathol.* 2008;2:231–235.

137. Taccagni G, Sambade C, Nesland J, et al. Solitary fibrous tumour of the thyroid: clinicopathological, immunohistochemical and ultrastructural study of three cases. *Virchows Arch A Pathol Anat Histopathol.* 1993;422:491–497.

138. Tanahashi J, Kashima K, Daa T, et al. Solitary fibrous tumor of the thyroid gland: report of two cases and review of the literature. *Pathol Int.* 2006;56:471–477.

139. Farrag TY, Micchelli S, Tufano RP. Solitary fibrous tumor of the thyroid gland. *Laryngoscope.* 2009;119:2306–2308.

140. Canos JC, Serrano A, Matias-Guiu X. Paucicellular variant of anaplastic thyroid carcinoma: report of two cases. *Endocr Pathol.* 2001;12:157–161.
141. DeLellis RA. Follicular dendritic cell tumour. In: DeLellis RA, Lloyd RV, Heitz PU, et al., eds. *Pathology and Genetics of Tumours of Endocrine Organs.* Lyon, France: IARC Press; 2004:120.
142. Biddle DA, Ro JY, Yoon GS, et al. Extranodal follicular dendritic cell sarcoma of the head and neck region: three new cases, with a review of the literature. *Mod Pathol.* 2002;15:50–58.
143. Kasajima T, Yamakawa M, Imai Y. Immunohistochemical study of intrathyroidal lymph follicles. *Clin Immunol.Immunopathol.* 1987;43:117–128.
144. Galati LT, Barnes EL, Myers EN. Dendritic cell sarcoma of the thyroid. *Head Neck.* 1999;21:273–275.
145. Kawasaki T, Watanabe G, Hasegawa G, et al. Multiple extranodal follicular dendritic cell tumors initially presenting in the soft tissue in the chest wall. *Pathol Int.* 2006;56:30–34.
146. Fonseca R, Yamakawa M, Nakamura S, et al. Follicular dendritic cell sarcoma and interdigitating reticulum cell sarcoma: a review. *Am J Hematol.* 1998;59:161–167.
147. Chan JK, Fletcher CD, Nayler SJ, et al. Follicular dendritic cell sarcoma. Clinicopathologic analysis of 17 cases suggesting a malignant potential higher than currently recognized. *Cancer.* 1997;79:294–313.
148. Favara BE, Jaffe R. The histopathology of Langerhans cell histiocytosis. *Br J Cancer Suppl.* 1994;23:S17–S23.
149. Writing Group of the Histiocyte Society. Histiocytosis syndromes in children. *Lancet.* 1987;1:208–209.
150. Willman CL. Detection of clonal histiocytes in Langerhans cell histiocytosis: biology and clinical significance. *Br J Cancer Suppl.* 1994;23:S29–S33.
151. Leahy MA, Krejci SM, Friednash M, et al. Human herpesvirus 6 is present in lesions of Langerhans cell histiocytosis. *J Invest Dermatol.* 1993;101:642–645.
152. McClain K, Weiss RA. Viruses and Langerhans cell histiocytosis: is there a link? *Br J Cancer Suppl.* 1994;23:S34–S36.
153. Mierau GW, Wills EJ, Steele PO. Ultrastructural studies in Langerhans cell histiocytosis: a search for evidence of viral etiology. *Pediatr Pathol.* 1994;14:895–904.
154. Thompson LDR. Langerhans cell histiocytosis. In: DeLellis RA, Lloyd RV, Heitz PU, et al., eds. *Pathology and Genetics of Tumours of Endocrine Organs.* Lyon, France: IARC Press; 2004:121.
155. Behrens RJ, Levi AW, Westra WH, et al. Langerhans cell histiocytosis of the thyroid: a report of two cases and review of the literature. *Thyroid.* 2001;11:697–705.
156. Chong VF. Langerhans cell histiocytosis with thyroid involvement. *Eur J Radiol.* 1996;22:155–157.
157. Dey P, Luthra UK, Sheikh ZA. Fine needle aspiration cytology of Langerhans cell histiocytosis of the thyroid. A case report. *Acta Cytol.* 1999;43:429–431.
158. el Halabi DA, el Sayed M, Eskaf W, et al. Langerhans cell histiocytosis of the thyroid gland. A case report. *Acta Cytol.* 2000;4:805–808.
159. Goldstein N, Layfield LJ. Thyromegaly secondary to simultaneous papillary carcinoma and histiocytosis X. Report of a case and review of the literature. *Acta Cytol.* 1991;35:422–426.
160. Kirchgraber PR, Weaver MG, Arafah BM, et al. Fine needle aspiration cytology of Langerhans cell histiocytosis involving the thyroid. A case report. *Acta Cytol.* 1994;38:101–106.
161. Lin CH, Lin WC, Chiang IP, et al. Langerhans cell histiocytosis with thyroid and lung involvement in a child: a case report. *J Pediatr Hematol Oncol.* 2010;32:309–311.
162. Mrad K, Abbes I, Ben SH, et al. Langerhans cell histiocytois of the thyroid: a rare disease not to be ignored. *Ann Pathol.* 2002;22:35–38.
163. Sahoo M, Karak AK, Bhatnagar D, et al. Fine-needle aspiration cytology in a case of isolated involvement of thyroid with Langerhans cell histiocytosis. *Diagn Cytopathol.* 1998;19:33–37.
164. Saiz E, Bakotic BW. Isolated Langerhans cell histiocytosis of the thyroid: a report of two cases with nuclear imaging-pathologic correlation. *Ann Diagn Pathol.* 2000;4:23–28.
165. Thompson LDR, Wenig BM, Adair CF, et al. Langerhans cell histiocytosis of the thyroid: a series of seven cases and a review of the literature. *Mod Pathol.* 1996;9:145–149.
166. Zhu H, Hu DX. Langerhans cell histiocytosis of the thyroid diagnosed by fine needle aspiration cytology. A case report. *Acta Cytol.* 2004;48:278–280.
167. Nezelof C, Basset F, Rousseau MF. Histiocytosis X histogenetic arguments for a Langerhans cell origin. *Biomedicine.* 1973;18:365–371.
168. Chu T, Jaffe R. The normal Langerhans cell and the LCH cell. *Br J Cancer Suppl.* 1994;23:S4–S10.
169. Lindley R, Hoile R, Schofield J, et al. Langerhans cell histiocytosis associated with papillary carcinoma of the thyroid. *Histopathology.* 1998;32:180.
170. Jamaati HR, Shadmehr MB, Saidi B, et al. Langerhans cell histiocytosis of the lung and thyroid, co-existing with papillary thyroid cancer. *Endocr Pathol.* 2009;20:133–136.
171. Lassalle S, Hofman V, Santini J, et al. Isolated Langerhans cell histiocytosis of the thyroid and Graves' disease: an unreported association. *Pathology.* 2008;40:525–527.
172. Licci S, Boscaino A, De PM, et al. Concurrence of marginal zone B-cell lymphoma MALT-type and Langerhans cell histiocytosis in a thyroid gland with Hashimoto disease. *Ann Hematol.* 2008;87:855–857.
173. Aleotti A, Cervellati F, Bovolenta MR, et al. Birbeck granules: contribution to the comprehension of intracytoplasmic evolution. *J Submicrosc Cytol Pathol.* 1998;30:295–298.
174. Valladeau J, Ravel O, zutter-Dambuyant C, et al. Langerin, a novel C-type lectin specific to Langerhans cells, is an endocytic receptor that induces the formation of Birbeck granules. *Immunity.* 2000;12:71–81.
175. Wohlschlaeger J, Ebert S, Sheu SY, et al. Immunocytochemical investigation of Langerin (CD207) is a valuable adjunct in the cytological diagnosis of Langerhans cell histiocytosis of the thyroid. *Pathol Res Pract.* 2009;205:433–436.
176. Mrad K, Charfi L, Dhouib R, et al. Extra-nodal Rosai-Dorfman disease: a case report with thyroid involvement. *Ann Pathol.* 2004;24:446–449.
177. Ladisch S, Gadner H. Treatment of Langerhans cell histiocytosis—evolution and current approaches. *Br J Cancer Suppl.* 1994;23:S41–S46.
178. Thompson LDR, Kahn LB. Rosai-Dorfman disease. In: DeLellis RA, Lloyd RV, Heitz PU, et al., eds. *Pathology and Genetics of Tumours of Endocrine Organs.* Lyon, France: IARC Press; 2004:119.
179. Rosai J, Dorfman RF. Sinus histiocytosis with massive lymphadenopathy: a newly recognized benign clinicopathological entity. *Arch Pathol.* 1969;87:63–70.
180. Powell JG, Goellner JR, Nowak LE, et al. Rosai-Dorman disease of the thyroid masquerading as anaplastic carcinoma. *Thyroid.* 2003;13:217–221.
181. Tamouridis N, Deladetsima JK, Kastanias I, et al. Cold thyroid nodule as the sole manifestation of Rosai-Dorfman disease with mild lymphadenopathy, coexisting with chronic autoimmune thyroditis. *J Endocrinol Invest.* 1999;22:866–870.
182. Deshmukh RR, Kumar V, Kumbhani D. Sinus histiocytosis of the thyroid with massive lymphadenopathy (Rosai-Dorfman disease). *J Indian Med Assoc.* 2003;101:597–598.
183. Ben GI, Naffati H, Khanfir M, et al. Disseminated form of Rosai-Dorfman disease. A case report. *Rev Med Interne.* 2005;26:415–419.
184. Cocker RS, Kang J, Kahn LB. Rosai-Dorfman disease. Report of a case presenting as a midline thyroid mass. *Arch Pathol Lab Med.* 2003;127:e197–e200.
185. Eisen RN, Buckley PJ, Rosai J. Immunophenotypic characterization of sinus histiocytosis with massive lymphadenopathy (Rosai-Dorfman disease). *Semin Diagn Pathol.* 1990;7:74–82.
186. Hage C, Willman CL, Favara BE, et al. Langerhans cell histiocytosis (histiocytosis X): immunophenotype and growth fraction. *Hum Pathol.* 1993;24:840–845.
187. Cimino-Mathews A, Illei PB, Ali SZ. Atypical granular cell tumor of the thyroid: cytomorphologic features on fine needle aspiration. *Diagn Cytopathol.* 2011;39:608–611.
188. Liu J, Krishnamouthy S. The importance of fine needle aspiration in conjunction with radiologic examination in the evaluation of granular cell tumor presenting as a thyroid mass: a case report. *Int J Clin Exp Pathol.* 2011;4:197–199.
189. Bowry M, Almeida B, Jeannon JP. Granular cell tumour of the thyroid gland: a case report and review of the literature. *Endocr Pathol.* 2011;22:1–5.
190. Cimino-Mathews A, Illei PB, Ali SZ. Atypical granular cell tumor of the thyroid: cytomorphologic features on fine needle aspiration. *Diagn Cytopathol.* 2011;39:608–611.
191. Espinosa-de-Los-Monteros-Franco VA, Martinez-Madrigal F, Ortiz-Hidalgo C. Granular cell tumor (Abrikossoff tumor) of the thyroid gland. *Ann Diagn Pathol.* 2009;13:269–71.
192. Chang SM, Wei CK, Tseng CE. The cytology of a thyroid granular cell tumor. *Endocr Pathol.* 2009;20:137–140.
193. Milias S, Hytiroglou P, Kourtis D, et al. Granular cell tumour of the thyroid gland. *Histopathology.* 2004;44:190–191.
194. Paproski SM, Owen DA. Granular cell tumor of the thyroid. *Arch Pathol Lab Med.* 2001;125:544–546.
195. Mahoney CP, Patterson SD, Ryan J. Granular cell tumor of the thyroid gland in a girl receiving high-dose estrogen therapy. *Pediatr Pathol Lab Med.* 1995;15:791–795.
196. Fanburg-Smith JC, Meis-Kindblom JM, Fante R, et al. Malignant granular cell tumor of soft tissue: diagnostic criteria and clinicopathologic correlation. *Am J Surg Pathol.* 1998;22:779–794.

Primary Thyroid Lymphoma

DEFINITION

Primary thyroid gland lymphoma is an uncommon neoplasm that encompasses a heterogeneous group of diseases.[1-4] Primary thyroid gland lymphomas are defined by their lack of systemic involvement, although regional lymph nodes may occasionally be affected by the process. Primary thyroid lymphoma is nearly always a B-cell lymphoma, with two subtypes accounting for most tumors. Using the World Health Organization (WHO) Classification,[5,6] the most common subtypes are diffuse large B-cell lymphoma (DLBCL) and extranodal marginal zone lymphoma of mucosa-associated lymphoid tissue (MALT lymphoma).[7-13] Approximately one-third of MALT lymphoma will coexist with DLBCL, and a separate diagnosis of DLBCL should be rendered rather than "high-grade MALT lymphoma." "Pseudolymphoma" is no longer acceptable as it does not accurately reflect current concepts of MALT-type B-cell lymphomas. MALT lymphoma is a low-grade tumor, which occurs in the gastrointestinal tract, salivary gland, thyroid, orbit, lung, skin, and breast, among others. MALT lymphoma is composed of a morphologically heterogeneous B-cell population including small lymphocytes, marginal zone (centrocyte-like) small cleaved cells, cells resembling monocytoid B cells with abundant cytoplasm, and scattered large transformed cells without formation of sheets.[14-16] Plasmacytic differentiation is a constant and frequently striking feature in MALT lymphoma of the thyroid gland, potentially confused with plasmacytoma.[3,17,18] Other rare primary thyroid gland lymphomas reported include follicular lymphoma (FL),[19,20] extraosseous (extramedullary) plasmacytoma (EOP),[21-26] classical Hodgkin lymphoma,[27] and Burkitt lymphoma.[10,28] Diagnosis of lymphomas in the current era requires a multiparametric approach and integration of morphologic features with the immunophenotype and, in some cases, genetic information (i.e., cytogenetic and/or molecular studies). These features are summarized in Table 17.1 by lymphoma subtype.

ETIOLOGY

Nearly all cases of thyroid gland lymphoma arise in the setting of chronic lymphocytic (Hashimoto) thyroiditis.[3,4,7,10,29-38] In fact, the estimated relative risk of developing a lymphoma is 67 to 80 in patients with chronic lymphocytic thyroiditis when compared with age- and sex-matched controls.[39,40] Chronic lymphocytic thyroiditis shows an infiltrate of lymphoid cells that can be nodular or diffuse, frequently associated with lymphoid follicle formation including germinal centers (GCs), fibrosis, and oncocytic metaplasia of the thyroid follicular epithelial cells (see Chapter 4). Fibrosis and squamous metaplasia frequently accompany the lymphoid infiltrate. The presence of serologic antithyroid autoantibodies is requisite for the diagnosis of Hashimoto thyroiditis. Three possible processes are postulated for the development of acquired MALT: an autoimmune process, an immune deficiency, or an inflammatory process. Although *Chlamydia psittaci* DNA has been identified in a subset of thyroid MALT lymphoma,[41] the etiologic agent responsible for chronic antigenic stimulation may not be known in all cases. Similar to their gastrointestinal, salivary gland, and lacrimal counterparts, there may be progression from a polyclonal, antigen-driven response to a monoclonal proliferation and subsequent development into an overt lymphoma. Interestingly, thyroid lymphomas may also show an increased ratio of CD8+ cells (suppressor/cytotoxic cell) to CD4+ cells (helper/inducer cell) as compared with lymphocytic thyroiditis alone, providing support for a difference in local immunologic conditions.[29,42]

PATHOGENESIS AND MOLECULAR GENETICS

Chronic lymphocytic thyroiditis is almost certainly a requisite for the development of lymphoma in the thyroid gland. Atrophy of the residual thyroid parenchyma and fibrosis supports the chronicity of the underlying process (acquired MALT) that is associated with the subsequent development of lymphoma.

The cytogenetic and molecular genetic features of MALT lymphoma of the thyroid gland have not been as extensively studied as in other sites. There seem to be anatomic site specific chromosomal frequencies, but three MALT lymphoma-associated translocations [t(11;18)(q21;q21), t(1;14)(p22;q32), and t(14;18)(q32;q21)] result in the constitutive activation of the nuclear factor-$\kappa\beta$ oncogenic pathway.[43,44] The t(11;18)(q21;q21) results in a chimeric fusion of the *API2* region on chromosome 11q21 with the *MALT1* gene on chromosome 18q21, yielding a product that may concomitantly work as a tumor suppressor gene and as an oncogene.[45] Although present in a large proportion of gastrointestinal and lung MALT lymphomas (24% to 53%), the t(11;18)(q21;q21) translocation is only rarely reported in thyroid lymphomas.[46-50] The t(3;14)(p14.1;q32) involving *IGH* and the forkhead box protein P1 (*FOXP1*) has been reported in up to 50% of thyroid MALT lymphoma and seems to be mutually exclusive of t(1;14), t(14;18), and t(11;18) rearrangements but may be accompanied by trisomy 3 or other aneuploidies.[50,51] The molecular mechanisms of this translocation and significance of deregulation of *FOXP1* expression have not been fully elucidated.

Microsatellite instability and loss of heterozygosity are not identified in thyroid lymphoma. Aberrant *p15*, *p16*, and *p73* promoter methylation is quite common.[36] *TP53* mutation followed by complete inactivation by the loss of the second allele may be associated with high-grade transformation. It is suggested that CD40 signaling in combination with Th2 cytokines is necessary for the development and progression of low-grade MALT lymphoma. T cells, which activate B cells in a CD40-dependent fashion, may contribute to lymphoma pathogenesis and may be identified in lymphocytic thyroiditis.[52] Epstein-Barr virus has been detected in thyroid lymphoma, but in a very limited number of cases, suggesting it is not a major etiologic agent.[53]

Several theories have been proposed about the putative cell of origin for MALT lymphoma. Carcinogenesis is a multistep, multifactorial process involving the progressive accumulation of genetic changes. The marginal zone of the B-cell follicle represents a well-defined compartment of the B area. Marginal zone–like B cells

Table 17.1

Morphologic, Phenotypic, and Genetic Features of Thyroid Lymphoma by Subtype

Lymphoma Subtype (%)	Typical Morphology	Usual Phenotype	Genetic Features
DLBCL (60%–70%)	Diffuse infiltrate composed of sheets of large lymphoid cells	CD20+, CD10–/+, BCL6+/–, IRF4/MUM1 –/+, CD5 –/+	Occasional *BCL6* rearrangements; *MYC* rearrangement in rare cases; Rare *BRAF* and *NRAS* mutations
Extranodal marginal zone lymphoma of MALT-type (20%–30%)	Destructive infiltrate of small lymphoid cells, usually with moderately abundant cytoplasm, often with follicular colonization, prominent plasmacytic component, and distinctive lymphoepithelial lesions ("MALT-balls")	CD20+, CD5–, CD10–, BCL2+, CD43–/+, +/– CD138+ plasmacytic component	t(3;14)(p14.1;q32) with *FOXP1-IGH*; Trisomy 3; +/– additional aneuploidies t(11;18) (q21; q21) with *API2-MALT1* rearrangement rare
FL (3%–10%)	Nodular proliferation of neoplastic lymphoid follicles composed of admixed centrocytes/centroblasts with variably prominent interfollicular and diffuse components. Diffuse areas composed predominately of centroblasts/transformed cells are considered DLBCL. Lymphoepithelial lesions may be present	Two subtypes: CD20+, CD10+, BCL6+, BCL2+ CD20+, CD10–, BCL6+, BCL2–	t(14;18)(q32;q21) with *IGH-BCL2* translocation May be absent in cases lacking BCL2 protein expression
Burkitt lymphoma (rare)[a]	Sheets of round, intermediate-sized lymphoid cells with several small nucleoli, moderate amounts of basophilic cytoplasm, and interspersed histiocytes with a "starry sky" appearance	CD20+, CD10+, BCL6+, BCL2–, TdT-IRF4/MUM1–, Ki-67 PI nearly 100%	t(8;14)(q24;q32) with *MYC-IGH*; less frequently *MYC* translocated to *IGL* (22q11) or *IGK* (2p12) *MYC* rearrangement is usually the sole abnormality[a]
Classical Hodgkin lymphoma (rare)[a]	HRS cells and variants identified within a polymorphous background of small lymphocytes, eosinophils, histiocytes, and plasma cells	CD30+, CD15+/–, PAX5 weak+, CD20–/weak+, IRF4/MUM1+, ALK–, Bob-1, and/or Oct-2–	No specific abnormalities[a]
Chronic lymphocytic leukemia/small lymphocytic lymphoma (rare)[a]	Destructive infiltrate of small lymphoid cells with pale areas corresponding to proliferation centers at low magnification	CD20+ (can be dim or –), PAX5+, CD5+, CD23+, FMC-7–, CD10–	del 11q, del 17p, trisomy 12, del 13q[a]

[a]The morphologic, phenotypic, and genetic features for Burkitt lymphoma, classical Hodgkin lymphoma, and chronic lymphocytic leukemia/small lymphocytic lymphoma are not thyroid specific.
PI, proliferation index; del, deletion.

"home" to an area outside the follicles of peripheral lymphoid tissues, such as the MALT tissues of the thyroid. These areas acquire organized lymphoid tissue as a result of chronic antigenic stimulation of lymphocytic thyroiditis. Its cellular composition is distinct from that of the follicle center while also distinct functionally in the immune response. Immunoglobulin (Ig) antigen receptor stimulation is thought to play an important role in clonal expansion of MALT lymphoma.[54] Ig heavy and light chain variable genes (VH and VL) expressed by MALT lymphoma show numerous point mutations in both VH and VL genes that are different relative to germ line genes. Furthermore, there is intraclonal sequence heterogeneity, indicative of ongoing somatic hypermutation. As Ig gene hypermutation is thought to occur at the post-GC stage of B-cell development, these findings suggest that the MALT lymphoma cell of origin is from post-GC, marginal zone B cells.[5,54–59] It is important to note, however, that gene rearrangements for Ig VH and VL and for T-cell receptor β-chain genes are detected in

lymphocytic thyroiditis, but to a much lesser degree.[32,60–62] Therefore, PCR detection of a rearrangement cannot be used for diagnosis without confirmation by immunohistochemistry and histology. There are sequence similarities between the clonal bands of cells from lymphocytic thyroiditis and cells from the subsequent lymphoma.[34] Interestingly, different families of VH genes are detected in different lymphoma types: DLBCL shows VH3, whereas MALT lymphoma shows VH4 and VH3.[63] With transformation into a DLBCL, peripheral B cells of either GC or post-GC origin may be the cell of origin.

 CLINICAL PRESENTATION

Primary thyroid gland lymphomas are estimated to represent up to 5% of all thyroid gland malignant neoplasms.[3–5,10,37] Lymphomas occur predominantly in middle to older aged women (mean age,

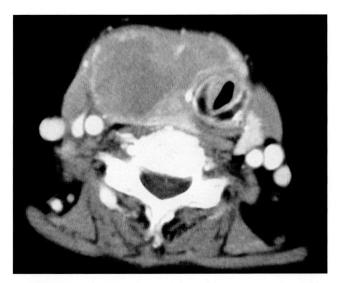

FIGURE 17.1. A CT image showing a large, heterogeneous mass in the right thyroid lobe. However, this change is nonspecific and is not specific for lymphoma.

60 to 65 years), although a wide age range at initial presentation is reported (14 to 90 years).[2–4,7,9,37,38,63–68] Lymphomas occur chiefly in women, with a female to male ratio of 3 to 7:1.[2–4,7,9,37,38,63–68] Patients present with a mass lesion or goiter (overall enlargement), often with recent enlargement (sometimes rapidly). The mass results in additional obstructive symptoms related to compression. Additional symptoms include pain, dyspnea, dysphagia, hoarseness, choking, coughing, and hemoptysis.[3,4,9,10,38,64,69] Symptoms are usually experienced for a limited time (mean, 6 months duration), but MALT lymphoma tends to be a chronic, long-term clinical disorder. Most patients do not have B symptoms (fever, profound night sweats, weight loss, and anorexia), but they may develop in patients with DLBCL or other high-grade lymphomas. Antithyroid serum antibodies are identified in most patients, a finding correlated with the histologic presence of chronic lymphocytic (Hashimoto) thyroiditis.[3,9,10] Many patients are euthyroid, but hypothyroidism is common; very rarely patients will have hyperthyroidism.[4,24,38,69,70]

Radiographic iodine uptake studies usually show a "cold" or "cool" nodule but can show diffuse areas of low uptake,[3,4,10,65,71] although [mTc]pertechnetate scintigraphy may show a "warm" nodule.[72] CT shows heterogeneous mass, sometimes with cystic change, whereas ultrasonographic features of primary thyroid lymphoma usually demonstrate a marked hypoechoic, asymmetrical pseudocystic mass compared with the residual thyroid tissue (Fig. 17.1).[38,73,74] By ^{18}F-Fluoro-deoxy-glucose positron emission tomography (FDG-PET), most lymphoma subtypes have high ^{18}F-FDG avidity with the exception of MALT lymphoma and small lymphocytic lymphoma.[75] However, ^{18}F-FDG PET may be more sensitive in MALT lymphoma with plasmacytic differentiation.[76] Incidental thyroid uptake with ^{18}F-FDG-PET is not uncommon although it is typically diffuse, and focal lesions require further workup.[77] In some cases, no significant radiographic abnormality is noted.

 STAGE

Most patients present with clinical and pathologic stage IE or IIE (extranodal) disease. Very few patients have stage IIIE or IVE disease, although patients with DLBCL are more likely to have higher stage disease at presentation than those with MALT lymphoma.[2–4,10,38,48,64,66,78–81]

 PATHOLOGY

Gross Presentation

There is a wide variation in tumor size, ranging from 0.5 to 19.5 cm in maximum dimension.[10,24] Tumors may involve either one or both lobes of the thyroid gland and have a variable macroscopic appearance. Tumors are soft to firm, lobulated, multinodular or diffuse, with solid and cystic areas. The cut surface is smooth or slightly bulging, pale tan, white-gray, or red with a fish-flesh appearance (Fig. 17.2). There may be a uniformly homogeneous or mottled appearance. Foci of hemorrhage or necrosis may be noted. Extension to adjacent adipose tissue or skeletal muscle is common.

Microscopic and Immunophenotypic Features

Extranodal Marginal Zone Lymphoma of Mucosa-Associated Lymphoid Tissue

Extranodal marginal zone lymphoma of mucosa-associated lymphoid tissue (MALT lymphoma) of the thyroid gland accounts for 20% to 30% of all thyroid gland lymphomas and occurs in the setting of chronic lymphocytic thyroiditis in almost all cases (Fig. 17.3).[3,7,10,65,78] There is a vaguely nodular or follicular to diffuse

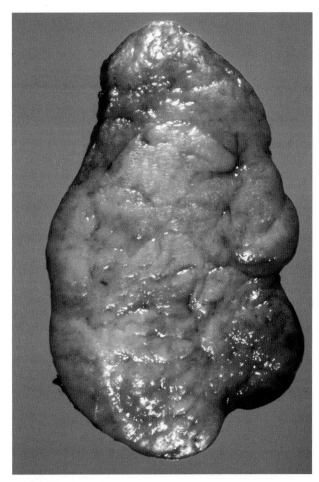

FIGURE 17.2. A "fish-flesh," nodular, cut appearance is characteristic of lymphoid lesions, although florid lymphocytic thyroiditis and lymphoma can have a similar appearance.

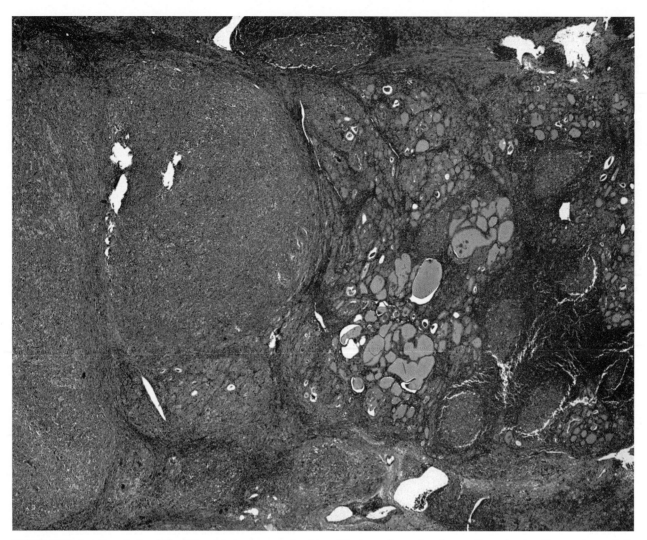

FIGURE 17.3. Lymphocytic thyroiditis with germinal centers on the right, while the malignant lymphoma effaces the thyroid parenchyma (left), arranged in a nodular and diffuse pattern.

pattern (Fig. 17.4A), composed of a heterogeneous B-cell infiltrate of small lymphoid cells, including marginal zone cells, monocytoid-like B cells, scattered large immunoblasts, and numerous plasma cells (Fig. 17.4B). Reactive GCs are invariably present, many of which are surrounded and infiltrated by neoplastic B cells colonizing the follicles. These cells often yield a darker zone within the follicles on low magnification and simulate follicle lysis (Fig. 17.5). Follicular colonization and the resulting nodular appearance may be prominent, and the histologic appearance may overlap with FL. Lymphoepithelial lesions, which represent infiltration of glandular (follicular) epithelial structures by neoplastic B cells, are a consistent feature (Fig. 17.6)[18] Lymphocytes within the epithelium can be seen in lymphocytic thyroiditis, but it is the destructive infiltration by the lymphoid cells that is critical for the diagnosis. In thyroid MALT lymphoma, the lymphoepithelial lesions may have a distinctive appearance as rounded balls or masses, filling and distending the colloidal space of the thyroid follicle ("MALT balls"; Fig. 17.7). Plasma cells and plasmacytoid cells with Dutcher bodies or cytoplasmic Ig ("Mott cells") may also be identified (Fig. 17.8). Sometimes crystal-storing histiocytes are noted (Fig. 17.8).[82] In some cases, the plasma cell population may predominate, simulating a plasmacytoma (Fig. 17.9). Perithyroidal extension into fat or skeletal muscle may be seen in approximately half of the cases. The monocytoid-like B cells are a monotonous population of atypical lymphoid cells with abundant,

pale cytoplasm with lobulated or kidney-shaped nuclei and occasionally form small nodules or sheets (Fig. 17.10). There may be single or multifocal zones of large cell transformation adjacent to the low-grade component (Fig. 17.11). Sheets of large lymphoid cells should prompt a second diagnosis of DLBCL in addition to MALT lymphoma. In many cases, areas of transition from low-grade to high-grade morphology is easy to identify.[83] In other sites, genetic evidence supports a transformation from low-grade to high-grade tumor by revealing identical gene rearrangements in both lesions from the same tumor.[84]

The B-cell immunophenotype of MALT lymphoma is confirmed by immunoreactivity for CD20 and/or CD79a (Fig. 17.12). The neoplastic cells are negative for the GC markers CD10 and BCL6. BCL-2 reactivity in the neoplastic, colonizing B cells (but not in the residual, reactive GC cells) is also characteristic. Follicular dendritic cell (FDC) markers (CD21, CD23, CD35) may be useful in highlighting the expanded FDC meshworks. In contrast to most chronic lymphocytic leukemias/small lymphocytic lymphomas and mantle cell lymphomas, the neoplastic cells are usually negative for CD5, although rare CD5+ MALT lymphomas have been reported.[85] Cyclin D1 negativity would tend to exclude mantle cell lymphoma. CD43 on the neoplastic CD20+ B cells may be seen in ~ 17% of thyroid MALT lymphoma (Fig. 17.13). An antibody to cytokeratin may be useful to highlight the epithelial remnants in the destructive lymphoepithelial lesions (Fig. 17.14). In general,

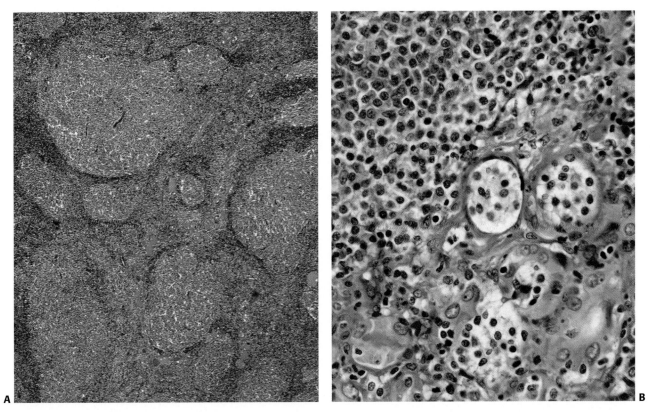

FIGURE 17.4. A: A nodular or "follicular" appearance is characteristic for MALT lymphoma in the thyroid gland, which can mimic FL. Isolated thyroid follicles can be seen. **B:** MALT lymphoma with a mixture of lymphocytes, monocytoid B cells, plasma cells, and rare transformed lymphocytes.

low-grade B-cell lymphomas, including MALT lymphoma, have a lower proliferation index, best highlighted with Ki-67 (MIB-1) immunoreactivity, as compared with high-grade lymphomas such as DLBCL.[86-88] However, it is important to be aware that this stain will demonstrate numerous positive GC cells in the reactive, non-neoplastic follicles within the infiltrate, and not to mistake these areas for large cell transformation.

Although most thyroid MALT lymphomas show a prominent plasmacytic component (67%), only 33% will show monotypic cytoplasmic Ig light chain expression.[18] Nevertheless, if present, Ig light chain restriction for either k or λ light chain is an extremely useful diagnostic adjunct as it serves as a surrogate for monoclonality (Fig. 17.15).[10] If fresh tissue is available, flow cytometric studies may be extremely useful to establish surface light chain restriction and the presence of a monotypic B-cell population. In difficult cases, molecular techniques to assess for a clonal *IGH* gene rearrangement may be useful, and PCR testing can be performed on paraffin-embedded tissue. However, these results need to be integrated with the morphologic and immunohistochemical information as entities in the differential diagnosis, such as Hashimoto thyroiditis, may also show clonal rearrangements.[32,60-62]

Diffuse Large B-Cell Lymphoma

Diffuse large B-cell lymphoma (DLBCL) accounts for ~ 60% to 70% of all thyroid gland lymphomas. Areas of infiltration by sheets of large, atypical lymphoid cells may occur in the absence of any recognizable low-grade areas. However, in many cases, areas of coexisting low-grade MALT lymphoma can be seen.[89] Depending on the biopsy size, fixation, and processing artifacts, it may be difficult to accurately distinguish from other lymphomas and malignant neoplasms of thyroid (such as carcinoma). Perithyroidal extension into fat or skeletal muscle is seen in most cases, along with areas of vascular invasion (Fig. 17.16). The large cells show

a spectrum of cytologic features that resemble centroblasts and immunoblasts and may show abundant cytoplasm and/or plasmacytoid features. The large cells are arranged in sheets, usually completely destroying any residual thyroid follicular epithelium (Fig. 17.17). Focal Reed–Sternberg-like (Fig. 17.17) or Burkitt-like cells that show brisk mitotic activity, apoptosis, and a starry sky pattern may be noted (Fig. 17.18). Atrophy of residual thyroid parenchyma and fibrosis are often noted. The intimate relationship and subtle areas of transition between the low-grade and high-grade regions give support to the notion of a large cell transformation of the low-grade component.[10,24,48,78,90]

The large lymphoid cells are positive for B-cell–associated markers such as CD20, CD79a, and Pax5. Gene expression profiling studies have identified two distinct subtypes of DLBCL, GC-like and activated B cell-like,[91] and some have shown that molecular profiling can predict survival with the GC subgroup showing the highest 5-year survival rate.[92] The Hans immunohistochemical algorithm, by defining CD10+ or a combination of BCL6+ and IRF4/MUM– staining pattern as GC subtype and all other combinations as non-GC subtype, strives to reproduce the molecular classification although it does not correlate perfectly, and is not currently incorporated into treatment algorithms.[93,94] Using this algorithm, most thyroid DLBCLs show a GC-phenotype.[48] In contrast to thyroid MALT lymphoma, deviated VH4 IGH usage is not found in thyroid DLBCL—in fact, in one case, the MALT lymphoma used the VH4 family, whereas the DLBCL component used the VH3 family, suggesting a de novo origin for the DLBCL.[63] Various cytogenetic abnormalities have been reported in thyroid DLBCL, including involvement of 3q27 (BCL6), *MYC* (8q24), as well as other aberrations.[48] Both reported cases of *MYC*+ thyroid DLBCL were CD10–, and one was BCL2+ unlike typical Burkitt lymphoma.[48,95] It is important to separate Burkitt lymphoma from DLBCL as Burkitt lymphomas receive more aggressive chemotherapeutic regimens.[94] Concurrent *MYC* and *BCL2* and/or *BCL6*

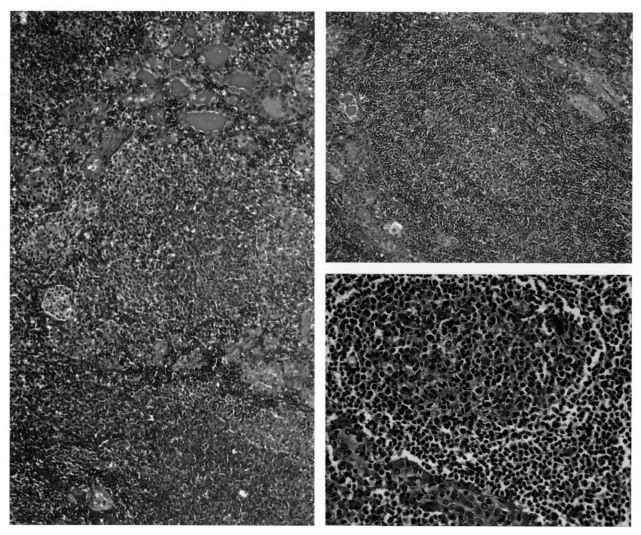

FIGURE 17.5. Left: MALT lymphoma cells surround and infiltrate follicles. **Right upper:** Infiltration of the GC by neoplastic B cells, simulating follicle lysis. Note the darker staining quality. **Right lower:** The neoplastic B cells are small in size with mature chromatin and scant to moderate amounts of cytoplasm.

rearrangements signify an extremely aggressive lymphoma and may be included within the new 2008 WHO category of "B-cell lymphoma, unclassifiable, with features intermediate between DLBCL and Burkitt lymphoma" depending on the morphologic and immunophenotypic characteristics. A subset of thyroid DL-BCLs also harbor genetic mutations characteristically found in thyroid carcinomas, such as *BRAF* and *NRAS* mutations.[96]

Follicular Lymphoma

Follicular lymphoma (FL) is considered a primarily nodal-based lymphoma that rarely occurs in the thyroid gland.[7,19,21,73,97] It is important to recognize that a follicular pattern can be seen in MALT lymphoma, and this by itself does not imply a *follicle center cell* lymphoma. The thyroid glandular architecture is replaced by back-to-back neoplastic GCs with attenuated or absent mantle zones. The neoplastic cells are a monotonous population of centrocytes and/or centroblasts typically without tingible body macrophages, especially in lower grade (grade 1 and 2) lesions. Several large transformed cells/high-power field (HPF) determine the grade with grade 1 and 2 showing 5 to 15/HPF and grade 3 showing >15/HPF.[98] Extrafollicular small centrocyte-like cells may be seen and may be extensive in some thyroid lymphomas.[20] Areas with extrafollicular sheets of large cells, however, would

warrant a separate diagnosis of DLBCL. Lymphoepithelial lesions may be seen and are not unique to MALT lymphoma.

FL expresses B-cell markers (CD20+, CD79a+), with two distinct subtypes described in the thyroid.[20] One group is typically grade 1 and 2, expresses GC markers CD10 and BCL6, is BCL2+, and harbors the t(14;18) *IGH-BCL2* translocation. These features are similar to nodal FL. The second group is often grade 3, is CD10– but BCL6+, lacks BCL2 expression as well as the t(14;18)/*IGH-BCL2* translocation, and remains localized to the thyroid. Some extranodal FLs from other sites share features with the second group, including those involving the testes[99] and skin.[100] If fresh tissue is available, flow cytometric studies may be useful to identify a monotypic B-cell population and characterize the immunophenotype (i.e., CD10+, BCL2+, CD5–). However, restricted κ/λ light chain ratios may be seen in GC B cells in Hashimoto thyroiditis without clinical, morphologic, or molecular evidence of lymphoma.[101] Therefore, the flow cytometric results need to be evaluated in the context of all available information.

Plasmacytoma

The thyroid gland is rarely the site of a plasma cell neoplasm, either solitary EOP or disseminated multiple myeloma (MM).[10,17,21–23,25,26,102] These tumors are indistinguishable histologically, but by definition,

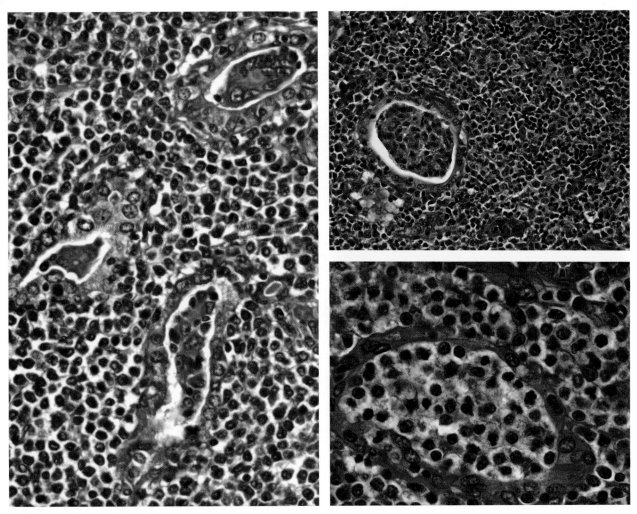

FIGURE 17.6. Lymphoepithelial lesions in MALT lymphoma. Left: Atypical lymphocytes infiltrate the thyroid glandular epithelium, destroying the parenchyma. **Right upper:** A lymphoepithelial lesion shows neoplastic cells within the lumen of the follicle. **Right lower:** Monocytoid-like B cells comprise this lymphoepithelial lesion that demonstrates a rim of glandular epithelium surrounded by similar-appearing neoplastic B cells.

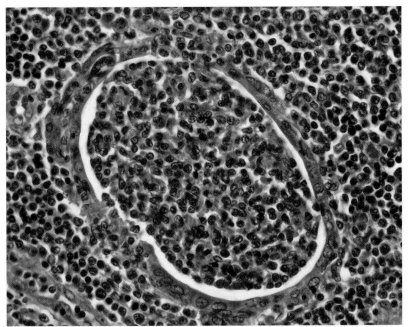

FIGURE 17.7. A lymphoepithelial lesion showing a mass or "ball" of neoplastic cells within a follicle ("MALT ball").

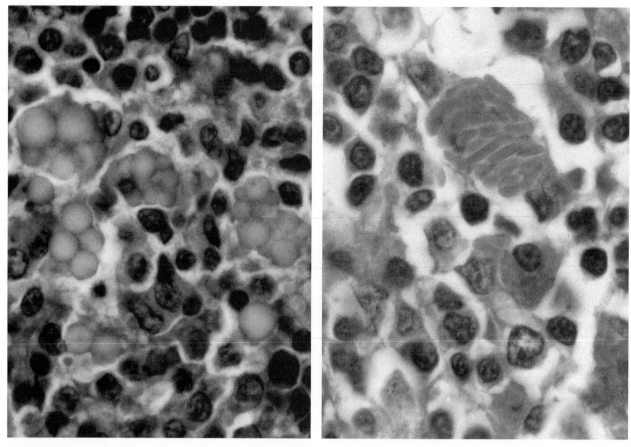

FIGURE 17.8. Left: Mott cells (Ig secretions) can be seen in mature plasmacytoid cells. **Right:** Intracytoplasmic crystals are also focally noted in MALT lymphoma.

EOP shows no evidence of bone marrow involvement, whereas MM is bone marrow based. EOP, representing 3% to 5% of all plasma cell neoplasms, affects women more commonly in thyroid gland disease, whereas men are affected more commonly in other anatomic sites. The tumors contain sheets of plasma cells (Fig. 17.19)

that may form nodules. Demonstration of cytoplasmic light chain restriction immunohistochemically would support a neoplastic plasma cell proliferation, but a monotypic plasmacytic component can be seen in MALT lymphoma. Demonstration of IgG heavy chain would tend to favor plasma cell neoplasm as lymphomas are

FIGURE 17.9. The plasmacytoid population predominates in this MALT lymphoma with extensive plasmacytic differentiation.

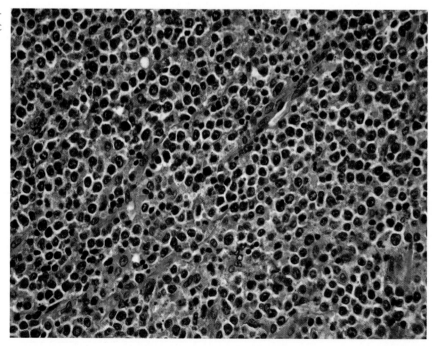

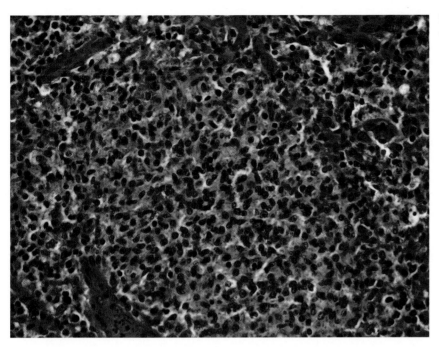

FIGURE 17.10. Sheets and nodules of monocytoid B cells are a prominent finding in MALT lymphoma.

typically IgM+, although exceptions may occur. Cyclin D1 positivity would exclude MALT lymphoma and support a plasma cell neoplasm, especially MM over EOP,[103] assuming other cyclin D1+ B-cell neoplasms such as mantle cell lymphoma and hairy cell leukemia are excluded. It may be difficult by morphology alone to distinguish a plasmacytoma from prominent plasma cell differentiation in a MALT lymphoma. In fact, it is our contention that true plasmacytoma is vanishingly rare, and these tumors should be thought of as MALT lymphoma with an extensive plasma cell component.[17,102] Interestingly, when described, they are often associated with a MALT lymphoma or DLBCL histologic or ultrastructural description, albeit called *histiocytic*, *large cell*, or *follicular* by earlier studies.[102] Accurate correlation of clinical, laboratory, radiologic, and pathologic

features is important to document the localized or systemic nature of the neoplasm and to determine treatment options.

Hodgkin Lymphoma

Classical Hodgkin lymphoma rarely involves the thyroid and is typically nodular sclerosis subtype. The prominent fibrosis may cause difficulty in establishing a definitive diagnosis, especially in limited specimens. The Hodgkin/Reed–Sternberg (HRS) cells and variants are found in a variably cellular background diathesis of small lymphocytes, plasma cells, eosinophils, and neutrophils.[27,64,104] These features can be seen in fine needle aspiration (FNA), but separation from lymphocytic thyroiditis is difficult. In

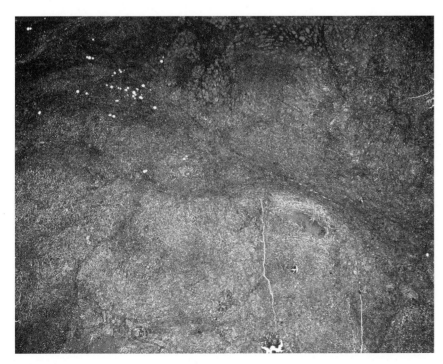

FIGURE 17.11. There are often areas of transformation or blending between low-grade and high-grade lymphoma. The top right shows lymphocytic thyroiditis, adjacent to areas of MALT lymphoma, which then blends into a DLBCL (lower field).

FIGURE 17.12. CD79a highlights the sheets of neoplastic cells. It also shows the neoplastic cells colonizing the reactive GC (lower left) in this MALT lymphoma.

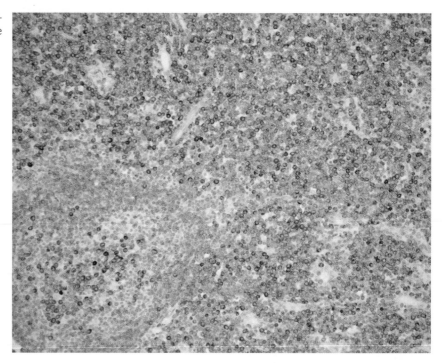

addition, a subset of thyroid Hodgkin lymphomas are associated with chronic lymphocytic thyroiditis, similar to other primary thyroid lymphomas.[27] Birefringent collagen banding (stromal fibrosis), nodular pattern, lacunar and mummified variant HRS cells, and epithelioid histiocytes can be seen (Fig. 17.20). HRS-like

cells may be seen in some non-Hodgkin lymphomas (NHLs), and immunophenotyping is recommended to establish the diagnosis. HRS cells will be CD45−, CD30+, and CD15+ (typically with a membrane and Golgi pattern) and show weak to absent staining for CD20 but weak positivity for the B-cell marker PAX5. In

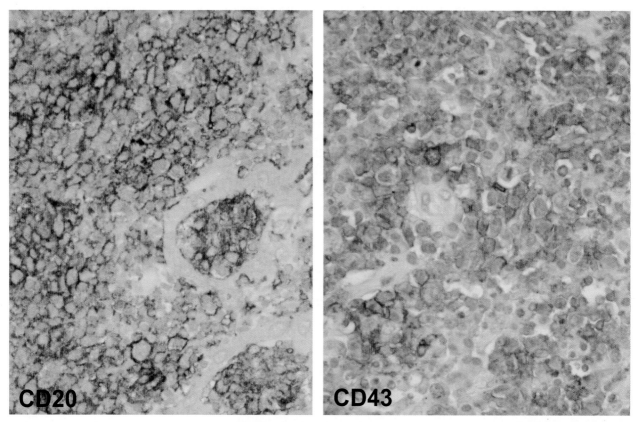

FIGURE 17.13. Left: CD20 highlights the neoplastic B cells, also noted here within the thyroid glandular epithelium. **Right:** Coexpression of CD43 is noted in this MALT lymphoma.

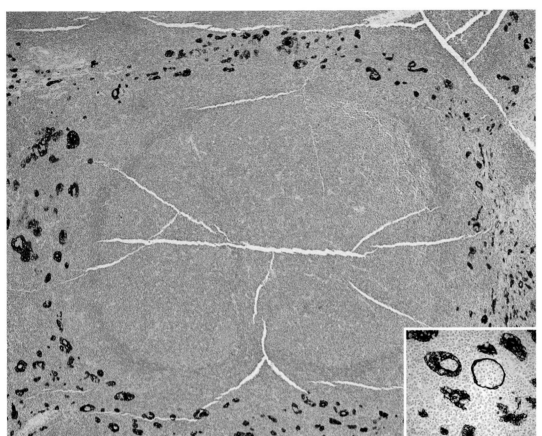

FIGURE 17.14. Keratin can be used to highlight the residual thyroid follicular epithelium, shown in this tumor to be completely destroyed in the neoplastic nodule in the center. The inset demonstrates the characteristic lymphoepithelial lesions, which have neoplastic lymphoid cells destroying the follicles.

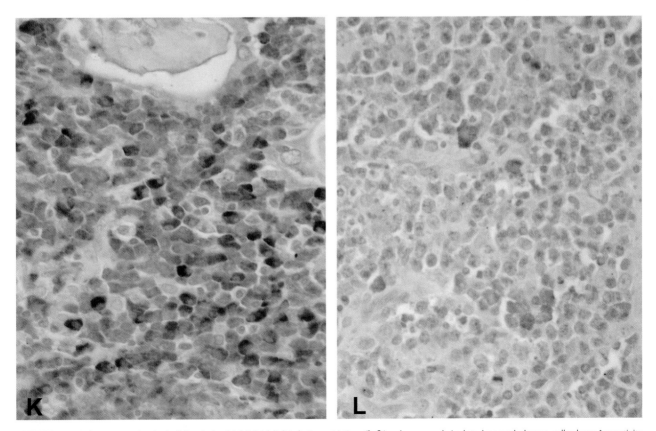

FIGURE 17.15. Immunostains for Ig light chains highlight *k* light chain restriction (**left**), whereas only isolated normal plasma cells show λ reactivity (**right**) in this MALT lymphoma.

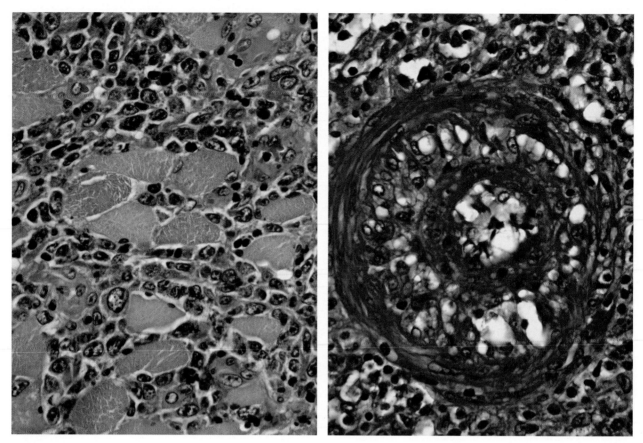

FIGURE 17.16. Left: Extension of the large cells into the adjacent skeletal muscle is common. **Right:** Vascular invasion with a perivascular distribution is noted in DLBCL.

difficult cases in which the differential diagnosis includes NHL, an expanded panel including Oct-2 and Bob-1 may be helpful as the HRS cells are Bob1– and/or Oct2–, whereas NHLs are typically positive for both. In limited specimens, strong staining for IRF4/MUM1 may be helpful to highlight the neoplastic cells, although this stain is not lineage specific and may be seen with other CD30+ lymphomas such as anaplastic large cell lymphoma. A cytokeratin stain may be useful in separation from sclerosing mucoepidermoid carcinoma with eosinophilia.[105]

Other Lymphoma Subtypes

Burkitt lymphoma may rarely involve the thyroid and presents as a rapidly growing mass,[28] although systemic disease is typically present.[1] Sheets of intermediate-sized cells with round nuclear contours, multiple small nucleoli, and occasional interspersed histiocytes impart a "starry sky" appearance. The neoplastic cells are CD20+ B cells with expression of GC markers (CD10, BCL6), are negative for BCL2 and TdT, and show a very high proliferative index of nearly 100%, as highlighted by Ki-67 immunostaining. Cytogenetic studies will show a *MYC* rearrangement, usually in the form of a translocation with *IGH, IGK,* or *IGL* [i.e., t(8;14), t(2;8), t(8;22)]. *MYC* gene rearrangements are not specific for Burkitt and may be seen with other lymphomas, and therefore, cytogenetic results always require correlation with the morphologic and phenotypic features.

Chronic lymphocytic leukemia/small lymphocytic lymphoma may rarely present in the thyroid as a primary neoplasm[1] or may be the first manifestation of systemic disease.[106] The morphologic and phenotype features are similar to those described at other sites. On low magnification, pale proliferation centers may be seen that are composed of admixed small lymphoid cells, intermediate sized prolymphocytes with small but distinct nucleoli,

and scattered large transformed cells (paraimmunoblasts). The neoplastic population is CD20+, although expression may be dim, and a PAX5 immunostain may be useful to confirm B-cell lineage. The B cells are CD5+ but, in contrast to mantle cell lymphoma, are cyclin D1– and usually CD23+. Depending on the clinical context, cytogenetic FISH studies may be useful, and deletion of 17p and 11p are adverse prognostic indicators.[94]

There are isolated case reports of primary thyroid T-cell lymphomas, including anaplastic large cell lymphoma and peripheral T-cell lymphoma.[13] The morphologic and immunophenotypic features are similar to those described at other sites. However, monoclonal gene rearrangements for T-cell receptor β- and γ-specific primers may be detected in chronic lymphocytic (Hashimoto) thyroiditis and may represent a reactive phenomenon.[2,60,107–110] Therefore, it is important to identify histologic, immunophenotypic, and molecular support for the diagnosis.

Cytopathology

In general, FNA is the study of choice for the initial evaluation of a nodule in the thyroid gland. Diffuse enlargement is not as amenable to this technique because a targeted approach cannot be undertaken. Overall, FNA can be used to screen for a lymphoma in the thyroid gland, although definitive diagnosis and lymphoma subclassification may require an excisional biopsy, especially at the time of initial diagnosis.[94] In general, FNA smears of a high-grade lymphoma are easy to interpret, but the cytologic diagnosis of a MALT lymphoma is much more difficult. In a DLBCL, the smears are highly cellular, with a population of large, monotonously atypical, noncohesive lymphoid cells. The cells are usually two to three times as large as mature lymphocytes. The nuclear chromatin is open and vesicular, with conspicuous nucleoli. The cytoplasm is ample, with a

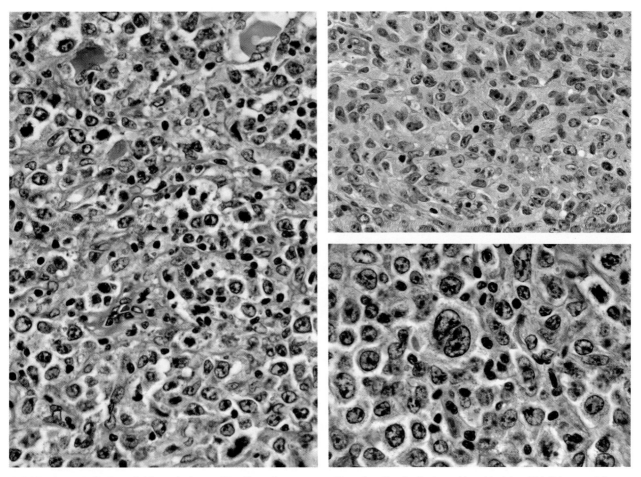

FIGURE 17.17. Left: Remarkably atypical centroblast-like cells are arranged in a sheetlike distribution, with residual thyroid follicles noted (upper field). **Right upper:** DLBCL composed of large lymphoid cells with abundant cytoplasm and nucleoli. **Right lower:** Reed–Sternberg-like variant can be seen in DLBCL.

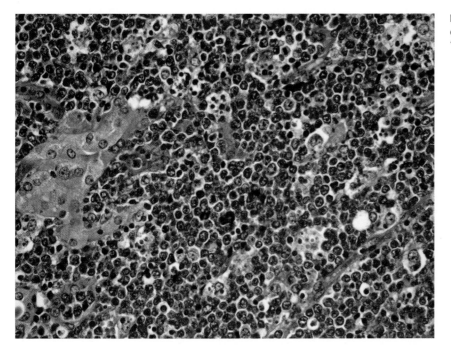

FIGURE 17.18. A high mitotic index with associated increased number of tingible body macrophages creates a "starry-sky" appearance, simulating a Burkitt lymphoma.

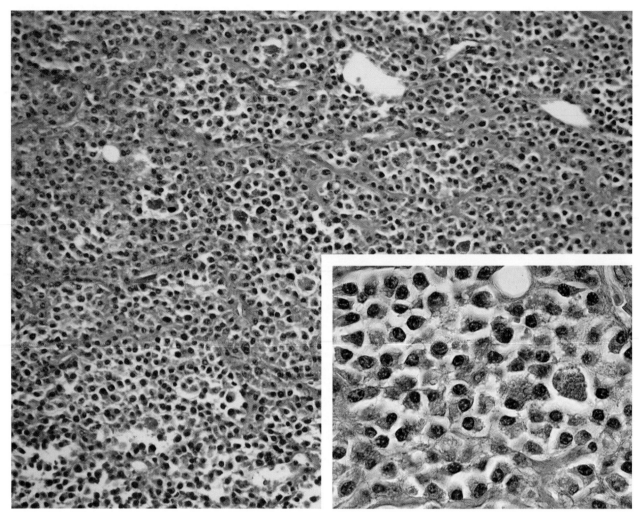

FIGURE 17.19. Sheets of atypical plasma cells are noted in this extramedullary plasmacytoma. The inset demonstrates the plasmacytic differentiation including Mott cells.

slightly basophilic quality. Naked nuclei and lymphoglandular bodies are easily identified in the background, helping to exclude epithelial neoplasms. Necrosis is sometimes present. Conspicuous by its absence is the lack of follicular epithelial cells in most aspirates. Smears from a MALT lymphoma show a heterogeneous lymphoid population, composed of small lymphocytes, plasma cells, immunoblasts, monocytoid cells, and large lymphoid cells. Most cells tend to be intermediate in size, the smears are cellular, and there are in general a lack of tingible body macropahges.[4,24,37,38,74,78,111,112] Immunohistochemistry, flow cytometry, and vectorette PCR–based Ig heavy chain gene rearrangements can be performed on aspiration material to help confirm the diagnosis.[58,113–115]

Differential diagnosis

The distinction between MALT lymphoma and lymphocytic thyroiditis may be difficult at times, and even more so on FNA smears. Although histologic evaluation remains the gold standard for diagnosis, immunohistochemical, flow cytometric, or molecular genetic analyses may be required. In both reactive follicular hyperplasia and MALT lymphoma, benign GCs are present, but in MALT lymphoma, the follicles are colonized by neoplastic B cells that express BCL-2. CD43 expression is seen in a subset of MALT lymphoma, in contrast to FL, which is generally CD43–. A dense, diffuse B-cell infiltrate, intranuclear inclusions (Dutcher bodies), cytologic atypia, and lymphoepithelial lesions are characteristically seen in MALT

lymphoma. The demonstration of light chain restriction by immunohistochemistry or flow cytometry supports the monoclonality of the B-cell lymphoma. PCR may be used to detect monoclonality for the Ig heavy chain gene in thyroid lymphomas and to distinguish this from chronic lymphocytic thyroiditis, although there may be cases where the technique does not work.[58,59,115,116] MALT lymphoma with prominent nodularity may simulate an FL. It is necessary, therefore, to distinguish the reactive, colonized GCs in MALT lymphoma from the neoplastic GCs in FL. Most cases of FL will show immunoreactivity for BCL-2 and will express the GC cell markers CD10 and BCL-6. In difficult cases, fluorescence in situ hybridization studies for the *IGH-BCL2* rearrangement may be useful, and these studies can be performed on paraffin-embedded tissue. As discussed above, however, a negative result would not necessarily exclude FL as a subset of primary thyroid FL will lack this abnormality. IgG4-related sclerosing disease is a mass-forming, steroid-responsive disease of possible autoimmune etiology that may enter into the differential diagnosis of MALT lymphoma. An extensive extranodal lymphoplasmacytic infiltrates accompanied by sclerosis, phlebitis, and increased IgG4+ cells are characteristic features. Although the criteria differ among studies, >50 IgG4+ cells/HPF and an IgG4/IgG ratio of >40% have been proposed.[117]

DLBCL may be indistinguishable from undifferentiated carcinoma or metastatic tumors by histology alone and may require a complete antibody screening panel, including CD45 (LCA), CD20, cytokeratin, TTF-1, thyroglobulin, and S100 protein to make the

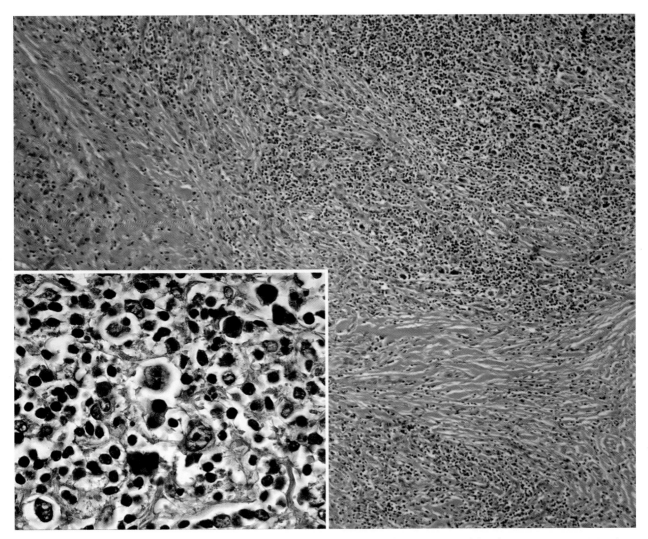

FIGURE 17.20. Classical Hodgkin lymphoma. Birefringent collagen bands separate the tumor into nodules. There are numerous HRS variants in the background, which shows eosinophils, plasma cells, and lymphocytes. The inset demonstrates a number of RS variants.

correct diagnosis.[71] Undifferentiated carcinoma does not really have a small cell pattern, a diagnostic category eliminated with enhanced ancillary studies. Ectopic thymoma will have T-cell antigens on the lymphocytes within the tumor. However, the presence of epithelial cells and inclusion of epithelial markers and CD5 should help make the distinction. FNA alone, however, may not make an accurate separation.[114,118,119] Sclerosing mucoepidermoid carcinoma with eosinophilia may histologically mimic Hodgkin lymphoma, although immunohistochemistry will usually separate these lesions.[105]

 ## TREATMENT AND PROGNOSIS

Thyroid lymphomas have been treated in the past with surgical excision, including thyroid lobectomy, partial or total thyroidectomy, and lymph node dissection. However, the current trend is toward adjuvant chemotherapy and radiation after appropriate classification through needle biopsy or limited surgery.[2,10,38,64,66,78,94,120–123] The management of thyroid DLBCL is combined modality with radiation therapy, cyclophosphamide, doxorubicin, vincristine, and prednisone chemotherapy.[38,67,78,121,124,125,126] Addition of rituximab, which targets the CD20 molecule, is a standard addition to most chemotherapy regimens for B-cell lymphoma.[94] Localized thyroid DLBCL with a

GC phenotype has a significantly better prognosis as compared with non-GC phenotype.[48,127] In disseminated cases, the most frequently involved sites are regional (cervical or perithyroidal) lymph nodes, followed by mediastinal and abdominal lymph nodes. Other uncommon sites of dissemination include bone marrow, gastrointestinal tract, lung, bladder, and liver.[128]

Most patients with MALT lymphoma of the thyroid gland present with stage IE or IIE disease.[9,10,64,120,121] The current management of stage I to IIE MALT lymphoma is more conservative as compared with DLBCL. The thyroid is one of the sites in which surgery could be considered, and therefore, the diagnostic biopsy could also be therapeutic if excisional.[94] Single modality radiation therapy may also be considered, especially in patients with positive margins. Radiation can be *involved field only* or *extended field radiotherapy*, the latter associated with lower rates of local recurrence or relapse.[67] This combined conservative treatment results in the lowest overall relapse rate and reduced distant recurrence rate[67,122] although also associated with the least side effects (mucositis, hypothyroidism, and radiation pneumonitis).[129] More advanced stage disease or relapses may necessitate systemic chemotherapy and/or immunotherapy. The prognosis of thyroid MALT lymphoma is very favorable in general, although it is dependent on advanced age (>65 years), gender (male), clinical stage, dysphagia (vocal cord paralysis), and tumor histology.[10,66,68,80]

Tumors that are localized (stage IE) at the time of presentation and demonstrate purely low-grade histology have an excellent prognosis, usually >90% 5-year survival.[2,7,9,38,48,64,68,81,120,121,130] Patients with either a diffuse large B-cell component or a higher stage disease seem to have a worse overall survival.[9,10,48,121,130] Extranodal primary thyroid gland FL has a better prognosis than nodal FL.[19] In particular, the CD10−, BCL2− subtype lacking the *IGH-BCL2* translocation is typically confined to the thyroid despite a high-grade histologic appearance.[20]

REFERENCES

1. Thieblemont C, Mayer A, Dumontet C, et al. Primary thyroid lymphoma is a heterogeneous disease. *J Clin Endocrinol Metab.* 2002;87:105–111.
2. Colovic M, Matic S, Kryeziu E, et al. Outcomes of primary thyroid non-Hodgkin's lymphoma: a series of nine consecutive cases. *Med Oncol.* 2007;24:203–208.
3. Compagno J, Oertel JE. Malignant lymphoma and other lymphoproliferative disorders of the thyroid gland. A clinicopathologic study of 245 cases. *Am J Clin Pathol.* 1980;74:1–11.
4. Hamburger JI, Miller JM, Kini SR. Lymphoma of the thyroid. *Ann Intern Med.* 1983;99:685–693.
5. Abbondanzo S, Aozasa K, Boerner S, et al. Primary lymphoma and plasmacytoma. In: DeLellis RA, Lloyd RV, Heitz PU, Eng C, eds. *Pathology and Genetics of Tumours of Endocrine Organs (WHO Classification of Tumours).* Lyon, France: IARC Press; 2004:109–111.
6. Swerdlow SH, Campo E, Harris NL, et al, eds. *WHO Classification of Tumours of the Haematopoietic and Lymphoid Tissues.* Lyon, France: IARC Press; 2008.
7. Anscombe AM, Wright DH. Primary malignant lymphoma of the thyroid—a tumour of mucosa-associated lymphoid tissue: review of seventy-six cases. *Histopathology.* 1985;9:81–97.
8. Ansell SM, Grant CS, Habermann TM. Primary thyroid lymphoma. *Semin Oncol.* 1999;26:316–323.
9. Aozasa K, Inoue A, Tajima K, et al. Malignant lymphomas of the thyroid gland. Analysis of 79 patients with emphasis on histologic prognostic factors. *Cancer.* 1986;58:100–104.
10. Derringer GA, Thompson LD, Frommelt RA, et al. Malignant lymphoma of the thyroid gland: a clinicopathologic study of 108 cases. *Am J Surg Pathol.* 2000;24:623–639.
11. Pedersen RK, Pedersen NT. Primary non-Hodgkin's lymphoma of the thyroid gland: a population based study. *Histopathology.* 1996;28:25–32.
12. Pledge S, Bessell EM, Leach IH, et al. Non-Hodgkin's lymphoma of the thyroid: a retrospective review of all patients diagnosed in Nottinghamshire from 1973 to 1992. *Clin Oncol (R Coll Radiol).* 1996;8:371–375.
13. Skacel M, Ross CW, Hsi ED. A reassessment of primary thyroid lymphoma: high-grade MALT-type lymphoma as a distinct subtype of diffuse large B-cell lymphoma. *Histopathology.* 2000;37:10–18.
14. Isaacson PG, Spencer J. Malignant lymphoma of mucosa-associated lymphoid tissue. *Histopathology.* 1987;11:445–462.
15. Isaacson PG. Lymphoma of the thyroid gland. *Curr Top Pathol.* 1997;91:1–14.
16. Bacon CM, Du MQ, Dogan A. Mucosa-associated lymphoid tissue (MALT) lymphoma: a practical guide for pathologists. *J Clin Pathol.* 2007;60:361–372.
17. Aihara H, Tsutsumi Y, Ishikawa H. Extramedullary plasmacytoma of the thyroid, associated with follicular colonization and stromal deposition of polytypic immunoglobulins and major histocompatibility antigens. Possible categorization in MALT lymphoma. *Acta Pathol Jpn.* 1992;42:672–683.
18. Rawal A, Finn WG, Schnitzer B, et al. Site-specific morphologic differences in extranodal marginal zone B-cell lymphomas. *Arch Pathol Lab Med.* 2007;131:1673–1678.
19. Goodlad JR, MacPherson S, Jackson R, et al. Extranodal follicular lymphoma: a clinicopathological and genetic analysis of 15 cases arising at non-cutaneous extranodal sites. *Histopathology.* 2004;44:268–276.
20. Bacon CM, Diss TC, Ye H, et al. Follicular lymphoma of the thyroid gland. *Am J Surg Pathol.* 2009;33:22–34.
21. Aozasa K, Inoue A, Katagiri S, et al. Plasmacytoma and follicular lymphoma in a case of Hashimoto's thyroiditis. *Histopathology.* 1986;10:735–740.
22. De Schrijver I, Smeets P. Thyroid enlargement due to extramedullary plasmacytoma. *JBR-BTR.* 2004;87:73–75.
23. Kuo CF, Chang HY, Hsueh C, et al. Extramedullary plasmacytoma of the thyroid. *N Z Med J.* 2006;119:U2005.
24. Lam KY, Lo CY, Kwong DL, et al. Malignant lymphoma of the thyroid. A 30-year clinicopathologic experience and an evaluation of the presence of Epstein-Barr virus. *Am J Clin Pathol.* 1999;112:263–270.
25. Mizukami Y, Michigishi T, Nonomura A, et al. Primary lymphoma of the thyroid: a clinical, histological and immunohistochemical study of 20 cases. *Histopathology.* 1990;17:201–209.
26. Chesyln-Curtis S, Akosa AB. Primary plasmacytoma of the thyroid. *Postgrad Med J.* 1990;66:477–478.
27. Wang SA, Rahemtullah A, Faquin WC, et al. Hodgkin's lymphoma of the thyroid: a clinicopathologic study of five cases and review of the literature. *Mod Pathol.* 2005;18:1577–1584.
28. Kalinyak JE, Kong CS, McDougall IR. Burkitt's lymphoma presenting as a rapidly growing thyroid mass. *Thyroid.* 2006;16:1053–1057.
29. Aozasa K. Hashimoto's thyroiditis as a risk factor of thyroid lymphoma. *Acta Pathol Jpn.* 1990;40:459–468.
30. Casparie AF, Ruitenberg HM. Non-Hodgkin lymphoma of the thyroid and Hashimoto's thyroiditis. *Neth J Med.* 1984;27:44–49.
31. Hsi ED, Singleton TP, Svoboda SM, et al. Characterization of the lymphoid infiltrate in Hashimoto thyroiditis by immunohistochemistry and polymerase chain reaction for immunoglobulin heavy chain gene rearrangement. *Am J Clin Pathol.* 1998;110:327–333.
32. Huo Z, Li Y, Zhong DR, et al. [Gene rearrangement studies in Hashimoto's thyroiditis and primary lymphoma of thyroid]. *Zhonghua Bing Li Xue Za Zhi.* 2006;35:344–347.
33. Hyjek E, Isaacson PG. Primary B cell lymphoma of the thyroid and its relationship to Hashimoto's thyroiditis. *Hum Pathol.* 1988;19:1315–1326.
34. Moshynska OV, Saxena A. Clonal relationship between Hashimoto thyroiditis and thyroid lymphoma. *J Clin Pathol.* 2008;61:438–444.
35. Scholefield JH, Quayle AR, Harris SC, et al. Primary lymphoma of the thyroid, the association with Hashimoto's thyroiditis. *Eur J Surg Oncol.* 1992;18:89–92.
36. Au WY, Fung A, Ma ES, et al. HLA associations, microsatellite instability and epigenetic changes in thyroid lymphoma in Chinese. *Leuk Lymphoma.* 2007;48:531–534.
37. Sangalli G, Serio G, Zampatti C, et al. Fine needle aspiration cytology of primary lymphoma of the thyroid: a report of 17 cases. *Cytopathology.* 2001;12:257–263.
38. Matsuzuka F, Miyauchi A, Katayama S, et al. Clinical aspects of primary thyroid lymphoma: diagnosis and treatment based on our experience of 119 cases. *Thyroid.* 1993;3:93–99.
39. Holm LE, Blomgren H, Lowhagen T. Cancer risks in patients with chronic lymphocytic thyroiditis. *N Engl J Med.* 1985;312:601–604.
40. Kato I, Tajima K, Suchi T, et al. Chronic thyroiditis as a risk factor of B-cell lymphoma in the thyroid gland. *Jpn J Cancer Res.* 1985;76:1085–1090.
41. Aigelsreiter A, Gerlza T, Deutsch AJ, et al. *Chlamydia psittaci* Infection in nongastrointestinal extranodal MALT lymphomas and their precursor lesions. *Am J Clin Pathol.* 2011;135:70–75.
42. Aozasa K, Tajima K, Tominaga N, et al. Immunologic and immunohistochemical studies on chronic lymphocytic thyroiditis with or without thyroid lymphoma. *Oncology.* 1991;48:65–71.
43. Du MQ. MALT lymphoma: recent advances in aetiology and molecular genetics. *J Clin Exp Hematop.* 2007;47:31–42.
44. Inagaki H. Mucosa-associated lymphoid tissue lymphoma: molecular pathogenesis and clinicopathological significance. *Pathol Int.* 2007;57:474–484.
45. Hu S, Du MQ, Park SM, et al. cIAP2 is a ubiquitin protein ligase for BCL10 and is dysregulated in mucosa-associated lymphoid tissue lymphomas. *J Clin Invest.* 2006;116:174–181.
46. Kobayashi Y, Nakata M, Maekawa M, et al. Detection of t(I 1; 18) in MALT-type lymphoma with dual-color fluorescence in situ hybridization and reverse transcriptase-polymerase chain reaction analysis. *Diagn Mol Pathol.* 2001;10:207–213.
47. Yang WX, Li GD, Zhou Q, et al. [Detection of API2-MALT1 fusion gene in extranodal B-cell lymphoma and its significance]. *Zhonghua Bing Li Xue Za Zhi.* 2006;35:92–96.
48. Niitsu N, Okamoto M, Nakamura N, et al. Clinicopathologic correlations of stage IE/IIE primary thyroid diffuse large B-cell lymphoma. *Ann Oncol.* 2007;18:1203–1208.
49. Streubel B, Simonitsch-Klupp I, Mullauer L, et al. Variable frequencies of MALT lymphoma-associated genetic aberrations in MALT lymphomas of different sites. *Leukemia.* 2004;18:1722–1726.
50. Streubel B, Vinatzer U, Lamprecht A, et al. T(3;14)(p14.1;q32) involving *IGH* and *FOXP1* is a novel recurrent chromosomal aberration in MALT lymphoma. *Leukemia.* 2005;19:652–658.
51. Joao C, Farinha P, da Silva MG, et al. Cytogenetic abnormalities in MALT lymphomas and their precursor lesions from different organs. A fluorescence in situ hybridization (FISH) study. *Histopathology.* 2007;50:217–224.
52. Greiner A, Knorr C, Qin Y, et al. Low-grade B cell lymphomas of mucosa-associated lymphoid tissue (MALT-type) require CD40-mediated signaling and Th2-type cytokines for in vitro growth and differentiation. *Am J Pathol.* 1997;150:1583–1593.
53. Tomita Y, Ohsawa M, Kanno H, et al. Sporadic activation of Epstein-Barr virus in thyroid lymphoma. *Leuk Lymphoma.* 1995;19:129–134.
54. Bahler DW, Miklos JA, Swerdlow SH. Ongoing Ig gene hypermutation in salivary gland mucosa-associated lymphoid tissue-type lymphomas. *Blood.* 1997;89:3335–3344.
55. Miwa H, Takakuwa T, Nakatsuka S, et al. DNA sequence of immunoglobulin heavy chain variable region gene in thyroid lymphoma. *Jpn J Cancer Res.* 2001;92:1041–1047.
56. Du M, Diss TC, Xu C, et al. Ongoing mutation in MALT lymphoma immunoglobulin gene suggests that antigen stimulation plays a role in the clonal expansion. *Leukemia.* 1996;10:1190–1197.
57. Takano T, Miyauchi A, Matsuzuka F, et al. Detection of monoclonality of the immunoglobulin heavy chain gene in thyroid malignant lymphoma by vectorette polymerase chain reaction. *J Clin Endocrinol Metab.* 2005;90:720–723.
58. Takashima S, Takayama F, Saito A, et al. Primary thyroid lymphoma: diagnosis of immunoglobulin heavy chain gene rearrangement with polymerase chain reaction in ultrasound-guided fine-needle aspiration. *Thyroid.* 2000;10:507–510.
59. Yamauchi A, Tomita Y, Takakuwa T, et al. Polymerase chain reaction-based clonality analysis in thyroid lymphoma. *Int J Mol Med.* 2002;10:113–117.
60. Katzin WE, Fishleder AJ, Tubbs RR. Investigation of the clonality of lymphocytes in Hashimoto's thyroiditis using immunoglobulin and T-cell receptor gene probes. *Clin Immunol Immunopathol.* 1989;51:264–274.
61. Matsubayashi S, Tamai H, Morita T, et al. Hashimoto's thyroiditis manifesting monoclonal lymphocytic infiltration. *Clin Exp Immunol.* 1990;79:170–174.
62. Tiemann M, Menke MA, Asbeck R, et al. Temperature gradient gel electrophoresis for analysis of clonal evolution in non-Hodgkin's lymphoma of the thyroid. *Electrophoresis.* 1995;16:729–732.

63. Sato Y, Nakamura N, Nakamura S, et al. Deviated VH4 immunoglobulin gene usage is found among thyroid mucosa-associated lymphoid tissue lymphomas, similar to the usage at other sites, but is not found in thyroid diffuse large B-cell lymphomas. *Mod Pathol.* 2006;19:1578–1584.

64. Brownlie BE, Fitzharris BM, Abdelaal AS, et al. Primary thyroid lymphoma: clinical features, treatment and outcome: a report of 8 cases. *N Z Med J.* 1994;107:301–304.

65. Burke JS, Butler JJ, Fuller LM. Malignant lymphomas of the thyroid: a clinical pathologic study of 35 patients including ultrastructural observations. *Cancer.* 1977;39:1587–1602.

66. DiBiase SJ, Grigsby PW, Guo C, et al. Outcome analysis for stage IE and IIE thyroid lymphoma. *Am J Clin Oncol.* 2004;27:178–184.

67. Harrington KJ, Michalaki VJ, Vini L, et al. Management of non-Hodgkin's lymphoma of the thyroid: the Royal Marsden Hospital experience. *Br J Radiol.* 2005;78:405–410.

68. Kanetake H, Toda M, Kawamoto Y. [Prognostic factors in primary lymphoma of the thyroid—a review of 74 cases]. *Nippon Jibiinkoka Gakkai Kaiho.* 1993;96:1105–1111.

69. Klyachkin ML, Schwartz RW, Cibull M, et al. Thyroid lymphoma: is there a role for surgery? *Am Surg.* 1998;64:234–238.

70. Doi Y, Goto A, Murakami T, et al. Primary thyroid lymphoma associated with Graves' disease. *Thyroid.* 2004;14:772–776.

71. Carcangiu ML, Steeper T, Zampi G, et al. Anaplastic thyroid carcinoma. A study of 70 cases. *Am J Clin Pathol.* 1985;83:135–158.

72. Honda N, Machida K, Inoue Y, et al. Scintigraphic findings of MALT lymphoma of the thyroid. *Ann Nucl Med.* 2002;16:289–292.

73. Kwak JY, Kim EK, Ko KH, et al. Primary thyroid lymphoma: role of ultrasound-guided needle biopsy. *J Ultrasound Med.* 2007;26:1761–1765.

74. Ota H, Ito Y, Matsuzuka F, et al. Usefulness of ultrasonography for diagnosis of malignant lymphoma of the thyroid. *Thyroid.* 2006;16:983–987.

75. Weiler-Sagie M, Bushelev O, Epelbaum R, et al. (18)F-FDG avidity in lymphoma readdressed: a study of 766 patients. *J Nucl Med.* 2010;51:25–30.

76. Hoffmann M, Wohrer S, Becherer A, et al. 18F-Fluoro-deoxy-glucose positron emission tomography in lymphoma of mucosa-associated lymphoid tissue: histology makes the difference. *Ann Oncol.* 2006;17:1761–1765.

77. Lin M, Wong C, Lin P, et al. The prevalence and clinical significance of (18) F-2-fluoro-2-deoxy-D-glucose (FDG) uptake in the thyroid gland on PET or PET-CT in patients with lymphoma. *Hematol Oncol.* 2011;29:67–74.

78. Mack LA, Pasieka JL. An evidence-based approach to the treatment of thyroid lymphoma. *World J Surg.* 2007;31:978–986.

79. Aozasa K, Ueda T, Katagiri S, et al. Immunologic and immunohistologic analysis of 27 cases with thyroid lymphomas. *Cancer.* 1987;60:969–973.

80. Junor EJ, Paul J, Reed NS. Primary non-Hodgkin's lymphoma of the thyroid. *Eur J Surg Oncol.* 1992;18:313–321.

81. Sasai K, Yamabe H, Haga H, et al. Non-Hodgkin's lymphoma of the thyroid. A clinical study of twenty-two cases. *Acta Oncol.* 1996;35:457–462.

82. Suarez P, el-Naggar AK, Batsakis JG. Intracellular crystalline deposits in lymphoplasmacellular disorders. *Ann Otol Rhinol Laryngol.* 1997;106:170–172.

83. Kuper-Hommel MJ, Snijder S, Jansen-Heijnen ML, et al. Treatment and survival of patients with thyroid lymphoma: a population-based study with clinical and pathologic reviews. *Clin Lymphoma Myeloma.* 2005;6:240–247.

84. Peng H, Du M, Diss TC, et al. Genetic evidence for a clonal link between low and high-grade components in gastric MALT B-cell lymphoma. *Histopathology.* 1997;30:425–429.

85. Ferry JA, Yang WI, Zukerberg LR, et al. CD5+ extranodal marginal zone B-cell (MALT) lymphoma. A low grade neoplasm with a propensity for bone marrow involvement and relapse. *Am J Clin Pathol.* 1996;105:31–37.

86. Llanos M, Alvarez-Arguelles H, Aleman R, et al. Prognostic significance of Ki-67 nuclear proliferative antigen, bcl-2 protein, and p53 expression in follicular and diffuse large B-cell lymphoma. *Med Oncol.* 2001;18:15–22.

87. de Jong D, Rosenwald A, Chhanabhai M, et al. Immunohistochemical prognostic markers in diffuse large B-cell lymphoma: validation of tissue microarray as a prerequisite for broad clinical applications—a study from the Lunenburg Lymphoma Biomarker Consortium. *J Clin Oncol.* 2007;25:805–812.

88. Insabato L, Di Vizio D, Tornillo L, et al. Clinicopathologic and immunohistochemical study of surgically treated primary gastric MALT lymphoma. *J Surg Oncol.* 2003;83:106–111.

89. Widder S, Pasieka JL. Primary thyroid lymphomas. *Curr Treat Options Oncol.* 2004;5:307–313.

90. Chan JK, Ng CS, Isaacson PG. Relationship between high-grade lymphoma and low-grade B-cell mucosa-associated lymphoid tissue lymphoma (MALToma) of the stomach. *Am J Pathol.* 1990;136:1153–1164.

91. Alizadeh AA, Eisen MB, Davis RE, et al. Distinct types of diffuse large B-cell lymphoma identified by gene expression profiling. *Nature.* 2000;403:503–511.

92. Rosenwald A, Wright G, Chan WC, et al. The use of molecular profiling to predict survival after chemotherapy for diffuse large-B-cell lymphoma. *N Engl J Med.* 2002;346:1937–1947.

93. Hans CP, Weisenburger DD, Greiner TC, et al. Confirmation of the molecular classification of diffuse large B-cell lymphoma by immunohistochemistry using a tissue microarray. *Blood.* 2004;103:275–282.

94. National Comprehensive Cancer Care Network (NCCN). 2.2011 Non-Hodgkin's Lymphoma Clinical Practice Guidelines in Oncology Web site. http://www.nccn.org. Accessed March 9, 2011.

95. Niitsu N, Okamoto M, Yoshino T, et al. t(8;14)(q24;q32) in two patients with CD10-negative primary thyroid diffuse large B-cell lymphoma. *Leuk Res.* 2007;31:707–711.

96. Aggarwal N SS, Ogilvie JB, Nikiforova MN, et al. Thyroid carcinoma-associated genetic mutations also occur in thyroid lymphomas. *Mod Pathol.* 2010;23:283A.

97. Isaacson PG, Androulakis-Papachristou A, Diss TC, et al. Follicular colonization in thyroid lymphoma. *Am J Pathol.* 1992;141:43–52.

98. Harris NL, Swerdlow SH, Jaffe ES, et al. Follicular lymphoma. In: Swerdlow SH, Campo E, Harris NL, Jaffe ES, Pileri SA, Stein H, Thiele J, Vardiman JW, eds. *WHO Classification of Tumours of the Haematopoietic and Lymphoid Tissues.* 4th ed. Lyon, France: IARC Press; 2008:220–226.

99. Bacon CM, Ye H, Diss TC, et al. Primary follicular lymphoma of the testis and epididymis in adults. *Am J Surg Pathol.* 2007;31:1050–1058.

100. Kim BK, Surti U, Pandya A, et al. Clinicopathologic, immunophenotypic, and molecular cytogenetic fluorescence in situ hybridization analysis of primary and secondary cutaneous follicular lymphomas. *Am J Surg Pathol.* 2005;29:69–82.

101. Chen HI, Akpolat I, Mody DR, et al. Restricted kappa/lambda light chain ratio by flow cytometry in germinal center B cells in Hashimoto thyroiditis. *Am J Clin Pathol.* 2006;125:42–48.

102. Buss DH, Marshall RB, Holleman IL Jr, et al. Malignant lymphoma of the thyroid gland with plasma cell differentiation (plasmacytoma). *Cancer.* 1980;46:2671–2675.

103. Kremer M, Ott G, Nathrath M, et al. Primary extramedullary plasmacytoma and multiple myeloma: phenotypic differences revealed by immunohistochemical analysis. *J Pathol.* 2005;205:92–101.

104. Hardoff R, Bar-Shalom R, Dharan M, et al. Hodgkin's disease presenting as a solitary thyroid nodule. *Clin Nucl Med.* 1995;20:37–41.

105. Solomon AC, Baloch ZW, Salhany KE, et al. Thyroid sclerosing mucoepidermoid carcinoma with eosinophilia: mimic of Hodgkin disease in nodal metastases. *Arch Pathol Lab Med.* 2000;124:446–449.

106. Shin J, Chute D, Milas M, et al. A rare case of chronic lymphocytic leukemia/small lymphocytic lymphoma presenting in the thyroid gland. *Thyroid.* 2010;20:1019–1023.

107. Abdul-Rahman ZH, Gogas HJ, Tooze JA, et al. T-cell lymphoma in Hashimoto's thyroiditis. *Histopathology.* 1996;29:455–459.

108. Koida S, Tsukasaki K, Tsuchiya T, et al. Primary T-cell lymphoma of the thyroid gland with chemokine receptors of Th1 phenotype complicating autoimmune thyroiditis. *Haematologica.* 2007;92:e37–e40.

109. Motoi N, Ozawa Y. Malignant T-cell lymphoma of the thyroid gland associated with Hashimoto's thyroiditis. *Pathol Int.* 2005;55:425–430.

110. Tiemann M, Asbeck R, Wacker HH. [Clonal B-cell reaction in Sjögren disease and Hashimoto autoimmune thyroiditis]. *Pathologe.* 1996;17:289–295.

111. Gupta N, Nijhawan R, Srinivasan R, et al. Fine needle aspiration cytology of primary thyroid lymphoma: a report of ten cases. *Cytojournal.* 2005;2:21.

112. Limanova Z, Neuwirtova R, Smejkal V. Malignant lymphoma of the thyroid. *Exp Clin Endocrinol.* 1987;90:113–119.

113. Lovchik J, Lane MA, Clark DP. Polymerase chain reaction-based detection of B-cell clonality in the fine needle aspiration biopsy of a thyroid mucosa-associated lymphoid tissue (MALT) lymphoma. *Hum Pathol.* 1997;28:989–992.

114. Ponder TB, Collins BT, Bee CS, et al. Diagnosis of cervical thymoma by fine needle aspiration biopsy with flow cytometry. A case report. *Acta Cytol.* 2002;46:1129–1132.

115. Takano T, Asahi S, Matsuzuka F, et al. Aspiration biopsy-nucleic acid diagnosis of thyroid malignant lymphoma by vectorette PCR: experience of eight cases. *Leuk Res.* 2008;32:151–154.

116. Takano T, Miyauchi A, Matsuzuka F, et al. Diagnosis of thyroid malignant lymphoma by reverse transcription-polymerase chain reaction detecting the monoclonality of immunoglobulin heavy chain messenger ribonucleic acid. *J Clin Endocrinol Metab.* 2000;85:671–675.

117. Cheuk W, Chan JK. IgG4-related sclerosing disease: a critical appraisal of an evolving clinicopathologic entity. *Adv Anat Pathol.* 2010;17:303–332.

118. Chang ST, Chuang SS. Ectopic cervical thymoma: a mimic of T-lymphoblastic lymphoma. *Pathol Res Pract.* 2003;199:633–635.

119. Oh YH, Ko YH, Ree HJ. Aspiration cytology of ectopic cervical thymoma mimicking a thyroid mass. A case report. *Acta Cytol.* 1998;42:1167–1171.

120. Cho JH, Park YH, Kim WS, et al. High incidence of mucosa-associated lymphoid tissue in primary thyroid lymphoma: a clinicopathologic study of 18 cases in the Korean population. *Leuk Lymphoma.* 2006;47:2128–2131.

121. Friedberg MH, Coburn MC, Monchik JM. Role of surgery in stage IE non-Hodgkin's lymphoma of the thyroid. *Surgery.* 1994;116:1061–1066; discussion 1066–1067.

122. Doria R, Jekel JF, Cooper DL. Thyroid lymphoma. The case for combined modality therapy. *Cancer.* 1994;73:200–206.

123. Meyer-Rochow GY, Sywak MS, Reeve TS, et al. Surgical trends in the management of thyroid lymphoma. *Eur J Surg Oncol.* 2008;34:576–580.

124. Wirtzfeld DA, Winston JS, Hicks WL Jr, et al. Clinical presentation and treatment of non-Hodgkin's lymphoma of the thyroid gland. *Ann Surg Oncol.* 2001;8:338–341.

125. Green LD, Mack L, Pasieka JL. Anaplastic thyroid cancer and primary thyroid lymphoma: a review of these rare thyroid malignancies. *J Surg Oncol.* 2006;94:725–736.

126. Onal C, Li YX, Miller RC, et al. Treatment results and prognostic factors in primary thyroid lymphoma patients: a rare cancer network study. *Ann Oncol.* 2011;22:156–164.

127. Watanabe N, Noh JK, Narimatsu H, et al. Clinicopathological features of 171 cases of primary thyroid lymphoma: a long-term study involving 24 553 patients with Hashimoto's disease. *Br J Haem.* 2011;153:236–243.

128. Evans TR, Mansi JL, Bevan DH, et al. Primary non-Hodgkin's lymphoma of the thyroid with bone marrow infiltration at presentation. *Clin Oncol (R Coll Radiol).* 1995;7:54–55.

129. Isobe K, Kagami Y, Higuchi K, et al. A multicenter phase II study of local radiation therapy for stage IEA mucosa-associated lymphoid tissue lymphomas: a preliminary report from the Japan Radiation Oncology Group (JAROG). *Int J Radiat Oncol Biol Phys.* 2007;69:1181–1186.

130. Aozasa K, Nara H, Ikeda H, et al. The influence of histologic type on survival in early extranodal non-Hodgkin's lymphoma in head and neck. *Oncology.* 1984;41:164–169.

Tumors Metastatic to the Thyroid

DEFINITION

Tumors developed in the thyroid gland as a result of lymphatic or hematogenous spread from distant sites are considered metastatic disease or secondary tumors.[1] Although not specifically discussed in this section, direct extension into the thyroid from the adjacent or contiguous structures (larynx, trachea, pharynx, esophagus, lymph nodes, soft tissues, mediastinum) may sometimes need to be included in the differential diagnosis of thyroid gland masses.[2,3] By convention, lymphomas and leukemias are not considered metastatic tumors, although the thyroid gland may be affected as part of systemic disease. Lymphomas are covered in a separate chapter (see Chapter 17).

ETIOLOGY

The exceedingly rich vascularity of endocrine organs predisposes to an increased likelihood of developing metastatic deposits.[1,4,5] The thyroid gland is affected by widely disseminated disease.[6] Curiously, the abnormal thyroid gland (affected by some other disease) tends to be more frequently affected than a normal gland, perhaps suggesting alterations in vascularity or blood flow may contribute to metastatic disease developing.[5,7]

CLINICAL PRESENTATION

Identification of metastatic disease in surgical pathology material is seen in up to 7.5% of thyroid glands,[7–9] although up to 25% of autopsied patients with disseminated malignancies will have thyroid gland metastatic deposits.[1,10,11] The apparent increase in cases recently may be related to advancement in radiographic studies, improved treatments resulting in prolonged survival, and increased frequency of fine needle aspiration (FNA) for thyroid gland nodules.[8,12,13] Patients of all ages are affected, although elderly patients are more frequently noted to have disease (mean age of 63.8 years for 340 reported cases) (Table 18.1).[5,7,9,10,12,14,15] There is a slight gender predilection (female > male, 1.1:1), but the gender differences are expected with breast and gynecologic primaries compared to prostate primaries.[4,5,7,8,10,15–18] The clinical presentation is usually a mass within the thyroid gland, although it may be masked by underlying thyroid gland disease.[1,5,8,10,12,13] Occasionally, a rapidly enlarging thyroid mass is seen.[19] Hoarseness (compression of the recurrent laryngeal nerve), dysphagia, dysphonia, neck pain, and even hemoptysis may also be noted.[5,14,15,19] In rare circumstances, hyperthyroidism may be the presenting symptom, apparently because of thyroid parenchymal destruction and hormone release.[15] The thyroid gland metastatic deposit is the initial presentation of an occult primary tumor in up to 40% of patients,[8,12] although this seems to be most frequently noted in kidney primaries.[5,20] This finding may help to direct the search for an unknown primary. Radiographic studies may help, with ultrasonographic studies exhibiting unilateral or bilateral, multiple, ill-defined, infiltrating, hypoechoic nodules with inhomogeneous

texture. There are no microcalcifications, although necrosis and hemorrhage can be seen.[12,13,15,16] Although nonspecific, bilateral, multiple nodules without microcalcifications may suggest metastatic disease in patients with a known nonthyroidal primary tumor (Fig. 18.1). FNA or core needle biopsy (often ultrasound guided) may help to confirm this impression and is the initial study of choice in this setting.[4,5,8,10–15,17]

The time to the appearance of metastatic disease from the identification of the primary tumor ranges up to 22 years, a finding suggesting an exceedingly careful clinical history is crucial to making an accurate diagnosis.[4–6,9,11,12,15] However, approximately 80% of metastases develop within 3 years of the primary tumor resection, with the exception of renal cell carcinoma that is notorious for having a long latency period.[4,5,7,9,10,12,14,15]

In clinical surgical pathology series, metastatic deposits are identified at a higher frequency in abnormal glands, such as, adenomatoid nodules, thyroiditis, and follicular-pattern neoplasms.[5,10,21] Interestingly, the metastatic deposits may be found within or adjacent to primary thyroid tumors (Figs. 18.2B and 18.3).[5,21,22] There is variability depending on whether the reported series is based on clinical or autopsy material. Carcinomas are most common (approximately 80%), with the most common primary sites in order of frequency being kidney, lung, breast, and gastrointestinal tract (esophagus, stomach, and colon); leiomyosarcoma (usually uterine, but gastrointestinal tract primaries are reported) and skin melanoma are the most common sarcomas (Table 18.1).[1,4–12,14–17,23] Isolated case reports from virtually every other organ have been reported, such as salivary gland, pancreas, bladder, tongue, nasopharynx, prostate, ovary, parathyroid, testes, and bone, to name just a few.[8,10,24,25]

GROSS PRESENTATION

Owing to high vascularity in the thyroid gland, multifocal and bilateral disease tends to be most common, but clinical evaluation is more likely to be initiated when there is a unilateral, solitary mass (Fig. 18.2).[1,5,10,15] In fact, metastatic renal cell carcinoma usually presents as a solitary mass (up to 80% of cases).[5,10] The metastatic foci range from microscopic up to 15 cm in greatest dimension.[5]

MICROSCOPIC FEATURES

Metastatic tumor tends to develop in two forms: small deposits within lymph-vascular spaces and larger, mass lesions.[1] Careful examination at the periphery of the thyroid gland, immediately adjacent to the thyroid gland capsule where the vasculature is the most dense, will help to identify intravascular metastatic deposits (Fig. 18.3).[5] When the tumor deposits form a mass lesion, they usually have an architecture and cytomorphology distinct from thyroid primaries. For the most part, the metastatic deposits histologically resemble the primary site, although frequently they are less differentiated.[10] Some exceptions exist, such as a poorly differentiated tumor and metastatic clear cell renal cell

Table 18.1

Literature Summary of Primary Sites Metastatic to the Thyroid Gland[4–12,14–16,18,19,22–26,28–33]

Characteristics	Number (n = 340)
Gender	
Females	180
Males	160
Age (years)	
Range	24–94
Mean	63.8
Anatomic site of primary (in order of frequency)	
Kidney (renal cell carcinoma; n = 88)	26%
Lung (n = 77)	23%
Not otherwise specified (n = 39)	
Squamous cell carcinoma (n = 17)	
Adenocarcinoma (n = 15)	
Neuroendocrine (small cell or large cell; n = 6)	
Breast (n = 39)	11%
Skin (n = 15)	4%
Melanoma (n = 14)	
Squamous cell carcinoma (n = 1)	
Esophagus (n = 14)	4%
Squamous (n = 11)	
Adenocarcinoma (n = 3)	
Stomach (n = 13)	4%
Adenocarcinoma (n = 12)	
Leiomyosarcoma (n = 1)	
Colon (n = 12)	4%
Uterus (n = 12)	4%
Leiomyosarcoma (n = 7)	
Cervix (squamous cell carcinoma; n = 3)	
Endometrium (n = 2)	
Larynx (n = 7)	2%
Bladder (n = 4)	1%
Salivary gland (parotid specifically; n = 3)	1%
Pancreas and biliary tract (n = 3)	1%
Soft tissue (angiosarcoma; n = 3)	1%
Nasopharynx (undifferentiated carcinoma; n = 2)	<1%
Oral (including tongue; n = 2)	<1%
Prostate (n = 2)	<1%
Ovary (n = 1)	<1%
Parathyroid gland (n = 1)	<1%
Miscellaneous or not specifically stated (n = 42)	12%

carcinoma. Specifically, metastatic neuroendocrine (small cell) carcinomas may resemble a medullary thyroid carcinoma, with both tumors possibly exhibiting thyroid transcription factor 1 (TTF1) and chromogranin immunoreactivity.[1,26] Clear cell renal cell carcinoma shows polygonal cells with clear cytoplasm, distinct cell membranes, and small compact eccentric nuclei within a rich vascular network (Fig. 18.4). A pseudoalveolar or pseudofollicular pattern of clear cell renal cell carcinoma may resemble

the clear cell variant of thyroid follicular carcinoma and adenoma. Metastatic tumor should be suspected based on rich vascularity, abundant extravasated erythrocytes, and pseudofollicular spaces filled with blood.

Metastatic adenocarcinoma from different locations, such as from lung, shows glandular differentiation, large tumor cell size, high nuclear to cytoplasmic ratio, coarse nuclear chromatin distribution, and prominent nucleoli, along with mitotic figures (Fig. 18.5).

Sarcomas can be primary or metastatic in the thyroid gland, sometimes requiring clinical and radiographic separation, as histologic and immunohistochemical features alone may not allow for a definitive diagnosis. Specifically, leiomyosarcoma, angiosarcoma, and malignant peripheral nerve sheath tumors can arise within the thyroid gland parenchyma (from native structures), arise from soft tissues adjacent to the thyroid gland, or metastasize from a distant primary.[19] Occasionally, the vessel or nerve origin may be identified, but this finding is infrequent.[27,28]

Tumors directly invading into the thyroid gland usually have a histologic appearance that is unique, accompanied by obvious clinical and radiographic findings to support a separate topographic primary site (Fig. 18.6).[2,3]

IMMUNOHISTOCHEMISTRY AND MOLECULAR DIAGNOSTICS

It is important to bear in mind that TTF1 can be seen in both thyroid gland (papillary, follicular, and medullary) and lung primaries (Fig. 18.7) as well as in small cell carcinomas from other locations. Likewise, chromogranin and calcitonin can be seen in medullary carcinoma and metastatic small cell carcinoma, although calcitonin is rarely identified in pulmonary tumors. Therefore, selected, pertinent immunohistochemical studies can aid in separating between primary versus metastatic tumors, keeping in mind overlapping positive results can be seen (Figs. 18.8 and 18.9).[1,20,26] In general, primary thyroid follicular tumors will be thyroglobulin, cytokeratin 7, TTF1, and TTF2 immunoreactive, whereas C-cell–derived tumors will be calcitonin, chromogranin, and carcinoembryonic antigen (CEA) reactive. Metastatic tumors are not expected to have immunoreactivity for thyroglobulin (Figs. 18.7 and 18.9).[5,20,22] Staining of entrapped thyroid follicles and the tumor cells due to the diffusion of thyroglobulin from surrounding thyroid parenchyma should not be considered as positive staining.

Molecular testing may be of help in some cases, especially when immunohistochemical studies are inconclusive (Fig. 18.10). Finding of BRAF, NRAS codon 61, HRAS codon 61, RET/PTC, or PAX8/PPARγ mutations strongly supports the diagnosis of primary thyroid carcinoma, although BRAF mutations also occur in melanoma, colorectal cancer, and ovarian cancer and with very low prevalence in lung adenocarcinoma and some other tumors. Finding of KRAS codon 12/13 mutations is more suggestive of metastatic carcinoma from the lung, colon, or other primary sites as they are exceedingly rare in thyroid tumors.[29] Loss of heterozygosity may also be used to search for specific regions of loss, such as for the VHL locus loss, which is common in renal cell carcinoma.

An exhaustive immunohistochemical panel and expensive molecular analysis can be avoided in many cases where a thoroughly investigated clinical history is available together with a knowledge of the findings on physical examination and in laboratory and imaging studies.

CYTOLOGIC FEATURES

FNA may be helpful in documenting the presence of metastatic tumor.[8,10–12,29–31] The smears are cellular, often showing two distinct cell populations. One is the uninvolved thyroid gland parenchyma,

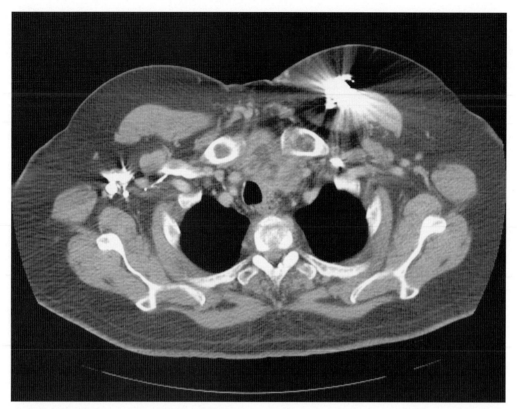

FIGURE 18.1. Metastatic transitional cell carcinoma to thyroid. This CT scan demonstrates a large heterogeneous mass, greater on the left than on the right. The artifact is from a pacemaker.

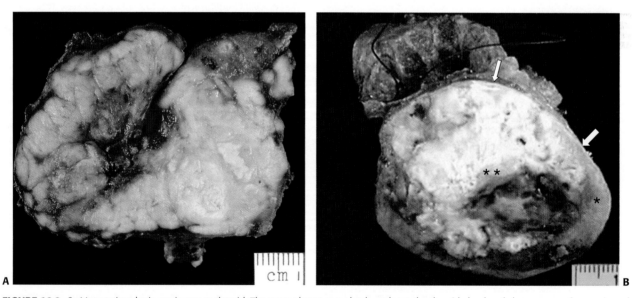

FIGURE 18.2. A: Metastatic colonic carcinoma to thyroid. The mass almost completely replaces the thyroid gland and shows areas of necrosis and hemorrhage. In addition to the main mass, smaller satellite tumor nodules are seen in the thyroid parenchyma (top right). **B:** Metastatic renal cell carcinoma to follicular variant of papillary thyroid carcinoma. Note an encapsulated nodule *(arrows)* of papillary carcinoma with homogeneous tan-brown tissue at the periphery *(*)* and a large ill-defined central area of metastatic renal cell carcinoma with extensive necrosis and hemorrhage *(**)*.

and the other is the metastatic neoplastic population. If there is a metastatic tumor to a primary thyroid gland neoplasm, separation may be more difficult, although adenocarcinoma and squamous cell carcinoma are distinctly different from usual thyroid gland primaries (Fig. 18.11). Sometimes a poorly differentiated

carcinoma metastatic to the thyroid gland can mimic a primary undifferentiated thyroid carcinoma. Furthermore, a significant bloody background with spindle cells can be seen in primary or secondary (direct extension or metastasis) angiosarcoma.[32] Therefore, FNA may be useful in identifying a neoplasm but not

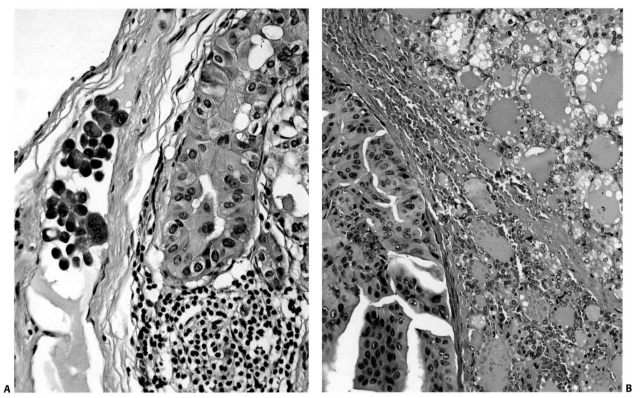

FIGURE 18.3. A: Metastatic lung adenocarcinoma within the vascular space, adjacent to a focus of papillary carcinoma. Note the different morphologies of the tumors. **B:** Metastatic breast adenocarcinoma to papillary thyroid carcinoma. Note the intravascular location of the metastatic breast carcinoma (left), whereas the follicular variant of papillary carcinoma comprises the right side of the illustration.

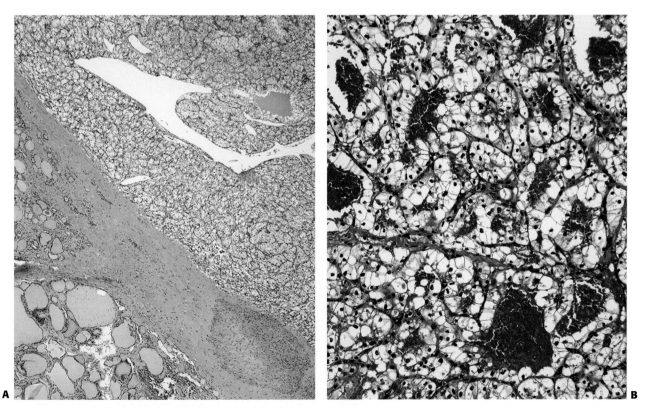

FIGURE 18.4. Metastatic renal cell carcinoma. A: This is a single "mass" lesion separated from the thyroid gland parenchyma by a fibrous connective tissue capsule. **B:** High-power view shows clear cytoplasm within prominent cell borders and small, hyperchromatic nuclear characteristic of renal cell carcinoma. Note the rich vascular plexus and pseudofollicular spaces filled with blood.

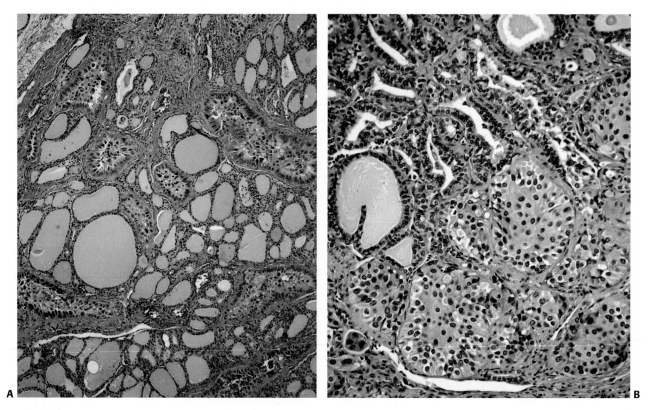

FIGURE 18.5. A: Metastatic lung adenocarcinoma to thyroid. There is a concentration of tumor within peripheral lymphatic spaces between unremarkable thyroid parenchyma. **B:** Metastatic urothelial carcinoma to a papillary carcinoma. Note the intimate blending of the tumor cells.

in the specific type of tumor present.[8,10,11,33] Renal cell carcinoma tends to be bloody, lacks colloid, and shows stripped nuclei with only occasional cells showing microvacuolated or clear cytoplasm.[4,17,20,30] Adenocarcinomas have gland formation and well-developed cell borders and tend to have coarse, heavy nuclear chromatin with prominent nucleoli. Necrosis and mitotic figures are frequently noted, findings uncommon in primary thyroid gland neoplasms.[33]

 DIFFERENTIAL DIAGNOSIS

In general, the multifocal nature of the process, often confined to interstitial lymphatic and/or blood vessel spaces, easily identifies metastatic disease. Sometimes the fibrous septa are expanded and more prominent in the setting of metastatic disease. A solitary metastatic renal cell carcinoma may be difficult to separate

FIGURE 18.6. An adenoid cystic carcinoma (ACC) arising from the minor salivary glands of the larynx directly invaded into the thyroid gland. Here you can see the collision of the ACC with a papillary carcinoma.

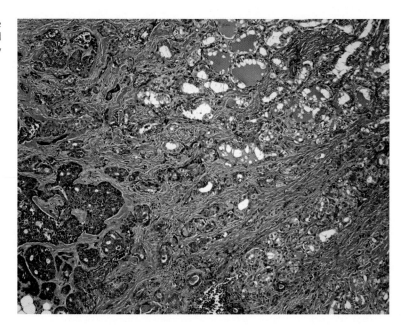

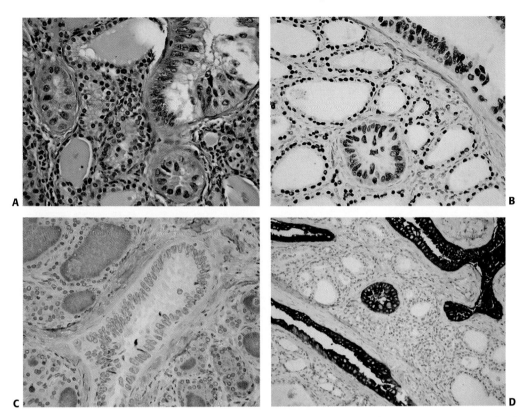

FIGURE 18.7. Metastatic lung adenocarcinoma immunohistochemistry. A: The metastatic tumor is confined to lymphatic spaces, with large cells and a high nuclear to cytoplasmic ratio compared with the surrounding paren-chyma. **B:** TTF1 reacts with both the thyroid and metastatic lung adenocarcinoma although with a different intensity and distribution. **C:** Thyroglobulin is present within the follicles but not in the metastatic tumor. **D:** CEA(m) is positive in metastatic lung adenocarcinoma but not in thyroid follicular epithelium.

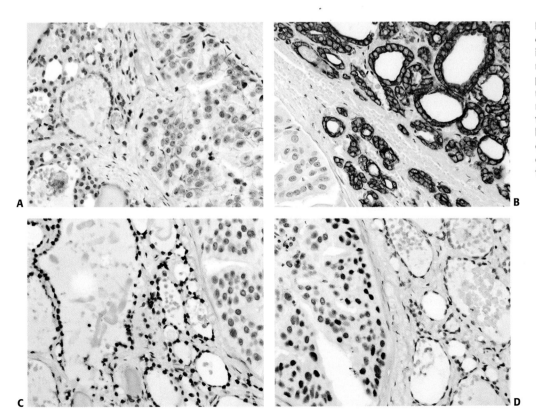

FIGURE 18.8. Metastatic breast carcinoma immunohistochem-istry. A: Her-2/neu membrane reaction (1+). **B:** Cytokeratin 7 is positive in native thyroid tissue but not in the metastatic breast carci-noma. **C:** TTF1 is positive in native thyroid tissue but not in metastatic breast carcinoma. **D:** Estrogen re-ceptor positivity in metastatic breast carcinoma but not in the adjacent follicles.

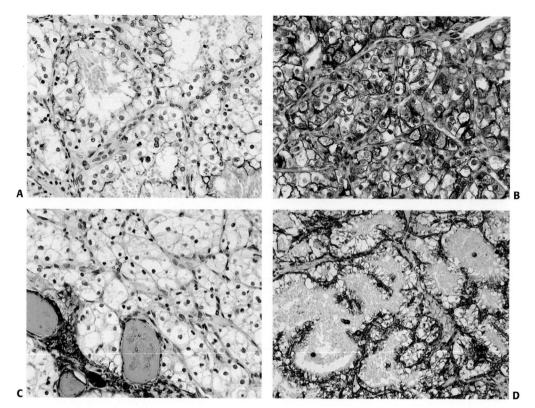

FIGURE 18.9. Metastatic renal cell carcinoma immunohistochemistry. A: Epithelial membrane antigen stains the membranes of the neoplastic cells. **B:** CD10 is strongly and diffusely immunoreactive, accentuated along the cell borders. **C:** Thyroglobulin is only positive in the entrapped thyroid follicles but not in the renal cell carcinoma. **D:** Vimentin accentuates the neoplastic cells and is positive in the vascular stroma.

from the clear cell change seen in follicular adenomas or carcinomas, and more rarely in papillary and medullary carcinoma. However, the prominent vascularity, pseudoglandular lumina filled with erythrocytes, sharp intercellular borders, and hyperchromatic nuclei favor a renal cell carcinomas.[4,5] The neoplastic cells are Renal cell carcinoma (RCC), CD10, and epithelial membrane antigen (EMA) immunoreactive, whereas they are nonreactive for TTF1 and thyroglobulin.[5] It is imperative that diffusion artifact of thyroglobulin is not overinterpreted as a positive result; sometimes the nuclear reaction of a TTF1 may be easier to interpret. However, TTF1 is positive in pulmonary tumors and small cell carcinomas from various locations. TTF2 and PAX8 immunostains may offer additional help. A recent study found strong nuclear reactivity for both markers in all follicular cell–derived tumors, whereas lung adenocarcinomas, squamous cell carcinomas, and large cell carcinomas were all nonreactive.[27] The specificity of these promising antibodies needs further validation. Small cell carcinoma or other neuroendocrine carcinomas metastatic to the thyroid gland tend to be predominantly within interstitial septa, show widespread thyroid gland involvement, have rosette formation, and are usually negative with calcitonin and CEA. Clinical information will often help to make

an accurate distinction between a metastatic versus a primary tumor. When considering the diagnosis of primary squamous cell carcinoma of the thyroid gland, direct extension from adjacent organs (larynx most commonly, followed by esophagus and tongue)[3,8] or metastases from another site (lung, uterine cervix) should be excluded before making a primary diagnosis.

 TREATMENT AND PROGNOSIS

The prognosis is determined by the underlying primary tumor and is usually poor by dint of metastasis alone.[1,7,10–15] Rarely, isolated metastatic deposits in the thyroid gland may herald the primary or be the only focus of metastasis. Under these conditions, surgery (lobectomy or total thyroidectomy) can result in prolonged survival.[4,6,12,17] In particular, renal cell carcinoma is well known to show unpredictable behavior.[4,5] Therefore, surgery is often advocated for metastatic disease, particularly when the tumor is slow growing or an isolated tumor, if only for palliation, to prolong disease-free interval (by about 10 months on average[9]) or to prevent the potential morbidity of another tumor recurrence in the neck.[5,7,11,13,14]

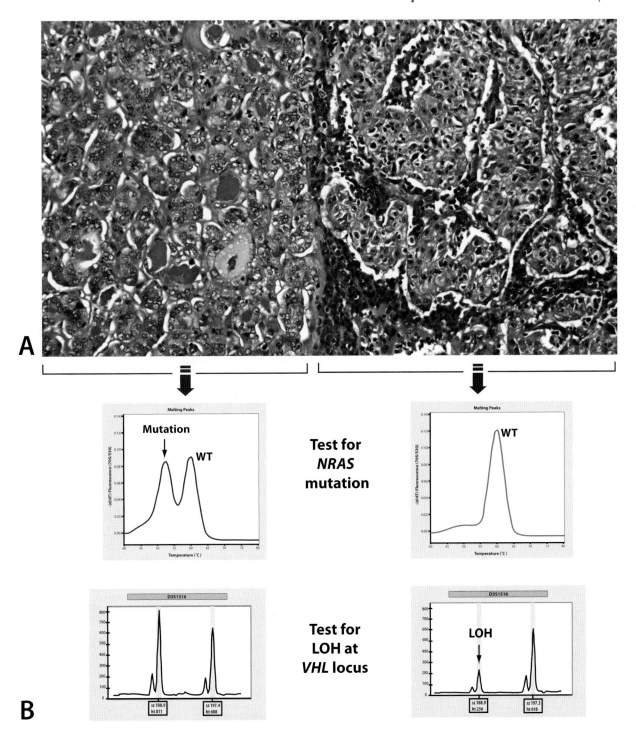

FIGURE 18.10. Molecular analysis of a thyroid tumor that revealed the areas of follicular variant of papillary carcinoma **(A, left)** intermixed with the differently appearing tumor areas **(A, right)**, which could be consistent with either dedifferentiation and progression to poorly differentiated carcinoma or a different tumor metastatic to the papillary carcinoma. Immunohistochemical analysis was inconclusive as the lack of thyroglobulin and TTF1 staining in the component in question could support both possibilities. **B:** Molecular testing revealed a *NRAS* codon 61 mutation in the papillary carcinoma but not in the second component and the presence of loss of heterozygosity for the *VHL* locus in the second component but not in the papillary carcinoma, indicating that these two tumors are of different origin and the second component most likely represents a metastatic renal cell carcinoma. The history of nephrectomy for renal cell carcinoma performed at a different institution was later obtained.

FIGURE 18.11. FNA of metastatic lung adenocarcinoma. A dual cell population is obvious. The thyroid follicular epithelium has slight hemosiderin pigment and is arranged in a sheet. The metastatic tumor is arranged in tight clusters of greatly enlarged cells with coarse nuclear chromatin and prominent nucleoli.

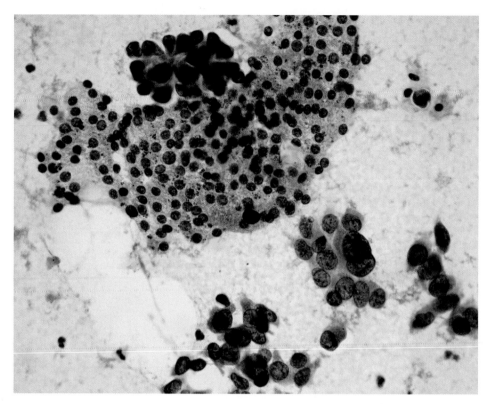

REFERENCES

1. DeLellis RA. Secondary tumours of the thyroid. In: DeLellis RA, Lloyd RV, Heitz PU, Eng C, eds. *Pathology and Genetics of Tumours of Endocrine Organs.* Lyon, France: IARC Press; 2004:122–123.
2. Watanabe I, Tsuchiya A. Secondary carcinoma of the thyroid gland. *Jpn J Surg.* 1980;10:130–136.
3. Nakhjavani M, Gharib H, Goellner JR, et al. Direct extension of malignant lesions to the thyroid gland from adjacent organs: report of 17 cases. *Endocr Pract.* 1999;5:69–71.
4. Chen H, Nicol TL, Udelsman R. Clinically significant, isolated metastatic disease to the thyroid gland. *World J Surg.* 1999;23:177–180.
5. Heffess CS, Wenig BM, Thompson LDR. Metastatic renal cell carcinoma to the thyroid gland: a clinicopathologic study of 36 cases. *Cancer.* 2002;95:1869–1878.
6. Ivy HK. Cancer metastatic to the thyroid: a diagnostic problem. *Mayo Clin Proc.* 1984;59:856–859.
7. Nixon IJ, Whitcher M, Glick J, et al. Surgical management of metastases to the thyroid gland. *Ann Surg Oncol.* 2011;18:800–804.
8. Michelow PM, Leiman G. Metastases to the thyroid gland: diagnosis by aspiration cytology. *Diagn Cytopathol.* 1995;13:209–213.
9. Papi G, Fadda G, Corsello SM, et al. Metastases to the thyroid gland: prevalence, clinicopathological aspects and prognosis: a 10-year experience. *Clin Endocrinol.* 2007;66:565–571.
10. Lam KY, Lo CY. Metastatic tumors of the thyroid gland: a study of 79 cases in Chinese patients. *Arch Pathol Lab Med.* 1998;122:37–41.
11. Nakhjavani MK, Gharib H, Goellner JR, et al. Metastasis to the thyroid gland. A report of 43 cases. *Cancer.* 1997;79:574–578.
12. Kim TY, Kim WB, Gong G, et al. Metastasis to the thyroid diagnosed by fine-needle aspiration biopsy. *Clin Endocrinol (Oxf).* 2005;62:236–241.
13. McCabe DP, Farrar WB, Petkov TM, et al. Clinical and pathologic correlations in disease metastatic to the thyroid gland. *Am J Surg.* 1985;150:519–523.
14. Dequanter D, Lothaire P, Larsimont D, et al. [Intrathyroid metastasis: 11 cases]. *Ann Endocrinol.* 2004;65:205–208.
15. Ferrozzi F, Bova D, Campodonico F, et al. US and CT findings of secondary neoplasms of the thyroid—a pictorial essay. *Clin Imaging.* 1998;22:157–161.
16. Chung SY, Kim EK, Kim JH, et al. Sonographic findings of metastatic disease to the thyroid. *Yonsei Med J.* 2001;42:411–417.
17. Czech JM, Lichtor TR, Carney JA, et al. Neoplasms metastatic to the thyroid gland. *Surg Gynecol Obstet.* 1982;155:503–505.
18. Selimoglu H, Duran C, Saraydaroglu O, et al. Prostate cancer metastasis to thyroid gland. *Tumori.* 2007;93:292–295.
19. Eng SP, Goh CH, Khoo JB, et al. Metastatic angiosarcoma to the thyroid. *Rev Laryngol Otol Rhinol.* 2005;126:111–114.
20. Halbauer M, Kardum-Skelin I, Vranesic D, et al. Aspiration cytology of renal-cell carcinoma metastatic to the thyroid. *Acta Cytol.* 1991;35:443–446.
21. Bohn OL, De las Casas LE, Leon ME. Tumor-to-tumor metastasis: renal cell carcinoma metastatic to papillary carcinoma of thyroid-report of a case and review of the literature. *Head Neck Pathol.* 2009;3:327–330.
22. Nabili V, Natarajan S, Hirschovitz S, et al. Collision tumor of thyroid: metastatic lung adenocarcinoma plus papillary thyroid carcinoma. *Am J Otolaryngol.* 2007;28:218–220.
23. Basu S, Alavi A. Metastatic malignant melanoma to the thyroid gland detected by FDG-PET imaging. *Clin Nucl Med.* 2007;32:388–389.
24. Puente S, Velasco A, Gallel P, et al. Metastatic small cell carcinoma to the thyroid gland: a pathologic and molecular study demonstrating the origin in the urinary bladder. *Endocr Pathol.* 2008;19:190–196.
25. Mattavelli F, Collini P, Pizzi N, et al. Thyroid as a target of metastases: a case of metastatic seminoma in a patient who died of a second cancer. *Tumori.* 2009;95:91–93.
26. Yamada H, Hasegawa Y, Mitsudomi T, et al. Neuroendocrine tumor metastasis to the thyroid gland. *Int J Clin Oncol.* 2007;12:63–67.
27. Thompson LDR, Wenig BM, Adair CF, et al. Primary smooth muscle tumors of the thyroid gland. *Cancer.* 1997;79:579–587.
28. Cruickshank JC. Leiomyosarcoma metastatic to the thyroid gland. *Ear Nose Throat J.* 1988;67:899–904.
29. Cozzolino I, Malapelle U, Carlomagno C, et al. Metastasis of colon cancer to the thyroid gland: a case diagnosed on fine-needle aspirate by a combined cytological, immunocytochemical, and molecular approach. *Diagn Cytopathol.* 2010;38:932–935.
30. Rizzo M, Rossi RT, Bonaffini O, et al. Thyroid metastasis of clear cell renal carcinoma: report of a case. *Diagn Cytopathol.* 2009;37:759–762.
31. Stoll L, Mudali S, Ali SZ. Merkel cell carcinoma metastatic to the thyroid gland: aspiration findings and differential diagnosis. *Diagn Cytopathol.* 2010;38:754–757.
32. Yu J, Steiner FA, Muench JP, et al. Juxtathyroidal neck soft tissue angiosarcoma presenting as an undifferentiated thyroid carcinoma. *Thyroid.* 2002;12:427–432.
33. Haraguchi S, Hioki M, Yamashita K, et al. Metastasis to the thyroid from lung adenocarcinoma mimicking thyroid carcinoma. *Jpn J Thorac Cardiovasc Surg.* 2004;52:353–356.

Gross Examination

INTRODUCTION

An understanding of the normal surgical thyroid anatomy is a requisite for accurate gross characterization of lesions. The fundamentals of thyroid anatomy are described in Chapter 1. These principles can be applied in a practical sense to the thyroid specimens that are commonly encountered at the gross bench. For neoplasms, many components of the gross examination are incorporated into tumor staging (see Chapter 7). A sample structured format for thyroid gross description is presented in Table 19.1.

Certain parameters are universal to all gross specimens.[1-5] First of all, the appropriate patient identification information and labeling should be confirmed. In addition, the "state" of the specimen (whether it is received unfixed, in saline or in formalin) on receipt should be documented as this may preclude ancillary molecular or flow cytometric studies. It is standard of care to provide overall specimen measurements along the X, Y, and Z axes in centimeters, and in the case of endocrine organs such as the thyroid, specimen weight in grams. These parameters not only are part of the documentation of the patient's procedure but also serve as the first indicators of a pathologic process.

THYROID SPECIMEN TYPES

Another key component of the thyroid gross examination is the identification of specimen type.[1-4] The proper orientation of a specimen based on anatomic and surgical landmarks provides a contextual framework for subsequent description of lesions. It allows for meaningful clinical and radiographic correlation and

---

Table 19.1

Sample Gross Description Structure

1st Paragraph (overall specimen description and measurement)
Patient and specimen identification
Specimen type
Measurements (X × Y × Z in cm) and weight (g)
Orientation sutures
Possible parathyroids and/or lymph nodes
Other features (capsular disruptions, attached skeletal muscle, etc.)

2nd to nth Paragraph (nodule description)[a]
Size (X × Y × Z in cm)
Location and distance from margin or capsular surface (in cm)
Configuration: infiltrative vs. well demarcated
   If well demarcated, presence or absence of capsule.
   Capsular thickness should be measured if >0.1 cm.
Nodule characteristics
   Color
   Homogeneous vs. heterogeneous
   Hemorrhage (pattern)
   Cystic change
   Calcification (pattern and location within nodule)

(n+1)th Paragraph (surrounding thyroid)[b]
Background disease—nodular or diffuse process

Final paragraph (ancillary procedures)
Photography, tissue frozen, submitted for electron microscopy, etc.

Ink code (inking scheme used)
   Black—right/left lobe
   Green—isthmus

Section code (designation of sections submitted)

[a]Each lesion should have its own paragraph. Multiple lesions can be arbitrarily designated as "lesion 1, 2, and so forth" for ease of dictation and interpretation.
[b]If there are no discrete lesions as in a completion thyroidectomy or a multinodular goiter, this becomes the second paragraph.

serves as a quality assurance checkpoint. The common thyroid specimens received for pathologic examination are as follows: the lobectomy, which consists of a thyroid lobe, often with some portion of the isthmus; and the total thyroidectomy, which contains the entire thyroid. The term *near-total thyroidectomy* is often used to describe specimens that consist of a thyroid lobectomy, isthmus, and a portion of the contralateral lobe with about 1 to 2 g of tissue left in the patient.[5,6] Occasionally, for locally aggressive processes, thyroidectomy specimens may be extended to include contiguous skeletal "strap" muscle and/or lymph node compartments. Other specimen types that may be encountered include excisions of substernal goiter. Intentional enucleation of nodules is no longer a standard practice, and these specimens will rarely be encountered, if at all.

 ORIENTATION

The correct orientation of a thyroidectomy can be ascertained in most cases in which the specimen is received intact. The surgeon may mark the superior pole of the thyroid with a suture or clip. This may be the only landmark for orientation in a severely distorted specimen. However, the orientation of most thyroidectomy specimens is readily apparent by gross examination even without a suture. This visual orientation should be performed even if the specimen is oriented by the surgeon, since sutures and clips may migrate and detach or even be incorrectly placed initially. In most situations, the superior pole of each thyroid lobe is longer and more tapered as compared with the rounded, bulbous inferior pole (Fig. 19.1A). The isthmus connecting the two lobes is typically situated inferiorly as well. The anterior surface of the thyroid is typically more convex and raised, whereas the posterior surface, which sits along the trachea, is more concave. The convergence of these surfaces results in a fairly sharp protuberant lateral border (Fig. 19.1B). Occasionally, the underlying pathologic process distorts the native contour of the thyroid gland to the point where orientation is very difficult or perhaps impossible. In these cases, orientation may still be salvaged, since the lateral border and superior poles of a lobe are more likely to retain their anteroposterior concave–convex configuration, even if the majority of the thyroid is massively distorted by a lesion (Fig. 19.1C). An additional gross clue in lobectomy specimens distorted by a lesion is the identification of roughened transected surface (typically with cautery) or fibrosis (from the site of prior surgery in a completion lobectomy specimen) as this would indicate isthmus where the specimen was transected (Fig. 19.1D). Finally, in extremely distorted specimens, if the location of a particular lesion is known based on imaging studies, the specimen can be oriented using the lesion as a landmark. For instance, if a dominant cystic nodule is noted inferiorly in the right lobe on ultrasound, once this lesion is identified in the specimen, it can be used to mark the right inferior pole.

 GROSS PATHOLOGY

Normal thyroid is surrounded by a smooth, semitranslucent capsule and displays a uniform, slightly gelatinous, red-brown parenchyma with delicate septae on cut surface. Initially, the outer surface should be inspected for parathyroid glands and lymph nodes. This will be nearly impossible after inking and sectioning. The parathyroid glands are typically found on the posterior surface as small brown ovoid masses.[3,5] Lymph nodes are often found near the isthmus. Before sectioning, the thyroid capsule should be inked as this capsule may not be readily discernible on histologic sections. Applying different colors to the lobes and isthmus (i.e., red, right; green, left; blue, isthmus), respectively, will allow for easier histologic interpretation. Microscopic extension of a tumor

to the capsular boundary can be more easily assessed with this ink. If grossly identifiable disruptions to the capsule are present, they should be noted and inked with a different color. These may be areas where a tumor extends through the thyroid capsule. Alternatively, these disruptions may be surgical. The most common and mundane example of this is the cauterized isthmus as noted above in a lobectomy specimen.

Pathologic processes are characterized not only by abnormal size but also by a deviation from this normal appearance. Thyroid gross pathology can be resolved into three main patterns: (1) one to a few discrete lesions such as nodules, cysts, or scars surrounded by unremarkable parenchyma; (2) a diffuse or multifocal global process; or (3) one to a few discrete lesions in the background of a diffuse process.

Nodules

There are two basic approaches to sectioning a thyroid lobe for the assessment of nodules: (1) serially sectioning each thyroid lobe from superior to inferior at close (2 to 3 mm) intervals (Fig. 19.2A) and (2) a single coronal slice, which in effect "bivalves" the specimen, followed by serial sectioning of the anterior and posterior halves at close (2 to 3 mm) intervals (Fig. 19.2B). The ability to histologically detect microscopic disease is also dependent on the ability to grossly detect lesions ranging 1 to 3 mm. From a practical standpoint, 2- to 3-mm intervals allow a prosector to place the tissue directly in a tissue cassette rather than having to split individual slices, a technique that is much more difficult and time consuming. This improvement in efficiency is important in the busy laboratories of today.

Both basic approaches have their advantages and disadvantages. Small nodules <2 cm are more amenable to the first method, namely direct serial sectioning. Retraction of the tissue capsule and time consumption are not as much of a concern for smaller lesions even in the intraoperative setting. A coronal slice will miss an eccentrically located lesion necessitating initial serial sectioning anyway. From an intraoperative standpoint, the resolution of the initial gross examination will be improved. Furthermore, histologic reconstruction of a lesion if a gross photograph is unavailable is simpler when serial sectioned alone, since the specimen will have been sectioned along only one plane and ideally submitted in sequence. Finally, since this approach yields complete cross-sections of a nodule within a cassette, the relationship of the lesion and the entire circumference of the capsule and the surrounding nonneoplastic thyroid can be displayed in one slice.

The second method of initial coronal section may be more advantageous for initial intraoperative evaluation of large nodules—an initial cut allows for rapid assessment of a lesion. Each half can then be serially sectioned after fixation with ease. When nodules are transected fresh, there is a tendency for these to bulge or protrude secondary to capsular retraction. This effect is more pronounced with larger nodules since with increasing size, volume increases more rapidly than capsular surface area. Having a single initial cut minimizes this effect. Moreover, as with most tissue, fixation homogenizes the consistency and allows for thinner and more even slices. Specimens sectioned coronally are more aesthetically pleasing and photogenic and allow for a more intuitive visualization of the location of a nodule and relationship to surrounding parenchyma. When two nodules are immediately adjacent to one another, the question often arises as to whether they represent one irregularly shaped nodule or two separate nodules. The coronal section is more likely to preserve this juxtaposition and allows a prosector to modify their sectioning approach. The region near the junction of two nodules should be sliced serially along a sagittal plane to most accurately demonstrate the relationship between the two nodules. Thus, this coronal section method is recommended for lesions >2 cm and for two or more nodules palpated adjacent to each other.

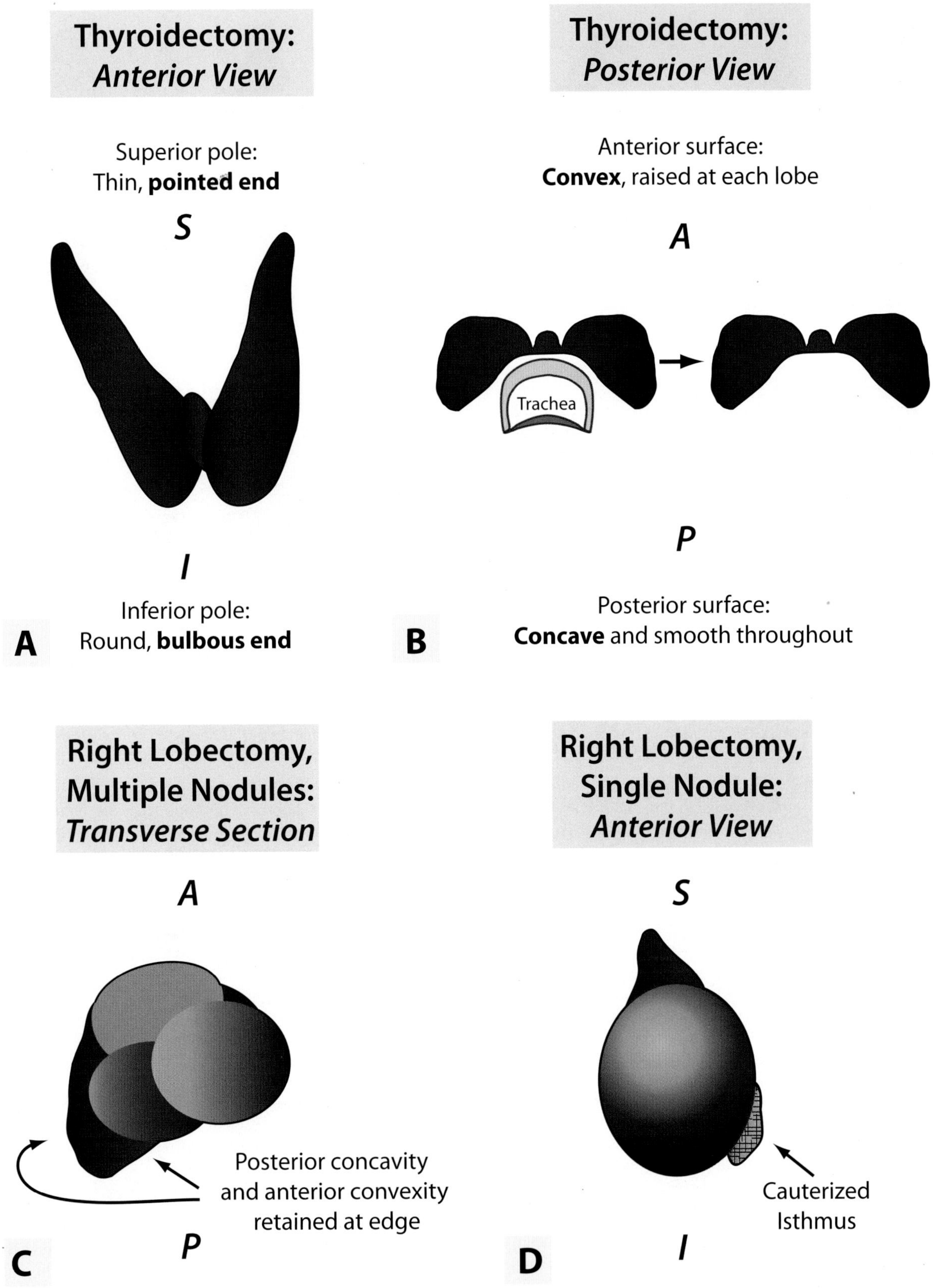

Thyroidectomy:
Anterior View

Superior pole:
Thin, **pointed end**

S

I

Inferior pole:
Round, **bulbous end**

A

Thyroidectomy:
Posterior View

Anterior surface:
Convex, raised at each lobe

A

Trachea →

P

Posterior surface:
Concave and smooth throughout

B

**Right Lobectomy,
Multiple Nodules:**
Transverse Section

A

Posterior concavity
and anterior convexity
retained at edge

C   *P*

**Right Lobectomy,
Single Nodule:**
Anterior View

S

Cauterized
Isthmus

D   *I*

FIGURE 19.1. A: Superoinferior orientation of the thyroid gland. The superior pole is longer with a tapered end, whereas the inferior pole is closer to the isthmus and demonstrates a more rounded bulbous end. **B:** Anteroposterior orientation of the thyroid gland. A schematic is shown "in situ" on the left in relation to the trachea. The anterior surface of each lobe is convex, whereas the posterior surface, which rests on the trachea, is concave. The confluence of these surfaces laterally results in a fairly sharp protuberant lateral border. **C:** Superolaterally, the normal contour is often retained even if most of the gland is distorted by a multinodular process, thus facilitation orientation. **D:** In lobectomy specimens, cautery at the isthmus may help orientation, since the isthmus is usually more inferior. S, superior; I, inferior; A, anterior; P, posterior.

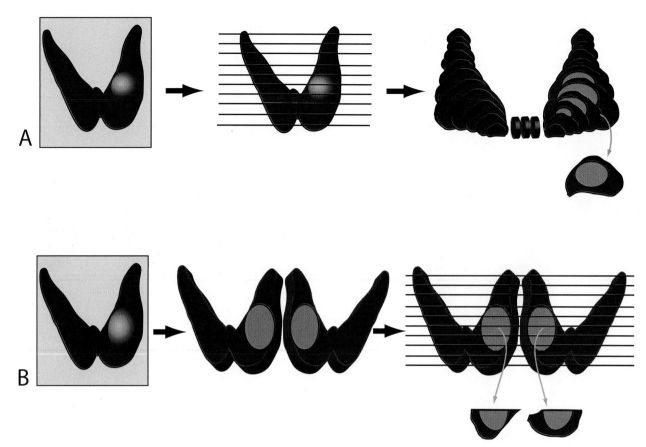

FIGURE 19.2. A: One-step procedure for sectioning thyroids. The thyroid is initially sectioned at 2- to 3-mm intervals transversely. This is simple and yields a high-resolution gross examination in the fresh state particularly for small lesions. **B:** Two-step procedure for sectioning thyroids. The initial cut is a coronal hemisection followed by transverse serial sectioning at 2- to 3-mm intervals of each half. The initial cut allows for rapid intraoperative evaluation of large lesions and preservation of the intact specimen for photography and more precise sectioning after fixation.

The goal of the aforementioned visualization and sectioning protocols is to assess the required gross components of a thyroid nodule. When these are well described, the histologic diagnosis can be suggested with great accuracy. First, the location of a lesion must be documented for clinical and radiologic correlation.[1,2] Second, the lesion must be measured in three dimensions ($X \times Y \times Z$). In addition, the distance from the thyroid capsule boundary or other margin should be documented for each nodule.

The nodule's shape or configuration is important as well. Nodules have either well-demarcated or infiltrative borders. Well-demarcated nodules generally suggest more indolent lesions, such as hyperplastic nodules or follicular adenomas; however, malignancies can present grossly in this fashion as well, and metastases to the thyroid can be deceptively well demarcated. If a lesion is well circumscribed, the presence or absence of a lesional capsule should be noted. By convention, follicular neoplasms are encapsulated, whereas hyperplastic nodules are not. When the capsule is thin, it is often difficult to make this assessment, and the term *possibly encapsulated* is acceptable. However, an encapsulated lesion with a thick capsule >0.1 cm is noteworthy and should be measured; thicker capsules are more suspicious for malignancy.[7]

Infiltrative or stellate nodules are more worrisome for malignancy, although degenerative change in multinodular goiter may present as an ill-defined scar as well. Occasionally, a lesion may be discernible as an infiltrative lesion with a central encapsulated nodule suggesting an antecedent adenoma.

In addition to shape and encapsulation, parameters such as color, heterogeneity, hemorrhage, cystic change, and calcification should be documented. Color and heterogeneity have a particular set of histologic correlates as depicted in Figure 19.3.

The distribution of hemorrhage and/or cystic change should be noted, since a linear pattern would suggest a fine needle tract. The distribution of calcifications may also yield valuable information. Thick nodular calcifications can be seen as a degenerative change in goiter, whereas punctuate irregularly distributed "gritty" calcifications are typical of papillary carcinoma.

Multinodular Process

In the setting of a multinodular process that yields several discrete lesions, each of those should be considered a unique nodule and described as per the above recommendations. When the lesions are not well demarcated, it may be difficult to decide whether a lesion should be considered discrete simply part of the multinodular process. In these situations, though somewhat arbitrary, any nodule that is significantly larger or has a different appearance (i.e., color, encapsulation) should be approached as a unique nodule.

Background Thyroid Parenchyma

A lengthy description of the background thyroid parenchyma is typically not necessary, though if the background thyroid parenchyma is abnormal, this should be noted as well. The change in color or consistency may be multifocal or diffuse.

SUBMISSION OF SECTIONS

Submission of sections for histologic examination is essentially grounded in the ideal mixture of "common sense" practicality and

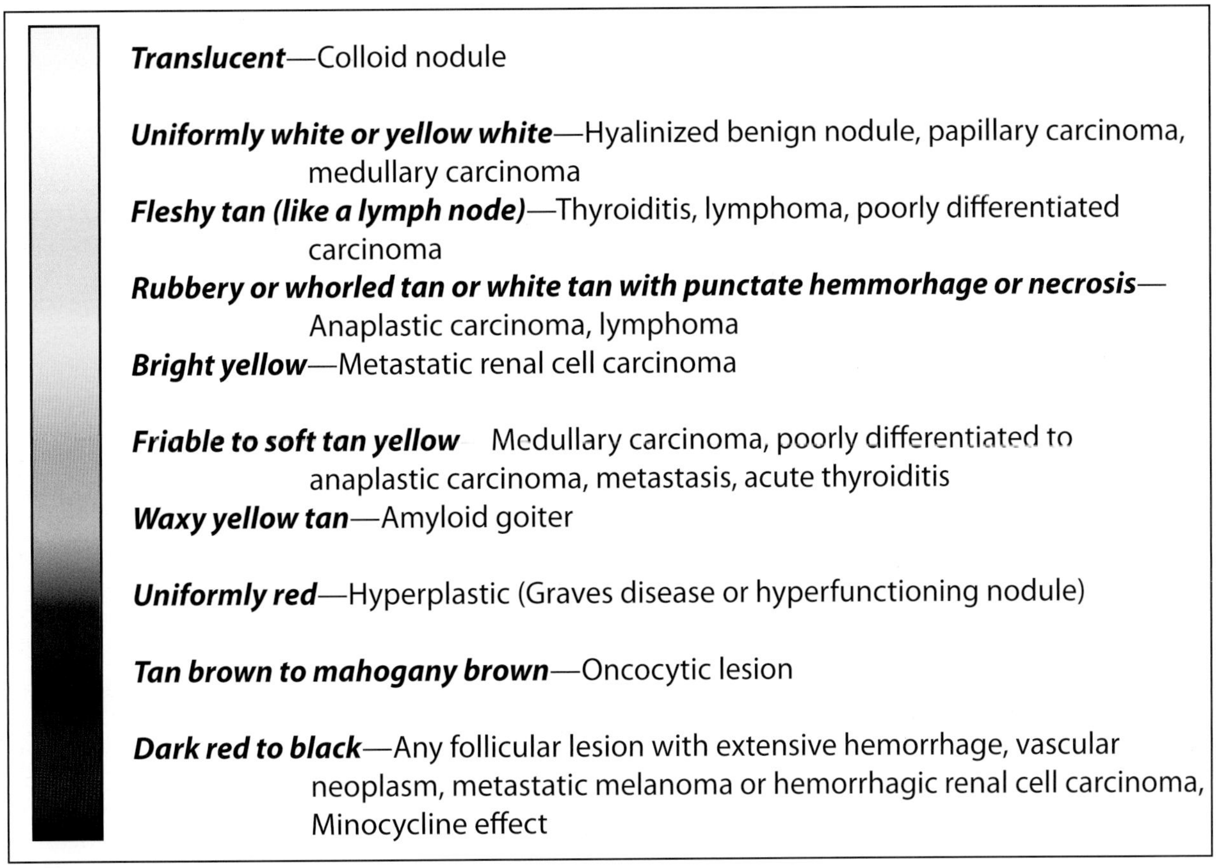

Translucent—Colloid nodule

Uniformly white or yellow white—Hyalinized benign nodule, papillary carcinoma, medullary carcinoma

Fleshy tan (like a lymph node)—Thyroiditis, lymphoma, poorly differentiated carcinoma

Rubbery or whorled tan or white tan with punctate hemmorhage or necrosis—Anaplastic carcinoma, lymphoma

Bright yellow—Metastatic renal cell carcinoma

Friable to soft tan yellow   Medullary carcinoma, poorly differentiated to anaplastic carcinoma, metastasis, acute thyroiditis

Waxy yellow tan—Amyloid goiter

Uniformly red—Hyperplastic (Graves disease or hyperfunctioning nodule)

Tan brown to mahogany brown—Oncocytic lesion

Dark red to black—Any follicular lesion with extensive hemorrhage, vascular neoplasm, metastatic melanoma or hemorrhagic renal cell carcinoma, Minocycline effect

FIGURE 19.3. Color/consistency correlates to various thyroid lesions. These gross descriptors when used in dictation should evoke certain set of differential diagnostic considerations.

thorough assessment of oncologically pertinent parameters. The approach of an institution with ample resources and academic interest will be different from an understaffed, private practice setting, but a minimum standard should be met. However, with a few exceptions,[7,8] most sectioning recommendations are not based on "hard" evidence from studies of gross sectioning. Submission guidelines are summarized in Table 19.2.

For nonneoplastic goiters, multinodular or diffuse without any discrete lesions, the goal is to document the underlying etiology and to examine for incidental disease, namely papillary microcarcinomas. The yield in terms of the latter objective will likely improve with an increased number of histologic sections submitted. However, the importance of finding "occult," extremely indolent disease should be weighed alongside the practical limitations of a laboratory's capacity to accommodate histologic sections and pathologist workload. As a good balance, if no discrete lesions are noted, 1 section per 5 g of tissue should be submitted up to a maximum of 10 per lobe and 2 for this isthmus, yielding a maximum of 22 sections per case. In practices where this is not feasible, alternative recommendations include one section per nodule up to five nodules in a nodular process and as few as three sections from each lobe, one from the isthmus (seven sections total) for a diffuse process.[3,5] In cases where a possible lymphoproliferative disorder is suspected (i.e., a fleshy tan cut surface), a portion of tissue should be set aside for ancillary studies.

Along similar lines, for discrete lesions of any type <2 cm, it is reasonable and practical to submit these entirely for histologic evaluation. For infiltrative or unencapsulated lesions >2 cm, particularly those with the preoperative diagnosis or gross appearance of a carcinoma, at least one section per centimeter size should be submitted, focusing on areas of

heterogeneity, the tumor-normal interface, and areas where the lesion approaches the thyroid capsular edge. For encapsulated lesions, the histologic assessment for capsular and vascular invasion is critical in distinguishing between adenoma and carcinoma. Thus, regardless of nodule size, ideally, the entire capsule should be submitted for histologic evaluation.[7] To minimize the number of blocks required to achieve this, each section should consist mostly of capsule and a small portion (2 to 3 mm) of the underlying nodule and of adjacent uninvolved parenchyma (Fig. 19.4). In this way, two to three sections can be placed in one cassette. An additional one to two sections of the center of an encapsulated nodule can be submitted for histologic evaluation as well. Although this is ideal, it may not be practical in many laboratories, since entire submission of a lesion's capsule may yield >50 slides in some cases. A study by Lang et al.[8] suggested that a minimum of 10 blocks were required to document evidence for malignancy. Although this study is retrospective and riddled with many flaws, most notably, the lack of a methodical comparison to a gold standard of total capsule submission, the prediction is that at least 97% of carcinomas are detected with 10 blocks. Hence, if total submission of a capsule of a nodule is not feasible, a minimum of 10 sections are recommended, focusing on areas of capsular thickening and grossly suspected invasion.

The surrounding thyroid parenchyma in a lesion should be sampled as well. If the background is a multinodular or diffuse goiter, then the submission guidelines for these process listed above should be followed. If the surrounding thyroid is unremarkable, one cassette per centimeter of lobe length should be submitted. In most cases, since normal thyroid slices are small, this effectively equates to total submission of surrounding parenchyma. Sampling the surrounding thyroid is particularly

Table 19.2

Section Submission Guidelines

Goiter (diffuse and multinodular with no discrete nodules)	*Ideal*: Nodular disease — one cassette per 5 g of thyroid weight focusing on nodular areas. Maximum 10 per lobe, 2 per isthmus (22 sections total). Diffuse disease — one cassette per 5 g of thyroid weight focusing on areas of heterogeneity (i.e., slightly more fibrotic, or hyperemic areas). Maximum 10 per lobe, 2 per isthmus (22 sections total). *Minimum*: Nodular disease — one section of each nodule up to five nodules. Diffuse disease — three sections each lobe, one isthmus (seven sections total).
Discrete infiltrative or unencapsulated lesion	<2 cm — submit entirely >2 cm — one section per cm, focusing on areas of heterogeneity and the tumor-parenchyma interface
Encapsulated lesion	<2 cm — submit entirely >2 cm — *Ideal*: entire capsule with at least 0.5-cm thick portion to include underlying lesion, capsule, and uninvolved parenchyma. *Minimum*: 10 cassettes of capsule focusing on thickened areas, calcification, and possible extracapsular extensions.
Normal thyroid (no gross lesions and no history of occult disease, e.g., incidental lobectomy attached to laryngectomy specimens)	One section per centimeter of lobe length
Occult disease, i.e., known positive lymph node in an otherwise unremarkable thyroid	*Ideal*: Submit until lesion is found or entirely, whichever comes first *Minimum*: 30 cassettes
Prophylactic MEN2 cases	*Minimum*: Superolateral two-thirds of each lobe (in practice, it is easier to submit thyroid gland in its entirety)

MEN2, multiple endocrine neoplasia type 2.

important in cases of papillary carcinoma, since the likelihood of finding several microcarcinomas that would not be grossly evident is increased.[9]

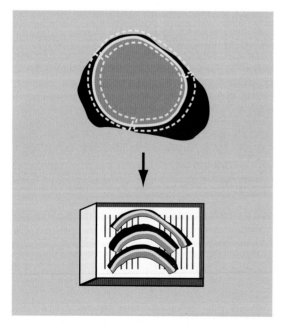

FIGURE 19.4. Sectioning of the capsule of a nodule. For large encapsulated nodules, a capsular section containing a 2- to 3-mm rim of underlying nodule and of overlying uninvolved parenchyma should be submitted. In this way, two to three sections can be placed in one cassette.

Thyroidectomy for preneoplasia or occult primary is unusual. One scenario is the incidental finding of a micrometastasis of thyroid carcinoma in a neck lymph node excised for other purposes.[10] The thyroid gland may be excised to find the primary. When the primary is grossly evident, standard procedure can be followed. However, more problematic is the absence of a grossly evident lesion. To ensure accurate staging, the entire thyroid should be submitted for histologic evaluation. Again this may not be feasible in some cases of multinodular goiter where the thyroid gland may weigh several 100 g. In addition, the benefit of finding a minute biologically indolent tumor[10] in this setting would likely be overshadowed by the exorbitant effort and resources spent to identify this tumor. Thus, it is recommended that 30 blocks be submitted for histologic evaluation.

The prophylactic thyroidectomy for multiple endocrine neoplasia type 2 (MEN2) cases is an example of thyroidectomy for preneoplasia. Even when gross lesions are not identified, c-cell hyperplasia and medullary microcarcinomas are frequently seen. Thus, it is essential to entirely submit the superolateral two-thirds of each lobe for histologic evaluation.[3] The region around the isthmus does not necessarily need to be submitted, since it is embryologically derived from the median anlagen and should not have C cells. In practice, it is usually easier to submit the entire thyroid for histologic evaluation than it is to spare the inferomedial portion of thyroid, and it does not dramatically alter the number of sections submitted for histologic evaluation.

REFERENCES

1. Sneed DC. Protocol for the examination of specimens from patients with malignant tumors of the thyroid gland, exclusive of lymphomas: a basis for checklists. Cancer Committee, College of American Pathologists. *Arch Pathol Lab Med.* 1999;123:45–49.

2. Association of Directors of Anatomical and Surgical Pathology. Recommended reporting format for thyroid carcinoma. *Mod Pathol.* 2000;13:1042–1044.
3. Lester SC. Thyroid and parathyroid glands. In: *Manual of Surgical Pathology.* Philadelphia, PA: Elsevier; 2006:569–575.
4. Fowler JC, Thompson LDR. Intraoperative consultation and grossing techniques. In: Thompson LDR, ed. *Endocrine Pathology.* Philadelphia, PA: Elsevier; 2006:351–357.
5. Rosai J. *Rosai and Ackerman's Surgical Pathology.* Edinburgh: Elsevier; 2004.
6. Ozbas S, Kocak S, Aydintug S, et al. Comparison of the complications of subtotal, near total and total thyroidectomy in the surgical management of multinodular goitre. *Endocr J.* 2005;52:199–205.
7. Yamashina M. Follicular neoplasms of the thyroid. Total circumferential evaluation of the fibrous capsule. *Am J Surg Pathol.* 1992;16:392–400.
8. Lang W, Georgii A, Stauch G, et al. The differentiation of atypical adenomas and encapsulated follicular carcinomas in the thyroid gland. *Virchows Arch A Pathol Anat Histol.* 1980;385:125–141.
9. Pacini F, Elisei R, Capezzone M, et al. Contralateral papillary thyroid cancer is frequent at completion thyroidectomy with no difference in low- and high-risk patients. *Thyroid.* 2001;11:877–881.
10. Ansari-Lari MA, Westra WH. The prevalence and significance of clinically unsuspected neoplasms in cervical lymph nodes. *Head Neck.* 2003;25:841–847.

Principles of Molecular Diagnostics in Thyroid Samples

GENERAL PRINCIPLES OF MOLECULAR BIOLOGY

Molecular diagnostics utilize the basic dogma of molecular biology that describes the relationship among DNA, RNA, and protein (Fig. 20.1). All genetic information in human cells is encoded in DNA, which is located in the nucleus of the cell. In order to decode genetic information and translate it into proteins, the DNA is copied (transcribed) into messenger RNA (mRNA) and then translated into protein.

DNA

DNA is a double-stranded molecule consisting of two complimentary strands of linearly arranged nucleotides: adenine (A), guanine (G), thymine (T), and cytosine (C). Two strands of DNA are held together through base pairing between adenine and thymine (A:T pairing) and guanine and cytosine (G:C pairing). As a result, the nucleotide sequence of one DNA strand is complementary to the nucleotide sequence of the other DNA strand.[1]

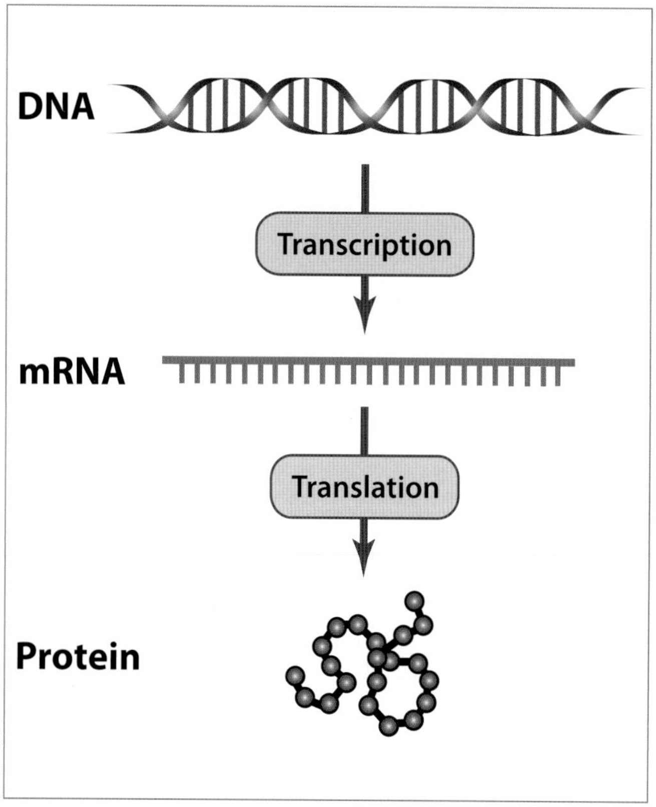

FIGURE 20.1 Basic dogma of molecular biology.

The human genome contains approximately three billion base pairs of DNA, which are compactly packed into chromatin by accessory proteins and divided among chromosomes. Each normal somatic cell contains two copies of 22 different chromosomes (one from each parent) and a combination of two sex chromosomes (X and Y).

Only a small portion of DNA (<5%) encodes a functional product, such as protein, transfer RNA (tRNA), ribosomal RNA (rRNA), microRNA (miRNA), and other small nuclear RNAs (snRNAs).[2] Most of human genome (>95%) is composed of noncoding DNA sequences that are mostly repetitive sequences either randomly repeated (minisatellites and microsatellites) or interspersed (short interspersed nuclear elements (SINEs) and long interspersed nuclear elements (LINEs)). Genes are segments of genomic DNA that encode functional products. Currently, around 25,000 distinct genes have been identified for a haploid genome. Each gene consists of protein-coding sequences, exons, and noncoding sequences, introns, which are located between the coding regions (Fig. 20.2).[3] In addition, genes also include regulatory regions, such as promoters and enhancers, which are used to facilitate processes of transcription or gene silencing.

RNA

RNA is a single-stranded molecule that is generally similar to DNA and consists of linearly arranged nucleotides on a sugar-phosphate backbone. However, the sugar in RNA is ribose rather than deoxyribose, and thymine is replaced by uracil. Owing to the irregular structure and additional hydroxyl group at the 2′ carbon of ribose, RNA is more vulnerable to chemical and enzymatic hydrolysis and is less stable than DNA.[4]

There are several types of RNA that are different in their structure, function, and location. Messenger RNA (mRNA) composes 1% to 5% of the total RNA. Each mRNA represents a copy of the genetic information from a specific gene and transfers this information from nucleus to cytoplasm, then serving as a "blueprint" for protein synthesis. The gene sequence is first transcribed into the primary RNA transcript by RNA polymerase. This transcript is an exact complimentary copy of the gene, including all exons and introns. Then, intron portions are spliced out from the primary RNA transcript, which is processed into mRNA and serves as a template for protein synthesis (Fig. 20.2).[5] Ribosomal RNA (rRNA) and transfer RNA (tRNA) compose up to 90% of the total cellular RNA. They are predominantly located in the cytoplasm and have important functions in protein synthesis. Other types of RNA include heterogeneous RNA (hnRNA) and small nuclear RNA (snRNA). Recently, several classes of short RNAs have been discovered, one of which is microRNAs (miRNAs). miRNAs are short (19 to 22 nucleotides), single-stranded molecules that function as negative regulators of the coding gene expression.[6,7]

Protein

Proteins are synthesized on ribosomes in the cell cytoplasm. mRNAs transfer genetic information from nucleus to cytoplasm and bind to the ribosomes. Ribosomes then direct the assembly of polypeptide chains by reading a three-letter genetic code on the

Gene

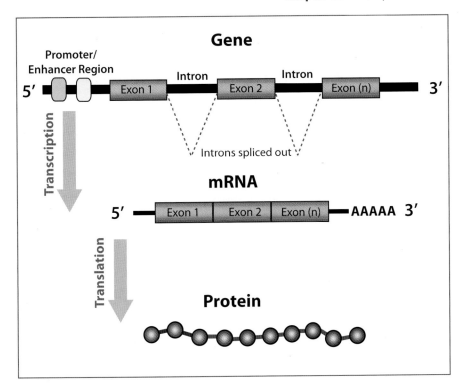

FIGURE 20.2 Gene structure and modifications during the process of transcription and translation. Genes consist of protein-coding regions (exons), noncoding regions (introns), and regulatory regions (promoter, enhancer). Mature mRNA has only protein-coding parts of the gene, which are used to build the protein.

mRNA and pairing it with a complementary tRNA that is linked to an amino acid. The three-nucleotide code, called codon, defines which specific amino acid is to be added by the tRNA to the growing polypeptide chain. Following the process of translation, the protein undergoes posttranslational modification, including chain cleavage, chain joining, addition of nonprotein groups, and folding into a complex, tridimensional structure.

Genetic Variations

Although DNA is highly conserved, the possibility of variation still exists. Allelic sequence variation (genetic polymorphism) is a difference in DNA sequences between individuals found in the general population at a frequency >1%. Polymorphism may be associated with a single nucleotide change, known as single nucleotide polymorphism (SNP), or with variation in several repetitive DNA sequences, such as minisatellites or microsatellites, which is known as length polymorphism. Usually, polymorphism is not a cause of the disease, but it results in subtle changes in the function of the protein as therefore is a predisposing factor.

A mutation is a permanent alteration of the DNA sequence of a gene and can be either germline, that is, present in all cells of the body, or somatic, that is, found in tumor cells only. *Somatic mutations* may provide a selective advantage for cell growth and initiate cancer development, but they are not transmitted to offsprings. In contrast, *germline mutations* will be passed on to the next generation. Mutations located in a coding sequence of a gene, in the regulatory elements of a gene, or at the intron–exon boundaries may affect transcription and/or translation and result in alteration of the protein structure and function. The sequencing of cancer genomes has revealed that most mutations occur in genes whose products affect signaling pathways that control important cell functions.[8] It is estimated that most mutations (90%) result in activation of the gene, typically forming an oncogene (such as *RET* and *RAS*), and smaller proportion of mutations (10%) lead to loss of function of a tumor suppressor gene (such as *TP53*).[8]

Current list of somatic mutations in cancer can be viewed at the Catalogue of Somatic Mutations in Cancer (COSMIC) database,

which documents somatic cancer mutations reported in the literature and identified during Cancer Genome Project (http://www.sanger.ac.uk/genetics/cgp/cosmic/). Not all somatic mutations have a clear biologic effect. Mutations that increase cell growth and survival and positively selected for tumor development are called "driver" mutations. Conversely, genetic alterations that do not confer a selective growth advantage to the cell and do not have functional consequences are defined as "passenger" mutations. They may be coincidently present in a cell that acquires a driver mutation and are carried along during clonal expansion, or occur during clonal expansion of a tumor. It is generally believed that only a small fraction of all mutations in a given tumor is represented by driver mutations. Thus, it has been estimated that a typical human tumor carries on average approximately 80 mutations that change the amino acid sequences of proteins, of which <15 are driver mutations.[9]

Finally, based on mutation size and structure, mutations can be classified into small-scale mutations (sequence mutations) and large-scale mutations (chromosomal alterations) (Table 20.1). Point mutations in coding sequences are termed nonsynonymous when they produce missense (altered amino acid) or nonsense (premature stop codon) changes. Point mutations that do not lead to amino acid change are termed synonymous or translationally silent mutations. Chromosomal rearrangements are generally less common than point mutations but similarly important in tumorigenesis. They lead to the fusion of DNA fragments from different chromosomal regions, either creating an abnormal fusion protein or leading to aberrant expression of a normal gene. Genetic alterations in thyroid cancer including well-characterized point mutations (such as *BRAF*, *RAS*, *PIK3CA*, *TP53*, *AKT*, *CTNNB1*, and *RET*) and chromosomal rearrangements (such as *RET/PTC*, *TRK*, *BRAF/AKAP9*, and *PAX8/PPARγ*), which are known to activate or inactivate important signaling pathways, therefore, are driver mutations. They are depicted in Figure 20.3. As of September 2011, the COSMIC database contains records of 29 genes with somatic mutations and rearrangements detected in different types of thyroid cancer.

Table 20.1

Classification of Mutations Based on Size and Structure

Mutation Type	Description
Small-scale mutations (sequence mutations)	
Point mutation	Single nucleotide substitution
Synonymous mutations:	
Silent mutation	Substitution of nucleotide(s) that does not change the amino acid
Nonsynonymous mutations:	
Missense mutation	Substitution of nucleotide(s) that leads to amino acid change and results in production of abnormal protein
Nonsense mutation	Substitution of a single nucleotide that results in a stop codon leading to truncated protein
In-frame deletion or insertion mutation	Addition or deletion of nucleotides divisible by three, which results in a changed number of amino acids
Frame-shift mutation	Addition or deletion of nucleotide(s) that is not divisible by three and cause a shift in the reading frame of the gene and eventually creating a premature stop codon
Large-scale mutations (chromosomal alterations)	
Numerical chromosomal abnormalities	Loss or gain of single or multiple chromosomes or large chromosomal regions
Chromosomal rearrangements (translocations and inversions)	Exchange of chromosome segments between two nonhomologous chromosomes or within the same chromosome, which frequently result in activation of specific genes located at the fusion point
Amplification	Multiplication of chromosomal region leading to increased dosage of the genes located within the region
LOH	Deletion of discrete chromosomal region with the loss of tumor suppressor genes residing in this area

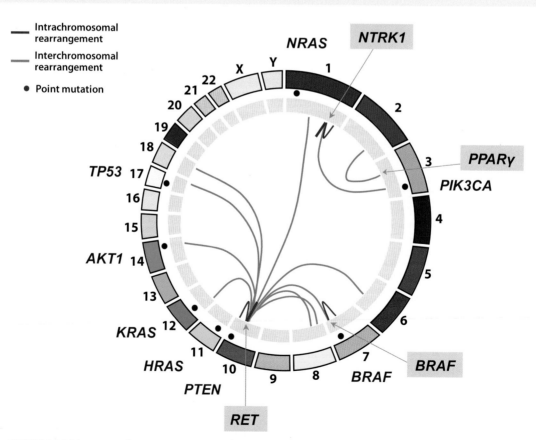

FIGURE 20.3 Ideogram of most common mutations in thyroid cancer. Chromosomes are shown and numbered in the outer ring. Point mutations (*blue dots*), intrachromosomal rearrangements (*red lines*), and interchromosomal rearrangements (*green lines*) are shown.

SAMPLES FOR MOLECULAR ANALYSIS

Molecular diagnosis of thyroid cancer can be performed on various clinical samples, such as fresh or snap-frozen tissue, formalin-fixed paraffin embedded (FFPE) tissue, fine needle aspiration (FNA) samples, blood or buccal swabs. Peripheral blood lymphocytes or cells from buccal swabs are typically used for the detection of germline mutations, for example, *RET* mutations in familiar medullary carcinoma. For the detection of somatic mutations, fresh or snap-frozen tumor specimens and freshly collected FNA specimens offer an ideal template, providing an advantage over fixed tissue or fixed cells due to the superior quality of isolated nucleic acids.

Detection of point mutations (i.e., *BRAF* and *RAS*), loss of heterozygosity (LOH) analysis, and clonality assays require the isolation of DNA. DNA is more stable than RNA and could be easily isolated from various specimens. Although fresh or frozen tissues are always preferable, FFPE specimens could be successfully used and will provide an acceptable quality and quantity of DNA. Ten percent neutral-buffered formalin (NBF) is a fixative that is most widely used. Formalin fixation leads to fragmentation of DNA, and therefore, molecular assays need to be optimized for the amplification of short DNA fragments (250 to 300 bp in length). However, prolonged (>24 to 48 h) fixation in 10% NBF adversely affects the quality of nucleic acids; therefore, specimens should preferably not be fixed for long time. Thyroid and other tissue specimens that were processed using bone decalcifying solution cannot be used for molecular analysis due to extensive DNA fragmentation.[10] Similarly, specimens exposed to fixatives containing heavy metals (e.g., Zenker, B5, acid zinc formalin) cannot be used for molecular testing due to inhibition of DNA polymerases and other enzymes essential for molecular assays.

When selecting a sample for molecular testing, a representative H&E slide of the tissue must be reviewed by a pathologist to identify a target and determine the purity of the tumor, that is, proportion of tumor cells and benign stromal and inflammatory cells in the area selected for testing. Manual or laser capture microdissection can be performed using unstained tissue sections under the guidance of an H&E slide to enrich the tumor cell population. The minimum percentage of tumor cells required for molecular testing depends on the methodology being used for analysis. In general, a minimum tumor cellularity of 50% and at least 300 to 500 tumor cells are required for Sanger sequencing.

Thyroid FNA specimens, either freshly collected or fixed, provide a good quality of DNA and are acceptable for testing. Additional information on collecting of thyroid FNA samples is provided in Chapter 21.

RNA is required for the detection of chromosomal rearrangements (i.e., *RET/PTC* and *PAX8/PPARγ*), gene expression profiling, and miRNA profiling. It is a less stable molecule than DNA and is easily degraded by various ribonuclease enzymes that are replete within the cell and environment. Therefore, freshly collected or frozen tissue and nonfixed FNA samples are considered to be reliable specimens for these techniques. RNA isolated from FFPE tissue is of poor quality and has to be used with great caution for clinical testing. The best alternative for the detection of rearrangements in FFPE tissue is of fluorescent in situ hybridization (FISH) technique, which provides reliable detection in most cases.

Conventional cytogenetic analysis requires fresh tissue. FISH can be performed on various specimens including fresh tissue sections, touch preps, paraffin-embedded tissue sections, and cytology slides.

COMMON TECHNIQUES FOR MOLECULAR ANALYSIS

Polymerase Chain Reaction

PCR amplification is the most commonly utilized technology in molecular diagnostics. It is a quick, sensitive, and reliable technique for the analysis of a DNA sequence of interest. The principle of PCR is based on exponential and bidirectional amplification of short DNA sequences through the use of oligonucleotide primers.[11]

The components of each PCR reaction are the DNA template to be amplified, two primers complementary to the target sequence, four deoxynucleotide triphosphates (dATP, dCTP, dGTP, and dTTP), thermostable DNA polymerase, and $MgCl_2$ mixed in the reaction buffer. The PCR primers are short (20 to 25 nucleotides), single-stranded DNA sequences that hybridize to the 5′-ends of the target DNA. Primers have to be completely complementary to the target DNA sequence in order to achieve sensitive and specific PCR amplification. There are three steps in the PCR cycle (Fig. 20.4A). The first step is DNA denaturation, where the reaction is heated to a high temperature (95°C) to separate the double-stranded DNA into single strands. The second step is the annealing of primers, where the reaction is cooled to 55°C (or a temperature in the range of 50°C to 65°C) to allow primers to attach to their complimentary sequences. The third step is DNA extension, where the reaction is heated to 72°C and DNA polymerase adds specific nucleotides to the attached primers and builds a new DNA strand. These three steps are repeated 35 to 40 times, and each newly synthesized DNA strand serves as a template for further DNA synthesis. This results in the production of 10^7 to 10^{11} copies of the DNA region of interest from a single DNA molecule. The PCR product can be visualized by standard gel electrophoresis (i.e., agarose and polyacrylamide) or by capillary gel electrophoresis if the PCR product is labeled with fluorescent dye (Fig 20.4B,C).

Efficiency of PCR amplification depends on the quality of the template, optimal primer design, and conditions for amplification, such as annealing temperature and Mg^{2+} concentration. PCR amplification of DNA isolated from fresh, frozen tissues allows amplification of long products (up to 3 to 5 kb). However, when dealing with DNA from fixed tissues, reliable amplification can be achieved of only relatively short DNA sequences (100 to 200 bp) due to the degradation of DNA during fixation. Amplification of longer DNA segments (300 to 400 bp) may be successful in some cases but should be generally avoided.

Reverse Transcription–PCR

Reverse transcription–PCR (RT–PCR) is used for the amplification of mRNA or small RNAs (miRNAs). In order to do this, RNA isolated from the tissue sample is converted to complementary DNA (cDNA) using a reverse transcriptase enzyme during a process called reverse transcription. This enzyme has the ability to synthesize cDNA from a single-stranded RNA, which will serve as a template for the subsequent PCR reaction. Initiation of the RT reaction requires primers that can be either nonsequence specific (mixture of random hexamers or oligo-dT primers) or sequence-specific primers designed to bind selectively to the mRNA molecule of interest. RT and PCR amplification can be performed as a two-step process in a single tube or as two separate reactions.[12]

RT–PCR technique is used for the analysis of gene expression and for the detection of gene rearrangements. Detection of gene expression is based on a measurement of the quantity of mRNA from a specific gene present in the sample relatively to mRNA of a housekeeping gene (e.g., GAPDH and PGK) and is frequently

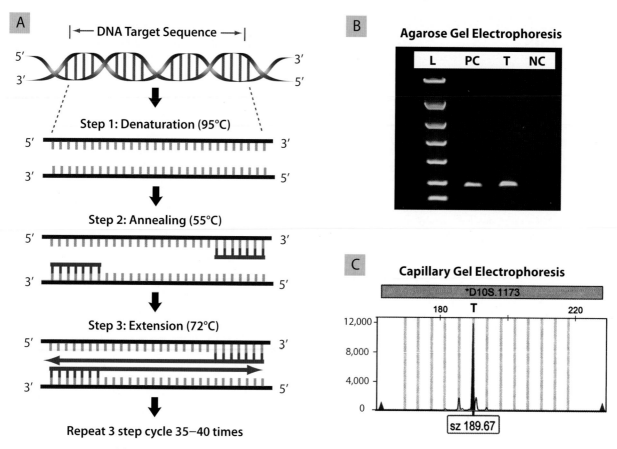

FIGURE 20.4 PCR amplification and amplicon detection. A: Schematic representation of the PCR. **B**: Example of agarose gel electrophoresis of PCR products. L-DNA ladder (DNA size marker); PC, positive control; T, tumor sample showing amplification product of the expected size; N-negative control with no input of DNA shows no amplification. **C**: Example of capillary gel electrophoresis of PCR products. Tumor sample amplified with fluorescently labeled primers shows a peak on capillary gel electrophoresis of 190 bp size.

performed by quantitative RT–PCR (qRT–PCR). Detection of gene rearrangements is easier to perform on the RNA level instead of DNA because most of fusion breakpoints are located in large size introns of genes and breakpoint site varies from tumor to tumor. During mRNA processing, the introns are spliced out, leaving the informative coding sequences intact and significantly shortening the product of amplification.

RNA is more difficult to handle in a laboratory, and strict laboratory techniques have to be applied to avoid RNA degradation.[13] The amplification of a housekeeping gene has to accompany each RT–PCR reaction to monitor RNA quality and quantity.

Real-time PCR

Real-time PCR is based on principals of conventional PCR amplification but detects and quantifies PCR products in *real time* as the reaction progresses. Real-time PCR should not be confused with RT–PCR: frequently, the RT–PCR reaction is also performed in *real time* to measure gene expression or to detect fusion transcripts.

In addition to all components of conventional PCR, real-time PCR utilizes either incorporation of fluorescent molecules (i.e., SYBR Green I) into the PCR product or annealing of fluorescently labeled probes (FRET hybridization probes, TaqMan probes, etc.) to the PCR product (Fig. 20.5A).[14] Special thermal cycling instruments (LightCycler [Roche], ABI 7500 [Applied Biosystems], etc.) record the increase in fluorescence generated during amplification of DNA sequences and construct an

amplification plot of fluorescence intensity versus cycle number. During the early cycles, the amount of PCR product is relatively low and fluorescence is not strong enough to exceed the baseline. As the PCR product accumulates and becomes detectable, the fluorescence signal will cross the baseline and will increase exponentially (Fig. 20.5B). At the end of the PCR reaction, the fluorescence reaches a plateau as most of the reagents are consumed.

LightCycler real-time PCR (Roche) utilizes fluorescence resonance energy transfer probes (FRET), which bind to the PCR product in a head-to-tail fashion. The 3′-end of one probe is labeled with a donor fluorophore and the 5′-end of a second probe is labeled with an acceptor fluorophore (Fig. 20.5A). When these two probes bind to the specific PCR product, the flourophores come into proximity, transferring energy from donor to acceptor fluorophore. This leads to an increase in fluorescence that is proportional to the amount of amplified product.[15] Unlike dual-labeled hydrolysis probes (i.e., TaqMan probes), FRET probes are not cleaved during the reaction and can be used for post-PCR fluorescence melting curve analysis. Melting curve analysis exploits the fact that even a single mismatch between the labeled probe and the sequence of interest will significantly reduce the specific melting temperature (T_m), which is defined as the temperature at which 50% of the double-stranded DNA becomes single-stranded. Thus, a probe that is bound perfectly to the target DNA (no mismatch) will separate (melt) at a higher temperature than a probe bound to the target DNA with one or more nucleotide mismatch (Fig. 20.5C). The melting curves are built upon the completion of the PCR reaction by gradual heating of the PCR product and measuring fluorescence at each temperature point. Hybridization probes are commonly used for the quantitation of gene expression and the detection of SNPs and point mutations.

TaqMan probes are most commonly used for real-time PCR or real-time RT–PCR on Applied Biosystems Real-Time PCR platforms (ABI 7300/7500/7900). The TaqMan probe is a short probe complementary to the internal sequence of the target DNA and is labeled at the 5′-end with the reporter fluorophore and at the 3′-end with the quencher fluorophore (Fig. 20.5A). Until two flouorophores are intact, flourescence will not be released. However, during the PCR reaction, the probe will be cleaved by DNA polymerase while building the complimentary DNA strand, resulting in a fluorescent signal increase proportional to the amount of amplified PCR product. TaqMan probes are excellent for quantitative assays and for the detection of fusion transcripts, but they cannot be used for the detection of mutations by melting curve analysis.

Real-time PCR with SYBR Green I fluorescent dye is the most flexible technique and can be performed on any real-time PCR platform. SYBR Green I fluorescent dye binds to double-stranded DNA nonspecifically during each annealing phase (Fig. 20.5A). After the dye is excited by a light source, SYBR green emission is increased proportionally to the amount of product amplified. SYBR Green PCR amplification is used for quantitative and qualitative PCR and requires only one pair of primers. However, because dye binds nonspecifically to DNA as opposed to probes that bind to the internal sequence of the amplified product, the specificity of the detection is lower. Post-PCR melting curve analysis may be used to improve specificity of the SYBR Green PCR format.

Real-time PCR is frequently utilized by clinical molecular diagnostics laboratories because it is a rapid, less laborious technique as compared with other methods and does not require processing of samples after PCR amplification, which minimizes the time of the procedure and the risk of contamination by previous PCR products.

PCR–RFLP Analysis

The principle of restriction fragment length polymorphism (RFLP) analysis is based on the ability of mutations to create or destroy a restriction site for a specific enzyme. After amplification, the PCR product is digested with the restriction enzyme and electrophoresed. The size of digested DNA fragments indicates the presence or absence of a mutation at the restriction site. This method is used for the detection of known sequence variations, both mutations and polymorphisms.[16]

PCR–SSCP Analysis

Single-strand conformation polymorphism (SSCP) analysis is a simple technique for the detection of randomly distributed

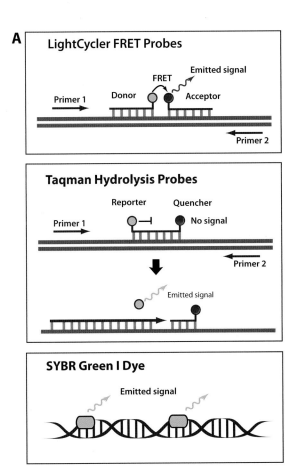
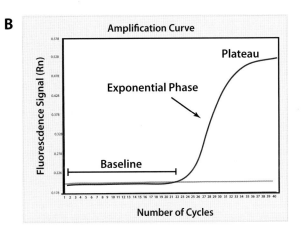
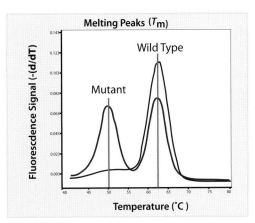

FIGURE 20.5 Real-time PCR. A: Schematic representation of the most common fluorescent methods used for real-time PCR. **B:** Amplification plot showing the low amount of fluorescence during the first cycles of amplification (baseline), exponential increase in fluorescence during the middle phase, and final plateau at the end of PCR reaction. **C:** Post-PCR melting curve analysis on LightCycler demonstrates higher melting temperature of the wild-type allele and lower melting temperature of the mutant allele due to a one nucleotide mismatch with the probe.

mutations. The region of interest is amplified by PCR, and the products are denatured by heat or by exposure to denaturing buffer and analyzed by polyacrylamide or capillary gel electrophoresis. The presence of a mutation will change folding conformation of the sequence and affect electrophoretic mobility of the PCR product, so that the wild-type and mutant bands will migrate differently in the gel. PCR–SSCP analysis can be used for screening for unknown mutations, including small deletions and insertions.[17] However, the method does not allow identification of the precise nucleotide change and requires an additional complementary method (such as direct sequencing) for confirmation.

Heteroduplex Analysis

Similarly to SSCP analysis, heteroduplex analysis is a method for identification of randomly distributed mutations. After amplification of the DNA sequence of interest, double-stranded PCR products are denatured by heat and slowly cooled to achieve random reannealing of the single-stranded DNA molecules and loaded into a gel for electrophoresis. A DNA strand without mutations can reanneal either to a complementary strand with no mutation (forming a homoduplex) or to a strand with a mutation (forming a heteroduplex). The presence of mismatched base pairs between the strands in heteroduplexes changes their structural conformation and forces them to migrate more slowly in a gel than homoduplexes, providing evidence for a mutation.

COLD-PCR

Coamplification at lower denaturation-PCR (COLD-PCR) is a recently developed modification of the PCR technique that utilizes the property of heteroduplexes to separate at lower temperature as compared with homoduplexes. COLD-PCR is performed at a reduced denaturation temperature that favors separation and therefore preferential amplification of heteroduplex templates while leaving homoduplex templates intact. This allows for enrichment in mutant sequences and leads to substantial increase in the sensitivity of mutation detection.[18,19] COLD-PCR can be coupled with different downstream detection methods, such as Sanger sequencing, real-time PCR/FMCA, and restriction enzyme digestion. A recently published real-time COLD-PCR/FMCA protocol for

detecting *BRAF* mutation in thyroid FNA samples demonstrated a 5% sensitivity of the detection.[20]

Allele-Specific PCR

Allele-specific PCR (AS-PCR) exploits the fact that PCR is critically dependent on the perfect base pairing of primers with template DNA in order to produce amplification. Under strict PCR conditions even one nucleotide mismatch at the 3′-end of the primer will prevent PCR amplification. Using AS-PCR, the amplification of target DNA is performed in two reactions: one reaction has primers complementary to a normal (wild-type) sequence and another reaction has a forward primer complementary to a mutant sequence and a reverse primer complementary to a normal DNA sequence. Detection of amplification is performed using gel electrophoresis or using real-time PCR. Normal alleles will show amplification with primers complementary to the normal sequence and no amplification with the mutant specific primer, whereas the mutant allele will show a reverse pattern of amplification. This method is sensitive, although it can be used only for the detection of a mutation with a fixed nucleotide substitution, such as the T to A mutation at nucleotide 1799 of *BRAF*.[21]

DNA Sequencing

DNA sequencing is a method used to determine the order of nucleotides in the target DNA sequence. The classic chain-termination or Sanger method is now used on automated platforms and requires a DNA template, primer, enzyme, and a mixture of regular nucleotides and chemically modified nucleotides (dideoxynucleotides) that terminate DNA strand elongation.[22] The incorporation of a dideoxynucleotide terminates extension of the DNA strand at a particular nucleotide, resulting in a mixture of DNA fragments of various lengths. Each of dideoxynucleotides is labeled with a different fluorescent dye, allowing their individual detection. The newly synthesized and labeled DNA fragments are separated by size using capillary gel electrophoresis. The fluorescence is detected using an automated sequence analyzer (i.e., ABI 3730), and the order of nucleotides in the target DNA is depicted as a sequence electropherogram (Fig. 20.6). The automated sequencing analysis is easy to perform and is used in many molecular diagnostic laboratories for the detection of mutations.

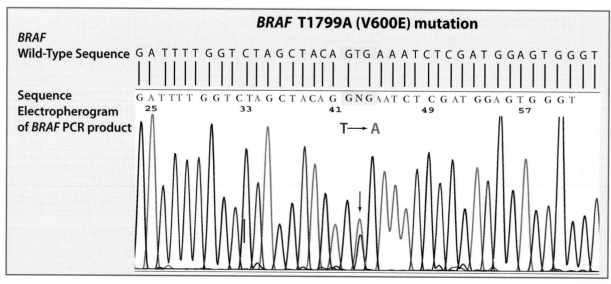

FIGURE 20.6 Sanger sequence electropherogram. It is generated using ABI 3130 Genetic Analyzer and demonstrates the presence of *BRAF* V600E mutation.

Recently, pyrosequencing has emerged as a new sequencing methodology.[23] It is based on the detection of the light emitted during synthesis of a cDNA strand. The addition of each nucleotide to a nucleic acid chain results in the release of an attached pyrophosphate (PPi) molecule, which is converted to ATP with production of light detected by the instrument. It is a fast and accurate technique but is limited to the analysis of short DNA sequences, as compared with classical nucleotide sequencing.

Introduction of next-generation sequencing platforms will enable simultaneous detection of multiple genetic alterations with high sensitivity, greater speed, and at lower costs. Several so-called second-generation sequencing platforms are now commercially available but are currently used predominantly as a discovery tool for detailed analyses of the cancer genome.

FISH

FISH utilizes fluorescently labeled DNA probes to provide a targeted approach to detect gene rearrangements or numerical chromosomal abnormalities in interphase or metaphase nuclei.

The method consist of four steps: the cellular DNA and the fluorescently labeled probe of interest are denatured by incubation at high temperature, the probe is added to the sample and hybridizes to the target DNA, a serious of posthybridization washes are applied to remove probe excess, and, finally, the background is counterstained and the probe signal visualized under a fluorescent microscope.

FISH is a versatile and highly sensitive technique and can be performed on various tissue specimens including fresh and frozen tissue, FFPE tissue sections, cytologic smears, and cultured cells. The resolution in the detection of small chromosomal deletions and rearrangements is higher than in conventional karyotyping, and it can be performed on interphase cell nuclei. However, FISH can only be applied toward the detection of known chromosomal alterations. In thyroid cancer, it can be used for the detection of *RET/PTC* rearrangements in papillary carcinomas, *PAX8/PPARγ* in follicular neoplasms, and numerical changes of chromosome 7 or other chromosomes in follicular adenomas and carcinomas.

The success and reliability of a laboratory-designed FISH assay depend on the probe design and quality of fluorescent labeling. The probes used for FISH should be relatively large in size, typically ranging from 50 to 200 kb. If probes are not commercially available, they are typically generated from cosmids, bacterial artificial chromosomes (BACs), P1 artificial chromosomes, and yeast artificial chromosomes. High-quality FISH probes for chromosome enumeration are commercially available and designed to hybridize to highly repetitive sequences of centromeric DNA and are ideal for detecting whole chromosome gains or losses. Probes for the detection of gene rearrangements, deletions, or amplifications have to be complementary to the gene of interest. Currently, there are no commercially available probes for detection of *RET/PTC* or *PAX8/PPARγ* rearrangements, but BAC clones are available and give good results.[24,25]

FISH assay for detecting chromosomal translocation may utilize two strategies: a break-apart probe design or a fusion probe design. The break-apart strategy uses either a large probe that corresponds to one of the translocation partner genes or two smaller probes located close to each other and surrounding the break point of the gene. In normal tissue, these probes produce a pair of signals (one per chromosome); however, in the case of translocation, each cell will have three signals (one normal signal and pair of split signals) (Fig. 20.7A).[26] In the fusion probe design, two probes are used, each spanning a translocation partner. This yields two pairs of signals (e.g., two green and two red signals) in normal cells but produces "fusion" yellow or red-green signals when these genes are brought together by translocation

(Fig. 20.7B).[24] The advantage of break-apart design is in its ability to detect all of the possible translocations for a particular gene, for example, all types of *RET/PTC* rearrangements for the *RET* gene; however, it does not identify the fusion partner. In contrast, the fusion probe design is useful for the confirmation of a specific type of translocation.

Appropriate controls and scoring criteria have to be used for accurate FISH diagnostics. The threshold level for positive results have to be established to avoid overinterpretation of small cell populations where signals are overlapping purely by chance due to two-dimensional FISH microscopy or where signals are lost due to the truncation of nuclei. For each individual assay, the normal control has to be evaluated for signal proximity and a threshold level has to be established. Normal tissue of the same cellularity and thickness should be used to establish a threshold.[27] For FISH translocation assays, the reported cut off for positive test results is between 8% and 30% depending on the probe design and the spatial proximity of genes participating in translocation.[24,28,29] Usually, fusion probe design requires higher cut off levels as compared with break-apart probes.

DETECTION OF POINT MUTATIONS

Multiple techniques for the detection of point mutations are available, and in practice the choice of method depends on the type of mutation, location of mutation (know hot spot vs. random distribution of mutation), required sensitivity of detection, specimen type, and test volume.

Detection of a point mutation at a specific hot spot with the same nucleotide substitution, such as *BRAF* T1799A (V600E) mutation, can be achieved using various molecular techniques including real-time PCR amplification and post-PCR melting curve analysis, allele specific PCR, direct nucleotide sequencing, restriction-fragment polymorphism analysis, and others[21,30–34] (Figs. 20.6 and 20.8A). All of these methods demonstrate reliable detection of *BRAF* mutation in different types of thyroid specimens. In one study, the comparison of probe specific real-time PCR, real-time allele specific PCR, direct sequencing, and colorimetric assay showed similar sensitivity in the detection of BRAF mutation in the archival FNA samples.[21] For *BRAF* testing in a clinical laboratory, the real-time PCR-based methods may be more preferable because they are rapid, easier to perform, and are run in a closed PCR system that reduces the risk of contamination. In addition, probe specific real-time PCR with post-PCR melting curve analysis allows to monitor DNA quality by simultaneous amplification and melting of the wild-type sequence.

The mutations with known hot spots but variable nucleotide substitutions at a particular codon, such as *RAS* mutations at codons 12, 13, and 61, can be successfully detected by probe specific real-time PCR amplification and post-PCR melting curve analysis or by direct nucleotide sequencing.[35,36] For real-time PCR amplification, two probes complementary to wild-type sequences are designed to span the mutation site for each mutational hot spot (codons 12/13 and 61) of *NRAS*, *HRAS,* and *KRAS* genes. If no mutation present, probes will bind perfectly to sample DNA and melt at a higher temperature, showing a single peak on post-PCR melting curve analysis. In contrast, if a heterozygous mutation is present, probes will bind to mutant DNA imperfectly, that is, with one nucleotide mismatch, and will melt (dissociate) earlier, producing two melting peaks (one for the wild-type allele and one for the mutant allele) or one melting peak at lower temperature if the mutation is homozygous. Each nucleotide substitution produces a melting peak at specific T_m (Fig. 20.8B). This method showed similar sensitivity in the detection of RAS mutation in thyroid tumors when compared with direct nucleotide sequencing as the "gold standard".[35]

A
Chromosome 10

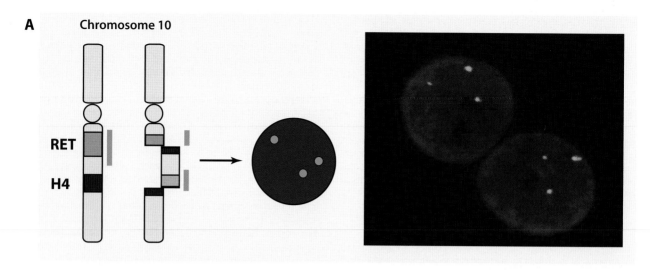

B
Chromosome 10

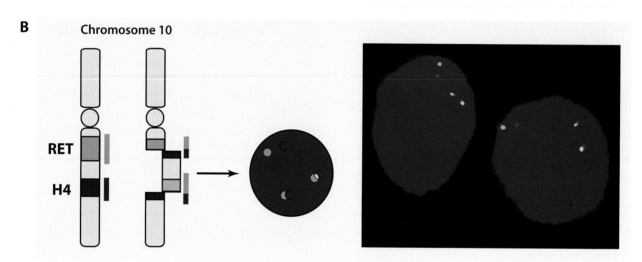

FIGURE 20.7 Fluorescence in situ hybridization (FISH). A: The break-apart design of the probe to detect *RET/PTC* rearrangement, which results in one green signal corresponding to the intact *RET* gene and a pair of signals corresponding to the rearranged *RET* gene. In this design, the *RET* translocation partner is not known. **B:** The fusion probe design that detects *RET/PTC1* type of rearrangement by showing a pair of green and red signals corresponding to the intact *RET* and *H4* genes and two fused signals corresponding to the fusion between the rearranged gene parts.

For the detection of point mutations with multiple hot spots, such as germline mutation in the *RET* gene, the most commonly used technique is direct nucleotide sequencing.[37,38] All exons known to harbor mutations have to be amplified in several PCR reactions, directly sequenced, and analyzed for the presence of a mutation. If the location of *RET* mutation is known from a test performed on other family members, the presence of this mutation can be tested for by RFLP-PCR.[16] Other techniques, such as SSCP and heteroduplex analysis, can also be used, although they may have lower sensitivity and are more labor intensive.[39,40]

DETECTION OF CHROMOSOMAL REARRANGEMENTS

The two most common approaches for the detection of *RET/PTC*, *PAX8/PPARγ*, and *TRK* rearrangements found in thyroid cancer are RT–PCR and FISH. RT–PCR is a reliable and sensitive technique for the detection of fusion transcripts in fresh or frozen tissue specimens and can be performed as conventional

or real-time RT–PCR (Fig. 20.9A–C).[24,41,42] For clinical testing, real-time RT–PCR has several significant advantages, as it is fast, is performed in a closed system with minimal risk of contamination, is more specific due to addition with internal probes, and allows quantitation of the amplified transcript. For the detection of gene rearrangements in FFPE samples, where RNA is severely degraded, FISH is the method of choice.[43] However, RT–PCR is more sensitive for the detection of chromosomal rearrangements in fresh or frozen tissue.[44]

Sometimes, to overcome the poor quality of RNA isolated from FFPE tissues, high sensitivity of detection was used by applying two rounds of PCR amplification or using sensitive hybridization with specific probes. These approaches carry an increased risk of detecting a false-positive product due to RT–PCR contamination or due to amplification of nonspecific sequences and requires rigorous use of negative controls.[45–47] In addition, these ultrasensitive techniques may result in the detection of rearrangements that are present in a small fraction of the tumor cell. This is particularly problematic for the detection of *RET/PTC* rearrangement, which may be quite heterogeneous and vary from involving almost all neoplastic cells (clonal *RET/PTC*)

BRAF V600E Mutation

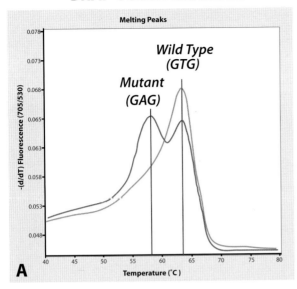

NRAS Codon 61 Mutations

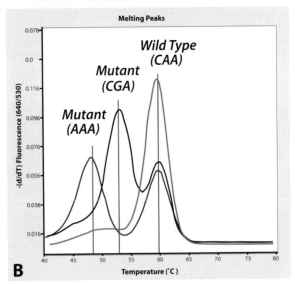

FIGURE 20.8 Detection of point mutations by LightCycler (Roche) real-time PCR amplification and melting curve analysis. A: The tumor sample with *BRAF* V600E mutation demonstrates T_m of 63°C for the wild-type sequence (GTG) and T_m of 58°C for the mutant sequence (GAG). The mutation is heterozygous because both the mutant and wild-type peaks are present. **B:** The tumor sample with *NRAS* 61 CAA CGA mutation has a melting peak at 53°C and another tumor sample carrying CAA AAA mutation shows a melting peak at 48°C, whereas the wild-type sequence has a melting peak at 60°C.

to being detected in a small fraction of tumor cells (nonclonal *RET/PTC*).[24] As only clonal *RET/PTC* is specific for papillary carcinoma, the establishing of cut off is particularly important in this situation. If detection is performed by RT–PCR, the fusion transcript has to be quantitated relatively to housekeeping gene and cut off for the detection of *RET/PTC* as a clonal event has to be established to ensure that >1% of tumor cells carry the rearrangement. As reliable quantitation cannot be achieved using RNA isolated from FFPE tissue, these samples should not be assayed for the RT–PCR detection of *RET/PTC* rearrangement for

clinical purposes. Instead, the FFPE samples should be tested by FISH. However, the appropriate cut-off levels have to be established for each probe design as well. In our experience, in order to detect a clonal *RET/PTC* rearrangement that is diagnostically relevant to papillary carcinoma, more than 17% of tumor cells should harbor this rearrangement.[24] Generally, it is not recommended to use ultrasensitive techniques on RNA isolated from fresh frozen tissue, and all unexpected results should be confirmed by independent techniques such as FISH, Southern blot, or cytogenetic analysis.

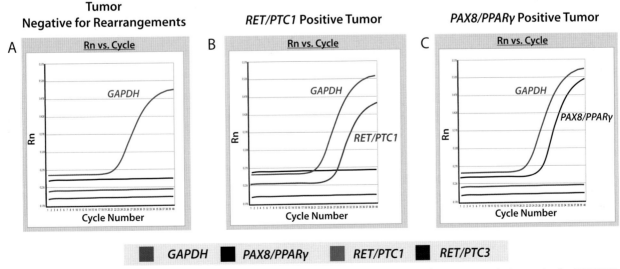

FIGURE 20.9 Detection of chromosomal rearrangements using real-time RT–PCR. A: The tumor sample is negative for *RET/PTC1*, *RET/PTC3*, and *PAX8/PPARγ* rearrangements (three flat lines on amplification plot) but shows strong amplification of the *GAPDH* housekeeping gene that confirms high quality of isolated RNA. **B:** The tumor sample shows amplification of the *RET/PTC1* fusion and *GAPDH* control. **C:** The tumor sample shows amplification of the *PAX8/PPARγ* fusion and *GAPDH* control.

Conventional Karyotyping

In molecular diagnostics of thyroid cancer, traditional cytogenetic analysis (conventional karyotyping) is useful for the detection of numerical chromosomal abnormalities and large structural rearrangements. The method is based on the visualization of stained metaphase chromosomes spread under brightfield microscopy. First, a fresh tissue specimen with viable cells is cultured in media with mitotic stimulants. After acceptable proliferation is achieved, cells are blocked in metaphase by exposure to colcemide, treated with hypotonic solution, and fixed on a slide. Finally, metaphase chromosomes are stained and visualized under the microscope.

The advantage of conventional cytogenetic karyotyping is in its ability to provide simultaneous evaluation of all chromosomal regions at once without previous knowledge of specific genetic alterations. However, this method requires fresh tissue and has low resolution for detecting small chromosomal deletions and translocations. An additional limitation of conventional karyotyping of thyroid tumors resides in the low-mitotic activity of tumor cells resulting in overgrowth of stromal fibroblast during culturing that can lead to erroneously normal karyotype.

COMPARATIVE GENOMIC HYBRIDIZATION

Comparative genomic hybridization (CGH) is an in situ hybridization method for evaluating the entire genome for chromosomal deletions and amplifications.[48–50] In thyroid, CGH analysis is used for the detection of chromosomal imbalances as a supplemental technique to conventional cytogenetics. It is based on hybridization of labeled tumor DNA and differently labeled normal reference DNA to normal human metaphase chromosomes (standard CGH) or to the BACs library (array CGH). The ratio of fluorescent staining between tumor and normal samples is scored for each chromosome, and the deviation in intensity of staining in the tumor versus paired normal tissue is identified as chromosomal gain or loss. Therefore, CGH allows in a single amplification to overview all DNA copy number changes in tumor specimens. It is more sensitive than conventional cytogenetics, with a resolution for the detection of chromosomal alterations down to 1 Mb, and it can be performed on DNA from paraffin-embedded archival tissues.[51]

DETECTION OF LOSS OF HETEROZYGOSITY

Loss of Heterozygosity (LOH) results from a deletion of small or large chromosomal regions and frequently correlates with the loss of important tumor suppressor genes residing in these areas. Detection of LOH is based on PCR amplification of microsatellite loci that are highly polymorphic, that is, frequently have different numbers of repeats in a population and, therefore, have a high probability of being different sizes on maternal and paternal alleles. They are excellent targets for the detection of LOH because they are inherited in a Mendelian codominant fashion, widely distributed in genome, and easily amplified using PCR techniques in fresh and archival tissue.[52]

For LOH detection, PCR primers are designed to flank the microsatellite region (Fig. 20.10A). PCR amplification of DNA isolated from normal (nonneoplastic) and neoplastic tissues is performed, and PCR products are subjected to polyacrylamide or capillary gel electrophoresis (Figs. 20.10B,C). PCR products from normal tissue are used to determine if patient is heterozygous for this locus, that is, has two alleles of different size and therefore is informative for LOH analysis. When a microsatellite marker is informative at a

particular chromosomal locus, it demonstrates two PCR products of different size (two peaks). A marker that is noninformative (homozygous) at this locus will show only one peak. For informative loci, an absence of amplification product of one of the alleles or a significant decrease in amplification product demonstrates LOH. Typically, a complete loss of one of the alleles is not seen due to the presence of some amount of nonneoplastic cells in the tumor specimen. Therefore, the quantitative calculation of LOH is based on the difference in ratios of two allelic peaks in normal tissue as compared with the same peaks in tumor tissue; allele ratios falling within the range of <0.5 and >2.0 are considered positive for LOH (Figs. 20.10B,C).[53,54]

Although, the LOH technique is reliable and simple, there are several aspects that have to be taken into consideration to achieve reproducible performance. In order to minimize "contamination" of tumor tissue with stromal and nonneoplastic cells that can mask allelic loss, tumor tissue microdissection

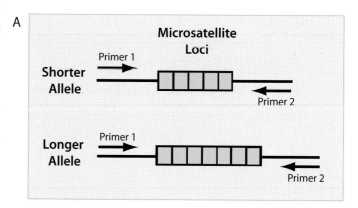

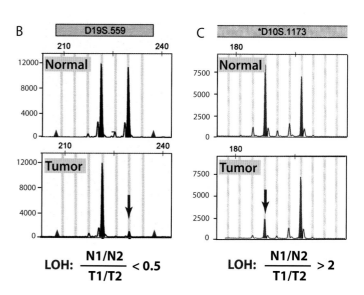

FIGURE 20.10 Detection of LOH. A: The primers are designed to flank a highly polymorphic microsatellite region. The allele containing a smaller number of microsatellite repeats will yield a shorter PCR product and one with a larger number of repeats will yield a longer PCR product. **B, C:** Two examples of capillary gel electrophoresis of PCR amplified regions of tetranucleotide repeats. The shorter size PCR products correspond to the first peaks on all electropherograms and the longer size products to the second peaks. The height of peaks corresponds to the amount of amplified product. For the calculation of LOH, the height of each peak in normal tissue (*N*) and in tumor tissue (*T*) is quantitated, and the ratio of normal peak heights is divided by the ratio of tumor peak heights. The final *N/T* ratio falling within the range of <0.5 (**B**) or >2 (**C**) are considered positive for LOH.

is typically performed. Normal tissue or other specimen types (blood, buccal swab, etc.) have to accompany the tumor tissue in order to provide the most reliable assessment of LOH. If testing is performed on FFPE tissue, primers have to be designed to produce PCR products <250 bp in size in order to increase the reliability of amplification. The DNA isolated from archival tissue has to be of optimal quantity to avoid random allele drop-outs and to demonstrate a reproducible result.[55,56] In addition, the coincidental presence of microsatellite instability that results from defects in the DNA mismatch repair genes can mimic patterns of allelic loss and LOH in this setting has to be interpreted with caution.

 ## DETECTION OF CLONALITY

According to the clonal model of carcinogenesis, neoplasm arises from a single cell that acquired somatic mutations and received growth advantage, that is, it is a monoclonal or clonal process, as opposed to normal tissue, which is polyclonal. In thyroid, determination of tissue clonality is used for the differentiation of neoplasms from polyclonal hyperplasic processes or to establish the independent origin of multiple tumor foci.[57-61]

There are two main approaches to determine tissue clonality: X-linked assays, the most common of which is human androgen receptor assay (HUMARA), and non-X-linked assays, such as LOH and detection of specific gene mutations or rearrangements.[62,63] The X-linked assays are based on random inactivation of one of the two X chromosomes in female cells. Inactivation of the X chromosome occurs by methylation early in embryogenesis and is stably transmitted in subsequent cell divisions. All normal tissues are expected to have an approximately equal mixture of cells with inactivation of maternal and paternal X chromosomes and are polyclonal (Fig. 20.11C). As neoplasm develops from a single cell, it is expected that the entire nodule will demonstrate inactivation of the same X chromosome. If two tumors developed in the same organ and show inactivation of different X chromosomes (i.e., one tumor of paternal chromosome and another of maternal), it can be concluded with high degree of confidence that they originated from different cells and represent independent tumors.[64]

The HUMARA assay utilizes a polymorphic locus of tandemly repeated CAG units (microsatellites) within the X-linked human androgen receptor gene to test the pattern of inactivation of the two X chromosomes. The most common version of this technique involves using a combination of treatment of DNA with methylation-sensitive restriction enzymes and subsequent PCR amplification of treated and nontreated DNA.[63,65] The PCR primers are designed to flank the region of CAG repeats and the restriction site of methylation-sensitive enzyme *HpaII* (Fig. 20.11A). Assuming the patient is heterozygous at this locus, PCR amplification of the original (nontreated) DNA will result in two products of different size, from the unmethylated (active) and from the methylated (inactive) X chromosomes. However, after enzymatic digestion with *HpaII*, only the methylated copy, which is protected from digestion, will remain intact and only one PCR product will be formed. The results of PCR amplification can be visualized by agarose or by capillary gel electrophoresis (Fig. 20.11B). If neoplasm is of a clonal origin, only one PCR band or peak can be seen on a gel, whereas a polyclonal process will manifest as two bands or peaks (Fig. 20.11C).

Although, HUMARA is considered to be a reliable technique for detecting clonality, it has some limitations. It can only be performed on tumors from female patients and the patient has to be heterozygous at the HUMARA locus (i.e., have different numbers of CAG repeats at this locus on maternal and paternal alleles). In addition, a patch size mosaicism can be a limiting factor for this assay. As X chromosome inactivation occurs early in embryogenesis and cells continue to proliferate, groups of mature cells originated from a single embryonic cell share the same pattern of X-chromosome inactivation are referred as patch size.[61] The patch size in normal thyroid tissue is expected to be relatively small, as in other tissues,[66] although some studies have suggested a large patch size, up to 48 to 128 mm².[67] Analysis of tissue samples smaller than patch size may erroneously demonstrate a clonal pattern of X-chromosome inactivation by HUMARA. Therefore, use of large tissue fragments or multiple samplings from different nodule areas are necessary to avoid this limitation of the clonality assay.

Non-X-linked assays for the detection of clonality are based on identification of the same genetic alterations, such as LOH, point mutations, or gene rearrangements in the majority of cells within a given tumor.[62,68,69] A genetic alteration detected within most cells in a lesion provides evidence that a single progenitor cell acquired this mutation and gave rise to the entire tumor, which supports its clonal origin. However, demonstration of only a few cells within the tumor carrying the mutation is not enough to conclude that the neoplasm is clonal.[70] Therefore, the detection of tumor clonality using this approach requires a quantitative assessment of cells with a particular mutation in a given lesion. Non-X-linked assays allow detection of clonality in tissues from male and female patients, and they are not affected by patch size.

 ## DETECTION OF DNA PLOIDY

Normal human cells are diploid, that is, contain two copies of each of the 22 autosomes and the 2 sex chromosomes. Aneuploidy, defined as a deviation from normal karyotype, reflects losses or gains of single or multiple chromosomes or large chromosomal regions, and it is an important feature of many cancers.[71] Assessment of DNA ploidy is typically performed either by flow cytometry or by static image cytometry.[72-74] In addition, it can be assessed by conventional cytogenetics, comparative genomic hybridization, and other molecular techniques.[75]

Flow cytometry offers a rapid, objective method for measuring the amount of DNA in cells and identifies the proportions of cells in different phases of the cell cycle. When DNA flow cytometry is performed, the tissue is placed in a solution that ruptures the cells, leaving only the nuclei. The nuclei are stained with a fluorescent dye that binds to the DNA and is analyzed on a flow cytometer. A focused light source (laser) excites the fluorescent dye bound to the DNA as nuclei pass one by one in a liquid stream. The intensity of fluorescence is proportional to the amount of DNA in the cell. This method can be performed on fresh frozen or FFPE tissues, but it does not permit morphologic confirmation. In contrast, static image cytometry is based on quantitative scanning of tissue sections and allows performing histologic evaluation of different areas of a tumor prior to the analysis.[76] For this method, cell nuclei are isolated on a glass slide and stained with special stain (Feulgen stain) that binds to the DNA. The intensity of staining is measured using a computer-assisted image analysis cytometry system, and the intensity of the stain is directly proportional to the amount of DNA present in the cells.

 ## GENE EXPRESSION ARRAYS

Gene expression arrays can qualitatively and quantitatively determine expression levels of multiple genes at once. There are several platforms for gene expression profiling, and the most common are GeneChip expression arrays from Affimetrix and Dual-Mode microarrays from Agilent Technologies. Both platforms utilize spotted microarray technology, where thousands

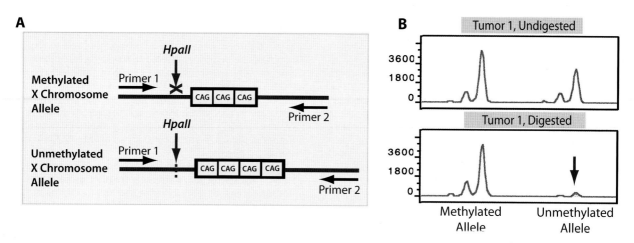

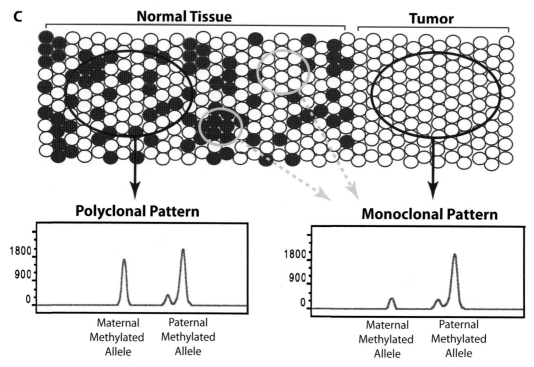

FIGURE 20.11 Detection of clonality using the X-linked human androgen receptor (HUMARA) assay. A: PCR primers are designed to flank the polymorphic CAG repeat locus and neighboring restriction site of the methylation sensitive *HpaII* enzyme. Treatment with the enzyme will result in digestion of DNA from unmethylated X chromosome leaving the methylated X chromosome intact. **B:** Capillary gel electrophoresis of the PCR products from the tumor sample without *HpaII* digestion (**top panel**) and with *HpaII* digestion (**lower panel**). The undigested tumor sample shows heterozygous amplification of two different size X-chromosome alleles. The digested tumor sample shows the amplification of only allele that was methylated and therefore protected from *HpaII* digestion. **C:** Schematic representation of normal female tissue with a random pattern of X-chromosome inactivation (depicted as a mixture of white and grey circles) and of tumor tissue that originates from a single cell. When large areas of normal and tumor tissue (red circles) are assayed, the normal tissue will demonstrate a polyclonal pattern of X-chromosome inactivation (two peaks) and the tumor tissue will show a monoclonal pattern (one peak). If the analysis is performed using a normal tissue fragment smaller than patch size, it may mistakenly demonstrate a monoclonal pattern of inactivation.

of oligonucleotide probes corresponding to known human genes are placed (spotted) onto a microarray surface at high density. For gene expression analysis, high-quality RNA has to be isolated from the tumor sample, converted into cDNA, and hybridized to the microarray chip. After hybridization, the microarray is washed to eliminate binding to nonspecific targets and is scanned. The measured intensity of hybridization signals is proportional to the expression level of genes in the tumor specimen.

Gene expression arrays are a great discovery tool for determining the unique gene expression signatures in thyroid cancer.[77] Their routine use in molecular diagnostic laboratories is still limited due to the high complexity of testing and difficulties in data analysis. However, with additional standardization and streamlining of protocols, they may evolve in the near future into powerful tool for molecular diagnostics.

REFERENCES

1. Watson JD, Crick FH. Molecular structure of nucleic acids; a structure for deoxyribose nucleic acid. *Nature.* 1953;171:737–738.
2. Lander ES, Linton LM, Birren B, et al. Initial sequencing and analysis of the human genome. *Nature.* 2001;409:860–921.
3. Chargaff E. Structure and function of nucleic acids as cell constituents. *Fed Proc.* 1951;10:654–659.
4. Shen LX, Cai Z, Tinoco I Jr. RNA structure at high resolution. *Faseb J.* 1995;9:1023–1033.
5. Sharp PA. Splicing of messenger RNA precursors. *Science.* 1987;235:766–771.
6. Bartel DP. MicroRNAs: genomics, biogenesis, mechanism, and function. *Cell.* 2004;116:281–297.
7. Ambros V. The functions of animal microRNAs. *Nature.* 2004;431:350–355.
8. Frates MC, Benson CB, Doubilet PM, et al. Prevalence and distribution of carcinoma in patients with solitary and multiple thyroid nodules on sonography. *J Clin Endocrinol Metab.* 2006;91:3411–3417.
9. Wood LD, Parsons DW, Jones S, et al. The genomic landscapes of human breast and colorectal cancers. *Science.* 2007;318:1108–1113.
10. Moore JL, Aros M, Steudel KG, Cheng KC. Fixation and decalcification of adult zebrafish for histological, immunocytochemical, and genotypic analysis. *Biotechniques.* 2002;32:296–298.
11. Mullis KB, Faloona FA. Specific synthesis of DNA in vitro via a polymerase-catalyzed chain reaction. *Methods Enzymol.* 1987;155:335–350.
12. Freeman WM, Walker SJ, Vrana KE. Quantitative RT-PCR: pitfalls and potential. *Biotechniques.* 1999;26:112–122, 124–115.
13. Micke P, Ohshima M, Tahmasebpoor S, et al. Biobanking of fresh frozen tissue: RNA is stable in nonfixed surgical specimens. *Lab Invest.* 2006;86:202–211.
14. Ginzinger DG. Gene quantification using real-time quantitative PCR: an emerging technology hits the mainstream. *Exp Hematol.* 2002;30:503–512.
15. Pryor RJ, Wittwer CT. Real-time polymerase chain reaction and melting curve analysis. *Methods Mol Biol.* 2006;336:19–32.
16. Dang GT, Cote GJ, Schultz PN, et al. A codon 891 exon 15 RET proto-oncogene mutation in familial medullary thyroid carcinoma: a detection strategy. *Mol Cell Probes.* 1999;13:77–79.
17. Nikiforov YE, Nikiforova MN, Gnepp DR, et al. Prevalence of mutations of ras and p53 in benign and malignant thyroid tumors from children exposed to radiation after the Chernobyl nuclear accident. *Oncogene.* 1996;13:687–693.
18. Milbury CA, Li J, Liu P, et al. COLD-PCR: improving the sensitivity of molecular diagnostics assays. *Expert Rev Mol Diagn.* 2011;11:159–169.
19. Mancini I, Santucci C, Sestini R, et al. The use of COLD-PCR and high-resolution melting analysis improves the limit of detection of KRAS and BRAF mutations in colorectal cancer. *J Mol Diagn.* 2010;12:705–711.
20. Nikiforov, YE et al. Impact of mutational testing on the diagnosis and management of patients with cytologically indeterminate thyroid nodules: a prospective analysis of 1056 FNA samples. *J Clin Endocrinol Metab.* 2011;96(11):3390–3397.
21. Jin L, Sebo TJ, Nakamura N, et al. BRAF mutation analysis in fine needle aspiration (FNA) cytology of the thyroid. *Diagn Mol Pathol.* 2006;15:136–143.
22. Sanger F, Nicklen S, Coulson AR. DNA sequencing with chain-terminating inhibitors. *Proc Natl Acad Sci U S A.* 1977;74:5463–5467.
23. Ronaghi M. Pyrosequencing sheds light on DNA sequencing. *Genome Res.* 2001;11:3–11.
24. Zhu Z, Ciampi R, Nikiforova MN, et al. Prevalence of RET/PTC rearrangements in thyroid papillary carcinomas: effects of the detection methods and genetic heterogeneity. *J Clin Endocrinol Metab.* 2006;91:3603–3610.
25. Kroll TG, Sarraf P, Pecciarini L, et al. PAX8-PPARgamma1 fusion oncogene in human thyroid carcinoma [corrected]. *Science.* 2000;289:1357–1360.
26. Nikiforova MN, Stringer JR, Blough R, et al. Proximity of chromosomal loci that participate in radiation-induced rearrangements in human cells. *Science.* 2000;290:138–141.
27. Tibiletti MG. Interphase FISH as a new tool in tumor pathology. *Cytogenet Genome Res.* 2007;118:229–236.
28. Bridge RS, Rajaram V, Dehner LP, et al. Molecular diagnosis of Ewing sarcoma/primitive neuroectodermal tumor in routinely processed tissue: a comparison of two FISH strategies and RT-PCR in malignant round cell tumors. *Mod Pathol.* 2006;19:1–8.
29. Tibiletti MG. Specificity of interphase fluorescence in situ hybridization for detection of chromosome aberrations in tumor pathology. *Cancer Genet Cytogenet.* 2004;155:143–148.
30. Sapio MR, Posca D, Troncone G, et al. Detection of BRAF mutation in thyroid papillary carcinomas by mutant allele-specific PCR amplification (MASA). *Eur J Endocrinol.* 2006;154:341–348.
31. Rowe LR, Bentz BG, Bentz JS. Detection of BRAF V600E activating mutation in papillary thyroid carcinoma using PCR with allele-specific fluorescent probe melting curve analysis. *J Clin Pathol.* 2007;60:1211–1215.
32. Hayashida N, Namba H, Kumagai A, et al. A rapid and simple detection method for the BRAF(T1796A) mutation in fine-needle aspirated thyroid carcinoma cells. *Thyroid.* 2004;14:910–915.
33. Nikiforova MN, Kimura ET, Gandhi M, et al. BRAF mutations in thyroid tumors are restricted to papillary carcinomas and anaplastic or poorly differentiated carcinomas arising from papillary carcinomas. *J Clin Endocrinol Metab.* 2003;88:5399–5404.
34. Kimura ET, Nikiforova MN, Zhu Z, et al. High prevalence of BRAF mutations in thyroid cancer: genetic evidence for constitutive activation of the RET/PTC-RAS-BRAF signaling pathway in papillary thyroid carcinoma. *Cancer Res.* 2003;63:1454–1457.
35. Nikiforova MN, Lynch RA, Biddinger PW, et al. RAS point mutations and PAX8-PPAR gamma rearrangement in thyroid tumors: evidence for distinct molecular pathways in thyroid follicular carcinoma. *J Clin Endocrinol Metab.* 2003;88:2318–2326.
36. Elenitoba-Johnson KS, Bohling SD, Wittwer CT, et al. Multiplex PCR by multicolor fluorimetry and fluorescence melting curve analysis. *Nat Med.* 2001;7:249–253.
37. Eng C, Mulligan LM, Smith DP, et al. Low frequency of germline mutations in the RET proto-oncogene in patients with apparently sporadic medullary thyroid carcinoma. *Clin Endocrinol (Oxf).* 1995;43:123–127.
38. Elisei R, Romei C, Cosci B, et al. RET genetic screening in patients with medullary thyroid cancer and their relatives: experience with 807 individuals at one center. *J Clin Endocrinol Metab.* 2007;92:4725–4729.
39. Kambouris M, Jackson CE, Feldman GL. Diagnosis of multiple endocrine neoplasia [MEN] 2A, 2B and familial medullary thyroid cancer [FMTC] by multiplex PCR and heteroduplex analyses of RET proto-oncogene mutations. *Hum Mutat.* 1996;8:64–70.
40. Ceccherini I, Hofstra RM, Luo Y, et al. DNA polymorphisms and conditions for SSCP analysis of the 20 exons of the ret proto-oncogene. *Oncogene.* 1994;9:3025–3029.
41. Nikiforova MN, Biddinger PW, Caudill CM, et al. PAX8-PPARgamma rearrangement in thyroid tumors: RT-PCR and immunohistochemical analyses. *Am J Surg Pathol.* 2002;26:1016–1023.
42. Nikiforova MN, Caudill CM, Biddinger P, et al. Prevalence of RET/PTC rearrangements in Hashimoto's thyroiditis and papillary thyroid carcinomas. *Int J Surg Pathol.* 2002;10:15–22.
43. Qian X, Jin L, Shearer BM, et al. Molecular diagnosis of Ewing's sarcoma/primitive neuroectodermal tumor in formalin-fixed paraffin-embedded tissues by RT-PCR and fluorescence in situ hybridization. *Diagn Mol Pathol.* 2005;14:23–28.
44. Ten Heuvel SE, Hoekstra HJ, Suurmeijer AJ. Diagnostic accuracy of FISH and RT-PCR in 50 routinely processed synovial sarcomas. *Appl Immunohistochem Mol Morphol.* 2008;16:246–250.
45. Schumacher JA, Jenson SD, Elenitoba-Johnson KS, et al. Utility of linearly amplified RNA for RT-PCR detection of chromosomal translocations: validation using the t(2;5)(p23;q35) NPM-ALK chromosomal translocation. *J Mol Diagn.* 2004;6:16–21.
46. Ivell R. A question of faith—or the philosophy of RNA controls. *J Endocrinol.* 1998;159:197–200.
47. Hill DA, O'Sullivan MJ, Zhu X, et al. Practical application of molecular genetic testing as an aid to the surgical pathologic diagnosis of sarcomas: a prospective study. *Am J Surg Pathol.* 2002;26:965–977.
48. Cowell JK, Wang YD, Head K, et al. Identification and characterisation of constitutional chromosome abnormalities using arrays of bacterial artificial chromosomes. *Br J Cancer.* 2004;90:860–865.
49. Forozan F, Karhu R, Kononen J, et al. Genome screening by comparative genomic hybridization. *Trends Genet.* 1997;13:405–409.
50. Kallioniemi A, Kallioniemi OP, Sudar D, et al. Comparative genomic hybridization for molecular cytogenetic analysis of solid tumors. *Science.* 1992;258:818–821.
51. Johnson NA, Hamoudi RA, Ichimura K, et al. Application of array CGH on archival formalin-fixed paraffin-embedded tissues including small numbers of microdissected cells. *Lab Invest.* 2006;86:968–978.
52. Koreth J, O'Leary JJ, J ODM. Microsatellites and PCR genomic analysis. *J Pathol.* 1996;178:239–248.
53. Johnson MD, Vnencak-Jones CL, Toms SA, et al. Allelic losses in oligodendroglial and oligodendroglioma-like neoplasms: analysis using microsatellite repeats and polymerase chain reaction. *Arch Pathol Lab Med.* 2003;127:1573–1579.
54. Marsh JW, Finkelstein SD, Demetris AJ, et al. Genotyping of hepatocellular carcinoma in liver transplant recipients adds predictive power for determining recurrence-free survival. *Liver Transpl.* 2003;9:664–671.
55. Farrand K, Jovanovic L, Delahunt B, et al. Loss of heterozygosity studies revisited: prior quantification of the amplifiable DNA content of archival samples improves efficiency and reliability. *J Mol Diagn.* 2002;4:150–158.
56. Sieben NL, ter Haar NT, Cornelisse CJ, et al. PCR artifacts in LOH and MSI analysis of microdissected tumor cells. *Hum Pathol.* 2000;31:1414–1419.
57. Kim H, Piao Z, Park C, et al. Clinical significance of clonality in thyroid nodules. *Br J Surg.* 1998;85:1125–1128.
58. Aeschimann S, Kopp PA, Kimura ET, et al. Morphological and functional polymorphism within clonal thyroid nodules. *J Clin Endocrinol Metab.* 1993;77:846–851.
59. Namba H, Matsuo K, Fagin JA. Clonal composition of benign and malignant human thyroid tumors. *J Clin Invest.* 1990;86:120–125.
60. Apel RL, Ezzat S, Bapat BV, et al. Clonality of thyroid nodules in sporadic goiter. *Diagn Mol Pathol.* 1995;4:113–121.
61. Thomas GA, Williams D, Williams ED. The clonal origin of thyroid nodules and adenomas. *Am J Pathol.* 1989;134:141–147.
62. Diaz-Cano SJ, Blanes A, Wolfe HJ. PCR techniques for clonality assays. *Diagn Mol Pathol.* 2001;10:24–33.
63. Shattuck TM, Westra WH, Ladenson PW, et al. Independent clonal origins of distinct tumor foci in multifocal papillary thyroid carcinoma. *N Engl J Med.* 2005;352:2406–2412.
64. Lyon MF. Some milestones in the history of X-chromosome inactivation. *Annu Rev Genet.* 1992;26:16–28.
65. Allen RC, Zoghbi HY, Moseley AB, et al. Methylation of HpaII and HhaI sites near the polymorphic CAG repeat in the human androgen-receptor gene correlates with X chromosome inactivation. *Am J Hum Genet.* 1992;51:1229–1239.
66. Novelli M, Cossu A, Oukrif D, et al. X-inactivation patch size in human female tissue confounds the assessment of tumor clonality. *Proc Natl Acad Sci U S A.* 2003;100:3311–3314.

67. Jovanovic L, Delahunt B, McIver B, et al. Thyroid gland clonality revisited: the embryonal patch size of the normal human thyroid gland is very large, suggesting X-chromosome inactivation tumor clonality studies of thyroid tumors have to be interpreted with caution. *J Clin Endocrinol Metab*. 2003;88:3284–3291.

68. Diaz-Cano SJ. Designing a molecular analysis of clonality in tumours. *J Pathol*. 2000;191:343–344.

69. Sieben NL, Roemen GM, Oosting J, et al. Clonal analysis favours a monoclonal origin for serous borderline tumours with peritoneal implants. *J Pathol*. 2006;210:405–411.

70. Pozo-Garcia L, Diaz-Cano SJ. Clonal origin and expansions in neoplasms: biologic and technical aspects must be considered together. *Am J Pathol*. 2003;162:353–354; author reply 354–355.

71. Silvestrini R. Relevance of DNA-ploidy as a prognostic instrument for solid tumors. *Ann Oncol*. 2000;11:259–261.

72. Lanigan D, McLean PA, Curran B, Leader M. Comparison of flow and static image cytometry in the determination of ploidy. *J Clin Pathol*. 1993;46:135–139.

73. Castro P, Eknaes M, Teixeira MR, et al. Adenomas and follicular carcinomas of the thyroid display two major patterns of chromosomal changes. *J Pathol*. 2005;206:305–311.

74. Christov K. Flow cytometric DNA measurements in human thyroid tumors. *Virchows Arch B Cell Pathol Incl Mol Pathol*. 1986;51:255–263.

75. Dudarewicz L, Holzgreve W, Jeziorowska A, et al. Molecular methods for rapid detection of aneuploidy. *J Appl Genet*. 2005;46:207–215.

76. Danque PO, Chen HB, Patil J, et al. Image analysis versus flow cytometry for DNA ploidy quantitation of solid tumors: a comparison of six methods of sample preparation. *Mod Pathol*. 1993;6:270–275.

77. Giordano TJ, Kuick R, Thomas DG, et al. Molecular classification of papillary thyroid carcinoma: distinct BRAF, RAS, and RET/PTC mutation-specific gene expression profiles discovered by DNA microarray analysis. *Oncogene*. 2005;24:6646–6656.

Molecular Testing of Thyroid FNA Samples

Molecular testing of thyroid fine needle aspiration (FNA) samples is gaining its use as an ancillary diagnostic tool for cancer diagnosis in thyroid nodules. Palpable thyroid nodules are common in adults and estimated to affect >100 million people in the United States.[1,2] Most of thyroid nodules are benign and can be managed conservatively, whereas approximately 5% to 15% of medically evaluated thyroid nodules are malignant.[3–7] A clinical challenge facing the physician is to accurately diagnose cancer in these nodules to ensure that each patient receives timely and appropriate treatment, while minimizing the risk of unnecessary thyroid surgery for benign disease.

Currently, the most common and reliable diagnostic tool for the evaluation of thyroid nodules is FNA cytology. FNA provides a definitive diagnosis of benign or malignant thyroid disease in most cases. However, in about 25% of nodules, FNA cytology cannot reliably exclude cancer and such cases are placed in one of the indeterminate categories.[1,3,8,9] This is because cytologic features of thyroid lesions with a follicular growth pattern are frequently not sufficiently different to distinguish between benign and malignant lesions.

The current Bethesda System for Reporting Thyroid Cytopathology recognizes three types of indeterminate cytological diagnosis: (1) atypia of undetermined significance/follicular lesion of undetermined significance (AUS/FLUS), (2) follicular neoplasm/suspicious for follicular neoplasm (FN/SFN), and (3) suspicious for malignant cells (SMC), with a predicted probability of cancer of 5% to 15%, 15% to 30%, and 60% to 75%, respectively.[10,11] Because FNA is unable to provide a definitive diagnosis for these nodules, most patients with indeterminate cytology undergo diagnostic surgery to establish a histopathologic diagnosis. However, only 10% to 40% of such surgically resected thyroid nodules will prove to be malignant.[4,11,12] The unneeded operations can be avoided if an FNA procedure allowed to reliably establish the diagnosis of a benign nodule. For patients diagnosed with cancer after

lobectomy, the standard of care is to offer a second operation to complete the thyroidectomy, with additional costs and increased morbidity. The improved diagnosis of cancer established preoperatively can lead to more optimal surgical treatment with a single "up-front" total thyroidectomy. Furthermore, *BRAF* V600E mutation has been associated with a substantially worse outcome, and nodal metastasis and the availability of this information preoperatively may be helpful to define the extent of surgery. Diagnostic use of mutational markers for thyroid FNA samples has been explored for a panel of mutations and for single genes.

TESTING FOR PANEL OF MUTATIONS

Testing for a panel of mutations is feasible in thyroid FNA samples and provides helpful diagnostic and prognostic information.[13–16] The panel includes most common mutations that collectively occur in approximately 70% of thyroid cancer, i.e. *BRAF* V600E, *BRAF* K601E, *NRAS* codon 61, *HRAS* codon 61, and KRAS codons 12/13 point mutations and *RET/PTC1, RET/PTC3*, and *PAX8/PPARγ* rearrangements, with the possible addition of the TRK rearrangement. The results of large and well-designed prospective studies performed in clinical molecular diagnostic laboratories demonstrate that detection of any mutation in an aspirated thyroid nodule was a strong predictor of malignancy irrespective of the cytological diagnosis.[13–16] Specifically, the presence of *BRAF, RET/PTC, or PAX8/PPARγ* was specific for malignant outcome in 100% of cases, whereas *RAS* mutations had a 74% to 100% positive predictive value for cancer (Table 21.1).

Testing for the panel of mutations is particularly helpful in nodules with indeterminate cytology, where it improves an

Table 21.1

Probability of cancer in thyroid nodules positive for specific mutations based on clinical studies that utilized a panel of mutations

	Cancer Probability in Nodules Positive for Specific Mutation			
	BRAF (%)	**RAS (%)**	**RET/PTC (%)**	**PAX8/PPARγ**
Nikiforov et al.[15]	100	88	100	100%
Cantara et al.[14]	100	74	100	n/a
Ohori et al.[16]	100	100	100	100%
Nikiforov et al.[13]	100	85	100	100%
Total	100	87	100	100%

NOTE: Total of 194 mutations (71 *BRAF*, 100 *RAS*, 17 *RET/PTC*, 6 *PAX8/PPARγ*) were detected in these studies.

assessment of cancer risk. In a prospective study of >1,000 thyroid FNA samples, identification of a mutation in specific categories of indeterminate cytology, that is, AUS/FLUS, FN/SFN, and SMC, conferred the risk of histologic malignancy of 88%, 87%, and 95%, respectively (Fig. 21.1).[13] The most common mutations found in these nodules were *RAS*, followed by *BRAF*, and *PAX8/PPARγ*, and the most frequent tumors carrying these mutations were follicular variant papillary carcinomas and follicular carcinomas, which are difficult to diagnose by FNA cytology. The risk of cancer in mutation-negative nodules was 6% in AUS/FLUS samples, 14% in FN/SFN, and 28% in SMC (Fig. 21.1).[13] In the AUS/FLUS group, among nodules negative for mutations, only 2.3% of cancers were invasive and only 0.5% had extrathyroidal extension.[13] Based on these data, combination of FNA cytology and molecular testing can result in a more refined clinical management of patients with thyroid nodules (Fig. 21.1).[13] Indeed, positive results of molecular testing, with the possible exception of *RAS*-positive nodules, should offer a strong indication for total thyroidectomy in all categories of indeterminate cytology. This will allow bypassing the repeat of FNA and eliminate the need for a two-step surgery, that

is, diagnostic lobectomy followed by completion thyroidectomy, for most patients with malignant nodules.

The mutation negative result does not completely eliminate the risk of cancer. Therefore, diagnostic lobectomy appears to be justified as initial surgical intervention for mutation-negative nodules with FN/SFN and SMC cytology. The appropriate approach for nodules with AUS/FLUS cytology that are negative for mutations is less clear. A 6% cancer risk in these nodules, with a risk of cancer extending outside the thyroid gland of <1%, raise a possibility of a more conservative management with clinical and ultrasound follow-up and repeat of FNA in appropriately selected patients.

The 2009 American Thyroid Association's management guidelines recommend to consider the mutational panel for nodules with indeterminate FNA cytology to help guide clinical management.[17]

 # TESTING FOR *BRAF* MUTATION

BRAF V600E is a highly specific marker for cancer diagnosis in thyroid FNA samples. A meta-analysis of the results reported in

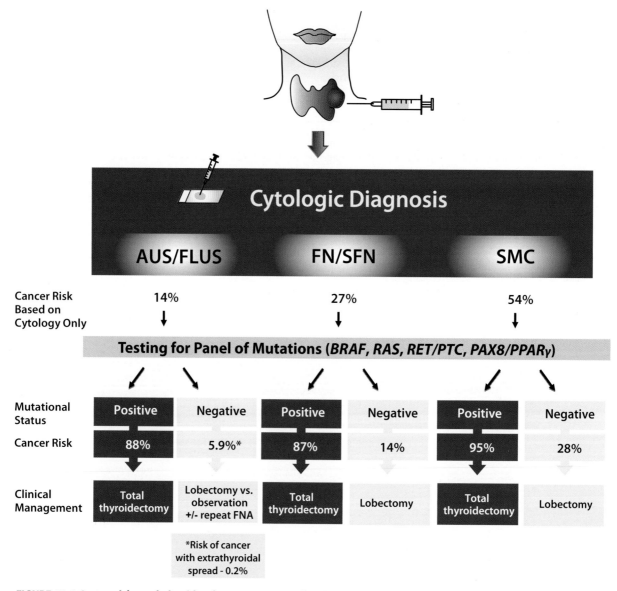

FIGURE 21.1 Cancer risks and algorithm for management of patients with cytologically indeterminate thyroid FNAs based on the results of mutational analysis combined with specific cytologic diagnosis.

22 studies[15,18–37] of thyroid FNA samples tested for *BRAF* V600E revealed that out of 1,117 nodules found positive for this mutation, 1,109 (99.3%) were diagnosed as papillary carcinomas on final histopathology.[38] Eight cases were false-positive as no cancer was found after surgery, of which five cases were reported in one study that used ultrasensitive detection of this mutation.[37] Even if these cases are accepted as true false-positive, *BRAF* mutation appears to be a highly accurate marker of cancer in thyroid nodules sampled by FNA, conferring the risk of malignancy above 99%. Importantly, 15% to 40% of samples tested positive for *BRAF* had indeterminate FNA cytology, indicating that *BRAF* can be of significant diagnostic value in these nodules.[15,25,29,32,35,37,39] Despite high specificity for cancer, testing for *BRAF* mutation alone misses many thyroid cancers that are negative for this mutation. The performance of molecular testing can be significantly improved by including in the analysis other frequently occurring mutations.

In addition to its diagnostic value, *BRAF* V600E is generally accepted as a reliable prognostic marker for papillary carcinoma. It has been associated in many studies with aggressive tumor characteristics such as extrathyroidal extension, advanced tumor stage at presentation, and lymph node or distant metastases.[40] Moreover, the association between *BRAF* V600E and tumor recurrence[18,41–44] and tumor-related mortality[41,45] has been shown. Tumors carrying this mutation require more often reoperation for the locally persistent or recurrent disease.[45–50] This suggests that patients with *BRAF* V600E-positive papillary cancer detected preoperatively may benefit from more extensive initial surgery.

OTHER POTENTIAL MOLECULAR TESTS

Resolution of mutational testing in thyroid FNA samples can be further improved by the addition of other genetic markers found in thyroid cancer at lower frequency, such as *PIK3CA*, *PTEN*, *AKT1*, rare types of *RET/PTC* rearrangement, and all types of *RAS* mutations.[38] It is not practical to test for these genetic abnormalities using currently available testing platforms. However, this may become possible with the introduction of new testing approaches (e.g. next generation sequencing, SNaPshot array, Sequenom analysis, etc.), which are expected to allow cost-efficient detection of multiple mutations. Additionally, the whole genome sequencing of thyroid cancer may lead to the discovery of novel mutations that can improve cancer detection in thyroid nodules.

In addition to gene mutations, expression of messenger RNA (mRNA) and micro RNA (miRNA) markers has also been explored for diagnostic use in thyroid FNA samples. A recent study tested the possibility of using expression levels of multiple genes for cancer detection in thyroid FNA samples.[51] Applying a proprietary classifier algorithm to a set of 48 thyroid FNA samples, the authors were able to distinguish benign and malignant nodules with the sensitivity of 92% and specificity of 84%, although the number of tested samples was relatively low.[51]

Several miRNAs, including miR-221, -222, and -146b, have been shown to be consistently overexpressed in papillary thyroid carcinomas and other thyroid cancers and can be of potential diagnostic use.[52–57] Their clinical utility has been recently explored in thyroid FNA samples where a panel of seven miRNAs (miR-187, -221, -222, -146b, -224, -155, and -197) was applied to discriminate benign thyroid nodules from malignant.[55] Upregulation of three or more miRNAs allowed to predict thyroid malignancy with the accuracy of 98%. This initial study demonstrates the feasibility of miRNA detection in preoperatively collected thyroid FNA samples and provides strong evidence for its possible diagnostic use.

MUTATIONAL TESTING OF FNA SAMPLES WITH NEGATIVE OR POSITIVE FOR MALIGNANCY CYTOLOGY

The main utility of mutational panel is in testing of nodules with indeterminate FNA cytology.[17] However, testing of FNA samples that are negative or positive for malignancy may also be considered in some cases.

Detection of mutations in nodules with negative cytology may decrease the rate of false-negative cytology. In one study, testing for panel of mutations decreased the rate false-negative cytology from 2.1% to 0.9%.[15] In another observation, molecular testing allowed to detect six out of nine cancers in 87 nodules with benign cytology.[14] However, whether molecular testing of all negative cytology samples is cost effective requires further investigation.

It remains to be established if molecular testing of FNA samples diagnosed as positive for malignancy should be performed and taken into account in the surgical and postsurgical management of patients with thyroid cancer. Molecular testing of samples diagnosed as malignant by cytology can identify *BRAF*-positive tumors, which, as discussed earlier, may require more extensive surgery. However, specific recommendations for the surgical management of thyroid cancer based on the mutational status have not been developed yet.

COLLECTION OF FNA SAMPLES FOR MOLECULAR TESTING

Samples collected directly for molecular testing during the FNA procedure are the best source of material for mutational analysis. Typical FNA procedure is conducted under ultrasound guidance, and thyroid cells are aspirated using a 23, 25, or 27 gauge needle for cytological evaluation. In most cases, 3 to 4 FNA passes are performed. Most of the aspirated sample from the first two passes (the most representative sample) can be used to make direct cytology smears, whereas the residual material in the needle and the needle wash from both passes can be placed into a tube containing nucleic acid preservative solution, for example, RNAlater (Qiagen), Nucleic Acid preservative solution (Roche), and Trizol (Invitrogen). Harvesting of cells directly into preservative solution prevents DNA and RNA degradation, provides excellent quality of nucleic acids, and allows to successfully test FNA samples that contain small quantity of thyroid cells. Using this approach, the collected material is sufficient for mutation detection in 90% to 98% of cases.[13,15] The collected FNA specimen can be frozen at –20°C or –80°C and stored until results of cytological evaluation become available. When molecular testing is required, the stored residual FNA material is retrieved and submitted for the analysis.

If collection of fresh FNA material is not possible, mutational testing can be performed on fixed FNA cytology preparations, i.e. stained cytology smears or cytology cell block. This approach is reliable for the detection of point mutations but is less effective for chromosomal rearrangements due to significant degradation of isolated RNA. In addition, it may require sacrificing of diagnostically important cytology slides.

ASSESSMENT OF SAMPLE ADEQUACY FOR MUTATIONAL TESTING

The adequacy of thyroid FNA samples for molecular analysis can be assessed based on (1) general quantity and quality of isolated nucleic acids and (2) proportion of thyroid epithelial cells within the sample.

The overall quantity and quality of isolated nucleic acids can be evaluated by spectrophotomeric measurements and by estimation of quantity and quality of PCR products. Real-time PCR platforms allow to determine adequacy of nucleic acids in a simple and cost efficient way via assessing amplification of the *RAS* or *BRAF* genes for DNA and amplification of the *GAPDH* housekeeping gene for RNA. We consider the quality and quantity of nucleic acids satisfactory when the PCR amplification cycle threshold (Ct) is 35 cycles or less.

In addition, the freshly collected FNA material into preservative solution submitted for molecular testing needs to be evaluated for quantity of epithelial (thyroid) cells present. FNA samples may contain several "contaminant" cells, that is, lymphocytes and other WBCs. Admixture of these cells may skew the mutational testing and lead to false-negative results.

Assessment of the proportion of thyroid epithelial cells within a FNA sample can be performed by comparing the expression of the universal housekeeping gene (*GAPDH*), which is uniformly expressed in all cell types, with the expression of genes that are expressed only in few distinct types of epithelial cells including thyroid cells. Examples of such genes are cytokeratin genes (*KRT7* and *KRT19*), the thyroid peroxidase (*TPO*) gene, thyroglobulin (*TG*) and others.[13,51] Recent study have validated the *GAPDH* and *KRT7* genes to assess the quantity of thyroid epithelial cells in freshly collected FNA samples.[13] Both genes were amplified using qRT-PCR and tested in surgically removed thyroid tissues and WBCs. Expression of *KRT7* and *GAPDH* was detected at similar levels in normal thyroid tissues, follicular carcinomas, and papillary carcinomas, whereas *KRT7* was expressed at a very low level in white blood cells (Fig. 21.2A). The increase in proportion of lymphocytes over thyroid papillary carcinoma cells was followed by a linear decrease in *KRT7* expression and unchanged *GAPDH* expression, with the difference in ΔCt of 3.5 corresponding to

approximately 10% of thyroid epithelial cells within the sample (Fig. 21.2B). This method was validated in a large series of freshly collected thyroid FNA samples.[13] The results showed that in FNA samples considered adequate by this approach, 95% of mutations subsequently found in the surgical samples from these nodules were detected. The limitations of this approach are related to the fact that *KRT7* expression is lost in thyroid anaplastic carcinomas, and FNA samples from these tumors will be found falsely inadequate for molecular testing. However, these tumors rarely contribute to indeterminate cytology results.

MUTATIONAL ANALYSIS

Clinically actionable detection of mutations should be performed in a certified clinical molecular diagnostic laboratory, and all molecular assays have to be validated according to the guidelines and regulations for molecular testing. Nucleic acids (DNA and RNA) can be isolated using various techniques. Most laboratories would offer separate isolation protocols for DNA and RNA. Isolation of total nucleic acids can be considered, particularly for small FNA samples, in order to minimize the nucleic acid loss during separate isolation procedures. Isolation of nucleic acids can be performed manually or using automated assays. Detection of *BRAF* V600E, *BRAF* K601E, *NRAS* codon 61, *HRAS* codon 61, and *KRAS* codons 12 and 13 point mutations can be performed by various assays and platforms including real-time LightCycler PCR and fluorescence melting curve analysis, Sanger sequencing, pyrosequencing, and other techniques as discussed in Chapter 20. Detection of *RET/PTC1, RET/PTC3,* and *PAX8/PPAR*γ rearrangements can be achieved using real-time RT-PCR or using FISH hybridization if testing is performed on fixed FNA sample. The sensitivity limits (known as analytical sensitivity) depend on a technique and vary from 10% to 50% of cells with heterozygous mutation for point mutations and from 1% to 20% for chromosomal rearrangements. As discussed in Chapters 11 and 20, the ultra-sensitive molecular assays with analytical sensitivity <1% should not be used because of the possibility of detection of non-clonal genetic abnormalities. The detection of very low-level mutations, which can be due to the error introduced during PCR amplification or due to genetic heterogeneity and presence of the mutation in a very small proportion of cells, has very limited diagnostic role and can lead to decreased clinical and analytical specificity of molecular testing.

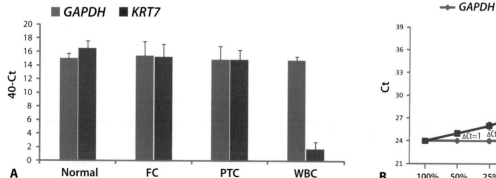

FIGURE 21.2 Evaluation of adequacy of collected FNA samples. A: Expression of *KRT7* and *GAPDH* is similar in normal thyroid tissues, follicular carcinomas (FC), and papillary carcinomas (PTC). However, *KRT7* was expressed at a significantly lower level in WBC, which are frequent contaminant of thyroid FNA samples. **B:** Serial dilution of RNA from thyroid papillary carcinoma tissue in RNA derived from normal WBC demonstrated a linear decrease in *KRT7* expression as compared with stable *GAPDH* expression with the ΔCt of 3.5 corresponding to approximately 10% of thyroid epithelial cells within the sample.

REFERENCES

1. Gharib H. Changing trends in thyroid practice: understanding nodular thyroid disease. Endocr Pract. 2004;10:31–39.
2. Mazzaferri EL. Thyroid cancer in thyroid nodules: finding a needle in the haystack. Am J Med. 1992;93:359–362.
3. Cooper DS, Doherty GM, Haugen BR, et al. Management guidelines for patients with thyroid nodules and differentiated thyroid cancer. Thyroid. 2006;16:109–142.
4. Mazzaferri EL. Management of a solitary thyroid nodule. N Engl J Med. 1993;328:553–559.
5. Kim DL, Song KH, Kim SK. High prevalence of carcinoma in ultrasonography-guided fine needle aspiration cytology of thyroid nodules. Endocr J. 2008;55:135–142.
6. Frates MC, Benson CB, Doubilet PM, et al. Prevalence and distribution of carcinoma in patients with solitary and multiple thyroid nodules on sonography. J Clin Endocrinol Metab. 2006;91:3411–3417.
7. Papini E, Guglielmi R, Bianchini A, et al. Risk of malignancy in nonpalpable thyroid nodules: predictive value of ultrasound and color-Doppler features. J Clin Endocrinol Metab. 2002;87:1941–1946.
8. Greaves TS, Olvera M, Florentine BD, et al. Follicular lesions of thyroid: a 5-year fine-needle aspiration experience. Cancer. 2000;90:335–341.
9. Sclabas GM, Staerkel GA, Shapiro SE, et al. Fine-needle aspiration of the thyroid and correlation with histopathology in a contemporary series of 240 patients. Am J Surg. 2003;186:702–709; discussion 709–710.
10. Ali SZ, Cibas ES. The Bethesda System for Reporting Thyroid Cytopathology. New York, NY: Springer; 2010.
11. Baloch ZW, LiVolsi VA, Asa SL, et al. Diagnostic terminology and morphologic criteria for cytologic diagnosis of thyroid lesions: a synopsis of the National Cancer Institute Thyroid Fine-Needle Aspiration State of the Science Conference. Diagn Cytopathol. 2008;36:425–437.
12. Baloch ZW, Fleisher S, LiVolsi VA, et al. Diagnosis of "follicular neoplasm": a gray zone in thyroid fine-needle aspiration cytology. Diagn Cytopathol. 2002;26:41–44.
13. Nikiforov Y. Impact of mutational testing on the diagnosis and management of patients with cytologically indeterminate thryoid nodules: a prospective analysis of 1056 FNA samples. J Clin Endocrinol Metab. 2011;96(11):3390–3397.
14. Cantara S, Capezzone M, Marchisotta S, et al. Impact of proto-oncogene mutation detection in cytological specimens from thyroid nodules improves the diagnostic accuracy of cytology. J Clin Endocrinol Metab. 2010;95: 1365–1369.
15. Nikiforov YE, Steward DL, Robinson-Smith TM, et al. Molecular testing for mutations in improving the fine-needle aspiration diagnosis of thyroid nodules. J Clin Endocrinol Metab. 2009;94:2092–2098.
16. Ohori NP, Nikiforova MN, Schoedel KE, et al. Contribution of molecular testing to thyroid fine-needle aspiration cytology of "follicular lesion of undetermined significance/atypia of undetermined significance". Cancer Cytopathol. 2010;118:17–23.
17. Cooper DS, Doherty GM, Haugen BR, et al. Revised American Thyroid Association management guidelines for patients with thyroid nodules and differentiated thyroid cancer. Thyroid. 2009;19:1167–1214.
18. Xing M, Clark D, Guan H, et al. BRAF mutation testing of thyroid fine-needle aspiration biopsy specimens for preoperative risk stratification in papillary thyroid cancer. J Clin Oncol. 2009;27:2977–2982.
19. Kumagai A, Namba H, Akanov, Z et al. Clinical implications of pre-operative rapid BRAF analysis for papillary thyroid cancer. Endocr J. 2007;54:399–405.
20. Xing M, Tufano RP, Tufaro AP, et al. Detection of BRAF mutation on fine needle aspiration biopsy specimens: a new diagnostic tool for papillary thyroid cancer. J Clin Endocrinol Metab. 2004;89:2867–2872.
21. Domingues R, Mendonca E, Sobrinho L, et al. Searching for RET/PTC rearrangements and BRAF V599E mutation in thyroid aspirates might contribute to establish a preoperative diagnosis of papillary thyroid carcinoma. Cytopathology. 2005;16:27–31.
22. Pizzolanti G, Russo L, Richiusa, P et al. Fine-needle aspiration molecular analysis for the diagnosis of papillary thyroid carcinoma through BRAF V600E mutation and RET/PTC rearrangement. Thyroid. 2007;17:1109–1115.
23. Sapio MR, Guerra A, Posca D, et al. Combined analysis of galectin-3 and BRAFV600E improves the accuracy of fine-needle aspiration biopsy with cytological findings suspicious for papillary thyroid carcinoma. Endocr Relat Cancer. 2007;14:1089–1097.
24. Sapio MR, Posca D, Raggioli A, et al. Detection of RET/PTC, TRK and BRAF mutations in preoperative diagnosis of thyroid nodules with indeterminate cytological findings. Clin Endocrinol (Oxf). 2007;66:678–683.
25. Jo YS, Huang S, Kim YJ, et al. Diagnostic value of pyrosequencing for the BRAF V600E mutation in ultrasound-guided fine-needle aspiration biopsy samples of thyroid incidentalomas. Clin Endocrinol (Oxf). 2009;70:139–144.
26. Zatelli MC, Trasforini G, Leoni S et al. BRAF V600E mutation analysis increases diagnostic accuracy for papillary thyroid carcinoma in fine needle aspiration biopsies. Eur J Endocrinol. 2009;161:467–473.
27. Jin L, Sebo TJ, Nakamura N, et al. BRAF mutation analysis in fine needle aspiration (FNA) cytology of the thyroid. Diagn Mol Pathol. 2006;15:136–143.
28. Cohen Y, Rosenbaum E, Clark DP, et al. Mutational analysis of BRAF in fine needle aspiration biopsies of the thyroid: a potential application for the preoperative assessment of thyroid nodules. Clin Cancer Res. 2004;10:2761–2765.
29. Salvatore G, Giannini R, Faviana P, et al. Analysis of BRAF point mutation and RET/PTC rearrangement refines the fine-needle aspiration diagnosis of papillary thyroid carcinoma. J Clin Endocrinol Metab. 2004;89:5175–5180.
30. Rowe LR, Bentz BG, Bentz JS. Utility of BRAF V600E mutation detection in cytologically indeterminate thyroid nodules. Cytojournal. 2006;3:10.
31. Marchetti I, Lessi F, Mazzanti CM, et al. A morpho-molecular diagnosis of papillary thyroid carcinoma: BRAF V600E detection as an important tool in preoperative evaluation of fine-needle aspirates. Thyroid. 2009;19:837–842.
32. Kim SK, Kim DL, Han HS, et al. Pyrosequencing analysis for detection of a BRAFV600E mutation in an FNAB specimen of thyroid nodules. Diagn Mol Pathol. 2008;17:118–125.
33. Hayashida N, Namba H, Kumagai A, et al. A rapid and simple detection method for the BRAF(T1796A) mutation in fine-needle aspirated thyroid carcinoma cells. Thyroid. 2004;14:910–915.
34. Chung KW, Yang SK, Lee GK, et al. Detection of BRAFV600E mutation on fine needle aspiration specimens of thyroid nodule refines cyto-pathology diagnosis, especially in BRAF600E mutation-prevalent area. Clin Endocrinol (Oxf). 2006;65:660–666.
35. Kim SK, Hwang TS, Yoo YB, et al. Surgical results of thyroid nodules according to a management guideline based on the BRAF(V600E) mutation status. J Clin Endocrinol Metab. 2011;96:658–664.
36. Nam SY, Han BK, Ko EY, et al. BRAF V600E mutation analysis of thyroid nodules needle aspirates in relation to their ultrasonographic classification: a potential guide for selection of samples for molecular analysis. Thyroid. 2010;20:273–279.
37. Kim SW, Lee JI, Kim JW, et al. BRAFV600E mutation analysis in fine-needle aspiration cytology specimens for evaluation of thyroid nodule: a large series in a BRAFV600E-prevalent population. J Clin Endocrinol Metab. 2010;95:3693–3700.
38. Nikiforov YE, Nikiforova MN. Molecular genetics and diagnosis of thyroid cancer. Nat Rev Endocrinol. 2011 30;7:569–580.
39. Cohen Y, Xing M, Mambo E, et al. BRAF mutation in papillary thyroid carcinoma. J Natl Cancer Inst. 2003;95:625–627.
40. Xing M. BRAF mutation in papillary thyroid cancer: pathogenic role, molecular bases, and clinical implications. Endocr Rev. 2007;28:742–762.
41. Elisei R, Ugolini C, Viola D, et al. BRAF(V600E) mutation and outcome of patients with papillary thyroid carcinoma: a 15-year median follow-up study. J Clin Endocrinol Metab. 2008;93:3943–3949.
42. Xing M, Westra WH, Tufano RP, et al. BRAF mutation predicts a poorer clinical prognosis for papillary thyroid cancer. J Clin Endocrinol Metab. 2005;90:6373–6379.
43. Kim TY, Kim WB, Rhee YS, et al. The BRAF mutation is useful for prediction of clinical recurrence in low-risk patients with conventional papillary thyroid carcinoma. Clin Endocrinol (Oxf). 2006;65:364–368.
44. Kebebew E, Weng J, Bauer J, et al. The prevalence and prognostic value of BRAF mutation in thyroid cancer. Ann Surg. 2007;246:466–470; discussion 470–461.
45. O'Neill CJ, Bullock M, Chou A, et al. BRAF(V600E) mutation is associated with an increased risk of nodal recurrence requiring reoperative surgery in patients with papillary thyroid cancer. Surgery. 2010;148:1139–1145; discussion 1145–1136.
46. Yip L, Nikiforova MN, Carty SE, et al. Optimizing surgical treatment of papillary thyroid carcinoma associated with BRAF mutation. Surgery. 2009;146:1215–1223.
47. Riesco-Eizaguirre G, Gutierrez-Martinez P, Garcia-Cabezas MA, et al. The oncogene BRAF V600E is associated with a high risk of recurrence and less differentiated papillary thyroid carcinoma due to the impairment of Na+/I- targeting to the membrane. Endocr Relat Cancer. 2006;13:257–269.
48. Durante C, Puxeddu E, Ferretti E, et al. BRAF mutations in papillary thyroid carcinomas inhibit genes involved in iodine metabolism. J Clin Endocrinol Metab. 2007;92:2840–2843.
49. Ricarte-Filho JC, Ryder M, Chitale DA, et al. Mutational profile of advanced primary and metastatic radioactive iodine-refractory thyroid cancers reveals distinct pathogenetic roles for BRAF, PIK3CA, and AKT1. Cancer Res. 2009;69:4885–4893.
50. Xing M. Prognostic utility of BRAF mutation in papillary thyroid cancer. Mol Cell Endocrinol. 2010;321:86–93.
51. Chudova D, Wilde JI, Wenge ET, et al. Molecular classification of thyroid nodules using high-dimensionality genomic data. J Clin Endocrinol Metab. 2010;95:5296–5304.
52. Mazeh H, Mizrahi I, Halle D, et al. Development of a microRNA-based molecular assay for the detection of papillary thyroid carcinoma in aspiration biopsy samples. Thyroid. 2011;21:111–118.
53. Chen YT, Kitabayashi N, Zhou XK, et al. MicroRNA analysis as a potential diagnostic tool for papillary thyroid carcinoma. Mod Pathol. 2008;21:1139–1146.
54. He H, Jazdzewski K, Li W, et al. The role of microRNA genes in papillary thyroid carcinoma. Proc Natl Acad Sci U S A. 2005;102:19075–19080.
55. Nikiforova MN, Tseng GC, Steward D, et al. MicroRNA expression profiling of thyroid tumors: biological significance and diagnostic utility. J Clin Endocrinol Metab. 2008;93:1600–1608.
56. Pallante P, Visone R, Ferracin M, et al. MicroRNA deregulation in human thyroid papillary carcinomas. Endocr Relat Cancer. 2006;13:497–508.
57. Visone R, Russo L, Pallante P, et al. MicroRNAs (miR)-221 and miR-222, both overexpressed in human thyroid papillary carcinomas, regulate p27Kip1 protein levels and cell cycle. Endocr Relat Cancer. 2007;14:791–798.

INDEX

In this index, page numbers in *italic* designate figures; page numbers followed by the letter *t* designate tables.